A
HISTORY OF THE
ARMY MEDICAL DEPARTMENT

A
HISTORY OF
THE ARMY MEDICAL
DEPARTMENT

Volume I

Lieutenant General Sir Neil Cantlie
K.C.B., K.B.E., M.C., MB.Ch.B., F.R.C.S.
Late Director General
Army Medical Service

CHURCHILL LIVINGSTONE
EDINBURGH AND LONDON 1974

CHURCHILL LIVINGSTONE
Medical Division of Longman Group Limited

Represented in the United States of America by
Longman Inc., New York, and by associated
companies, branches and representatives throughout
the world.

First published 1974

ISBN 0 443 01066 8

Printed in Great Britain

CONTENTS

ILLUSTRATIONS

MAPS

LARGE MAPS

CONTRACTIONS

A.G.   Adjutant General
A.A.G.   Assistant Adjutant General
A.Q.M.G.   Assistant Quartermaster General
A.H.C.   Army Hospital Corps
B.M.J.   British Medical Journal
C. in C.   Commander in Chief
C.O.   Commanding Officer
D.G.   Director General
D.I.G.H.   Deputy Inspector General of Hospitals
D.N.B.   Dictionary of National Biography
D.S.G.   Deputy Surgeon General
G.O.C.   General Officer Commanding
G.S.W.   Gun Shot Wound
H.E.I.C.   Honourable East India Company
I.G.H.   Inspector General of Hospitals
I.M.D.   Indian Medical Department
I.M.S.   Indian Medical Service
K.C.B.   Knight Commander of the Bath
K.C.S.I.   Knight Commander Star of India
L. of C.   Lines of Communication
M.O.   Medical Officer
P.M.O.   Principal Medical Officer
M.S.C.   Medical Staff Corps
N.C.O.   Non Commissioned Officer
P.R.O.   Public Record Office
Q.M.G.   Quartermaster General
R.M.O.   Regimental Medical Officer
S.G.   Surgeon General
S.M.   Surgeon Major
S.M.O.   Senior Medical Officer
W.O.   War Office

PREFACE

It was the story of the Crimean War which first awakened my interest in medical history. When I considered the numerous accounts of the inefficiency of the medical arrangements in that war it struck me that the true facts ought to be studied and represented. It was also, I felt, a reflection upon the medical service that alone amongst the corps of the army no comprehensive history had ever been written except the interesting account by Surgeon General A. A. Gore under the name of 'The Story of Our Services under the Crown' published in 1879. From this source I found valuable help, and I must pay further tribute to the noteworthy researches of the late Major H. A. L. Howell, R.A.M.C., and the late Lieut. Colonel G. A. Kempthorne, R.A.M.C. which made my task so much easier. But neither of these officers had the time or the opportunity to provide more than the many interesting articles which were published in the Journal of the Royal Army Medical Corps. As Garrison says, 'If we are to have a clear view of the panorama of medical history we must necessarily stand upon the shoulders of our predecessors.'

My interest in the Crimean War led me on to attempt to write an account of the Army Medical Department from the time of the institution of the Standing Army in 1660 to the formation of the Royal Army Medical Corps in 1898.

I can speak I am sure for many of our officers when I say that we are ignorant of many of the problems which our predecessors had to face partly from the absence of any comprehensive account, apart from those I have already mentioned, and partly from the absence up to the present time of the necessary instruction in our training.

On the financial side it is due to the great generosity of the Trustees of the Wellcome Foundation that I have been able to undertake my task. In addition I have to thank the Officers of the Royal Army Medical Corps and the members of the Knott Trust for their generous help in so liberally providing financial assistance.

Surgeon James Mouat (6th Dragoons), 25th October, 1854 — Balaclava, Crimea.

Assistant Surgeon Thomas Egerton Hall (7th Fusiliers) 8th September 1855 — Crimea.

Assistant Surgeon Henry Thomas Sylvester (23rd Regiment), 8th September 1855 — Crimea.

Surgeon Herbert Taylor Reade (61st Regiment), 14th and 16th September 1857 — Indian Mutiny.

Surgeon Joseph Gee (78th Regiment), 25th September 1857 — Indian Mutiny.

Assistant Surgeon Valentine Munbee McMaster (78th Regiment), 25th September 1857 — Indian Mutiny

Surgeon Anthony Dickson Home (90th Regiment), 26th September 1857 — Indian Mutiny

Assistant Surgeon William Bradshaw (90th Regiment), 26th September 1857 — Indian Mutiny.

Assistant Surgeon William Temple (Royal Artillery), 20th November 1863 — New Zealand.

Assistant Surgeon William George Nicholas Manley (Royal Artillery) 26th September 1864 — New Zealand.

Assistant Surgeon Campbell Millis Douglas (24th Regiment) 17th December 1867 — Andaman Islands.

Surgeon Major James Henry Reynolds (Army Medical Department), 22nd January, 1879 — Rorke's Drift, South Africa.

Lance Corporal Joseph John Farmer (Army Hospital Corps) 27th February 1881 — Majuba, South Africa.

Surgeon Captain Ferdinand Simeon Le Quesne (Medical Staff), 4th May 1889 — Burma.

Surgeon Major Owen Edward Pennefather Lloyd (Medical Staff) 6th January 1893 — Burma.

Introduction

'He who neglects the lessons of history is condemned to repeat them.' So wrote George Santayana. In applying the truth of this saying to the medical service of the British Army we have attempted to record its history from the time of the creation of the Standing Army in 1660 to the foundation of the Royal Army Medical Corps in 1898. To provide a background on which to build our story it is however an essential prelude to give an account of the medical arrangements of earlier times.

Prior to 1660 physicians and surgeons served with the army during all the campaigns which were fought both at home and overseas. They were called to arms from civil life and their services ended when peace was declared. Only from the date of the creation of the Standing Army was a permanent regular medical service instituted.

Colonel Walton the author of the *History of the British Standing Army* begins the chapter which deals with the Medical Service with these words: 'There are two branches of administration which unlike the other administrative branches just treated of are not absolute essentials to an army, although the army that should be without them or imperfect in them would be said to be sadly incomplete. These branches are the Medical and Religious branches. An army could exist without either.'[1]

Without doubt an army could exist without the Medical branch, but the question arises for how long? Walton wrote his book in 1909 and had he wished he would have found ample evidence to refute this irresponsible statement. Had he never heard of the disastrous Walcheren expedition when the campaign had to be abandoned due to malaria? Had he never heard of the epidemics of yellow fever in the West Indies during the Napoleonic Wars when the drain on the lives of the thousands of troops which were poured into these islands had a major effect upon the strategy of the war in Europe? Had he never heard of typhoid fever in South Africa, and cholera in India? It is true that until science had revealed their secrets in the second half of the nineteenth century the causation of many diseases was unknown and treatment was on an empirical basis, but even so did he really believe

I

that without the Medical Department the results would have been equally successful? Armies would have melted away due to wastage from sickness unless hospitals had been provided to cure and return men to duty. And what of the moral aspect? History reveals that prompt medical aid for the wounded has a great psychological stimulus to the fighting spirit of combat troops.

Strong evidence in support of an efficient medical service was revealed in Burma during the Second World War when malaria would have wiped out the army within a few months had not special treatment hospitals been pushed up to the forward areas to cure cases and return them to the firing line. Many commanders in the field have had no doubts about the role the medical service has played in contributing to victory. Wellington in the Peninsular War gave credit to James McGrigor his Principal Medical Officer for helping to win the battle of Vitoria because thousands of men had been returned from hospitals to the ranks after the disastrous retreat from Burgos. Viscount Montgomery after the Second World War wrote from Berlin on the 28th September 1945 a message which reads thus. 'To the Royal Army Medical Corps with admiration and high regard to a Corps whose contribution to victory has been beyond all calculation.'[2]

It has been the fate of the medical service that certain military officers in war have belittled its role, and during campaigns many commanders leave the medical branch ignorant of impending operations, often from lack of appreciation of the role they can play rather than deliberate intention. Why, they say, do doctors want to know? On occasion it is because they regard medical officers as bad security risks and so withhold secret information. They do not appreciate the fact that the medical branch in battle is a front line service and unless information is received in advance, the positioning of field units in time to receive casualties will not be possible and men's lives will be sacrificed unnecessarily. Examples of this neglect will be seen as the history unfolds.

For most of the period covered by this history there were two distinct branches of medical officers—the regimental branch and the medical staff branch. In the regimental branch the medical officer was granted a commission in the regiment with the approval of the commanding officer. He wore the regimental uniform, and was responsible to his colonel for the regimental hospital and its administration. Some medical officers spent their whole army career with the regiment and never rose above the rank of regimental surgeon.

The medical staff branch was composed of medical officers who served in the general hospitals, or acted as garrison surgeons or as administrative officers both in hospitals or at the headquarters of military formations. General hospitals in peacetime were few because the regimental hospitals carried out medical treatment to finality. Soldiers lived or died in their regimental hospitals under the care of the regimental surgeon. But when war broke out, general hospitals were formed for the expeditionary force which went overseas, and they were staffed by physicians, surgeons, apothecaries, and subordinate assistants who were either promoted from the regimental surgeons, or were civilian doctors newly commissioned. When the war ended these staff officers were for the most part relegated to half pay, with a liability to be recalled to the colours when another war occurred.

The service was controlled by a physician general and a surgeon general who might either be selected senior regular medical officers or chosen from eminent members of the civil medical profession. The latter had little or no army experience and were often employed on a part time basis. To these was added an apothecary general who controlled the supply of medicines. In the middle of the eighteenth century an inspector of regimental infirmaries was appointed. He was an officer of the regular service, and the physician general the surgeon general and the inspector of regimental infirmaries composed the Army Medical Board which concurrently directed affairs.

In the year 1809 the Army Medical Board was dissolved and an Army Medical Department came into being under a director general. This department from its institution until after the Crimean War was a civil and not a military department. It then became a part of the War Office organization and was ultimately placed under the Adjutant General's branch.

The Cardwell system of army reorganization came into effect in the 1870's and its impact upon the Medical Department was the establishment of what is known as the 'unification' system. The regimental medical officers then ceased to exist as a part of the regimental establishment and they were united with the medical staff officers to form one corps. Those medical officers who carried out the duties of regimental medical officers were now only 'attached' for duty with the regiment, and were supervised and controlled by officers of their own service.

Up to the period of the Crimean War in 1854 there was no rank and file branch of the medical service. The nursing in both regimental and general hospitals was carried out by men who were seconded from units for hospital duty. Although in regimental hospitals these orderlies from long experience acquired a degree of medical knowledge, those who were sent for duty in general hospitals in time of war were entirely unskilled and were generally the worst characters in the unit whom commanding officers were glad to be rid of. This also applied to the hospital stewards, ward masters, office staff, and cooks. Moreover these men could be changed at will by their commanding officers. It can be appreciated that the efficient administration of general hospitals under such conditions presented almost insuperable difficulties.

The first corps of other ranks came into being in the early days of the Crimean War and has existed since then under various changes of name. From that time the first orderlies trained in ward nursing and first aid take their origin.

The history will describe the gradual rise in the status of the medical officer and the fight for equality of rank *vis-a-vis* combatant officers. Until the last quarter of the nineteenth century medical officers were not given executive rank and were forbidden to exercise command over their orderlies or their patients. To execute this role, combatant officers were appointed as directors of general hospitals and as officers in command of orderlies. It will be seen that the attainment finally of substantive military rank brought recognition that the Department was an integral part of the armed forces. Their duties now comprised not only professional competence as doctors but as administrators and commanders of medical units.

Throughout this time the medical officers were quite separate from the rank and file who formed the Army Hospital Corps, later renamed the Medical Staff Corps. It was not until 1898 that the two branches were united to form the Royal Army Medical Corps.

As its chief task the history records the administrative aspect, but it includes accounts of the principal diseases which plagued the army throughout the centuries and the general treatment of wounds. It deals with the department problems arising from the campaigns in which the British Army has been engaged in all theatres of war, and to appreciate these problems the broad outlines of the strategy and tactics of these campaigns and an account of the various battles has been described.

Apart from the valuable assistance I have obtained from the writings of the late Surgeon General Gore, the late Major Howell, and the late Lieut. Colonel Kempthorne I am greatly indebted to Major E. W. Sheppard, O.B.E., M.C., for his advice and his work in revising and correcting the manuscript, and to Dr. Ruth G. Hodgkinson of the Wellcome Institute of the History of Medicine for her review and many valuable suggestions. Major General A. Maclennan, O.B.E., R.A.M.C. (retd.), Curator of the R.A.M.C. Historical Museum has given me much help in reading the manuscript and supervising the maps. Amongst others I have to thank are Dr. P. O. Williams, F.R.C.P., Director and Secretary to the Wellcome Trust; Dr. F. N. L. Poynter, Director of the Wellcome Institute of the History of Medicine; Mr. E. Gaskell of the Wellcome Library; the Commandant Royal Army Medical College for facilities placed at my disposal, and Mr. Davies the librarian for much practical assistance; the late Major General E. E. Barnsley, C.B., M.C., R.A.M.C.; Brigadier Sir John Boyd, O.B.E., F.R.S., M.D. F.R.C.P., R.A.M.C. (retd.), the late Director of Pathology, War Office; Lieut. Colonel A. B. Fountain, R.A.M.C.

(retd.), and Major General R. W. Galloway, C.B.E., D.S.O., R.A.M.C. (retd.); Mr. Charles Terrot for permission to quote from Miss Terrot's diary in the Crimea. I have also to thank Mr. Machin and Miss Walshaw for making the maps and Mr. Tonbridge for preparing the illustrations.

REFERENCES

[1] Walton. *History of the British Standing Army*, p. 852.
[2] The statement is preserved in the Royal Army Medical Corps Historical Museum.

ERRATUM

Vol. 1, page 5, line 4.
'Walshaw' should read 'Walsham' and 'Tonbridge' should read 'Troubridge'.

Chapter 1

THE NEW MODEL ARMY

From the earliest records available of military operations some provision was always made for the care of the sick and wounded in battle, and during the wars of ancient Egypt and Greece there are references to surgeons who were skilled in the treatment of wounds. In Egypt the healing art was in the hands of the priesthood; in Greece it was so highly esteemed that Aesculapius was looked upon as a son of the gods and honours almost divine were paid to him. But Grose tells us, 'the military surgeons of ancient times are very rarely mentioned in history; perhaps they were not in very great estimation, the superstitious abhorrence of what was deemed a violation of the dead prevented their having an accurate knowledge of the human frame, which is only to be acquired by frequent dissections'.

In the Roman armies each legion of 6,000 men had at least one surgeon, for we read that in A.D.138 the Emperor Antoninus personally communicated with the surgeon of the 2nd Legion[1], and there were also subsidiary or assistant surgeons with each cohort or tenth of a legion, for on the Roman Wall in Britain there is a memorial to Anicius Ingenuus—medical officer of the Tungrian cohort. There are, in fact, no less than forty-six different inscriptions giving the name, the rank, and the unit of some sixty Roman army surgeons, scattered over a wide range of countries of the old Roman Empire, evidence in itself of the extensive medical organization.[2] From Roman historians we learn that after great battles the wounded were received in the private houses of the Patricians where they were attended by surgeons, but when warfare was carried into unknown and distant lands each standing camp had a well founded *valetudinarium* with wards and sick attendants. Moreover, invalids rendered incapable of further active service were provided for at the public expense. The Romans were also very attentive to the preservation of the health of their soldiers, for we learn from Vegetius that they took great care that they should be well supplied with good water and 'not use bad or unwholesome water of marshes, for bad water was very productive of disease'. It was advised that camps should never be located near unwholesome marshes, or on dry uncovered ground in summer; nor remain too long on the same ground

6

in summer or in autumn. Orders included rules on marching and exercise, for exercise did a great deal more for the preservation of health than the art of physic. Officers were instructed to see that the sick had regular meals and were well looked after by the surgeons.[3]

Following the Roman occupation of Britain which lasted for 400 years it is a distinct probability that any medical arrangements of the armies in Saxon times followed more or less the Roman pattern, but the earliest mention of army surgeons comes to light in the so called *medici* of the Welsh. An early account from Italy tells us that in the ninth century Pope Leo VI had in addition to surgeons, cavalrymen called *deputati*, who had two stirrups on the left side of the saddle which were used to pick up wounded men behind them and carry them off the field.[4] They also carried water to relieve the sufferings of the wounded and are expressly mentioned as a necessary adjunct to an army, furnished as they were with field medicines and surgical materials.

By the settling of the Moors in Spain, Arabic medicine was introduced into Europe. At Salerno in Italy the first medical college in Europe was founded in the year 808, and was the first establishment to grant medical degrees after a prescribed course of five or six years study. The influence of its teaching was felt by the then embryo medical service of armies. When the Arabs were driven from Spain in the fifteenth century the Saracenic schools of medicine declined, the fountains of science dried up, and an intellectual darkness lasted for some 300 years, until the study of anatomy by dissection became permissible, and the circulation of the blood was discovered. The mediaeval physician and surgeon pursued his task with a feeble glimmer of empirical illumination which the army surgeons helped to keep alight, for as our story unfolds many instances will come to light where the knowledge and experience gained in campaigns have benefited contemporary medicine and surgery.

Largely due to their knowledge of Arabic, many of the physicians in Europe at the close of the tenth century were Jews, but the clergy were at this time trying to rival them as practitioners in physic and claiming that the practice of medicine was their peculiar privilege. A cannon law was passed declaring that no Jew might be a physician or treat a Christian. Consequently, in England as in most countries the practice of medicine at this early period lay in the hands of the clergy and the monks, and it was in the shelter of their religious houses that both military and civilians received treatment. Surgery ranked much below medicine, and the practice of this branch suffered a further serious decline when the celebrated Edict of Tours was promulgated in 1163. This forbade the clergy to shed blood, and Pope Honorious III directed that they should refuse their benediction to those who practised it. This split medicine and surgery wide apart, for while the priests and monks continued to practise medicine, surgery was relegated to their former lay assistants whose primary duty was shaving the monks' heads. The medical service of armies suffered particularly, for the treatment of wounds and injuries was undertaken by the more ignorant amongst the followers of the healing art. As a result the quacks and the charlatans were attracted to practise their unskilled craft with disastrous effects upon the common soldiery. In this unforeseen way too, the barber surgeons came into existence as an offshoot of clerical medicine, and this explains the link between the Church and the medical profession. An Act was passed in England in 1511 that no one could practise as a physician or surgeon in the City of London or within seven miles of it until he had first been examined and approved by the Bishop of London or the Dean of St. Paul's. This relationship existed as late as 1601, for according to Manningham's Diary, 'one Tristram Lyde, a surgeon, admitted to practice by the Archbishops, later was tried at Rochester Assize for killing divers women by annoytinge them with quicksilver'. Moreover the Archbishop of Canterbury exercised his power of conferring the degree of M.D. as lately as 1854.

It took some 400 years before the need for a comprehensive study of healing spread from Italy to England and medicine began to rid itself of the barbarism and superstition which up to now had surrounded it. It was not until the end of the twelfth century that the first college was founded at Oxford for the faculty of medicine, while in 1386 we read that on the foundation of New College by William Wykeham permission was given to follow 'the new study of medicine'. Henceforward we find army doctors being derived from two sources. The first were the educated class who had graduated in the University and were given the senior appointments in the medical department attached generally to the princes and nobles who commanded the army; the second source which provided the bulk of military surgeons were derived from the barber surgeons of inferior status who had acquired their skill by practical instruction and experience.

The military expeditions to the East which are known as the Crusades took place between the eleventh and thirteenth centuries. The Crusaders seemed to have forgotten the hygienic measures of the Romans, and in the insanitary conditions which prevailed in the heat of Palestine the three great afflictions of armies, dysentery, fever, and typhus caused considerable losses; moreover, both smallpox and leprosy were introduced into Europe. After the battle of Jaffa in 1192, the putrefying carcasses of thousands of horses and dead men 'made the air corrupt, and King Richard I of England and our army were much distressed and fell ill to such an extent that they almost all died'. 'The King lay very sick in his camp, the typhus continued, and the leeches were whispering about the great semitertian fever. They began to despair, and the wild despair spread over the camp.' King Philip of France too became seriously ill with fever, and we read that he 'sent to sick leeches to whom he gave fair jewels, praying for their advice on the best way of curing his malady. The leeches took counsel together and God gave them His grace, so that he recovered of his ailment.'[5] In the absence of organized hospitals or medical attendants the sick and wounded were of necessity treated by their comrades, and 'many a gallant knight who had escaped the dangers of the battlefield fell victim to disease, performing the humblest offices of a hospital nurse amongst his plague stricken comrades.'[6]

On the other hand Arabian doctors were renowned for their skill and knowledge, and Saladin's army appears to have been better served than the Crusaders. Even the principles of hygiene were practised to some degree, for we hear from Abd-el-Atif, a physician of Baghdad, that there were in the camp 'more than a thousand baths'[7], which were probably connected with the Mohammedan cult for religious cleanliness; the cost of a bath was a piece of silver.

Prince Edward of England in 1272 had 'chirurgeons' with his forces in Palestine, and when he was attacked and severely wounded by a follower of that leader of the Assassins 'the old man of the mountain', the weapon was regarded as poisoned, and the Master of the Templars administered what was considered a certain antidote which proved useless; an English chirurgeon was rash enough to come forward and promise a cure, which he was able to accomplish after making deep incisions and cutting away the mortified flesh.

The zealous work performed by surgeons in the Crusades is said to have impressed King Louis IX of France so favourably that in 1268 he founded a college or confrère of surgeons in honour of St. Cosme and St. Damien, and gave orders that all sick and wounded were to be medically treated at all churches dedicated to these saints on the first Monday of each month.[8]

We cannot pass over the period of the Crusades without mentioning the Knights of St. John of Jerusalem or the Hospitallers. This great military medical organization originated from a hospital founded in Jerusalem in 1023 by some rich merchants of Amalfi who had won favour with the Egyptian caliph, and was intended for the treatment of sick amongst the Christian pilgrims to Jerusalem. In 1113 their original endowment was added to by a Bull of Pope Paschal II and shortly afterwards in 1130 the order was organized on a military basis similar to the Knights Templars. It will be appropriate here to anticipate the further fortunes of the Order which was constituted of knights, chaplains, and serving brothers under a Grand Master. By 1331 there were branches throughout most of the European countries; the English branch was under two Grand Masters—one for England and one for Ireland—with headquarters at Clerkenwell in London. In King Stephen's reign they acquired further properties and became very wealthy. Many of the possessions of the Templars after their suppression in 1312 passed to the Hospitallers who later took part in the defence of Christendom against the Turks. Driven from Palestine they went to Cyprus, and thereafter conquered Rhodes where they were established for 200 years. Expelled from Rhodes by Soleyman the Magnificent in 1512, they came to Malta, where they remained until their Grand Master surrendered to the French in 1792. In describing the merits of this great order it will be appropriate to mention the formation of the St. John Ambulance Brigade in Britain in the nineteenth century, which, with its men and women trained in first aid and nursing, has rendered in time of war such devoted service in the ranks of the army medical service.

In the English feudal system the armoured knights and the men at arms constituted the principal strength in offensive warfare, while the footmen consisted of archers and Welsh spearmen. The latter received little medical attention in war—'he was bought to be sacrificed, he was used while in health and when sick or wounded left to die'.[9] Moreover, as Hart says, the scope of the military surgeon was limited by the policy of discharging soldiers who were unfit rather than treating them, a policy based on the cynical though economic fact that it cost more to cure a soldier than levy a recruit. What medical attention there was available was devoted to the treatment of the nobles and knights who were often accompanied by their wives. These ladies, who until they were married were usually educated in nunneries, were expected to have a good knowledge of the healing art and their office was to make salves and attend to the wounded, 'they shared with the monks in the knowledge which the age possessed of vulnerary medicaments'.[10]

The earliest account of English army surgeons occurs in the year 1223 when Henry III invaded France to attempt the reconquest of Normandy. It was in the form of a recommendation from the Chief Justice to the Bishop of Chichester of 'one Master Thomas, an army surgeon, who knows how to cure wounds, a science particularly useful in the siege of castles'. When Edward I invaded Scotland in 1298 he was accompanied by no fewer than seven medical men, including 'a King's physician and two juniors, a King's surgeon and two assistants, and a simple surgeon'. That they found plenty to do is indicated by the fact that the chief surgeon got compensation for three horses killed in Scotland 'on the King's service'[11]. The King's physician and surgeon of superior university status each received a knight's pay of 2s. a day, the 'simple' surgeons ranked as esquires and drew 1s. a day, and the assistants of leeches of inferior status like the 'medici' of the Welsh were paid 6d. a day. This points to three grades of military surgeons.

The number of these superior surgeons and physicians were few, for in Edward II's reign from 1307 to 1327 there were none upon the muster rolls.[12] But in the wardrobe account there are records of the payment of chirurgeons or leeches, who must have been of the barber surgeon type, for they ranked low in the military hierarchy with other trades such as farmer, blacksmith, butcher or merchant.

Edward III's reign was conspicuous for the two great victories in France of Crécy in 1346 and Poitiers in 1356. At Crécy the fight was largely won by the pitiless torrent of arrows poured upon the French horse by the long bowmen of England, although Fortescue says that equal credit must go to the valiant fight of the men at arms. The French left 11 great lords, 83 bannerets, 1,200 knights and thousands of common soldiers dead on the field, but the English losses are not quoted by Fortescue. It is certain they were not excessive and this is perhaps just as well as the name of only one surgeon is recorded, that of John Arderne, who in virtue of his appointment as sergeant surgeon to the King was attached to the staff of the Prince of Wales. He was one of the most distinguished surgeons of these early years, operated for fistula *in ano*, devised improvements in the technique of trepanning, and wrote *De Arte Medicinal*. Grose explains this apparent shortage of surgeons by the facts already noted, that in addition to the superior surgeons there were also inferior surgeons or barbers who were taken from the ranks and therefore paid and mustered as private soldiers. The latter rendered first aid to the common soldiery in the fight, and after treatment the slightly wounded were sent to the nearest monastery or religious house where they were attended by monks or nuns, and those men whose wounds required a considerable time to recover were dismissed with a small pecuniary provision to carry them home.[13] For the severely wounded who had no chance of recovery, it was customary for their comrades to quietly slit their throats on the field of battle and put them out of their pain. Soldiers who were permanently disabled and unfit for further service were sent to a religious institution to be there supported either for a time or for life.

Ten years later the victory of Poitiers was gained by the Black Prince, when both men at arms and archers fought superbly although outnumbered ten to one by the French army of 60,000 men. With the Welsh spearmen who fought in this battle were the first army surgeons to be distinguished in the field by wearing a baldrick as part of their uniform. This distinctive mark was a cross belt passing over one shoulder and under the opposite arm and may have been used to carry a pouch containing dressings for wounds.

In Edward's reign there is also the first mention of a form of army medical establishment in the accounts of the Treasurer to the King's household, for Grose says: 'There is one surgeon for the King's household troops; four physicians and one surgeon for the army of North Wales; two physicians and one surgeon for that of South Wales.' The pay of the sergeant surgeon to the King was 12d. a day with 8 marks per annum. But 12d. was only the same pay as that accorded to ushers, servers and butlers, so the majority of the profession was still regarded as of slight account. But Lanfranc who in the late fourteenth century wrote the *Science of Chirurgerie* gives a very different picture of the qualities of a surgeon of the superior or university class—'needful it is that a surgeon be of a complexcioun well proporciound, and that his complexcion be temperat'. One whose face is not seemly is impossible to have good manners. 'A surgeon must have hands well schape, long small fingers, and his body nought quakynge, and all his limbs able to fulfill good workings of his soule. He must be a sutyl wytt.' Referring then to both physicians and surgeons, he says—he must not be a glutton or a niggard but be pleasant in his manners to the sick. He is generally advised even in desperate cases to promise recovery, but to tell the patients' friends the truth, to abstain from self praise and from blaming other physicaians. He is to be well educated with a knowledge of philosophy, logic, grammar, rhetoric, physics, medicines and the science of mixtures. Going on to describe the treatment of surgical and medical complaints, he tells us that simple wounds were treated by binding them up with compresses so as to bring the parts of the wound together, and using a powder composed of frankincense, two parts of dragon's blood, and three parts of quicklime; larger wounds were stitched with stitches deep enough to leave no hollows in the wound; purulent wounds were to be well cleaned. Broken bones must be placed in apposition, and if an open wound is present it is not to be allowed to close until the bone has united. A good description of trepanning is given, and the noise affecting the patient during the operation was to be diminished by blocking up the ears. For hernia, a pad, a plaster, and a bandage was applied, the patient was dieted, violent exercise forbidden and constipation avoided. Hydrocele was treated by open incision; dropsy by diuretics, and ascites by tapping.

Turning now for a moment to the Continent, Guy de Chauliac published a work in 1363 on the healing of wounds which was probably the first of its kind and gives us an insight into the general treatment then adopted particularly in France and Germany. He classified surgeons into five groups—the first applied poultices to all wounds and abscesses; the second used wine only; the third treated wounds with ointment and soft plasters; the fourth, who attended to the armies, promiscuously used charms, potions, oil and wool; the fifth were old women and ignorant people who in all cases had recourse to the saints. De Chauliac himself recommended the German method of wound treatment which comprised exorcism, oil, wool and cabbage leaves.

Some fifty years later, when Henry V invaded France in 1415 at the head of an army of some 30,000 men, medical provision was on a more extended scale. There were two principal medical officers, Nicholas Colnet, a physician and William Morestede, a surgeon. Colnet was engaged for one year and attended closely on the King, with three men classified as archers as his attendants or assistants who were obviously barber surgeons and were paid 6d. a day together with 'regards'[14]. Colnet himself received 40 marks a year which was equal to the pay of an esquire in the same expedition. He was treated also as a combatant in receiving a share of plunder, but if his booty exceeded £20 he was to give up one-third to his Majesty[15]. Morestede was designated King's surgeon, and accompanying him was another principal surgeon William Bradwardyne by name, each of them with nine additional surgeons in their train, making a score in all[16]. Henry regarded their services as so important that he paid their salary a quarter in advance, 'and that they might always have security for the next quarter, the King engaged to put into their hands by way of pledges as many jewels or other articles as might be equal to one quarter's pay and subsistence'.[17]

Originally there was to have been a contingent of forty-eight surgeons under Morestede, for Rymer tells us that he was to procure by press, 'as many surgeons, and other artisans as were needful to make certain surgical instruments, as were required'.[18] But for some reason compulsion does not appear to have produced this number in sufficient time, for there were only fifteen present at the battle of Agincourt. They were as usual classed as tradesmen, amongst miners, gunners, armourers, painters, pavilion men, surgeons, grooms, purveyors, smiths and saddlers.[19] They were subject to military discipline, this list including 'soldiers, shoemakers, tailors, barbers (surgeons), physicians and washerwomen'.[20]

At the siege of Harfleur which preceded Agincourt the army was decimated by such a severe epidemic of dysentery that 2,000 men died, including many of the senior officers, and 5,000 had to be sent back to England to recover. But by the aid of cannon which was here used by the English forces for the first time, Harfleur surrendered after a month. Henry however was not content with this relatively small success, and although after losses from disease, casualties, and garrisoning Harfleur, he could only muster some 9,000 men, he set out with these on the march to Calais. At Agincourt, north of the river Somme his progress was barred by a French army 60,000 strong, and the great victory which followed was won by the outstanding success of the English bowmen. There is no information of the medical arrangements for the battle where Morestede acted as the principal medical officer, and was provided with 1 waggon and 2 sumpter horses presumably to carry medical equipment. The disposal of the wounded[21] must have followed the methods with which we are already familiar, the majority being admitted to the religious houses in the vicinity and left to the care of the monks, while the severely wounded presented no medical problem for 'on the following morning, the English troops, in marching off the field, killed all the hopelessly wounded, for the humane purpose of putting them out of pain'.[22]

In Henry's reign an attempt was made to purge the profession of many unqualified persons who practised surgery and by their rude methods brought it into disrepute. 'No one shall use the mysterie of fysyk, unless he hath studied it in some university, and is at least a bachelor in that science.' So ran the Act of Parliament 9th Henry V. 1422.[23]

During Edward IV's reign Jacobus Fryle was King's physician at 2s. a day with two assistants at 6d. a day each, while William Hobbs as surgeon of the King's body had 1s. 6d. a day. Engaged to serve the King in France there were in addition to these principal medical officers 7 surgeons at 1s. a day, and 5 inferior surgeons or barbers at 6d. a day.[24]

We have already mentioned the employment of cannon at the siege of Harfleur when 'men are martyrized and cut down at more than half a mile distance by those furious and thundering engines of great cannon'. We have now to study the unusual problems which army surgeons had to face in treating wounds of an entirely new type. At first the general opinion was that wounds were poisoned by the powder used or by the heat generated by the projectiles' passage through the air. This provoked serious discussion on gun shot wounds by the early writers who included the most famous French surgeon of the time, Ambroise Paré, the inventor of the ligature. The initial treatment adopted for these 'poisoned' wounds was to kill the poison by heat in the form of boiling oil, and this was reinforced by prayers, incantations, exorcism and charms as necessary adjuncts to cure. But Paré was the first to reject this 'poison' theory and abandon boiling oil and the cautery. Further it was by chance that he stumbled on the new treatment which was to make history.

'Now I was at this time a fresh water soldier; I had not yet seen wounds made by gunshot at the first dressing. It is true I had read in John de Vigo's first book *Of Wounds in General* eighth chapter, that wounds made by firearms partake of venemosity by reason of the powder, and for their cure he bids you cauterize them with oil of elders scalding hot mixed with a little treacle; and to make no mistake, before I would use the said oil, knowing this was to bring great pain to the patient, I asked first before I applied it, what the other surgeon did for the first dressing; which was to put the said oil, boiling well, into the wounds, with tents and setons, wherefore I took courage to do as they did. At last my oil ran short and I was forced instead thereof to apply a digestive made of the yolk of eggs, oil of roses and turpentine. In the night I could not sleep in quiet, fearing some default in not cauterizing, that I should find the wounded to whom I had not used the said oil dead from the poison of their wounds; which made me rise very early to visit them, where beyond my expectations I found that those to whom I had applied my digestive medicament had but little pain, and their wounds without inflammation or swelling, having rested fairly well that night, the others to whom the boiling oil was used, I found feverish, with great pain and swelling about the edges of the wounds. Then I resolved never more to burn these cruelly poor men with gunshot wounds. While I was at Turin I found a surgeon famed above all others for his treatment of gunshot wounds into whose favour I found means to insinuate myself, to have the recipe of his balm, as he called it, wherewith he dressed gunshot wounds. And he made me pay my court to him for two years before I could possibly draw the recipe from him. In the end, thanks to my gifts and presents, he gave it to me: which was to boil in oil of lilies young whelps just born and earth worms prepared with Venetian turpentine. Then I was joyful and my heart made glad, that I had understood his remedy which was like that I had obtained by chance. See how I learned to treat gunshot wounds; not by books.'[25]

We have in this account anticipated the chronology of our story for it happened in the year 1536. Although much fun has been made of the oil and puppy dressing, Clifford Allbutt says that, 'from this time the receptive mind of Paré perceived venom and burn were figments both, and that a gunshot wound was just a contusion or combination like another'.[26] Sir William MacCormac in his Hunterian oration of 1899 summed up the benefits to surgery which this remarkable man was able to achieve. 'The surgery of the Middle Ages,' he said, 'was a trade; Ambroise Paré and Jean Louis Petit converted it into an art; John Hunter elevated it to the rank of a science.'

We must turn back to some important events in medical history which occurred between the fourteenth and sixteenth centuries. The superior or qualified surgeons or the master surgeons by which name they were sometimes designated, many of whom had seen army service, formed themselves into a separate guild in 1368-9. Fifty years later in the year 1421 they combined with the physicians. The barber surgeons who carried out the tasks of venesection, cupping, application of leeches, giving enemas and extracting teeth obtained a separate charter in 1462 in the reign of Edward VI and became a city company 'the better to protect the King's lieges from going the way of all flesh through the ignorance and negligence of various unskillful barbers and other practioners in surgery'.

The union of the physicians and master surgeons was not a happy one and it was dissolved some fifty years later when Linacre, one of Henry VIII's physicians, obtained through Cardinal Wolsey letters patent from the King incorporating physicians in one body. This body formed in 1518 was the forerunner of the Royal College of Physicians, and one of its chief privileges was the power of preventing anyone taking up the practice of physic within 7 miles of London except by special licence. This was followed by the master surgeons becoming incorporated in a fellowship which was accorded a grant of arms, ultimately leading in 1540 to amalgamation with the barber surgeons. Holbein's famous picture shows the formation of the Company of Barbers and Surgeons with Henry presenting the charter.

The monopoly given to the College of Physicians was a bitter bone of contention between physicians and surgeons for many years, the former endeavouring to prevent the surgeons giving internal remedies, and as late as 1632 the physicians obtained an Order in Council forbidding surgeons to perform major operations unless a physician was present.

These important advances in the organization of the profession are of interest because the improvement in status which affected all doctors would it was hoped be reflected in advancing the position of the army surgeons in their relationship with their combatant comrades.

Thomas Gale was the most noted army surgeon of Henry VIII's reign and served in the expeditions which Henry undertook in accordance with his alliance with the Emperor Charles I. He was present as principal medical officer at the siege of Montreuil in 1554, and at St. Quentin three years later, where in a force of some 5,000 Horse and Foot and a train of artillery, Gore tells us there were no fewer than fifty-seven surgeons.[27] This unusually large number may be accounted for by a change which was taking place in army organization. The infantry company consisting of 100 men under a captain, was now emerging as the tactical unit, and to each company a surgeon was to be attached. In addition all senior officers were more than adequately provided for, for we learn that there were 2 surgeons for the General, 1 for the Lieutenant General, 1 for the High Marshall, 1 for the General of Horse, 1 for the General of Foot, and 1—a new appointment—for the Master of Ordnance or artillery train. There had been great difficulty in providing sufficient surgeons for this force and Gale had written to Queen Elizabeth—'I have myself helpe to furnish out of London in one year seventy-two surgeons who were good men, which served by sea and land, and were well able to serve, and all Englishmen. Now there are not thirty-four of the whole company of Englishmen, and yet the most part of them be in noblemen's service, so that if we should have need I do not know where to find twelve sufficient men.'[28] This shortage appears to be due to two causes; first, the provision of a surgeon to each company increased enormously the number required and was a shocking waste of medical manpower, and secondly, the attachment of so many surgeons to the staff or noblemen's service as Gale describes it. It was obviously asking too much of the recently constituted Company of Barbers and Surgeons in the twenty-five years of its existence to provide competent surgeons on this scale. Inevitably, the way lay open for charlatans and quacks to prey upon the soldiers. 'When I was at the wars of Muttrel,' Gale tells us, 'there was a great rabblement there that took upon them to be surgeons. Some were sow gelders and horse gelders, with tinkers and cobblers.' These quacks made such pretentious claims to cure that the Duke of Norfolk, hearing that many men had died at their hands, made Gale investigate their claims. He quickly exposed their malpractices. Such trash as grease for horses' heels, shoemakers' wax, and rust from old pans was used for what they termed a 'noble salve', and this 'worthy rabblement' as Gale terms them, 'were committed to the Marshalsea prison'.[29]

Neither had the low status of the army surgeons been improved, for we read in a code of 'instructions for forming camps' that 'the servants, the physicians and the chirurgeons of the court are classed together in the allotment of ground'. This appears strange when Henry's support of the doctors' charter is remembered; and moreover the amateur practice of medicine was a common habit amongst the higher nobility. Henry VIII himself is said by Froude to have been one of the first physicians of his kingdom and dabbled in pharmacy, for amongst the Sloane manuscripts in the British Museum is one termed 'A booke of plaister, spasmdrops, ointments, etc. devysed by the King's Magestie, Dr. Burts, Dr. Chambers, Dr. Cromer and Dr. Augustine.'

His wide experience provided Gale with a sound knowledge of the treatment of gunshot wounds, (*An excellent treatment on wounds made with Gunneshot, 1563.*) and in spite of their livid appearance, he condemned the theory that they were poisoned, and denied that bullets acquired heat whilst in motion so that the wounds appeared to have been cauterized. Accordingly, he agreed with Paré and said it was entirely wrong to treat them as if they were venomous snake bites by the application of boiling oil and the cautery. Instead, he advised the use of a styptic powder made of a mixture of alum, lime, arsenic and strong vinegar applied by means of tow covered with white of egg. Fortescue tells us how much the boiling oil treatment was feared and resented. 'Wise men took refuge in the virtues of cold water and kept the surgeons at a safe distance.'[30] 'Trust a doctor and he will kill you, mistrust him and he will insult you,' wrote a Frenchman who had suffered much from the profession.[31] In recognition of his services he was made Sergeant Surgeon to Queen Elizabeth, an appointment which carried a retaining fee as salary on the condition that he attended the Sovereign on active service in the field.

Ralphe Smith was another writer who tells us that for forty years from 1559 to 1603 the unsatisfactory position occupied by army surgeons, largely due to the inferior social class from which they were recruited, attracted frequent attention. A remedy was attempted by improving the necessary qualifications, and a code of rules was drawn up laying down the attributes which medical men should possess. 'Surgeons should be men of sobriety, of good conscience, and skilful in that science; able to heal all sores and wounds, especially to take out a pellet of the same.'

The company organization with a surgeon employed for each company was as we have pointed out excessively wasteful of medical manpower, but the detached role the company was called on to play made some form of medical aid essential, especially in conditions such as prevailed in Ireland. These surgeons drew pay at 1s. a day, and still had the task of hair cutting and trimming for which they were paid 2d. a month by each soldier as 'regards'. But this money did not go into the surgeon's pocket. The tight fisted Treasury had no intention of providing medicines for the troops while this source of revenue lay to hand. So the surgeon was made to buy his drugs and dressings locally as best he might;—'that the surgeon be truly paid his wages, and all money due to him for cures, that by the same he maye be able to provide all such stuffs as to him is needful' and 'readily employ his industry upon the sore and wounded soldiers'.[32] On the captain lay the responsibility that his surgeon should have 'all oyles, balms, salves, instruments, and necessary stuffs to them belonging', and he had to provide for their transport. So the wretched soldier was by his 'regards' indirectly paying for his own medicines.

It was in Queen Mary's reign that a material benefit was first made for her disabled soldiers, for in her will she left provision for a house in London with an endowment of 400 marks a year. This at least was the beginning of a humanitarian outlook for the long neglected soldier, but the numbers of the disabled soon far exceeded the accommodation, and in Elizabeth's reign they were relegated to the care of their respective parochial authorities.

Although the pay in general was now being gradually increased there were many fluctuations at different times, and the remuneration depended largely on the decision of the different commanders. This is revealed by the remarks of John Harvey, an army surgeon in the previous reign of Henry VII. He repeats the fact with which we are now familiar that there were several different grades of surgeons differentiated by their training and professional skill, and we are here introduced for the first time to the system of patronage which was to last until the end of the eighteenth century. 'He that will be a surgeon in the war must select and choose him a captain or some noble liberal man that loveth well men and know that he will allow his surgeon a dey(?). If he be a noble man that is your captain he will allow you as other noble men do, that is 2s. a day unto the chief surgeon, unto the second surgeon 20d. a day, the third surgeon 16d. a day, the fourth surgeon 12d. a day, his servant 6d. and a groat apiece of every soldier every month.'[33] Ralphe Smith says in a manuscript quoted by Scott that the army surgeon's pay should be augmented by 2d. from every soldier at pay day 'as in tymes past hath been accustomed, in consideration whereof the surgeon ought readilie to employ his industrie upon the soare and wounded souldiers, not intermedlinge with any other cures to them noysome . . . such surgeons muste wear their baldricks, whereby they may be known in the tyme of slaughter; it is their charter in the field.'

That baldricks were indeed the mark of the surgeon is evident from the account of a march past of the London contingent of the Militia held in 1539 when the surgeons of the city appeared 'without harness in white coates with their bandes of white and green baldrick wise, and their splatters over the bende in good order and apparell'.[34]

It was in Elizabeth's reign that the growing importance of an efficient medical service received the attention of military writers, and the sudden deluge of military pamphlets which burst over the country from 1587 onwards. Barnaby Rich wrote *Pathway to Military Practice* in which he affirmed that 'a good and skilful chirurgeon is a necessary man to be had in a companie, such a one as should work according to art, not practising new experiments upon a poore souldier, by means whereof many have been utterly maymed by a chirurgeon's practice, that otherwise might have done very well'. The need to provide amb- ulance transport for the casualties was stressed in another pamphlet by Digges in his '*Stratiocon*'. 'It were convenient,' he says, 'to appropriate certain carriages and men of purpose to give their attention in every skirmishe and encounter to carry away the hurt men to such place as surgions may immediately repayre unto them, which shall not only greatly incourage the souldier, but also cause the skirmish to be better maintained when the souldiers shall not need to leave the field, to carry away their hurt men.' This sensible proposal to save manpower and improve morale was, it should be noted, made by a combatant and not by a medical officer, but nothing whatever was done by the authorities, and even as late as the period of the Crimean war in 1854 we will see that positive orders had to be given by commanders that the fighting ranks must not be depleted by wounded men being carried out of action by their comrades. Such utter disregard to the provision of special bearers for the wounded compelled them to remain helpless on the field of battle until the action was over, and it is impossible to calculate the sacrifice of life and limb which resulted from the neglect of these wretched victims of war.

The whole pattern of war was now changing. Firearms and pikes were now replacing the bill and the long bow. Regiments now appeared comprising a variable number of companies temporarily united under the command of a lieutenant colonel. At regimental headquarters a surgeon major was appointed to co-ordinate the duties of the company surgeon.

In Elizabeth's reign there was continuous trouble in Ireland, there were constant disorders on the Scottish border, and there were wars against France and Spain. The operations in Ireland were carried out in a country largely covered with dense forests and bogs. It became impossible to feed the troops from local sources and rations were supplied in part payment of the troops wages. The lack of good food and the constant exposure, in spite of the provision of tents, brought on attacks of dysentery, while the natural dampness of the Irish climate rendered intermittent fever as great a pest as dysentery, and there were scattered outbreaks of bubonic plague. Owing to the suppression of the monasteries and abbeys and the dispersion of the monks the hospitals and houses of entertainment which they had been in the habit of maintaining had closed, and there was almost complete dearth of local medical assistance. There is no exact record of the number of medical officers serving with the army over the long period of forty-five years which covered Elizabeth's Irish wars, but when we come to the year 1597 we find that under Lord Mountjoy there were sixteen surgeons with a principal medical officer in charge and one physician serving with a force of 12,000 men located on the Ulster border. There was in fact a shortage of physicians, and a soldier of fortune wrote to Lord Burghley from Drogheda, 'I have my Lord, thank God, recovered my health, having no other physytyne nor ffrende to looke to but Hym,'[35] and a letter is extant from one Barnaby Googe describing how 'comynge syck from sea, my lodgyng on the ground, the sudden change of my dyett and the barbarous relief I have had brought me the country disease, (dysentery)'. He ascribes his recovery to drinking water out of a 'rusty skull'. There was at this time only one apothecary in all Ireland, one Thomas Smythe of Dublin, to whom in 1566 was given an agreement to receive 'the yearly sum of one day's pay of the Lord Deputy, and whole army in Ireland, and also twenty shillings of each sworn councillor, in order to encourage the said Smythe to continue in the discharge of his ministry in Ireland.'[36]

Sick and wounded officers were always carried to the nearest towns, where Gore tells us that some would die of gangrene a year after the receipt of their wounds. But the common soldiery had to endure less preferential treatment, and when they could not be transported to the nearest town or castle had to be left behind to the tender mercy of the enemy, whose own wounded were chiefly tended in caves and other secret localities by the young leeches or physicians who followed the fortunes of their tribes. The guerilla tactics adopted by the Irish meant that constant guard over the sick and wounded was essential.

We must turn now to the important field of operations in the Low Countries where English troops first set foot in 1572 to help the Dutch in their fight against the Catholic overlords of Spain.

As principal medical officer to the forces in the Netherlands went William Clowes, a surgeon of prominence who was originally a naval surgeon, and accompanying him came William Godorus the Queen's Sergeant Surgeon. In Holland we are faced once more with the ever present complaint of surgeons of poor quality, tending the sick to 'the great distress of the army'. 'It is most truly said,' writes Clowes, 'there is no coine so current but hath in it some counterfeits, which make it suspicious; so it is there is no profession so good but hath also some counterfeits, which breed in it disgrace; and none so much I suppose as there bee in some these daies, that take upon them the honest title and name of travelling surgeons . . . they have beene and daily are entertained to be principal surgeons of ships of war, and charge of numbers of men . . . truly, many a brave soldier and mariner hath perished.'[37] This was in a work which he published in 1596 under the title *A Profitable and Necessary Book of Observation for all those that are Burned with the Flames of Gunpowder and also for the Curing of Wounds made with Musket, and Caliver, Shot, etc.* Clowes followed Paré's treatment of using emollient applications; in checking haemorrhage after amputation he applied 'buttons' of absorbent styptic material to the bleeding vessel sustaining them in position by means of tow and lint under strong pressure; although acquainted with Paré's methods of ligature he never found it necessary to employ them.

We know nothing more of the medical arrangements of these wars except the names of certain individuals, and amongst them we mention Peter Lowe who for four years was Chirurgeon Major to the Spanish regiment in Paris. He published a book on the whole *Art of Chirurgie* His method of amputation was simply to chop the limb off by the use of a hatchet and check haemorrhage with red hot irons to the stump.

John Woodall makes his first appearance as army surgeon in 1589 under Lord Willoughby in the Low Countries and we will come across him later serving under the Stuart kings. He rose to direct the medical service both of the navy and of the East India Company, travelled extensively, including a voyage to India, and was noteworthy in being the first to recommend lime juice in the treatment of scurvy. He regarded it as a disease of the spleen and treated it by lime juice 'each morning two or three spoonfulls, and fast after it two hours, and if you add one spoonful of aqua vitae thereto to a cold stomach it is better'. In 1617 he wrote *The Surgeon's Mate* which gives a list of instruments, utensils, and medicines of a naval surgeon's chest, and deals with fractures, dislocations, and amputations. By some he is credited with inventing the trephine. Woodall followed the example of his contemporary Paré in ligaturing vessels after amputation. 'If the leg be taken off above the knee there is the more danger, also there is great care to be had of the great vein and artery, namely that thou take them up and pierce them threw, and make strong ligature about them, which must be speedily done if thou canst do it.' His experience of the plague in the epidemics of 1625 and 1636 induced him to write a treatise on the *Plague and Pestilential Fever.*

In James I and Charles I's reigns troops continued to serve both in the Low Countries and in Germany. In 1624 the final breach with Spain occurred, and a force of 16,000 men, levied by press, was sent to serve in the Netherlands under Prince Maurice of Nassau. The list of medical officers dispatched shows at last that there was a substantial increase in pay for the more senior ranks 'in the General's trayne', 'with two physicians at 6s. 8d. a day each, two surgeons at the same rate of pay and two apothecaries at 3s. 4d.'. Every regiment of foot now consisted of twelve companies of 150 men, with a surgeon major at 4s. *per diem*, (equal to the pay of a captain), and a surgeon to each company at 1s. a day (the pay of an ensign). The staff of the General of Cavalry included one chief surgeon at 4s. a day, and every troop of 100 men had a surgeon at 2s. 6d. a day. In medical charge of the ordnance and pioneers there was a surgeon at 2s. a day and two under-surgeons at 6d. a day each.

In the wars in Scotland the force dispatched in 1639 included 2 physicians, 2 surgeons and 2 apothecaries attached to the Lord General's train, and these acted as specialists in the treatment of the medical and surgical cases which the regimental surgeon major and his company surgeons were unable to treat. 'In everie companie there must be a chirurgeon to attend which are sick, to dress the wounds of such as are hurt (being as an assistant to the chirurgeon of the regiment) having proper remedies to staunch the blood, to hinder inflammation, and to assuage the pain.'[38]

It is noteworthy that field hospitals did not appear in the English army until the end of the seventeenth century and they make their first appearance in William III's campaign in Ireland in 1690. In this we were far behind the Continent, for both in Spain and France they had existed for many years. It is in fact in the year 1484 that there is a record of the first field hospital accompanying troops during active operations, and this took place in Spain in the reign of Queen Isabella. In France the first movable hospital was established at the siege of Amiens in 1597, and in January 1629 an ordinance of Richelieu authorized the first stationary hospitals in the rear of armies in the field. During the reign of Louis XIV military hospitals were established in increasing numbers in many garrison towns and in support of armies in the field.

It is perhaps hardly necessary to remind the reader that all physicians and surgeons serving with the armies were employed only for the duration of hostilities and received their discharge when the campaigns ended.

The New Model which came into being in 1645 was the creation of Oliver Cromwell during the Civil War between Royalist and Roundhead. It was the precursor of the Standing Army. The New Model was composed of 12 regiments of foot and 11 regiments of horse with artillery and engineers, in all some 30,000 strong. For the first time it was clothed in scarlet tunics, a colour which was to become the traditional uniform of the 'red coats'. For each regiment there was now a regular medical establishment consisting at first of one regimental chirurgeon, assisted by one barber-chirurgeon with each company, whose task was to cut the soldiers' hair as well as giving first aid. But when the companies were reduced in size and number in 1655 these barber-chirurgeons were abolished, and from then on the establishment for a regiment of Foot was one chirurgeon and one chirurgeon's mate, and for a regiment of Horse one chirurgeon. The withdrawal of these barber-chirurgeons was not universally approved, for Elton wrote in 1659: 'In every Company there ought to be a barber-chirurgeon for the trimming of the soldiers' hair, who ought likewise to have some skill in chyrygery, so that he may be at hand in the absence of the chirurgeon of the regiment to bind up and dress the hurt and wounded men.' This was equivalent to a first aid dresser in each company.

With the creation of the regimental medical establishment came the origins of the regimental hospital equipped with beds for the sick and wounded which in due course was standardized to treat up to forty patients. Soldiers from the regiment were detailed as hospital orderlies and subordinate staff. Inevitably they were raw and untrained and were generally assigned because of their unsuitability as fighting soldiers rather than for their ability as sick attendants. There was invariably female help available from the wives of the soldiers, a proportion of whom were always allowed to accompany their husbands to the wars, but they were usually employed on washing and culinary duties.

It was hoped that the creation of a regular army with its prospect of long and continued service would overcome the constant shortages of regimental surgeons which had hitherto prevailed. In the beginning of Charles I's reign it had been so difficult to provide sufficient surgeons on a voluntary basis for the forces employed in the war against France and Spain that Orders in Council were issued by the King in 1626 to the Company of Surgeons of London ordering them to impress medical officers for the expeditions.

The Company of Surgeons was at this time deeply involved in service matters and acted as the administrative head of both the army and the navy; not only were they ordered to undertake the impressment of all surgeons, but to control and supply both medicines and surgical materials for the surgeons' chests. The arbitrary power of impressment given to the Company was that of forcing members or freemen of their Corporation who had undergone the ordinary examinations to qualify them to practice in London to serve with the army. At this time the guiding spirit of the Surgeon's Company was John Woodall, who proceeded to point out the inducements offered to young doctors to join the army. 'I acquaint the younger sons of surgeons,' he said, 'with these special favours which it then (1626) pleased our most gracious King Charles to bestow upon our Corporation in particular . . . for the good of his soldiers and seamen, and our encouragements thereby to animate and enable us the more heartily to serve him.' We learn that the pay of surgeons was to be 30s. a month and the pay of surgeons' mates 20s. a month. These miserly rates would never attract well trained doctors, so extra allowances were offered as an inducement as Woodall points out, 'Also His Majesty allowed to each surgeon 2s. 6d. the day which is £3 15s. 0d. the month, and to each mate £3 a month, and moreover alloweth and gave to each surgeon appointed to 250 men a surgery chest of £17 valew free of account.' This meant that the total pay for a surgeon was 5 guineas a month and for a mate £4 a month. For a senior surgeon (or surgeon major as he was called) the pay was to be 5s. a day, and two mates under him were to receive 4s. a day each, while 'His Majestie alloweth to the surgeon major a store chest or a magazine chest of £48 valew for a supply to furnish upon all wants and occasions.' These allowances were not ungenerous but in the case of the regimental surgeon and mate they were not to last, for the surgeon's pay was subsequently fixed at 4s. a day and the mate's pay at 2s. 6d., and these rates were to last for the next 100 years. When the expedition to Rochelle was planned in 1628, the King issued the following mandate: 'These shall be to will and require you the Master and the Wardens of the Company of Chirurgeons forthwith to impress and take up . . . sixteen able and efficient chirurgeons, and that you take special care that they be such in particular as are best experienced in the care of wounds made by gun shot, and likewise that their chests be sufficiently furnished with all necessary provisions requisite for the said employment, and that you charge them upon their allegiance as they will answer the contrary at their perils to repair to Portsmouth by the 10th of July, to go along with such commanders whose company they shall be appointed to serve.'[39]

In the New Model Army a similar obligation on the Company to provide surgeons continued if volunteers were not forthcoming, for there is an extract from the journal of the House of Commons for 12th October 1644: 'Ordered that it be referred to the Master and Wardens of the Apothecaries and Surgeons to make choice of able and fit men for surgeons to be sent to My Lord General's army; and if such as be chosen and appointed by them shall refuse to go . . . that they give orders to the pressing of them for the said service.'[40]

Although the compulsion to service was chiefly directed to surgeons, for the need of them was so essential, physicians were not exempt, for on the 1st July 1643—the House of Commons 'Ordered that Dr. Paul de Laune and Dr. Nathalean Chamberlaine, Physicians, be forthwith sent to the Army for the service of the Army . . . and this House doth declare that whatever physicians or surgeons shall be employed by the House, shall have the same allowances as others formerly have had . . . And the two surgeons now to be employed shall have their chests furnished with medicine each of them to the value of £20.'[41]

Medicines at this time were divided into internal and external and were in fact what the names imply. It was only the medicines for internal use which were to be provided by the State to stock the surgeons' two chests or panniers which were carried on a pack horse. External medicines such as materials for fomentations, liniments, dressings for ulcers, ointments, etc. were on the other hand to be supplied by the surgeon, but the cost of them was in fact borne by the soldiers themselves from the compulsory stoppage of 2d. a month levied from their pay. By this regulation the Treasury saved money and laid the cost of treatment on the poorly paid soldier.

On the Headquarters Staff of the Army the medical appointments in which we are interested comprised a physician who was personal medical attendant to the Commander, 1 army physician, 1 apothecary, 1 chirurgeon, and 2 mates. They were classified as staff officers and drew higher rates of pay.[42] Their task was to treat the sick and wounded which the regimental chirurgeons were unable to cope with in their regimental hospitals. In the absence of a field military hospital they were expected to give their services wherever they were most required, usually by collecting the sick and wounded in some private house or institution where an *ad hoc* hospital would be formed with bedding and other items of furniture provided under local arrangements. As these officers were the first holders of medical staff appointments, their names deserve to be mentioned; the physicians were Doctors Payne and Strawhill; the apothecary who drew such an unusually high rate of pay was Mr. Webb, and the chirurgeon Mr. Firth.

Apart from the headquarter organization for the regiments of Foot there was a separate headquarters for the eleven regiments of Horse to which a chirurgeon and mate were appointed whose task as staff officers was of a similar nature.

The titles of physician general, surgeon general, and apothecary general make their first appearance during the Civil War, although they do not officially appear as officers of the Headquarters Staff until King William III's campaign in Flanders in 1691,[43] and on the Home Establishment until 1717.[44] But it is known that Manchester, one of the Parliamentary generals had Dr. Henry Glisson as Physician General; in General Monk's army in Scotland it was Dr. Samuel Barrow, and in Cromwell's army in Ireland there were Dr. John Waterhouse and Dr. William Petty. All were paid at the rate of 10s. a day. The next appointment to be made was the apothecary general who was required to supply the internal medicines which the physicians and regimental surgeons needed and he was paid at the rate of 6s. 8d. a day. Lastly came the chirurgeon general—Cromwell had one by the name of Mr. James Winter, but as his pay was only 4s. a day he was obviously not of high professional standing.

There was in fact a great difference in the medical training of physicians and surgeons. Physicians justifiably considered themselves the *élite* of the medical profession for they were graduates of the universities of Oxford or Cambridge, while the great majority of surgeons were not graduates but qualified to practice medicine after a series of lectures and attendance in the wards of a civil hospital. Mates were drawn from the class of apprentices to general practitioners.

We must now describe the medical aspects of the Civil War and the arrangements for the care of the sick and wounded. In the absence of any military hospitals with the armies in the field, casualties were admitted to civil hospitals or treated in private houses or other accommodation. On the Parliamentary side the arrangements to use civil hospitals were made by the Parliamentary Commissioners who exercised all the administrative functions of the medical service, and we find some of the greater hospitals in London utilized, including St. Thomas, St. Bartholomew, Bridewell and Bethlehem. During the siege of Reading in 1643, the Earl of Essex sent his wounded to these hospitals, but in the course of time owing to the numbers under treatment the cost became so great—St. Bartholomew's alone had 1,122 'maimed soldiers'—that in 1644 Parliament compounded by freeing the hospitals from taxation. The pressure of numbers however continued so that it became necessary finally to establish military hospitals in different parts of the kingdom. In London two were opened, one at the Savoy in November 1644, and another at Ely House for 350 patients in 1648; in Dublin two more were established for the Irish campaign in 1649; and in Scotland where outbreaks by Royalist sympathizers led to a campaign by General Monk to reduce the Highlands in 1654, Heriot's Hospital was opened in Edinburgh. At Heriot's there is a record of the patient's diet; on four days each week patients had $1\frac{1}{2}$ lbs. of meat, 2 lb. of bread, and one Scots pint of beer; on the other three days, 5 oz. of butter and 5 oz. of cheese, and a pint of milk or gruel. The cost was 4s. per patient per week, while convalescents fed themselves out of hospital on an allowance of 3s. 6d. a week. The total cost of running this hospital ranged from £1,300 in 1655 to £587 in 1659, but we are not told whether the staff in the military hospitals were military or civilian. Female nurses, however, were employed in all of them at pay between 4s. and 4s. 6d. a week; with one nurse to every five patients in Edinburgh to one to every twelve patients in London. If a sick soldier broke the hospital rules he was fined and expelled after the third offence. Nurses also were expelled if they neglected their duties, and marriage between nurses and patients was forbidden.

In 1642 Parliament published a declaration to provide for disabled soldiers, their wives and families, and soldiers' widows and orphans; in 1648 £100 was paid to soldiers blinded at the battle of Marston Moor.

To deal with casualties in the field the policy adopted was to reinforce the medical staff officers with civilian surgeons sent from London, and this occurred after the battle of Naseby where the wounded were collected at Northampton and some fifty or sixty local inhabitants who had received wounded men in their houses were paid for the attention they had given to the cases. During an attack on Nottingham Castle by the Royalists, the Commandant of the besieged Roundheads complained that 'not so much as a surgeon was amongst them'. But the Governor's wife supplied the want, having some 'excellent balsams and plasters in her closet, with the assistance of a gentleman who had some skill, dressed all their wounds, whereof some were dangerous (being all shots) with such good success that they were all cured in convenient time'.[45] When a distinguished soldier was sick or wounded a special consultant from London was sent to attend him; thus when Cromwell fell ill in Edinburgh in 1651 Drs. Wright and Bates were sent from London; in such cases liberal fees were paid by Parliament.

In the Irish campaign Cromwell's forces were indifferently supplied with medical assistance. At the siege of Clonmel, Cromwell wrote to Lord Craighill that 'he was in a miserable condition before Clonmel where his army was suffering from the bloody flux'.[46] When General Monk took over command he was careful and solicitous of his men's welfare, although they were ill shod and without clothes, he 'took charge himself of the soldiers' food, did his best to provide them with quarters, watched over them in difficulties, and even had, when necessary, his remedies and prescriptions'.[47] As the only hospitals with the army in the field were the small regimental hospitals which were constantly on the move and ill equipped to deal with severe cases, these were treated by the medical staff officers in the military hospitals which had been opened in Dublin with civilian nurses as attendants. But there were many occasions when the casualties received treatment locally as in the incident recorded of the Viscountess Thurles; after the fight at Archestown she tended the wounded and kept them for many weeks, when they were returned 'well cured and refreshed with supplies of money and provisions'.[48]

Cromwell's conquest of Ireland brings the name of Dr. William Petty to our notice. In 1651 he was appointed Physician General to the army in Ireland with pay at the very high rate of 20s. a day, and being heartily dissatisfied with the arrangements for the supply of medicines he usurped the task of the Apothecary General and determined to take on the supply himself. The result was that he deprived the Apothecary General of his legitimate perquisites by saving the sum of £500 a year. To quote his own words: 'the vast and needless expense of

27

medicaments, and how the Apothecary General of the army with his three assistants did not spend their time to the best advantage; and forthwith, to the content of all persons concerned, with the stated bare disbursement of £120, he did save them £500 per annum of their former charge; and furnished the army hospitals, garrisons and head-quarters with medicaments without the least noise or trouble, reducing that affair to a state of easiness and plainness which before was held a mystery, and a vexation to such as laboured to administer it well'.[49]

Petty was a remarkable character. A self-made man, he studied medicine at Utrecht, Leyden, and Paris, before taking a degree at Oxford University, and becoming a member of the College of Phys-icians. After the conquest of Ireland the rebel lands were divided up amongst the officers and soldiers as compensation for their arrears of pay, and the officers had such confidence in his ability that he was appointed to supervise the survey of the forfeited lands in the process of which he did so well for himself that he left the army and settled in London where he became well known in the city. One of the original founders of the Royal Society, he was knighted by Charles II in 1662 when that body was incorporated. Amongst other activites he invented a 'velocipede', and wrote a book on political economy; a friend of Christopher Wren and Evelyn, the latter said that he had 'never known such another genius', and he was called 'the Most Versatile Man of his Age'. By the marriage of his daughter with Thomas Fitzmaurice he became the ancester of Lord Lansdowne.

So much for the Roundheads; let us see how the Royalists fared. Dr. Wilson was personal physician to the King during the war and accompanied him to Hampton Court where he shared his captivity; the illustrious William Harvey the discoverer of the circulation of the blood, was with the King's forces in his capacity as a physician.

After the defeat of the Parliamentarians at Newbury in September 1643 the extent of the Royalist success was made evident by the booty captured, and a correspondent of the *Mercurius Anglicus* writes 'a further evident argument of the victory His Majesty's Army obtained over the Rebels, that they were forced to leave behind them heavy carriages, with many barrels of Whiskey and Pistoll Bullets, and very many chirurgeons' chests full of medicaments'.[50] The King celebrated it by giving orders to make every effort to extend generous treatment to the Roundhead wounded. 'Our will and command is that you forthwith send into the towns and villages adjacent, and bring hence all the sick and hurt souldiers of the Earl of Essex's army, and though they be rebels and deserve the punishment of Treators yet out of our tender compassion upon them as being our subjects, Our will and pleasure is that you carefully provide for their recovery as well as for those of Our own Armay, and then to send them to Oxford.'[51] After the second battle of Newbury when the Royalists were defeated, their wounded were left behind at Donnington Castle and it is hoped they received equally humane treatment.

The most noted surgeon on the Royalist side was Richard Wiseman, who for his services was later made Sergeant Surgeon to Charles II. His experiences are still extant in eight surgical treatises which contain detailed accounts of some 600 cases of wounds, and he was an advocate of primary amputation immediately after receipt of the injury. Wiseman not only exercised an important influence on English surgery by his efforts to make its practice dependent on scientific principles, but raised the social status of practitioners. Surgeons were joining together in closer union as a fraternity and were adding to their knowledge by the establishment of anatomical dissections and lectures on surgical practice at Barber Surgeons Hall. They were, too, demanding higher education in their apprentices. They had long been kept in a state of subservience to the more highly educated and more learned fraternity of the Doctors of Medicine, and were now trying to throw off the physicians' domination, and show that a scientific education was as essential for a good surgeon as for a good physician.

Let us now look at the diseases to which the armies were subject. Dysentery and typhus were the two great scourges and the principal causes of sick wastage. Dysentery or the bloody flux usually occurred in the summer months and was an infective enteritis caused by flies contaminating food, but a winter type also occurred due to exposure to wet and cold made worse by poor or defective clothing and unsuitable food. The first regiments ordered to Ireland had amongst them many 'boon companions, old blades, stout men and well nerved'[52] who were very discontented it is said on finding no beer or cheese, the food they largely lived on in England. Typhus occurred chiefly in the winter months when men were crowded together for warmth, for then the body louse which was the carrier of the disease had easy access to fresh victims; but as their clothing was constantly infested with lice it was liable to attack the troops at all times. While the mortality from dysentery was relatively small, typhus in the worst epidemics could cause a death rate of up to 75 per cent. Gore tells us we often read of soldiers dying of 'fever little less than a plague; many also died on their return from the attacks, being found dead in the woods and towns they passed through'.[53] Apart from dysentery and typhus there was an even more deadly enemy in the shape of bubonic plague which claimed many victims in the operations at Limerick.

It is now time to mention the foreign wars of the Protectorate which although little remembered launched the army on its long career of tropical conquest and victory in Europe. The war against the Dutch need not detain us, for it was purely a naval war, although some

2,000 red coats served in the ships. When a force of 6,000 men under General Venables, escorted by a squadron under Admiral Penn sailed across the Atlantic to attack Spain's West Indian possessions, it proved an expensive fiasco for it lost heavily in an unsuccessful attack on San Domingo (the present Cuba). The hazards encountered in the tropical heat of the jungle while dressed in thick scarlet tunics, in drinking polluted water, and in eating fresh fruit torn from the trees, evoked attacks of diarrhoea and dysentery which laid hundreds low.

San Domingo having been abandoned because of incompetent tactics and the ravages of disease the war was carried to the neighbouring island of Jamaica, which thanks to a speedy naval landing quickly fell into our hands. But here a new enemy appeared in the shape of yellow fever, which in the years to come was to lay low tens of thousands of red coats; within a short time men were dying at the rate of twenty a day, and during the next eighteen months three of the force commanders died in succession and two-thirds of the men. Reinforcements to take their place were hurried out only to meet the same fate.

In 1657 Cromwell formed an alliance with France and an expeditionary force of 6,000 troops was sent to the Spanish Netherlands and in the following year Dunkirk was invested and fell after a Spanish attempt to relieve it had been repulsed. Other towns were also captured including Ypres in September 1658.

After the fight at Dunkirk there were 700 casualties to provide for, and under the orders of General Sir William Lockhart a hospital was opened in a building in the town and nuns engaged to provide nursing care and food at the cost of one styver ($\frac{1}{2}$d.) a day for each patient. This arrangement, however, broke down, doubtless because the collection of wounded from different units under one roof caused difficulties and confusion in attendance and treatment when every regimental surgeon was determined to look after his own cases. Instead a number of regimental hospitals were opened, a sutler was hired to provide food, and 'a convenient number of women to wait upon them.'

Before the capture of Ypres Cromwell was dead, and on General Monk's suggestion Charles II was invited to return to London and assume the Crown.

REFERENCES

[1] *Fonblanque.*
[2] Garrison. *History of Military Medicine*, p. 64. Saunders, London (1929).
[3] Quoted by Gore. *Our Services under the Crown*, p. 8. Balliere, Tindall & Cox, London (1879).
[4] Meyrick. Vol. I, p. 73 quoted by Gordon. *Army Surgeons and Their Works*, p. 12 Lewis, London (1870).
[5] Archer. *The Crusade of Richard I* quoting *L'Histoire d'Eraeles.*
[6] *Fonblanque*, p.25.
[7] *Cornhill Magazine*, p. 84.

[8] Milligan. *Medical Experiences, vol. II*, p. 13.

[9] *Fonblanque*, p. 26.

[10] Mills. *History of Chivalry, vol. II.*

[11] Withington. *Medical History*, p. 223-224 quoted by Garrison. *History of Military Medicine*, pp. 89-90.

[12] Grose. *Military Antiquities, vol. II*, p. 274, and *Scope of Military History*, p. 367. T. Egerton, London (1801).

[13] Milligan. *Medical Experiences, vol. II*, p. 13.

[14] This was money paid by each soldier for shaving and hair trimming by the barber surgeon and amounted to 2d. each pay day.

[15] Hennen. *Military Surgery*, p. 5. Longman Hurst Rees Orme and Brown, Edinburgh (1818).

[16] 3 Henry V.

[17] Grose.

[18] Rymer Feodora.

[19] Nicolas. *Agincourt*, p. 387.

[20] Grose.

[21] Varying accounts put the number as a ew hundred up to 1,600.

[22] Chevers. *Moral and Social Condition of the British.*

[23] Petyt's MSS.

[24] From a MS. quoted by Grose.

[25] Ambroise Paré. *The Journey to Turin in 1536*, quoted by Garrison. *History of Military Medicine*, p. 112.

[26] Allbutt. Op. cit. 83.

[27] Gore. *Our Services under the Crown.* p. 41. Balliere Tindall & Cox, (1879).

[28] Gore. *Our Services under the Crown*, p. 41. Balliere Tindall & Cox, (1879).

[29] Gore. *Our Services under the Crown*, p. 36. Balliere Tindall & Cox, (1879).

[30] Fortescue. *History of the British Army*, book II, chapter I, p. 103. Macmillan, London (1910).

[31] Tavannes.—ed. Petitot, vol. I, p. 304.

[32] Ralphe Smith MSS.

[33] This refers to the system of 'regards' to the surgeon.

[34] Dr. Cecil Wall—quoted by Barnsley. *Mars and Aesculapius*, p. 3. Muniment Room, R.A.M. College.

[35] Gore. *Our Services under the Crown*, p. 43. Balliere Tindall & Cox, (1879).

[36] Gore. *Our Services under the Crown*, p. 42. Balliere Tindall & Cox, (1879).

[37] Gore. *Our Services under the Crown*, p. 46. Balliere Tindall & Cox, (1879).

[38] Lord of Praissac. *Art of Warre under head of Chirurgeon.*

[39] Gore. *Our Services under the Crown*, p. 54. Balliere Tindall & Cox, (1879).

[40] Gore. *Our Services under the Crown*, p. 54. Balliere Tindall & Cox, (1879).

[41] Gore. *Our Services under the Crown*, p. 55. Balliere Tindall & Cox, (1879).

[42] Their daily pay was as follows: General's physician 6s. 8d., physician 6s. 8d., apothecary 10s., chirurgeon 4s., mate 2s. 6d.

[43] Common Journals.

[44] Common Journals.

[45] Gore. *Our Services under the Crown*, p. 57. Balliere Tindall & Cox, (1879).

[46] Gore. *Our Services under the Crown*, p. 50. Balliere Tindall & Cox, (1879).

[47] Wortley quoted by Gore. *Our Services under the Crown*, p. 50. Balliere Tindall & Cox, (1879).

[48] Prendergast quoted by Gore. *Our Services under the Crown*, p. 51. Balliere Tindall & Cox, (1879).

[49] Gore—quoted from Down's *Survey*. Balliere Tindall & Cox, (1879).

[50] Gore. *Our Services under the Crown*, p. 55. Balliere Tindall & Cox, (1879).

[51] Gore. *Our Services under the Crown*, p. 55. Balliere Tindall & Cox, (1879).

[52] Gore. *Our Services under the Crown*, p. 57. Balliere Tindall & Cox, (1879).

[53] Gore. *Our Services under the Crown*, p. 57. Balliere Tindall & Cox, (1879).

Chapter 2

THE STANDING ARMY

With the restoration of the Monarchy in 1660 the New Model Army of the Commonwealth was disbanded and the Standing Army came into being. The Coldstream Guards, the Life Guards, and the Grenadier Guards, were the first of the new regiments to be formed, followed in succeeding years by the 4 senior regiments of Foot, and 3 of Horse. These formed in all a force of some 5,000 men embodied by the authority of the Crown and paid out of the Civil List.

The direction of military affairs was organized on lines similar to the New Model but on a reduced scale because of the smaller numbers involved. On the medical side we find civilians of high professional attainments appointed as physician general, surgeon general, and apothecary general; and it was the surgeon general who received the first commission when John Knight, Sergeant Surgeon to Charles II, became 'Surgeon General of all the forces in England and Wales' on the 16th December 1664.[1] Knight, who was then a naval surgeon, had attended Charles on the occasion of his voyage from The Hague to Dover, being accompanied by 'Dr. Quaterman, physician, and Mr. Richard Billing'. In 1661 he had become Principal Surgeon to the King for a fee of £26 6s. 8d. a year and a pension of £150, and later in the same year First Principal Surgeon and First Sergeant Surgeon with an annuity of £150.[2] He appears afterwards to have controlled the medical arrangements both of the navy and the army and moreover carried out this task single handed. In July 1666 it was agreed by Lord Arlington that 'no surgeons have their commissions signed till allowed by him as Surgeon General; also that all orders for chests and medicines be directed to him, to see that they are sufficient both in quality and quantity'.[3]

But Knight was not the first medical officer to receive the title of Surgeon General in the Standing Army. This distinction goes to Alexander Eristy who was made 'Surgeon General of Hospitals' at Dunkirk on the 4th March 1662. The use of the term 'general' in this and other instances does not necessarily mean that the individual is of the seniority we now associate with the rank. The term was used to indicate that he was graded as an officer of the staff, and held the superior authority in that particular area.

The first Physician General to the Standing Army as reported in Johnston's Roll[4] was Dr. Thomas Lawrence who did not receive his commission until the 24th June 1685 which is twenty-five years later.

Richard Whittle was appointed the first Apothecary General on the 1st January 1686 but previously he had received a commission as the first apothecary to the Standing Army on the 24th January 1673 and in that position must have carried out similar duties but with less pay and rank. Both the Surgeon General and Physician General received pay of 20s. a day, the Apothecary General 10s. a day.

In addition to the senior medical appointments authorized in England there was at this time and for many years to come a separate army establishment for Ireland. Here Dr. William Currer was appointed Physician General as early as the 3rd July 1660 (although his patent was not issued until 1663), while James Fountaine became 'Chirurgeon General' on the 5th April 1661. Even before Currer's appointment, a Dutchman Arnold Boate is reputed to have been Physician General[5] but his patent is not in the Patent Rolls. In Scotland too a Physician General was appointed later and Dr. David Mitchell was the first holder of the post in 1696.[6]

The first physician appointed by Charles II appears to have been Dr. Henry Wyatt on 14th November 1661 as 'Physician to the Garrison of Dunkirk and Forces in Flanders'[7] followed on 7th March 1663 by Dr. Tim Clarke, Physician in Ordinary to the King who was appointed 'Physician to the new raised forces within the Kingdom'.[8]

Following the pattern of the New Model there was a chirurgeon[9] to each regiment of Horse and Foot, although the Life Guards had at first a chirurgeon to each troop, and not until 1673 was a chirurgeon's mate added to each infantry regiment. The chirurgeon held a commission granted by the Sovereign and was paid 4s. a day, with 2s. a day for forage allowance for a horse to carry his medical equipment which comprised two regimental medicine chests, containing instruments, dressings, medicines, and medical comforts such as brandy.

The regimental surgeon's commission was, like all combatant commissions, either acquired by purchase or obtained by influence, as all regiments of Horse and Foot were raised by men of rank or position or by distinguished officers. But even at this early stage there was difficulty in procuring enough regimental surgeons due to the poor rates of pay offered by a tight-fisted Treasury, and over the centuries the fight for more pay and better conditions of service has engaged the constant attention of the heads of the medical services. When in 1670 war was declared against Holland and the number of regiments were increased there was such a shortage of medical officers volunteering for appointments as regimental surgeons that the King in 1672 was compelled to direct the Company of Barber Surgeons of London to provide 'twenty chirurgeons and twenty chirurgeons' mates for military duty'. This, in fact, was the last impressment of surgeons made on the College. Once the surgeon had joined the regiment he became a regimental officer, often spent his whole army career in its ranks, and owed loyalty to no one but his colonel. He was independent of any control by his medical superiors except with regard to the professional care of his patients.

With the poor pay which surgeons received this kind of life only appealed to doctors who were attracted by the excitement and adventure of an army career, or enjoyed the camaraderie of army life, or the facilities which it provided for sport and pleasure. It is true it did not often attract the keen professional men, for the work was anything but arduous, but there was always a sprinkling of good and well qualified doctors amongst the regimental surgeons. As it was not essential to possess a medical degree the applicants for commissions varied widely in their professional standards, from graduates of the Scottish and Irish universities to those who only had certificates of attendance at lectures and clinical instruction in the London hospitals, or were members of the College of Surgeons. Money was certainly not the attraction, for out of 4s. a day pay, 3s. went to provide subsistence, and there were other deductions, some of a disgraceful nature, which will be referred to later, leaving less than 1s. a day for the surgeon to spend on himself. No self-respecting doctor would join the army with such miserable prospects, and to their credit their fellow officers recognized their poverty and various subterfuges were adopted to help them financially. General Monk, the famous Restoration figure, was most anxious to improve their lot, and invented the quite illegal practice of allowing them to draw the pay of a non-existent private soldier which added 8d. or 9d. a day to their pay; in some regiments it was the custom of the officers to come to their assistance by subscribing a guinea a year from the lieutenants to 10 guineas from the colonel; and finally there was the policy authorized by government of allowing the surgeon to hold a double commission by purchasing an ensign's commission in the regiment; this added an extra 3s. a day, but under these circumstances government stepped in and restricted him drawing more than 2s. 6d. a day for his medical duties; he was excused guards and picquets, while if promotion occurred either the combatant or the medical commission had to be given up. This authorization of holding a double commission continued until it was cancelled by regulations in the year 1783. Unfortunately all these various expedients to augment their income only served to encourage the Treasury to withhold a proper living wage.

Regimental mates were ranked only as warrant officers and their selection was the prerogative of colonels of regiments. The Surgeon

General had no control over their appointments. As they were not made to pass any examination on entry their professional standards were often low; the best amongst them had been apprenticed to a medical practitioner or surgeon following attendance at lectures and some instruction in the wards of a London hospital; in others, even this amount of training was overlooked when the C.O. of the regiment chose a mate for his social qualities rather than for his professional attainments. The mate's low status was emphasized when as a result of his rank he became liable to all the punishments to which warrant officers were subject, and could actually be flogged, put in irons, and dismissed from the service at the will of the commanding officer.

With the growth of the army and the wider distribution of troops both garrison physicians and surgeons were appointed. Dr. Gideon Harvey was made physician to the Tower of London and there was one at Portsmouth, the principal port for troops arriving from or departing overseas; these physicians were paid at the rate of 10s. a day. Garrison surgeons made their first appearance in 1666 and were located in Scilly, Tangier, Berwick, Hull, Gravesend, Plymouth, and Sheerness, drawing pay at the rate of only 2s. 6d. a day.

Charles II had married Catherine, Princess of Portugal, whose dowry brought him half a million of money and the cities of Bombay and Tangier, the latter a troublesome possession because it was in constant peril of recapture by the Moors and required a garrison to protect it. This gave the Standing Army its first taste of active service and the medical service its first hospital abroad. In 'our establishment of the Forces raised the 10th day of October 1661 for His Majesty's service in the Kingdoms of Sus, Fez, and Morocco under the command of His Excellence Ye Earl of Peterborough' we find amongst 'the Field and Staff Officers of His Excellency's owne Regiment of Foote' a chirurgeon and mate. This regiment was 1,000 strong and there were three other regiments varying between 500 and 1,000 men, each with their own medical officers. Amongst the 'Field and Staff officers of Horse' there was a chirurgeon; and with the 'General Officers of the Trayne, two physicians', and an apothecary, who constituted the staff of the military hospital.

The hospital staff were constantly employed dealing with the casualties from the frequent skirmishes against the Moors and the many victims of dysentery and fever which originated in this subtropical climate, and within a year of the forces' arrival there were 250 wounded under treatment and there had been 250 deaths from sickness. In May 1664 the Earl of Teviot when making a reconnaissance in force some miles into Moroccan territory fell into an ambuscade and lost 'nineteen commissioned officers, fifteen gentlemen and volunteers, the doctor (Dr. White) together with 396 N.C.O.'s and men'. Only nine men escaped.

The same year complaints were made of the way the soldiers 'die apace' for want of proper food, and in 1668 the garrison was reduced to 1,400 Foot and half a troop of Horse. The men were falling sick at the rate of ten a day, and this kept the hospital physicians and apothecary fully employed, for the apothecary being a medical officer not only made up the prescriptions but acted as an assistant to the physicians in the wards. It is not until 1674 that we read of a chirurgeon and mate being added to the staff. The cost of running the hospital amounted to between £600 and £700 a year and Pepys' accounts for the period 12th May 1666 to the 11th June 1669 came to £2,019 14s. 9d.; which included the payment of the medical officers.[10]

Reinforcements of a battalion of Guards, the Royal Scots, and six troops of Horse were sent out in 1680, and in September of this year the force of 4,000 attacked the Moorish camp and effectively defeated 15,000 of the enemy. This was the last major engagement, for Parliament, after twenty-two years of occupation, seemed to be tired of a venture which had cost thousands of lives, although it had been on the whole a fine feat of arms. After refusing to provide further funds the garrison was withdrawn in 1684.

In 1673 new regulations for the supply of medicines were instituted. Up to this date they had been supplied by the Crown, but it was now decided to adopt a policy of granting the regimental surgeon an allowance, undoubtedly with the idea of saving the Treasury money. Medicines as before were divided into internal and external, and for the Foot Guards the Apothecary General was to supply the internal medicines at a cost of 40s. a year, while the external medicines were found by the regimental surgeon himself on an allowance of 40s. a year for each company, which with ten companies in the regiment would amount to £20 a year[11] and a total of £22. For regiments of Foot other than the Guards the responsibility for providing all medicines lay entirely in the hands of the regimental surgeon; his allowance for each company of sixty men and over was, for internal medicines 20s. a year, and for external medicines 40s. a year,[12] a total of £30. Claims for repayment of money expended against the value of these allowances are common in the accounts for Tangier; £20 in one case for the surgeon at Charles Fort for medicines and instruments; £32 9s. in another instance for quarters and care of the sick and wounded of the Earl of Plymouth's regiment; and £50 2s. 7d. again in a third for two chests of old linen and one chest of medicaments.

A more important event than the skirmishes in Tangier now engaged the Government's attention, for in 1665 war was declared against the Dutch Federation due to their interference with trade both in Africa and the East Indies. In America, New Amsterdam was captured and was given the now famous name of New York, and James, Duke of

York, won a splendid naval action off Lowestoft. Then in 1666 Louis XIV threw in his lot with the Dutch and declared war against England, but two years later Charles ranged England beside France and both declared war on Holland. Six thousand English troops under James, Duke of Monmouth, served with Turenne the French Commander in Chief.

This is a campaign which we will not follow but there are some medical aspects of the war which deserve mention. The first is the setting up of the Commission for the Sick and Hurt which was empowered to nominate surgeons to treat the sick and wounded at the various ports where they might land, and as there were no military hospitals in the kingdom to which they could be admitted except the Savoy which had been reopened in 1665, they were authorized to reserve one half of the civil hospital beds in the country, of which St. Thomas' Hospital in London was a notable inclusion. Notwithstanding these extensive arrangements many cases according to the old custom continued to be boarded out in taverns where, as John Evelyn the diarist who was one of the Commissioners said, they suffered from being badly fed, they were attended with difficulty by the surgeons, and were 'tempted to debaucherie'.[13] In the course of duty Evelyn visited Margate on the 25th March 1672, 'here', he writes, 'we had abundance of miserably wounded men, His Majesty sending his chief chirurgeon, Sergeant Knight, to meet me'. As a result of these war experiences he suggested constructing a hospital at Gravesend, but the money—for Charles was as usual in acute financial straits—was not forthcoming, and the project fell through, although it is said the King had spent £34,000 on the sick, wounded, and prisoners during the war.

It was too during the Dutch war that Charles put forward his edict to the Barbers and Surgeons Company for the impressment of twenty chirurgeons and a similar number of mates, and these were needed not only for the ports in England where the sick and wounded landed, but for duties abroad in the various stations of the fast growing Empire. Between Charles II's accession in 1660 and his death in 1685, a span of twenty-five years, the total number of commissions granted to medical officers amounted to 109—an average of only just over four a year—a figure which shows the slow growth in the army strength. The rates of pay over these years were by no means constant except in the case of the regimental chirurgeon and mate which never exceeded 4s. and 2s. 6d. respectively, and it was unfortunately destined to remain at this level for many years to come. The pay of the senior ranks is confusing because there were physician and surgeon generals not only at Army Headquarters but on the Headquarters of Commands in both Ireland and Scotland and to some of the expeditionary forces which fought overseas. Generally speaking the Army and Command appoint-

37

ments received pay at 20s. a day, while the senior officers to other forces received 10s. a day.

The picture then at this time is that each regiment of Foot had a regimental chirurgeon and mate; the Guards had a regimental chirurgeon and two mates, the regiments of Horse had a chirurgeon only. There were garrison physicians and chirurgeons and there were the senior appointments of physician, surgeon and apothecary general at Army Headquarters, at the headquarters of the establishments in Scotland and Ireland, and at headquarters of overseas expeditions when these were mobilized.

It will be noticed that there is so far no reference to military hospitals. The reason is that such units did not exist, and as we shall see later only made their first appearance in 1689. The only hospitals were the regimental hospitals capable of treating up to two score of patients under conditions which can only be described as primitive, situated as they were in a hired house or leaky barn; often cold and cheerless without means of heating they were anything but conducive to the recovery of the sick. The nursing of patients suffering from severe illnesses could hardly be said to exist; reliance had to be placed either on untrained orderlies from the regiment or the hire of a nurse who was probably the wife of a soldier. It was under these conditions that the sick soldier lived or died. A fuller account of the typical regimental hospital will engage our attention later.

This then was the picture in time of peace. We pass on now to the year 1689 when under William III the first field hospitals were created during the invasion of Ireland, the first major military operation in which the Standing Army was engaged. The regimental hospitals in war were constantly on the move and had to be relieved of their sick and wounded; instead of leaving them in private houses or civil hospitals to be looked after as best they might by the local doctors and inhabitants field hospitals were now formed to take them over. To staff these hospitals we find a whole new range of medical officers being commissioned who possessed higher professional attainments and greater skill than the regimental surgeons possessed. So at the beginning of a campaign we find the following appointments of medical officers for the hospitals; directors, physicians, master surgeons, surgeons, master apothecaries, apothecaries, purveyors, deputy purveyors, surgeons or hospital mates, and apothecaries' mates.

In general all physicians appointed in war were of necessity civilians. There were two reasons for this. The first was because physicians did not exist in peacetime at home, except for the two we have already mentioned. The second reason and an important one was that army surgeons were not allowed to become physicians, because the former did not possess the necessary professional qualifications. Physicians were regarded with justice as the *élite* of the profession, and there was bitter rivalry between them and the surgeons, for the physician styled himself a *medicus purus*, although in fact he was often a sterile pedant and a coxcomb.[14] They were all university graduates, and those commissioned in the army by the Physician General were licentiates, members, or fellows of the College of Physicians of London. The surgeons on the other hand were members of the Company of Barber Surgeons of much inferior status. Physicians' pay was commensurate with their higher education and standing and was usually double that of the surgeons. The Physician General jealously guarded the privilege of recommending physicians for commissions, but instances occasionally occurred when surgeons or apothecaries were made physicians on the recommendation of a Commander-in-Chief in the field, for he possessed the privilege of appointing medical officers on the spot to fill vacancies. These appointments the Physician General was sometimes unwillingly forced to accept but on other occasions he was able to have them revoked, even though the medical officer held the degree M.D. or was willing to sit the examination for entry to the College of Physicians. It was customary in war to appoint a physician as the personal medical attendant of the Commander-in-Chief in the field, and on one occasion at least he rose from this position to be Physician General to the Force. Physicians were never numerous in the army and as late as the end of the eighteenth century seventeen is the highest number recorded as serving at one time.

Surgeons selected to serve on the staff of the military hospitals were promoted from the best of the regimental surgeons or were appointed from civil life. They were chosen for their operating ability, and one was selected as master surgeon who acted as consultant in the most difficult cases. Both the surgeons of the hospital staff and the garrison surgeons were nominated by the Surgeon General and were under his jurisdiction; in contrast, the regimental surgeons were responsible to their commanding officer alone.

Apothecaries were in charge of the medicines, dressings and instruments, which were supplied to the field hospitals by the Apothecary General. They were responsible for the dispensary and supervised their mates in making up the complex prescriptions which were so common. The master apothecary like the master surgeon was the senior apothecary to a force in the field, but both these appointments ceased in the early years of the eighteenth century.

A purveyor was first appointed in 1690, and initially he was 'to perform the duty of butler for distributing the provisions to the sick and wounded'.[15] He acted in fact as the commissariat officer who was responsible for contracting for the supply of food; later however his responsibilities were greatly increased and were extended to the provision and care of equipment, and of pay. Purveyors were well reimbursed in the hope that they would avoid the temptation of peculation and not feather their nests in the matter of contracts, probably a vain hope at a time when government corruption was rampant. Both apothecaries and purveyors at this period were nearly always promoted regimental surgeons, both appointments being much sought after for the reasons of promotion and the higher pay.

The director of hospitals was at first either a military officer or a civilian, but their lack of knowledge of hospital matters soon became so apparent that from the middle of the eighteenth century a medical officer held the position, sometimes combining this appointment with that of purveyor and so adding the control of hospital contracts to his administrative duties. But as a medical officer was without executive power he could not be the commanding officer, for he was unable to punish either the patients or the subordinate staff for disobedience of regulations; a military officer, therefore, was always present in the hospital to control discipline, and sometimes combined this duty with the command of the hospital guard.

As military hospitals were only in existence during the war years the hospital staff officers were made redundant when peace came, and either had to resign from the service altogether or were placed on half pay. Half pay was instituted by Royal Warrant on the 17th July 1689 for the benefit of the officers who were dismissed from the old Irish Army for their Protestant sympathies; the rates of half pay for the physician general and surgeon general were 14s. 9d. a day, for physicians 11s. 9d. a day, and for regimental surgeons of Horse and Foot 3s. and 2s. a day respectively.

It was some twenty years after Charles had come to the throne that the first steps were taken to provide some means of support for the infirm and maimed soldiers who had fought or served in Tangier, in Flanders, and the West Indies. A contemporary epigram aptly records their distress:

> 'Our God and soldiers we alike adore
> When at the brink of ruin, not before,
> After deliverance both alike requited,
> Our God forgotten and our soldiers slighted.'[16]

The discharge of men when they became unfit was regulated by a code in the Articles of War which stated—'If any Souldier shall be sick, wounded or maimed in Our Service, he shall be sent out of the camp to some far place for his recovery, where he shall be provided for by the Officers appointed to take care of sick and wounded Souldiers, and his wages or pay shall go on and be duly paid till it does appear that he can be no longer serviceable to Our Army, and then he shall be sent by pass to his Countrey, with money to bear his charges in his travel.'[17]

Public opinion now voiced the feeling that something further should be done for these old soldiers after they had returned to their homes where they were thrown on the scrap heap and made to beg their bread or starve. Their sympathy found fulfilment in the establishment of two institutions—Kilmainham Hospital in Dublin which was opened in 1680, and the Royal Hospital at Chelsea in 1691. Dean tells us: 'There was nothing original in these institutions, which were simply a logical development of the ancient almshouses . . . which were usually open to old soldiers, and a few were exclusively devoted to their relief.'[18]

The Royal Hospital at Kilmainham was constituted by Letters Patent dated the 27th October 1679 for the infirm and maimed soldiers who in the language of the time, 'having honestly served the King from the time of their youth, and being arrived at old age, which rendered them incapable of further service, they could not properly be continued any longer in the same; and they by their constant service therein having neglected all other ways of procuring a livelihood by arts or trades, must of necessity starve, if dismist'.[19] Within two months of the charter being granted, 10 officers and 100 of the rank and file had been admitted.

The Royal Hospital at Chelsea owes its origin to the philanthropy and forethought of Sir Stephen Fox, a Treasury Commissioner, when at his own expense he purchased the property known as Chelsea College from the Royal Society. Fox made a considerable fortune when Paymaster of the Army by charging poundage at the rate of a shilling in the pound. Owing to the inadequate revenue, payment was always in arrears, but Fox agreed to pay the troops weekly by obtaining the necessary credit from the bankers. It was on the 14th September 1681 that John Evelyn describes how he: 'Din'd with Sir Stephen Fox, who proposed to me the purchasing of Chelsea College which His Majesty had some time since given to our Society, and would now purchase it again to build an Hospital or Infirmary for Souldiers there, in which he desired my assistance as one of the Council of the Society.'[20]

It is perhaps unfortunate that history does not confirm the legend that Charles had promised the site to his mistress Nell Gwynne, and that her generous feeling for the old soldiers inspired her to give it up for their benefit. The facts are more prosaic, and contemporary documents show quite conclusively that the property was bought from the Royal Society and that Charles was directly influenced by a desire to promote the welfare of those who had been maimed or had grown infirm in his service. The building was begun in 1682, but it was nine years later in August 1691 before the Royal Hospital was opened. To help pay for it, two-thirds of the Army poundage fund was allocated for the purpose, a sum at that time of over £60,000.

By a regulation brought in on the 1st January 1685 compensation for injuries was introduced if certified by the Surgeon General. There was a King's bounty of one year's pay for the loss of an eye or limb or the total loss of the use of a limb, with bounties for other wounds in proportion. For those soldiers who were temporarily disabled by wounds a daily pension was paid varying from 5d. for a private to 11d. for a sergeant of infantry; for horse and dragoons it was 6d. to 1s. 6d.; and for gunners 7d. to 1s. 2d. In William III's reign these benefits were extended to all soldiers of over twenty years' service or those who had been rendered unfit.

When William of Orange came to the throne in 1689 he was confronted with a war in Ireland, a war in Flanders, and the practical certainty of insurrection in Scotland. In view of these threats to the security of the country the Army was increased to a strength of 87,000 men and 4 cavalry and 9 infantry regiments were added to the establishment with the standard allotment of chirurgeons and mates.

When William had landed in England, France had declared war against Holland, and Lord Marlborough was ordered to ship 4 battalions of Guards and 6 of the Line to Flanders pursuant to our treaty obligations with the Dutch. The fighting in this campaign of 1689 was negligible, but there were reports of the men being sickly and undisciplined, with defective clothing and bad footwear.

Before he was driven from the throne James II had prepared Ireland as a place of refuge and he landed there in March 1689. With help of French officers who came from France in his train he had organized the Irish levies, and with the inclusion of Roman Catholics, several thousand Protestant veterans were dismissed, including some regimental surgeons and mates. The siege of Londonderry by James' troops reduced the garrison to the last extremity of starvation and sickness before it was relieved on the 30th July 1689 by troops from England, but Enniskillen more than held its own, and the Irish Army was defeated at Newtown Butler. Meanwhile in Scotland, Claverhouse, Marquis of Dundee had rebelled and had won the battle of Killiecrankie.

The invasion of Ireland was now undertaken with a force of nearly 19,000 men under Marshal Schomberg, a polyglot army of English, Dutch, Protestant French refugees, Scots, Danes, and a new regiment of Irish Protestants—the Enniskillen Regiment. On the medical side Schomberg's principal medical officers were Dr. Thomas Lawrence the Physician General, who was commissioned on the 20th July 1689 'Physician General to the Army now going to Ireland, and to be Director of the Hospital attending the same',[21] Mr. Paul de Buissière the Surgeon General, and Mr. Isaac Teale the Apothecary General.

On the 13th August this polyglot army landed at Bangor, captured Carrickfergus, and pushed on to Dundalk where Schomberg entrenched. Owing to corrupt administration it was not long before he was in desperate straits from lack of provisions, and by the middle of September

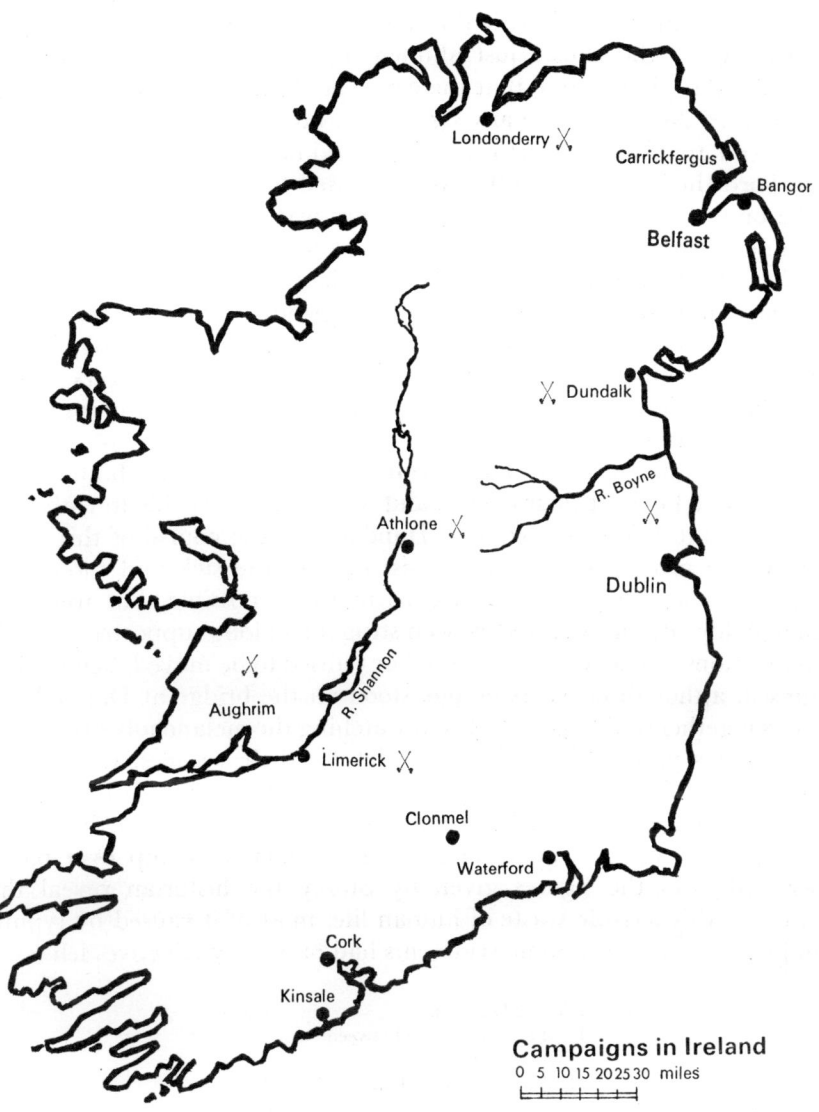

Campaigns in Ireland
0 5 10 15 20 25 30 miles

the men began to perish by hundreds not only from starvation but from exposure, while sickness was made worse when the defenders of Londonderry joined the army and brought with them the contagion of typhus. The officers' behaviour was disgraceful. 'The lions in Africa', wrote one who was on the spot, 'are not more barbarous than some of our officers are to the sick.'[22] In this low lying unhealthy camp site, ill clothed, starved and exposed to the bad weather, it is little wonder that the men were struck down with fevers and 'fluxes'; and there were no medical arrangements worthy of the name. Wright tells us that there were 'surgeons well furnished against all the accidents of active war,

43

but totally unprovided with the medicines necessary for the diseases generated by the causes just alluded to, and that disease spread to such an alarming degree that the camp at Dundalk seemed like a vast hospital'.[23] Nor was there any sign of the hospital to which Lawrence had been appointed Director because it did not exist. This was because Harbord the Treasurer to the Army refused to provide a penny for it. The only shelter for these poor wretches was in the poorly equipped regimental hospitals which were only collections of sick huddled together in a tent or hut. Harbord was a shameless rascal, who by some jobbery had contrived to obtain an independent troop of cavalry for which he drew pay as though it were complete, though the troop in fact consisted of himself, two clerks whom he put down as officers, and a standard which he kept in his bedroom. This was the only corps which was regularly paid.[24]

By November the rain had become so intolerable that both armies were obliged to quit their camps, and Schomberg was able to withdraw his men into winter quarters at Dundalk. In the course of this move the whole army appeared to consist only of the sick and those who attended them; waggons carried as many as possible, but were not enough for all; many sick were seen struggling along supported by their companions, others were left behind or refused to be moved. Schomberg himself, although 80 years of age, stood on the bridge at Dundalk for hours together in the wind and cold watching the melancholy procession of waggons pass, and thanking the sick for their services. Eventually, those left behind were taken by sea to the civil hospital in Belfast where in the absence of any field hospital with the army, the medical staff officers were concentrated. Out of 14,000 men in camp over 6,000 perished, and the figures given by Storey the historian reveal the extent of this terrible waste of human life, most of it caused by typhus and camp dysentery. Some regiments had only sixty effectives left.

Died at Dundalk	1,700
Died on board ship between Dundalk and Belfast	870
Died in hospital at Belfast	3,762
	6,332

The deporable conditions underlying this illhealth were largely due to the shameless neglect and duplicity of Shales the Commissary and Harbord; the latter admitted afterwards that if he had known as much about hospitals at the beginning as at the end of the campaign he might have saved two-thirds of the men who died.

For the campaign of 1690, 27,000 seasoned troops, 17,000 of them British and the remainder Dutch and Danish were brought over from England and Holland. The medical and especially the hospital arrangements were entirely reorganized, and for the first time in our history military hospitals accompanied a force taking part in active operations. These field units were described as 'The Marching Hospital' and 'Fixed Hospital' and Royal Warrants authorizing their establishment were issued in March 1690.[25] As these are the first hospitals of their kind and represent the types which were to accompany our armies in the field for many campaigns it is necessary to look at them in some detail. In the course of time their names were to change, the Marching Hospital became the Flying Hospital, and the Fixed Hospital became the General Hospital.

The Marching Hospital, as its name implies, was designed to move with the army, and possessed its own waggons and tentage. Its task was to open up as close to the regimental hospitals as the tactical situation allowed, receive and treat their sick and wounded, and either keep them until recovery or evacuate them back to the Fixed Hospital in the rear. As the range of cannon fire was at this period limited the hospital could be sited within a mile of the front line. In the establishment[26] there were 17 hospital staff officers; 1 physician, 1 master surgeon and 8 surgeons' mates, 1 master apothecary and 3 apothecaries' mates for dispensing duties and the care of medical stores, and 3 purveyors for commissariat duties.[27] Included in the strength we find the principal medical officers who accompanied the Commander-in-Chief in the field, and the physician general, surgeon general, and apothecary general are in the list. For the subordinate staff only female nurses or 'tenders' as they were called, are mentioned for ward duties and there were no male orderlies or ward masters. But it was quickly found that many of the ward tasks under active service conditions were too heavy for women to undertake, and male orderlies were then added; these were either soldiers detailed from regiments or they came from the men of the hospital guard which under an officer was always provided, both to guard the hospital during hostilities against enemy incursions, and to control the patients, prevent absenteeism and drinking, and preclude unauthorized visitors. The guard was an essential part of hospital administration as medical officers possessed no executive powers and could not punish staff or patients who disobeyed the hospital rules; this duty often devolved on the officer in charge of the guard. It is as well to point out that these male orderlies had no training whatever and were constantly and often daily changed by their own commanding officers.

The hospital governor or director was in administrative charge and controlled the various hospital departments, such as the clerical side, the accounts, the pack store for patients' arms, the number of orderlies and nurses, the pay and the transport, while under him the purveyor supervised the cooking and feeding and the equipment. The director if a civilian could not exercise any powers of punishment.

45

The number of beds for which the Marching Hospital was equipped was flexible, but generally in the region of 300.[28] Bedsteads were rarely carried but bedding rolls provided each containing a palliasse, blankets, sheets and a coverlet or rug; and there were ward utensils such as bed pans and urinals. To make it self-contained as regards transport there were twelve waggons to carry the equipment and stores, and a farrier was included in the staff. This then is the establishment of the first military hospital designed to move with the army.

We come now to the establishment of the Fixed Hospital.[29] In active operations this was sited in buildings in a town situated at a convenient distance from the front. It had no transport of its own and no tentage. The same categories of hospital staff officers and sub-ordinate staff are included as in the Marching Hospital but with additional surgeons and more nurses. Here again the work in the wards was reinforced by the inclusion of soldiers detailed from units or from the hospital guard. The equipment was similar to the Marching Hospital but often included some form of bedstead, sometimes obtained locally, sometimes improvised; and if these were unobtainable the palliasses in the bedding rolls had to be used. The number of equipped beds was generally about 500 but there was no rigid establishment, and at the commencement of every war they varied in size and in the number of staff according to circumstances.

If the rates of pay are referred to the nurses with 2s. 6d. a day appear generously paid when the surgeons' mates were only receiving 3s. We are not told the source from which these female nurses were recruited but from their high rate of pay it seems they must have had previous training perhaps in civil hospitals, for the soldiers' wives were only paid 6d. a day for working in regimental hospitals and were confined to the simpler duties of washing linen, cooking and feeding the sick.

Marshal Schomberg remained in winter quarters around Dundalk until March 1690. Health had now improved with only some 300 patients in the Belfast hospital. There were also according to Howell smaller hospitals in the towns where troops were stationed[30] and with the efficiency of these units Schomberg was seriously concerned when he wrote to the King on the 3rd March. He made favourable comments on the services of Paul de Buissière his Surgeon General but the other hospital officers came in for his general condemnation. Probably as a result of these criticisms, the King in April 1690 authorized Dr. John Hutton his First Physician in Ordinary to visit, and 'to inspect the hospitals and to enquire into the qualifications of all who pretend to the employment of physicians, surgeons and apothecaries, and to see that all care is taken of the sick and wounded, and that all necessary medicines, nursing and attendance are provided, and to reform and amend what is found amiss and defective'.[31] It seems unnecessary to have introduced another civilian to carry out this duty when already the Physician General and Surgeon General were on the spot, but Hutton was obviously highly trusted.

In June 1690 William himself landed at Belfast with further reinforcements of Horse and Foot bringing the strength up to 37,000 men. The battle of the Boyne fought on the 1st July brought a resounding victory to William with few casualties on either side, but was marked by the death of Schomberg. James now considered his cause was in jeopardy and soon afterwards embarked at Kinsale for France, while William entered Dublin in triumph.

Dublin was chosen as the best location for the Fixed Hospital and two sites seem to have been used. One was the Royal Hospital of Kilmainham, and the second site was in James Street in the city. Dr. Patrick Dun, a physician of Dublin who had been made Physician General to the Army in Ireland in 1688, now joined William's force in place of Dr. Lawrence who returned to London as Physician General to the Army. Dun was with the army at the capture of Waterford and during the advance to Limerick proceeded with the Marching Hospital which was opened at Clonmel. Limerick itself was defended stoutly and a siege of the city had perforce to be undertaken. But now the weather broke down, and there was not a scrap of shelter for the besiegers. To add to these hardships the clothing was defective, the soldiers were without pay so that food was hard to purchase, and Count de Solmes, who had assumed command, for William had returned to England, had to give orders for food to be provided, 'as I cannot seen them die of starvation'.[32] No wonder the Marching Hospital became inundated with sick and the siege had to be raised, 'We have to move a great many men into the hospitals', wrote Solmes in September, 'and on account of the sickness doctors are wanted.'[33] In the Guards 50 men had died within a short space of time, while in Belcastle's regiment there were not more than 10 men capable of bearing arms.

While the operations at Limerick were suffering this setback a landing had been made on the south coast by a force under Marlborough, and within a month it had captured Cork and Kinsale. Here too there were administrative troubles. Only 100 pairs of shoes existed amongst 500 men, and the rations were so short that Marlborough said his troops must either conquer or starve. A Marching Hospital was opened in a large private house in Kinsale for the numerous sick which these hardships had caused and Marlborough was entreated 'to lend or sell coals for the use of the hospital, the charge to be defrayed by way of a rate on the inhabitants of the town'.[34]

Scarcely six months had elapsed since the hospitals had taken the field when criticism started and it was said that the funds had been 'very ill applied'. These teething troubles we see reflected in a good many complaints, both as to the quality of the doctors and the treatment of the sick and wounded, which are recorded in the State Papers of the time. In a 'Memo. of abuses and faults observed in the Army in Ireland' the quality of the medical officers is scornfully attacked. 'The men in charge of the hospital pass for doctors, but they are not so; the hospitals must be governed differently. Many officers and men have perished for want of doctors and proper care being taken of them in the hospitals'.[35] There were too bitter complaints at the new regulations for hospital stoppages which made the wounded pay for their hospital treatment, and again de Solmes wrote to the King: 'Both officers and men complain of the manner in which the hospitals are conducted.' These stoppages from the men's pay to which they so strongly objected was ordered by the authorities to cover the cost of food while they were patients in the field hospitals, and was deducted at the rate of 3d. a day for a Horse soldier and 2d. a day for the Foot.[36]

Moreover the fixed allowance paid to regimental surgeons in accordance with the Royal Warrant of 1673 to provide both internal and external medicines when put to the test of war was found open to abuse because surgeons were tempted to make money out of it. The Secretary at War therefore assumed the responsibility of ordering the medicines which were then forwarded through the Apothecary General and he thus became security for the payment of them. But unfortunately the Secretary never took the pains to make any proper arrangements for their transport, custody, and repayment, and when each regiment in Ireland received two chests of medicines a dispute arose whether the colonels or the surgeons were to be liable for the cost of carriage; the consequence was that in those regiments where the surgeon had not money enough to purchase and maintain a pack horse the chests were left behind, and the troops marched on active service without a drug or plaster, because a civilian was at the head.[37] There is no doubt the supplying of medicines both to regiments and hospitals whether on recharge to government or on a fixed allowance was regarded as a good pecuniary speculation, for in 1691 the Adjutant General in Ireland petitioned to be allowed to find the supply as a perquisite attaching to his office. Further, the surgeons of regiments had great difficulty under the old regulations of recouping their expenses on medicines from the Treasury, and the surgeon of the 23rd Foot put forward a bill for £44 4s. which was in excess of his allowance on the reasonable plea that every surgeon should always have a chest of medicaments ready for service.

All these complaints culminated in a committee of army physicians being set up under the chairmanship of Colonel Venner the Director of Kilmainham and new proposals were approved by the King in April 1691 when he directed 'that the said hospitals be forthwith established and settled, and fit persons appointed for that service. And you (the

Lord Justices) are to appoint such a salary as you shall judge suitable to that employment.'

There were now to be two Fixed Hospitals. While the main hospital and the depot of medicines and equipment was to be established as before in Dublin, a second advanced Fixed Hospital was to be sited in a town nearest to the scene of operations to take in cases from the Marching Hospital or direct from the adjacent camps. There was to be a redistribution of staff on the following lines—1 physician, 1 master surgeon and 1 apothecary were to be allotted to each of the three hospitals, and the Surgeon General himself with another master surgeon was to be stationed at the Marching Hospital, and ready to be moved elsewhere as ordered by the G.O.C. Eighteen surgeons' mates and six apothecary's mates would be distributed between the hospitals, and there would be one purveyor to each 'who shall be obliged to perform the duty of butler for distributing the provisions to the sick and wounded.'[38] Finally, 40 nurses and 15 washerwomen were allotted as required.

For the greater comfort of the patients wooden beds were now introduced into the tented wards of the Marching Hospital. Each tent was $8\frac{1}{2}$ feet broad and 20 feet long, and four beds were allotted to each tent 'each bed to be four feet wide, or a little more, that it may hold two sick or wounded men'.[39] There were twenty-five of these tents in the equipment, with a total capacity of 200 patients 'which may be sufficient for this campaign'.[40]

Experience gained in these few months showed that female nurses alone could not do the heavier tasks, and twenty-five of them were replaced by soldiers who could help to put up the tents and do the general fatigues and duties. Transport too was increased to 12 carts to carry the tents and convey the sick and wounded to the Fixed Hospital, and 8 waggons for equipment and medical supplies.

General Ginkell who had now assumed command opened the campaign of 1691 in June with the siege and capture of Athlone. Here Storey tells us at the Marching Hospital there were 'a great many large tents set up in form of a quadrangle with quilts and other conveniences for every soldier'.[41] The stay in winter quarters had in great measure restored the troops' health; as early as the previous November de Solmes had informed the King 'the enemy are dying apace and our men are in good health'.[42] In July was fought the desperate battle of Aughrim when the Irish army was heavily defeated, leaving, it is said, 4,000 dead on the field and losing altogether between 6,000 and 7,000 men. The battlefield was so strewn with white corpses that it was described as looking like a pasture covered with flocks of sheep. Limerick was then besieged for the second time and although again the sick and wounded suffered many hardships from the lack of shelter the town was finally captured in October. Many of the Irish wounded found in the city had never been dressed, although the shortage of Irish medical officers had been helped by the addition of twenty-four French surgeons who had arrived as reinforcements. In fact nine of the Irish regiments were without surgeons at all, which must have been a cause of concern to James' principal medical officers, Dr. Archibald[43] who was Physician General, and Mr. Patrick Archibald who was Surgeon General.

But the end of the war was now in sight, for the final capture of Limerick saw the termination of this unhappy conflict.

The conclusion of peace in 1691 allowed the remains of James' army, some 19,000 men in all including many of the surgeons, to leave their native country for France to form the famous Irish Brigade. One of the clauses of the peace treaty states: 'The General will cause provision and medicine to be furnished to the sick and wounded officers, troopers, dragoons, and soldiers of the Irish Army who could not pass into France at the first embarkment and after they are cured will order their ships to pass into France if they are willing to do so.[44]

Storey's figures for the losses of the English army in the three years of the war amount to 10,297 made up as follows:

Officers killed: 140
Soldiers killed in the field: 2,037
Murdered by the Rapparees: 800.
English and foreign officers who died during the three campaigns: 320.
Soldiers who died: 7,000.

The sick wastage of certain units was very considerable; for example the 13th Foot in 1691 had 216 in hospital at one time out of a strength of 678, a rate of 31 per cent. As we have already recorded, the deaths from disease in 1689 amounted to 6,332 so that the figures for 1690 and 1691 amounted only to 988 and Storey confirms this when he says that in the last two campaigns, 'few died except recruits and such as died of their wounds'.[45] The remarkable drop in the death rate from 33·3 per cent in 1689 (6,332 deaths in a strength of 19,000) to 2·6 per cent in 1690 and 1691 (988 deaths in a strength of 38,000) is a striking testimony to the improved hospital facilities which the field hospitals provided after their initial teething troubles. Of the records of treatment there are none, but we refer later to the general principles which were common to the period. One curious prescription of Dr. Dun's for General Ginkell may be mentioned. 'Chester ale, claret, potted chicken and geese. This is the physic I advice you to take. I hope it will not be nauseous or disagreeable to the stomach. A little to be taken on a march.'

Although the Irish war is an unhappy episode let us remember that it is a landmark in the history of the medical department by the creation of the field hospitals.

Before the war in Ireland had been brought to a successful conclusion William as we have seen had left the country to turn his attention to the conflict with France which had begun in 1689 with Louis XIV's declaration of war against Holland. France had the finest and strongest army in the world, well trained, well equipped and well organized. Opposed to them were the Allies—England, Holland, Austria, Spain, some German states and Denmark, and troops from all these countries were gathered under King William's command. The French frontier lay along the boundary of the Spanish Netherlands.

For the campaign of 1691 Parliament voted 70,000 men, 50,000 of them British. The campaign was unfavourable to the Allies for the French invested and captured Mons, but there was little serious fighting. In 1692 a force of 23,000 British troops crossed the Channel, the most important army sent to the Continent since the days of Henry VIII.

The responsibility for making the medical arrangements for the force was in the hands of Dr. Lawrence the Physician General who had recently returned from service in Ireland, and the Surgeon General, William Van Loon, appointed in 1689 and obviously one of William's Dutch nominees. No fewer than six Fixed Hospitals were formed for service overseas, and the number of hospital staff officers required to staff these field units totalled 89, made up of 6 physicians, 8 master surgeons, 8 staff surgeons, and 38 surgeons' mates or hospital mates as they were afterwards designated; there was a master apothecary, 8 apothecaries' mates, and 3 supernumerary apothecaries' mates, and 17 supernumerary surgeons' mates. If to these are added the regimental surgeons and their mates the total strength must have been in the neighbourhood of 120, which for a force of 23,000 gives one medical officer for every 200 soldiers in the field—probably the most generous allotment that any British force on the Continent was to have for the next 100 years.

The original small force which had gone to Flanders in 1690 had taken a hospital with them, for an unsigned report available condemns it for its bad organization and poor medicines. 'The medicine has arrived and is worthless, it will rather kill those it is meant to cure, than cure them. The master of the hospital is incapable. Want is everywhere apparent.'[46]

Such criticism of the neglect of the sick and wounded was not confined to Flanders, for when those who were unfit for service in the field were shipped back to England nothing was done for them. Distressing accounts are given of their condition when landed at Rochester in November 1690. 'Complaints about sick seamen and soldiers increase, partly from ill payments which make people refuse to lodge them, partly from their great number. Within a few days two or three have died in the streets for want of quarters and many more would have laid down and died had not the Mayor lodged them in the Town House on straw, and private charity relieved them. A surgeon might be appointed to take charge of them and then the lives of many brave men might be saved.'[47] As many as 700 of these poor wretches were found begging in the streets and from house to house.[48] There was in fact no organization of any kind to deal with the sick when they were sent over from Flanders and it appears this contingency had never even been thought of. Continental warfare was a new venture. There were no military hospitals in the country and it appears it was no concern of the medical service.

The Transport Commissioners were responsible for the sick on transports and what happened to them on landing no one seemed to know or care. The Commissioners for the Sick and Hurt appear to have been completely inactive.

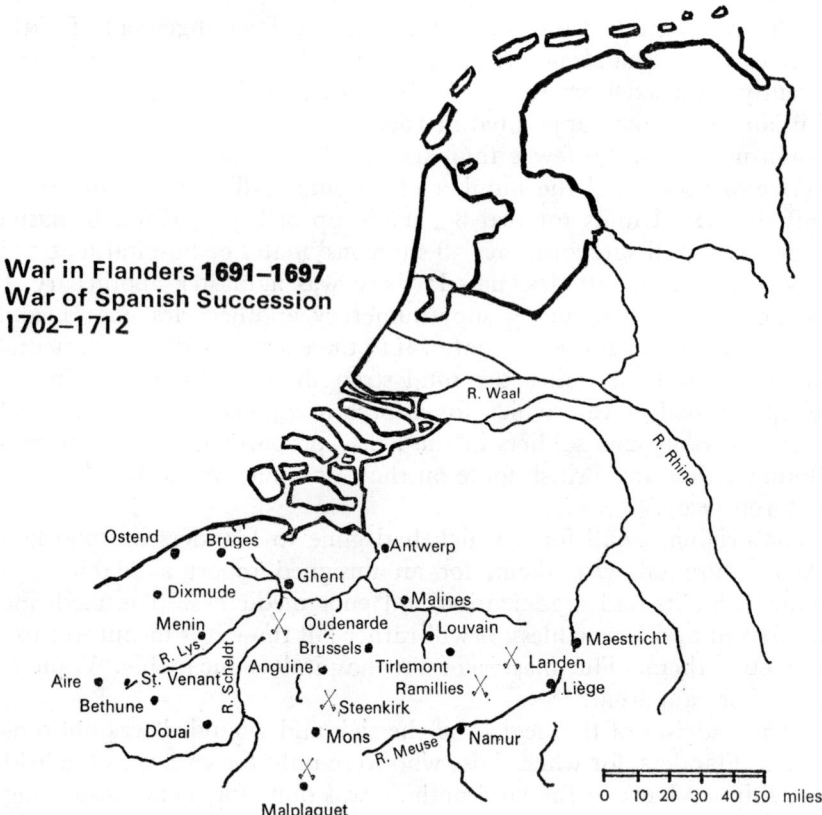

War in Flanders 1691–1697
War of Spanish Succession
1702–1712

When the campaign of 1692 opened the French army as usual was first in the field, and Namur was invested and captured in June. This was followed by the battle of Steenkirk which resulted in an Allied defeat although Fortescue says the British troops never fought a finer action. Casualties were heavy on both sides and those of the Allies

52

amounted to 3,000 killed, 3,000 wounded and 1,300 prisoners most of whom were wounded. The medical arrangements were quite extensive with Fixed Hospitals at Ghent, Dixmude, Bruges, Brussels, Namur, and Liege, all under the direction of Colonel Venner formerly Hospital Director at Dublin. Further hospitals at Louvain, Malines and Tirlemont functioned for periods when the tactical situation required. After the battle, many of the wounded were treated at a Flying Hospital at Anguine, before being evacuated later to Brussels. Here the hospitals of the different Allied contingents were soon so crowded with cases that many wounded were left lying in the streets awaiting attention. The story is told how the Princess de Vaudemont finding them in this distressing condition made many journeys with her coach to pick them up and carry them off to her own residence where, with the help of her ladies, they were dressed and looked after. Throughout the war extensive use was made of civil hospital buildings to accommodate the Fixed Hospitals, and the civilian nurses who were almost exclusively 'religieuses', provided excellent help in the wards. This was the case at Malines which was used for military purposes from the 17th May until the 22nd October 1692 and the rent paid for the building and the nuns' salaries are on record. The same applied to the St. Elizabeth hospital at Louvain where 604 florins were paid 'for the soldiers entertained there this year'. In Brussels the Hospitals of St. Jean and St. Giles by Bethlehem were both taken over and here the nurses were paid 10 stivers (about 5d.) a day.

Because of the previous complaints of poor administration a new plan was adopted in 1692 of appointing a contractor for the hospitals who would supply all food and other requirements, which in the following year even included the pay of the medical officers and nurses.

When the campaign of 1693 opened the French adopted their usual plan of besieging fortress towns, and William, alarmed by these tactics, weakened his army by detaching troops to reinforce Liege and Maestricht, and the garrisons on the Meuse. Luxemburg had hoped for and had foreseen this possibility, and hastened to bring William's army to battle at Landen on 29th July. Once again the Allied army was defeated and the casualties on both sides were very severe, the French losing about 8,000 and the Allies 15,000. Out of the 19 British battalions engaged 135 officers were either killed, wounded or prisoners, but the losses of the British rank and file are not known, but must have been considerable. The Fixed Hospital at Liege some twenty-five miles away was the nearest to the scene of action. This campaign closed with the surrender of Charleroi and the gain by the French of the whole line of the Sambre.

As 1694 brought no operations of importance we pass to 1695, when William undertook the siege of Namur. The major part of the French army was locked up in the defence of a vast system of fortified lines which stretched from Namur to the sea. William masked his intention by a series of feints and then marched swiftly to the Meuse and invested Namur. The British were largely concerned in capturing the outworks, the town itself, and finally the citadel, though at a cost of 1,556 killed and 2,205 wounded.

Although comprehensive sick returns are not available we can get a picture of the general state of health by the study of occasional reports. Monthly regimental states were furnished for the King and those dated 4th September and 4th October 1695 show the following figures for a total of twenty-eight British regiments.

	4th September	4th October
Sick in camp	282	169
Sick in hospital	3,005	2,889
Fit for service	14,446	13,765
Effectives	18,722	17,887
Missing or prisoners	73	51
Dead	11	18
Deserters	8	3

If the number of sick are calculated against the effective strength, this gives 17·5 per cent for the September figures, and 17 per cent for the October figures, a moderately high rate of sickness.

We also have the figures for admissions to the six large military hospitals for the whole of 1695.

Hospital	Admissions
Ghent	3,351
Dixmude	1,061
Bruges	985
Brussels	2,800
Namur	2,087
Liege	3,332
Total	13,616

As the strength of the troops in 1695 was 30,000 it means that 45 per cent of the troops were admitted to hospital during the year where their average stay was twenty-one and a half days. The total deaths amounted to 910 including 217 men who died of wounds, an overall mortality rate of 6·7 per cent, but from sickness alone of 5·1 per cent, a figure which shows at least that the troops were untroubled by any serious epidemics of either typhus or dysentery.

Some details of hospital staff and administration have come down to us. A Warrant for 1st April 1695 now gives the strength of medical staff officers in Flanders as 3 comptrollers of hospitals, 4 physicians, 3 master apothecaries, and 9 apothecaries mates, 3 master chirurgeons and 24 chirurgeons' mates.

Hospital stoppages were charged at the rate of 3 stivers (about $1\frac{1}{2}$d.) a day up to 1694 but were then increased to 5 stivers. This, however, was not sufficient to cover the hospital expenses which amounted to over 9 stivers ($4\frac{1}{2}$d.) a day and the Government therefore advanced for each patient daily the sum of over 4 stivers. The total hospital expenses for the year including the pay of medical officers and staff amounted to 194,723:$18\frac{1}{2}$ florins, to which the hospital stoppages contributed 72,409:10 florins, leaving 122,314:$08\frac{1}{2}$ florins to be found by the Treasury. Mr. Patrick Lamb, who was the contractor for victualling, asked for an additional $\frac{1}{2}$ stiver per patient per day for succeeding campaigns because of the rise in the cost of food, and he was, he said, unable to obtain civilian servants for work in the hospital at the low rates offered; the nurses' pay alone came to £1,500 a year and as the rate for a nurse was about 6d. a day it meant that some 166 nurses were employed in the six military hospitals, an average of nearly 28 in each hospital. Parliament voted £25,000 for the hospitals in Flanders for the year 1695; and in 1696 the hospital charges amounted to £22,304 10s. $1\frac{1}{2}$d. Lamb petitioned the Treasury in June for £16,000 on account as the 'English hospitals in those parts (Flanders) were reduced to the greatest straits'. He got £4,000 in August to pay the hospital staff officers who had had none since they were given a two month's advance before they left England! Arrears of pay were a common complaint, and the case of Sir Patrick Dun, the Physician General in Ireland may be mentioned, who was still arguing over pay fifteen years after the Irish war was over. In another instance Theophilus Allen, a surgeon, was still asking the Treasury in July 1691 to reimburse him the sum of £80 8s. 6d. paid by him for the sick of Colonel Luttrell's and Sir John Guise's regiments after nearly two years had been spent trying to get payment. It was not only the officers who suffered, the soldiers' pay was two months in arrears, and it is reported that a detachment in the West Indies had had none for seven years.

The cost of medicines and dressings supplied each year came to between £4,000 and £6,000. In 1694 the arrears 'unpaid and payable' for 'physick for the army' was £4,000; for 1696 Mr. Teale, the chief apothecary, applied for payment of £5,888 2s. 2d., a claim which My Lords of the Treasury chose to cut down by £1,000; in 1697 it was £5,348 13s. 10d., the items provided including a magazine of drugs and medicines, and ninety-five pairs of regimental chests for the use of the hospitals and forces in Flanders to be subject to the goodness and prices of Dr. Hutton the Physician General.

With the capture of Namur in 1696 ended the first stage of the great conflict which was to be waged against Louis XIV. In 1697 the Treaty of Ryswick was signed, a treaty which the French nation, reduced to exhaustion by the war, was glad to conclude.

With the conclusion of peace the standing army was cut down to a total of 7,000 men, and the medical establishment suffered a corresponding reduction with the relegation of all hospital officers and some regimental surgeons to half pay.

Although there are no specific reports on the treatment of wounds during the wars of William III the general trends of surgery in the seventeenth century will be sufficient to convey the principles which were in common use. This was the great period of amputating limbs and it was done with reckless profusion by the regimental surgeons, many of whom had little skill, and by the surgeons of the field hospitals who were expected to have a great deal more. Garrison says that 'wholesale lopping off of limbs often times resulted in the speedy death of the patient from shock and haemorrhage and filled the cities with mendicant cripples'.[49] Wiseman's practice of primary amputation while the patient was free from fever was generally accepted, while in 1679 the first case of flap amputation was carried out by James Yonge.[50] In France, Morel had introduced the tourniquet in 1674 and this was successfully applied in ligating the femoral artery in 1688. Primary debridement of wounds was common, all surgeons were keen on the removal of the bullet, and they were only too ready to explore wounds with dirty fingers. The cautery was in common use to check haemorrhage after amputation, and the pain of the operation was sometimes lessened by giving the patient a sponge to breathe which was steeped in a mixture of opium, hyoscyamus and belladonna. All wounds suppurated, made worse by the practice of stuffing them with charpie,[51] dilating them with tents, and by the surgeons active interference. Wound dressings consisted of salves or ointments compounded of ingredients which were often of strange and nauseating origin, and boiled with turpentine or camphor. When inevitably fever occurred as the result of suppuration, blood letting was practised and often repeated to excess.

Turning now to the diseases which caused the greatest sick wastage in the armies during the seventeenth century there are three principal causes—dysentery, fever and typhus. Added to these there were occasional outbreaks of smallpox and bubonic plague.

Dysentery or camp dysentery as it was called occurred both in summer and winter. The summer variety was an enteritis due to fly borne infection, while in winter the effects of wet, cold, exposure, and lack of suitable food and clothing produced the symptoms of the 'bloody flux'.

Fever was divided clinically into intermittent, remittent, and continuous varieties and was due to a multiplicity of undiagnosed causes. These included malaria in the Low Countries, typhoid fever and relapsing fever in most of the countries of Europe. Typhus fever, however, was beginning to be recognized as a specific entity and was known as jail fever because of its frequency amongst criminals who were crowded together in prison.

Outbreaks of smallpox occurred all over England in the years 1666 to 1675 and almost the entire population suffered from its effects at one time or another, while bubonic plague killed 69,000 people in the Great Plague of London in 1665. Sydenham was the foremost of the physicians of the period and the remedies he and others employed were often made up of the most loathsome ingredients usually compounded from parts of different animals. The medical chests provided for the army which now came into use contained a huge consortium of remedies; Garrison quotes one which contained 284 different items including oil of vipers and angle worms, beetles, earwigs, and powdered mummy.

REFERENCES

[1] *Calendar of State Papers*, Domestic, Charles 11, but Walton gives the date of the first chirurgeon general as 1669.

[2] *Calendar of State Papers*, Domestic, Charles II.

[3] *Calendar of State Papers*, Domestic, Charles II.

[4] Johnston. *Roll of Commissioned Officers in the Medical Services of the British Army*, Introduction. p. XXII. Aberdeen University Press (1917).

[5] Cameron. *History of Royal College of Surgeons, Dublin.*

[6] Dalton. *English Army Lists and Commission Registers 1661–1685.*

[7] P.R.O. Military Entry Books—see also Dalton.

[8] P.R.O. Military Entry Books.

[9] The word chirurgeon is from the Greek KEIR—a hand, and ERGON—work, that is one who works cures by external manipulation or operation. Chirurgeon and surgeon are synonymous.

[10] Physician at first 10s. and then 15s. a day, apothecary 5s., chirurgeon 4s. and mate 2s. 6d.

[11] See Appendix A.

[12] See Appendix B.

[13] Dean. *The Royal Hospital, Chelsea*, p. 19. Hutchinson. London (1950).

[14] Garrison. *Notes on the History of Military Medicine*, p. 119. Saunders, Washington (1922).

[15] *Calendar of State Papers*, Ireland. *King's Letter*, book I, p. 110.

[16] Francis Quarles (1592–1644) quoted by Dean. *The Royal Hospital, Chelsea*. Hutchinson, London (1950).

[17] Dean. *The Royal Hospital, Chelsea*, p. 18. Hutchinson, London (1950).

[18] Dean. *The Royal Hospital, Chelsea*, p. 15. Hutchinson, London (1950).

[19] Gore. *Our Services under the Crown*, p. 63. Balliere Tindall & Cox, (1879).

[20] Dean. *The Royal Hospital, Chelsea*, p. 29. Hutchinson, London (1950).

[21] Howell. Journal *R.A.M.C.*, vol. XVII, p. 651.

[22] Fortescue. *History of the British Army*, book V, chapter I, p. 345. Macmillan, London (1910).

[23] Gore. *Our Services under the Crown*, p. 67. Balliere Tindall & Cox, London (1879).

[24] Fortescue. *History of the British Army*, book V, chapter I, p. 346. Macmillan, London (1910).

[25] Harleian Manuscripts 7439.

[26] See Appendix C.

[27] Apothecaries and purveyors were medical officers.

[28] P.R.O., W.O. 24/884.

[29] See Appendix D.

[30] Howell. Journal *R.A.M.C.*, vol. XVII, p. 650.
[31] Howell. Journal *R.A.M.C.*, vol. XVII, p. 652.
[32] *Calendar of State Papers*, Domestic 1690.
[33] *Calendar of State Papers*, Domestic 1690, p. 120.
[34] Wolseley. *Life of Marlborough*. R. Bentley & Son, London (1894).
[35] *Calendar of State Papers*. Domestic. King William's Chest II, No. 20.
[36] Harleian Manuscripts. 29th July 1689. MSS 7439.
[37] Walton. *History of the British Standing Army*, p. 758. Harrison & Sons Ltd. (1894).
[38] Howell. Journal *R.A.M.C.*, vol. XVII, p. 656 quoted from Clarke MSS.
[39] *Calendar of State, Papers* Ireland. King's Letter Book I.
[40] *Calendar of State, Papers* Ireland. King's Letter Book I.
[41] Walton. *History of the British Standing Army*, p. 756. Harrison & Sons Ltd. (1894).
[42] Howell. Journal *R.A.M.C.*, vol. XVII, p. 655.
[43] Howell. Journal *R.A.M.C.*, vol. XVII, p. 653.
[44] Gore. *Our Services under the Crown*, p. 72. Balliere Tindall & Cox, (1879).
[45] Gore. *Our Services under the Crown*, p. 68. Balliere Tindall & Cox, (1879).
[46] *Calendar of State Papers*, Domestic.
[47] *Calendar of State Papers*, Domestic. King William, p. 170.
[48] Morley to Sir Joseph Williamson. *Calendar of State Papers*, *S.P.* Domestic W. & M.3, No. 49.
[49] Garrison. *Notes on the History of Military Medicines*, p. 128. Saunders, Washington (1922).
[50] Garrison. *Notes on the History of Military Medicines*, p. 128. Another source says Lowdham at Oxford was the first. Saunders, Washington (1922).
[51] Charpie is linen separated into short threads about 2–3 inches long and made from old bed linen.

Chapter 3

WAR OF SPANISH SUCCESSION

During the first half of the eighteenth century there were many changes and advances in military medicine: barracks for troops were begun, a common daily ration was introduced, regular orders for the administration of military hospitals came into force, the medical examination of recruits was initiated, limited periods of enlistment were tried, standardized uniforms and equipment for soldiers and colours for regiments were provided. As far as surgery is concerned the advances we should note are the invention of the screw tourniquet by Petit in 1718, while operation for strangulated hernia was performed for the first time.

The direction of medical affairs lay in the hands of the Physician General and the Surgeon General whose duties were merely part time and their pay of £1 a day only a small part of the income which they earned in private practice. In times of peace their task was minimal for it was only concerned with the administration involved in the selection of regimental surgeons and the new class of garrison surgeons which were coming into being, and in 1718 Gore estimates the total strength of regular officers as 170. The outbreak of war brought a burst of activity and the first half of the century was marked by the important campaigns of the War of the Spanish Succession 1701–1712, the war against Spain 1739–1742, the War of the Austrian Succession 1742–1748, while there were many less extensive operations to which reference will be made including the short-lived rebellion of Prince Charles Edward Stuart the Young Pretender in 1745. For these campaigns marching and fixed or general hospitals as they were later called had to be organized, and their stores, equipment and medicines provided, and medical officers of different grades to staff them had to be selected and appointed.

It was the Surgeon General who shouldered the major responsibilities for the overseas expeditions, the Physician General being chiefly concerned with the selection of physicians and advising on the treatment of disease. The earlier apothecary generals such as Whittle and Teale were holders of office only in a commercial sense and it was in 1710 that an Act of Parliament was passed 'to the end that Her Majesty's Forces

59

might be supplied with good and wholesome medicines internal and external, and for preventing the loss and suffering of many officers and soldiers for want thereof'.[1]

We now record the names of those who had the direction of the medical service in their hands during the first half of the century:

Physician Generals

Thomas Lawrence	24th June 1685
Sir Samuel Garth, Bart	15th October 1714
Thomas Gibson	23rd January 1719
Sir Hans Sloane, Bart	3rd June 1722
John Hollinges, F.R.S.	10th October 1727
Charles Peters	14th May 1739
Sir Edward Wilmot, Bart, F.R.S.	27th April 1746

Surgeon Generals

John Knight	16th December 1664
Thomas Gardiner	1st October 1701
Alexander Inglis	25th December 1710
John Pawlett	27th January 1737
David Middleton	3rd March 1748

Apothecary Generals

Richard Whittle	1st January 1686
Benjamin Teale	1710 and 28th January 1715
Thomas Graham	18th May 1727
Isaac Garnier	15th May 1733
George Garnier	7th March 1736

With regard to the Physician Generals the chief point to emphasize is that none of them were regular medical officers but were selected by the Sovereign on account of their eminence in the civil profession. Few of them had ever seen war service, although Lawrence had served in Ireland and Sir Hans Sloane had been to Jamaica on the staff of the Duke of Buckingham as personal physician, but Hollinges, Peters and Wilmot had no army experience whatever. They were, however, all Physicians or Physicians Extraordinary to the Sovereign, two were Fellows of the Royal Society, and of course all were Fellows of the College of Physicians. There was no limit to their tenure of office and most of them served until they died. Wilmot who was appointed Physician General in 1746 served for no less than forty years, and he died in 1786 still holding office at the age of 93! In addition to recommending physicians for commissions the Physician General exercised control over the apothecaries, advised on the treatment of medical diseases in the hospitals, and presided over the examination of candidates for hospital mate.

The Surgeon Generals on the other hand were men of a different stamp with considerable military experience who had started their army career either as regimental surgeons, or were commissioned in the rank of surgeon to general hospitals in war. Inglis, Pawlett, and Middleton were all regular officers: Inglis had been Surgeon to the Queen's Horse (King's Dragoon Guards) in 1702 and was present at Blenheim and Malplaquet; Pawlett was a mate at Blenheim with the train of artillery and later was Surgeon to the Horse Guards; Middleton, also Surgeon to the Horse Guards, had distinguished war experience, for he was Chief Surgeon in Flanders in 1743, Director of Hospitals in 1744, and in 1756 was made Sergeant Surgeon to the King. On the whole they were well fitted by their training and experience for their task. As there was no retiring age all continued in office until they died, and remarkable as it may seem all carried out their duties without any office establishment or deputies to assist them.

The Apothecary General purchased the medicines and dressings from civil chemists and fitted out the regimental surgeons' chests once a year at Apothecaries' Hall, where they were examined and certified by the Master and Warden of the Apothecaries as well as by the Physician General and Surgeon General. In peacetime, medicines and dressings were paid for by the regimental surgeons out of the medicine money stopped weekly from the pay of the N.C.O's and men of the regiment,[2] their annual expenditure in this respect being around £40 to £45, varying with the regimental strength. In wartime medicines were supplied by the government. When the Garniers assumed office, the family in 1735 somehow managed to acquire a patent to hold the appointment in perpetuity. This patent was renewed on the 19th January 1747 in favour of George Garnier 'to obey the King and his superior officers for the time being and to furnish good and wholesome medicines to the Army'.[3] It was to prove a lucrative post, for besides the pay of 10s. a day Garnier was entitled to a percentage of the contracts entered into for the supply of medicines by civil firms, and we shall see that some seventy years later the Government became considerably disturbed by the profits which went into the pocket of the Apothecary General and tried without success to limit it.

As the regimental hospitals provided all the care and treatment required there were no general hospitals in peacetime. Neither in wartime did they exist in Britain until towards the end of the century, and the omission to provide them (which was purely on the grounds of expense) led to disgraceful lack of treatment for the sick and wounded soldiers after disembarkation from overseas expeditions.

During the greater part of this century the pay of the regimental surgeon was 4s. a day and his mate 2s. 6d. His total emoluments are given in the following table.

	Surgeon	Mate
Daily pay	4s.	2s. 6d.
Yearly pay	£73	£45 12s. 6d.
Subsistence	3s. a day	2s. a day
	or £54 15s. a year	or £36 10s. a year
Poundage	£3 13s.	£2 5s. 8½d.
Royal Hospital Chelsea: one day's pay	4s.	2s. 6d.
Agency	12s. 2d.	7s. 7½d.
Warrants	9s. 4d.	8s.
Arrears	£13 7s. 10d.	£6 7s. 8½d.

This for the surgeon was less pay than that of the lieutenant, the quartermaster or the chaplain. With so inadequate a reward the custom already referred to arose whereby he was allowed to add to his pay by the purchase of an ensign's commission.

All commissions were signed by the Secretary of State for War or the local Commander-in-Chief abroad, and candidates for regimental surgeons from the year 1666 had to be approved by the Surgeon General, and in 1691 after complaints of 'negligence and ignorance', he was directed to examine them personally. Regimental mates had their warrants signed by the colonels of regiments; hospital and garrison mates by the Surgeon General,[4] while apothecary's mates for some reason received commissions.

A dispute arose between the Barber Surgeons' Company and retired medical officers who had been placed on half pay after the termination of hostilities and set up in practice for themselves without obtaining the diploma of the Company. The officers declared themselves to be acting under an Act passed in 1728 entitled 'An Act to enable such officers, mariners and soldiers as have been in His Majesty's Service since his accession to the throne to exercise trades.' This dispute went on for some fifty years before in 1782 the Company of Surgeons stated a case for consideration of the Law Officers of the Crown and a decision was entered against them.[5]

During Queen Anne's reign (1701–1714) there were several Articles of War for the forces overseas which provided for assistance to disabled soldiers. All plunder taken before the enemy was entirely beaten was forfeited for the use of the sick and maimed soldiers, and after the battle one-tenth part of the spoil was to be laid apart towards the relief of the sick and maimed. There was also an Article of War which laid down that every soldier neglecting to attend Divine Service should become liable to a fine of 12d. which was applied to the relief of sick soldiers. Marshall says this regulation was in force up to 1846.[6]

In 1702 the Royal Hospital at Chelsea was in such financial difficulties that the time-honoured custom of making the army pay was adopted, and one day's pay per annum was levied from all officers and men including medical officers; this was supplemented later by a Government grant, the Duke of Marlborough taking an active interest and using his personal influence to make a success of this institution for old soldiers who had suffered disabilities acquired in the service of their country. Two classes existed, In Pensioners and Out Pensioners; the In Pensioners lived in the Royal Hospital and were organized into Companies of Invalids each commanded by a disabled officer, while their medical care devolved upon a staff comprising a physician, a surgeon, an apothecary and a surgeon's mate. The holders of these appointments included many distinguished doctors who had had army service, Wintringham and Pringle amongst the physicians, and Ranby amongst the surgeons. When Ranby became medical Superintendent the Hospital had a reputation as 'a perfect model of everything that is right for hospital management, cleanliness and order, and the treatment of sores and wounds'.[7]

As always, political consideration governed the strength of the army. When war was declared it was temporarily increased and reduced as soon as peace came. The army was in fact very unpopular, and 'No Standing Army' was the cry, for Cromwell's military despotism had left a memory which rankled deeply. A further reason was the wretched quality of the soldiers who were often recruited from the dregs of the population.

In George I's reign of thirteen years (1714–1727) there was little to disturb the peace except the Jacobite rebellion of 1715, and an expedition to capture Vigo, when war was declared against Spain in 1719, and where the medical arrangements were purely regimental. In 1722 Walpole who was then Prime Minister fixed the peace establishment at 22,000 men. Enlistment was for life, few soldiers getting their discharge except through age, infirmity, disablement by wounds, or chronic incurable disease. The greatest hardship for troops was the long period of service in foreign stations. One regiment remained in the West Indies for nearly 60 years, another in Gibraltar for 28 years, another continuously on foreign service from 1717 to 1763. Even invalid soldiers in the West Indies could not be brought home because of lack of funds, and pensioners were sent to Gibraltar to serve. As a result of such harsh conditions there was much desertion, and as a punishment these men when recaptured were sent overseas.

The year 1716 saw the establishment of the Royal Artillery as a regiment, and the Master General of the Ordnance appointed the first surgeon and mate to the new corps in 1727, while in course of time we shall see the Ordnance Medical establishment becoming independent with its own Director and with its own hospitals.

After George II came to the throne in 1727 the regiments of Foot were increased from the 42nd to the 70th Regiment, and fifteen second battalions were added. By 1740 the strength was over 28,000 exclusive of the troops in Ireland where a separate army establishment was set up in April 1728. Here the direction of the medical service lay in the hands of a Physician General and Surgeon General at Dublin who were quite independent of control from Headquarters at the Horse Guards.

War of Spanish Succession

It was the death of Charles II of Spain in 1700 which led to the War of the Spanish Succession. Louis XIV of France accepted the provisions of the will of Charles II which left the crown of the vast Spanish Empire to Louis' son Philip of Anjou under the title of Philip V. But previous to his death two Treaties of Partition had been entered into by France, England, and the Netherlands, agreeing to the division of these possessions. When Louis accepted the provisions of Charles II's will these Treaties went for naught, and accordingly the Emperor of Austria contested Louis XIV's acceptance of the will and its vast inheritance, and Austria was supported by William III and Holland.

The foundations of the Grand Alliance of England, Holland and Austria which fought the war against France from 1701 to 1712 were laid by the Duke of Marlborough, and the years of costly strife ended with the Treaty of Utrecht in 1713. Louis XIV struck first in 1701 by pouring troops into the Spanish Netherlands and occupying the Dutch barrier fortresses. This invasion of Holland by a great power was always a threat to which England reacted with vigour, and moreover we were bound by treaty to provide a force of 6,400 men to come to the aid of the Dutch in an emergency. Accordingly in June 1701 twelve battalions were shipped off to Holland under the command of John Churchill, later Duke of Marlborough, and this was followed by an agreement that England should furnish a contingent of 40,000 men, 18,000 of them British and the remainder foreigners. The French had some 200,000 men under arms, and the field of operation was Flanders, the cockpit of Europe. Military movements were slow and deliberate as befitted an age when admirals wore full bottomed wigs, and siege warfare constituted the most important part of military science. The object of a campaign was not necessarily to seek out an enemy and destroy him. To live in enemy territory and subsist on the country and destroy all that could not be consumed was considered highly successful, although a shot was never fired. To keep the enemy marching and counter-marching for weeks without striking a blow was equally to be commended, for when recruits to replenish the ranks proved difficult to get, commanders sought rather to avoid than invite deliberate encounters. In all this, however, Marlborough was to prove exceptional, and his hammer blows were to prove decisive.

We have seen that for William III's campaigns two forms of hospital were organized, and it is certain that Marching and Fixed Hospitals must have existed under Marlborough. Moreover the constant manoeuvring which characterized the operations must have made it extremely difficult at times to prevent the hospitals from falling into enemy hands unless they were continually on the move behind and close to the army. Only in winter quarters could they remain static.

At the Horse Guards the conduct of the medical arrangements depended on the three heads of branches—Dr. Lawrence the Physician General, Mr. Gardiner the Surgeon General, and Mr. Whittle the Apothecary General. It was on the Surgeon General that the chief responsibility lay for the medical organization of the campaign; and the provision of hospital equipment and the selection of medical officers to staff them was in his hands. The appointment of physicians was the only exception to this rule for this was the prerogative of the Physician General. Although the Surgeon General had the power to select a capable regimental surgeon to be a hospital surgeon, for the most part the hospital officers were recruited from the civil profession and served only for the duration of the campaign.

The general hospital which was planned to go overseas with Marlborough had Mr. Hudson as Commissary or Director. Johnston says that like his predecessors under William III he was not a medical man, and the first medical director of hospitals was not to be appointed until 1727.[8] His duties were strictly administrative—equipment, rations, moves, transport. With Mr. Hudson there was a team of physicians, surgeons, apothecaries, and hospital mates. Of trained subordinate staff there was none, and this was the difficulty which handicapped all general hospitals throughout the centuries. The ward duties and bed making, the cooking and washing and other hospital duties had to depend upon what labour could be supplied from regiments or by employing the soldiers' wives who accompanied their husbands and followed the drum. These so called 'nurses' were given a few pence a day as payment and although they were destined to get a bad name because of the fondness for drink—yet they played a worth while part in looking after both the sick and the wounded of many a campaign. The soldiers who worked in the wards as ward masters or orderlies or on the hospital departments as cooks or stewards were either men detailed from regiments or were patients who had recovered to the convalescent stage. As the men from regiments could be changed every twenty-four hours at the whim of their commanding officer it meant there was a continual procession of untrained men passing through the wards which made it well nigh impossible to preserve a semblance of order or continuity of treatment.

The regimental medical establishment consisted of the regimental surgeon and his mate with a pack horse carrying the two panniers of medical and surgical equipment. The establishment also included the bedding and equipment of a regimental hospital of forty beds.

Two further appointments must be mentioned, one a physician and the other a surgeon appointed to the headquarters staff. Each drew pay at the rate of 10s. a day, a circumstance which is unusual as the physician usually drew higher pay than the surgeon.

We pass now to the details of the campaigns. In July 1702 the Allied army of 60,000 men, comprised of 12,000 British troops, the rest Dutch and German, was concentrated in South Holland. Apart from Marlborough's superiority in tactics which the year revealed, the opportunities to defeat the French were thwarted by the Dutch civilian deputies who accompanied the army. In 1703 the number of British troops in the Low Counties was 18,000, raised in 1704 to 22,000; added to this number there were 28,000 German mercenaries, a total of 50,000 men. Interference by the Dutch deputies again thwarted Marlborough's efforts, and apart from the capture of Bonn there was no major engagement. But in 1704 he decided to leave Flanders to the protection of the Dutch and carry the war into the heart of Germany.

From winter quarters on the Meuse, 16,000 British troops set out in May 1704 for their long march to the Danube. Marlborough's aim was to defeat the armies of the Elector of Bavaria and the French, which were ready to strike a blow at Vienna. Behind the army the general hospital was carried up in boats on the Rhine bringing the bedding and equipment, the medical stores and provisions, all of which were pushed forward 'with all imaginable care and haste' first to Coblentz and thence to Mainz. Here a temporary halt was made while the hospital opened to treat the sick who had fallen out on the march, happily few in number, for in spite of their exertions and the bad weather, the troops were healthy largely due to Marlborough's care and forethought. After joining up with the army of Prince Louis of Baden at Ulm, Marlborough was ready for operations. The general hospital was now close behind at Geislingen; it had been carried up the Rhine from Mainz to Mannheim, disembarked and brought forward on waggons the 80 miles to its new destination. On the 22nd June, Marlborough ordered General Churchill to open a small hospital at Heidesheim 'send them thither in carts with an able surgeon and a mate or two'[9] but the main hospital he wanted at Nordlingen, 'and being returned (from Prince Louis' quarters) about ten at night he (Marlborough) sent an express to the Commissary of the Hospital to hasten him away to Nordlingen and to march day and night till he had settled with it there. This express was followed by two more to hasten the apothecaries and surgeons, his Grace sending them a recommendation . . . "to the magistrate and inhabitants of the place for all manner of necessaries".'[10]

The victory of Schellenberg near Donauworth was followed by the decisive battle of Blenheim fought on the 2nd August. Here the Allied losses amounted to 4,500 killed and 7,500 wounded, of which the British share was 670 killed and 1,500 wounded. The French losses fell little short of 40,000 men, 11,000 of whom were prisoners, with 129 colours, 171 standards, and 124 guns and mortars.

Marlborough's humanity and consideration was clearly shown in the interest he displayed in the medical arrangements and care of the wounded. Before the battle he selected the position of the regimental hospitals. Sergeants from every regiment were sent out to collect their own casualties, and temporary shelter was found for them in the tents captured from the French. Dr. Hare tells us, 'The moment the action was ended it grew dark and rained violently. This proved very fatal to the wounded of which we had great numbers. All his Grace's care was now employed about sending the wounded away to the Hospital and as there was a particular hand of Providence directed him in all his marches and designs, so it was very remarkable in the happy arrival of the apothecaries, surgeons, and medicaments, at Nordlingen in the time of the action.'[11] For transport 'he orders all the country round about him to bring in waggons and carriages upon pain of military executions'.[12] We can thus appreciate the truth when Marlborough writes, 'Ever since the battle I have been so employed about our own wounded men and prisoners, that I have not had one hour's quiet.'[13]

There were nine surgeons in the Nordlingen hospital and they must have been immensely busy dressing and carrying out amputations on these 1,500 casualties. The staff officers present included Dr. Lawrence the Physician General and it appears that he took an active part in the campaign. It will be convenient here to follow up the final disposal of these cases at Nordlingen. Many were still undergoing treatment during September, but with the approach of winter all who could be moved were evacuated in waggons to Mainz, and in October sent down the Rhine in boats to join their respective regiments. The few remaining had medical officers left with them, and Marlborough— meticulous as always in doing the right thing—thanked the inhabitants for their liberality on behalf of the patients, not omitting at the same time to express his gratitude to his own surgeons.

Like all great commanders Marlborough paid the closest attention to the welfare of his men. He won their hearts not only for his care and concern but because they trusted his ability and his genius to lead them to victory, and morale was always high. Any tendency to intemperance and licentiousness was suppressed, and their sense of duty and the need of restraint constantly impressed upon the men by moral and religious instruction. 'By these means,' wrote a contemporary biographer, 'his camp resembled a quiet well governed city.'[14] The daily march was usually begun about 3 a.m., and after covering 14 to 16 miles the infantry halted around 9 a.m. Beef and bread were the rations on which the army chiefly subsisted, and herds of cattle were driven along with the troops as the source of fresh meat. Supplies were carried ahead to the camping area where the troops had only to pitch their tents, boil their kettles and lie down to rest.

In the campaign of 1705 Marlborough's chief success was gained in July when he broke through the centre of the fortified French lines which extended from near Namur right through to Antwerp. From this point of penetration he swept north-westwards nearly as far as Louvain, but once again further successes were thwarted by refusal to move on the part of the Dutch general, and the opportunity to complete the defeat of the French and even to end the war was lost. In this campaign there is only one mention of the general hospital at Neierbach, but its movements must certainly have conformed closely to that of the army, and maximum use must have been made of the many rivers and canals both in moving the hospital and in bringing back sick and wounded from the regimental hospitals. Of sickness we know nothing except that typhus had occurred during winter quarters in the Moselle area, so it is little wonder that in June we hear of the inhabitants fleeing in terror before the troops for fear of acquiring the 'distemper'.

It was in 1706 that the battle of Ramillies was fought. Marlborough began the campaign at Maestricht in May with 60,000 men under his command, including 20,000 British troops, and when a fortnight later he came up with Villeroy at the village of Ramillies he decided to attack. British losses were few, but the total Allied casualties amounted to between 4,000 to 5,000 men, the Dutch and Danish troops suffering most heavily. The French lost some 15,000 in killed, wounded and prisoners. The sole information about the casualties tells us that the medical organization was so poor that some wounded had to be left upon the field for days before they were dressed, but by Marlborough's orders the casualties of both sides received equal attention, first in tents captured from the enemy, and later in hospital which was pro-bably at Maestricht some 35 miles distant, which had been the seat of winter quarters. The effect of this victory was instantaneous. Louvain, Brussels, and Malines soon fell, followed by Ghent, Bruges and Antwerp, and within a fortnight the French had fallen back to their own frontier. Then came the siege and capture of Ostend and the surrender of Menin, so that within a single month Marlborough's arms were triumphant from the Meuse to the sea.

As the year 1707 went by without major engagements of importance our story passes on to the year 1708, when the battle of Oudenarde was fought on the 11th July. Here again the loss of British troops was small, amounting only to 4 officers and 49 men killed and 17 officers and 160 men wounded, although the total Allied loss amounted to some 3,000. The French lost 6,000 killed and wounded and 9,000 prisoners. For these operations we read for the first time of two general hospitals being open, one at Ghent and another at Brussels. Unfortunately the loss of Ghent meant that the hospital with the medical officers and patients were captured. Vendome the French commander offered to hand over the sick and wounded, and in exchange Marlborough sent 150 French wounded then in our hospital at Brussels to Ghent, and the barges brought our own cases back to Brussels.[15]

The Allied commanders now decided to lay siege to Lille, one of the strongest fortresses in the world, fortified by Vauban with his utmost skill. After an obstinate resistance the town capitulated. The five British infantry regiments engaged in the first assault lost 350 killed and wounded, but of the 5,000 British troops committed for the next attack, casualties are not ascertainable. A feature of the siege was the daring exploit of a British sergeant who was foremost in swimming a stream to a French post and letting down the drawbridge for the assault. The captured sick and wounded were sent to a general hospital which had now been opened at Douai, and were treated with as much consideration as our own casualties.

In July 1709, the Duke had besieged and captured Tournay, another of the strongest fortresses in France, and four British regiments bore their share in this work and suffered heavily in the course of it. In anticipation of the casualties Marlborough had given orders to open a general hospital in Lille and before commencing the siege he had written to the magistrates at Lille and arranged for a commodious building to be set aside, asking them at the same time to give the hospital officers every assistance in carrying out their duties.

At the battle of Malplaquet, fought on the 31st August 1709, the French under Marshall Villars held a strong position, and the Allied victory cost them 20,000 casualties and the French 12,000. The British loss amounted to 1,900 including 1,200 wounded. The fighting was so desperate and the losses so severe that many slightly wounded were seen returning 'though pale and bleeding, to take again their places in the ranks, and support their gallant comrades'.[16] Marlborough was almost distracted by the numerous appeals made by the officers of the different nations for relief of the wounded, and two days were spent in searching the woods in which 3,000 casualties lay concealed. Before Malplaquet had been fought, the Allied had invested Mons, and the siege of this fortress was resumed after the battle. The weather was bad, the ground swampy, and the regimental hospitals full of sick, but with its capitulation on the 9th October the season's operations ended.

The campaign of 1710 was confined to the siege and capture of Douai, Bethune, Aixe and St. Venant, which cost the Allies some 15,000 men killed and wounded, besides a considerable wastage from sickness.

It was in the following year that Eugene was ordered to withdraw the Austrians from the Allied army, and although there was no major engagement, Marlborough's superb tactics which completely deceived the enemy enabled him to penetrate the French lines at Arleux and capture Bouchain. It was to be his last campaign, for he fell into disfavour with Queen Anne and was replaced as commander-in-chief in 1712 by the Duke of Ormonde. The Government opened negotiations with Louis XIV and Ormonde had instructions to engage neither in a battle nor a siege. In fact it was not long before suspension of hostilities with France was announced and Britain withdrew from the Alliance, and by the Treaty of Utrecht in 1713 Fortescue tells us that every object for which the war was fought was sacrificed.

There are no sources of information which tell the amount of sickness, but experience tells us that the common causes of sick wastage were the usual dysentery, fever and typhus.

Fever was both of the intermittent and continuous variety, the former of malarial origin and the latter no doubt including typhoid fever. Most of Flanders was low lying and mosquito breeding areas were widespread in the summer and autumn months. Putrid malignant fever or typhus fever frequently broke out in overcrowded hospitals and was the most dreaded of all diseases because of its high mortality. As one would expect there were chest complaints during the winter months of the nature of bronchitis and pneumonia, and many of the older soldiers suffered from rheumatism. But of the treatment of wounds it must be recorded that we have no knowledge, for no historian has been found to enlighten us.

It was not only in Flanders that the War of the Spanish Succession was waged, for operations which involved British troops were also taking place at the same time both in Portugal and Spain. Among the Spanish people there were many adherents to the Austrian cause who favoured placing the Archduke Charles of Austria, otherwise Charles V on the Spanish throne, and the British Government decided to support them by sending expeditions to both countries in the Peninsula.

The first operation was the capture of Gibraltar by a British fleet in July 1704 and although the troops who were landed were besieged by some 12,000 Spaniards and French, Gibraltar remained safely in our hands. Subsequently in 1705 Lord Peterborough led the expedition to Catalonia in Eastern Spain and Lord Galway commanded the force chosen to land at Lisbon. In both areas British troops were destined to fight campaigns for six long years.

In the expedition to Catalonia Peterborough with a force of 6,500 men which included six British battalions landed at Barcelona in October 1705 and captured the city. The hospital staff which accompanied him comprised 2 physicians, 2 master surgeons, 2 apothecaries and 4 hospital mates. In charge of the general hospital which was opened in Barcelona was Mr. Watkins the Director who was also the purveyor or commissary, a position similar to that held by Mr. Hudson in Flanders.[17] This was an age when the public conscience of officers did not prevent them lining their own pockets at government expense, and the pay of 15s. a day of the Director was given in the hope that this would lessen the temptation to peculate. With the expedition came hospital bedding and equipment, and medicines to the value of £500 had been supplied by the Apothecary General.

In Portugal the force sent amounted to some 3,000 British, but with Dutch and Portuguese troops Lord Galway had 19,000 men under his command. With this expedition there came a master surgeon, 6 surgeons and 4 hospital mates, all of whom had been hurried off to Lisbon as early as July 1704 with the equipment and medicines for a general hospital.

Peterborough, after capturing Barcelona, fought an audacious campaign against a more numerous enemy in eastern Spain the following year. By consummate trickery he was able to capture Valencia in January, and after returning to drive away a French army which was besieging Barcelona, the road to Madrid lay open. There appears to have been no correlation of strategy between the two British commanders and Galway had already forestalled him by entering Madrid on the 27th June. Here he was joined by Peterborough in August bringing with him the Archduke Charles who was proclaimed King.

The object of the war now seemed to have been fulfilled, but the success did not last long; the country rose in revolt; sickness reduced the combined force to 14,000 men, and Galway remained inactive in Madrid until a retreat became inevitable. His lines of communication with Lisbon were cut and he decided to fall back on Valencia where he took up quarters for the winter under the protection of the British fleet.

In 1706 a further reinforcement of some 7,000 Horse and Foot arrived at Lisbon from England, but after a delay there of two months due to bad weather the mortality on board the overcrowded transports when finally they landed at Valencia in 1707 was so frightful that their numbers had been reduced by half from typhus fever.

Galway's polyglot army now numbered 15,000, of which a bare third were British, the rest Portuguese, Dutch, German and Huguenot, and he was rash enough to fight the battle of Almanza on the 25th April against superior numbers. Within two hours Galway had lost 4,000 killed and wounded and 3,000 prisoners; the British alone lost 88 officers killed and 286 captured of whom 92 were wounded. Galway drew off his remaining troops as best he could and returned to Barcelona and in 1708 left Catalonia for Lisbon. The following year the British were again defeated at the battle of the Caya River, and Galway vowed he would never fight in company with the Portuguese again.

After the establishment of the hospital at Barcelona in October 1705 the medical arrangements are shrouded in mystery, but when Galway brought his troops to Valencia in the winter of 1706/7 the general hospital must have moved to the same city. Of the hospital arrangements for the battle of Almanza we are equally ignorant but in view of the mountainous nature of the country it can only be assumed that a flying hospital accompanied the force. On Galway's return to Barcelona the hospital must have returned there, and we hear of fresh supplies of medicines arriving for it in 1709 which included over a hundred different kinds of drugs, including a supply of Peruvian bark at a cost of 16 guineas. Mr. Neilson, who had been one of the surgeons sent with Peterborough's force, had succeeded Watkins as Director, and was promoted to 'Physician to the Hospitals in Spain'.

Meanwhile, Field Marshal von Staremberg had succeeded Peterborough in command of the troops left in Catalonia, but his army being very inferior in numbers to the French, under Marlborough's advice he sailed off with the fleet and captured Sardinia and Minorca. Returning to Catalonia in 1710 he received a reinforcement of 4,200 British troops. But typhus fever on the voyage had again played havoc, and of a detachment of 300 men only 100 reached their regiment.[18] A private of the First Guards summed up his experience of a troop ship as 'continual destruction in the fore top, the pox above board, the plague between decks, hell in the forecastle, and the devil at the helm'.[19] However, with German as well as British reinforcements a force of 20,000 foot and 5,000 horse was assembled and after a victory at Saragossa, Madrid was regained. A much reinforced French army now advanced from the north and Staremberg had to evacuate Madrid, his army much weakened by an outbreak of autumnal fever which was undoubtedly malarial in origin. Apart from some petty operations in 1711 this for practical purposes ended the war. Spain had been lost, although Barcelona and Tarragona were still kept for the Austrian side.

These campaigns in Portugal and Spain were unpopular amongst the soldiers not only because of the ill health from fever and dysentery which were endemic in every town in the Peninsula, but also from the discomforts and long confinement of the sea voyage when they sickened and died miserably from typhus. The Transport Commissioners who controlled the sea voyages had had many complaints directed against them about the salt provisions and the weevily biscuits, but by 1702 this had been largely improved; no one, however, cared or interfered when men were left for weeks or sometimes months waiting to sail, and when fever and typhus was causing a shortage of medicines and medical supplies of all kinds it was no concern of the medical branch at the Horse Guards.[20] Neither on their return from service overseas was any provision made for the soldiers' care or comfort; a ship's load of men from Portugal were turned adrift in the streets of Penryn penniless and reduced to beg for charity, and as for the sick and wounded it was only in the fourth year of the war that the Commissioners for Sick and Hurt were appointed to make them their special care and take over these duties from the Transport Commission.[21]

There were still British troops in Lisbon in 1712, and the indifference and neglect of the Horse Guards was such that there was not a penny for the payment of hospital expenses. There were 300 sick lying in the Misericorde hospital attended by our own surgeons who could not be embarked as the Portuguese authorities refused to let them go until the proper charges had been paid. A further 300 were lying in the King of Portugal's own hospital because the Portuguese refused to co-operate and no other accommodation existed. Neilson who, as we have pointed out, was Director of Hospitals and now Physician General to the Forces in Portugal complained bitterly that he was so short of money that he had to spend his own pay and pledge his own credit, for the Portuguese had said that the hospital must shut if money was not forthcoming. Moreover, General Pearce the Commandant in Lisbon grumbled that there had been no pay for the officers for four months 'and a great many poor gentlemen have had to beg their way home, many of which are in the campayne and with the hospital, where there are many sick men'.[22]

It was, however, not only in the Peninsula that troops were exposed to conditions which were nothing short of scandalous. There were units serving in New York, in Bermuda, and in Newfoundland, and there were four to six battalions in the West Indies all of which seem to have been neglected and forgotten. No provision was made for their pay or clothing and those colonels who looked after their men's welfare were compelled to borrow money to save them from starvation and naked-ness, while those colonels who didn't care came home to England and left their men to shift for themselves.[23] In the Mediterranean garrisons of Minorca and Gibraltar things were little better, for the latter was a hot bed of sickness due to malaria which struck down half the garrison in 1706; and this was not the only cause for complaint; exposure due to lack of fuel and housing was severe but barracks were not built until four years later, and even in 1711 the men were obliged to burn their own miserable quarters from want of fuel.[24]

In 1727 the Spaniards unsuccessfully besieged Gibraltar for a period of five months. The Spaniards lost 3,000 men, while our losses in action were 75 killed and 202 wounded, but the wastage from sickness espec-ially from scurvy was very heavy: 'twas chiefly by sickness . . . so that by the lists (of casualties) which are most exact and true, about eight times as many died from distemper, occasioned it is thought by want of provisions.'[25] The absence of fresh vegetables for a period of five months brought on scurvy. As this is one of the early accounts of the disease it is appropriate to say a few words about it. The symptoms, usually insidious in origin, were gradual weakness, petechial haemorrhages over the body and brawny swellings in different parts due to effusions of blood; the gums became swollen and spongy, bled easily, and the teeth loose. Later, the patient had a bloated look, was markedly breathless on exertion and liable to fits of syncope; haemorrhages might occur from any of the mucous surfaces and there might be ulceration of the skin. Death occurred from exhaustion, anaemia, syncope, pneumonia or haemorrhage.

James Lind a Scottish naval surgeon who gained the title of 'The Father of Nautical Medicine' made his epoch-making experiment on the cure of scurvy by lemon juice in 1753. This was the first controlled dietary experiment on record and given to the world in his 'Treatise of the Scurvy'.[26] But it was to be forty years before the Admiralty in 1795 authorized the issue of lemon juice after its efficacy had been proved in many naval voyages. These effects were so dramatic that in the last four years of the Napoleonic war only two cases were treated in Haslar Hospital.

Under Walpole as Prime Minister there was peace in Europe until 1739 when war was declared against Spain. For fifty years the British and Spanish nations had been at variance over the right of free trade with the latter's possessions in South America. Walpole did his best to avert war, but a burst of democratic patriotism following on the incident of Captain Jenkins and his famous 'ear',[27] a patriotism which was encouraged by the Opposition in the hope of turning out the Government, imposed on Walpole the choice of resignation or war, and to his shame he chose war. But no account had been taken of the state of the armed forces, and the Opposition had for years consistently voted to reduce the strength of the army—the same Opposition which was now clamouring for war. The rich Spanish possessions in the West Indies were prizes of the first importance and under Admiral Vernon's instigation an expedition of 6,000 men under Lord Cathcart was ordered to assemble in the Isle of Wight in April 1740.

The hospital staff officers appointed for the expedition were twelve in number, with Dr. John Cathcart as Director and Purveyor. The senior physician Dr. George Martin was named Physician General, and Mr. Thomas Mascie, Surgeon General; there was a chief surgeon, 5 surgeons and surgeons' mates, an apothecary and 2 apothecary's mates.

From the very start of the expedition things went wrong. It had been agreed that in view of the seasonal prevalence of sickness in the West Indies it ought to sail in June; it left in fact in November after official blundering and contrary winds had delayed it for months. The soldiers had been embarked at Spithead in August, and here they remained cooped up on board ship for month after month, for to allow leave ashore was to risk desertion. After six weeks most of the victuals intended for the voyage had been consumed, and with nothing but salt rations to eat, scurvy had already caused sixty deaths by the time the expedition started. 'Surely', said General Cathcart, 'some fresh meat might be given to the troops,'[28] but the authorities had never thought about it. On the voyage a further 100 deaths took place, and of the 600 marines transferred for seamen's duty to the men-of-war, hardly one was fit for duty. Cathcart died of dysentery the day after the expedition had reached Dominica, and the command passed to the hands of Brigadier Wentworth. Removal from the intolerable atmosphere of the troop decks where the men had lain 'suspended in rows fourteen inches apart, deprived of the light of day and breathing nothing but the noisome atmosphere exhaling their own excrements and diseased bodies'[29] is said to have wrought a marvellous improvement among the sufferers from scurvy. The ultimate rendezvous was Jamaica, where Admiral Vernon's squadron lay, and here the expedition received reinforcements of 3,000 newly enlisted American Colonial troops who lacked the discipline of regiments of the Line and were both disorderly and mutinous. In the Jamaican climate all alike were soon the victims of fever and dysentery so that by the end of the year 600 men had died and 1,500 more were on the sick list.

It was Admiral Vernon who decided that Carthagena, a town on the Caribbean (in modern Colombia), was the most promising object of attack. The town lay on a low sandy island which with another island Terra Bomba to the south formed a great natural harbour; it was also a favourite breeding area for mosquitoes, and both yellow fever and malaria were endemic. This was a combined operation of the navy and the army, and to ensure success there had to be close collaboration between Vernon and Wentworth. The Admiral, rightly impressed with the need for rapid action for tactical reasons, and well aware of the risk of health entailed by delay urged Wentworth to pursue 'vigorous measures as most conducive to the preservation of men's lives from the Ravaging Hand of Sickness, the most fatal enemy'.[30] But before the fleet could enter the harbour the fort at the entrance had to be overcome. Wentworth however was determined not to take any operational risks, and the fort, which undoubtedly would have been captured by an immediate and determined attack, only fell after days of methodical preparation.

After this belated success the fleet entered the harbour and the troops were disembarked to capture the city itself. The Admiral urged Wentworth to attack the city because the yellow fever season was starting and the ever present dysentery and the ubiquitous malaria had already seriously affected the troops' health with 600 men on the sick list and 250 deaths. But Wentworth refused to be rushed into action so that relations between him and Vernon became extremely strained. It was now decided to attack Fort San Lazar on the outskirts of the city, but the preparations ran into difficulties for the troops had been landed without tents or tools. Vernon as before urged an immediate assault but Wentworth hesitated for day after day until after delays which gave the defenders ample warning, the assault was fixed for the 20th April. It was, however, repulsed with severe loss. Added to this disaster yellow fever had now appeared in camp, and already by the 13th April great numbers of sick had been sent aboard the transports and after the failure of the attack there was nothing for it but to break off the operation. On the 28th April the soldiers were re-embarked. It was indeed high time. Between the 18th and the 21st April their numbers had dwindled from 6,600 to 3,200. After embarkation the transports lay idle for ten terrible days in harbour while over 3,000 sick and wounded suffered indescribable horrors in these so called 'hospital ships' which were merely transports converted for hospital use. Smollett the naval surgeon and author was present in a ship of the line and described the conditions in these words. 'They were squeezed into certain vessels which obtained the name of hospital ships, though me thinks they scarce deserved such a creditable title seeing that few of them could boast of their surgeon, nurse or cook, and the space between decks was so confined that the miserable patients had not room to sit upright in their beds. Their wounds being neglected contracted filth and putrefaction, and millions of maggots were hatched amidst the corruption of their sores, which had no other dressing than that of being washed by themselves in their own allowance of brandy. Nothing was heard but groans, lamentations and the language of despair invoking death to deliver them from their miseries. What served to encourage their despondency was the prospect of those poor wretches who had strength or opportunity to look around them, for there they beheld the naked bodies of their fellow soldiers and comrades floating up and down the harbour affording prey to the carrion crows and sharks who tore them in pieces without interruption and contributed by their stench to the mortality that prevailed.'[31] Officers and men died together. All discipline on transports came to an end.

This scene of chaos and neglect was largely due to the embittered relations between Vernon and Wentworth, for in these combined operations the army expected the navy to help with their surgeons and the use of naval ships as well as with medical and food supplies. But because they were not on speaking terms the Admiral would not proffer any assistance by his naval surgeons unless he was asked, and as Wentworth was too proud to do so the men perished from want of care and attention. Smollett says every ship could have lent one surgeon to assist and it is a distressing thought that these naval officers stood by while the dozen hospital staff officers and the ten or a dozen regimental surgeons grappled with over 3,000 cases until death effectively thinned the ranks of the sufferers. No medical planning which could have been foreseen would have been adequate to cope with these numbers as some sixty doctors would have been needed. Nor did the breakdown apply to medical officers alone, for the nursing care if it was to be effective needed trained attendants by the hundred. Of these there were none. The only female 'nurses' were the wives of the soldiers who went on the expedition—'nurse tenders' as they were called, and these no doubt played their part as they always did in every general hospital or hospital ship which accompanied our oversea expeditions. In every campaign the treatment in all general hospitals was bedevilled by the absence of skilled attendants or orderlies; the argument against them was that as general hospitals only existed in war and not in peace such attendants were only needed in war and could not be provided on a permanent basis.

As yellow fever was destined to haunt every expedition to the West Indies, we take the opportunity to record here the contemporary definition of the disease. 'A bilious fever attended with such a putrefaction of the juices that the colour of the skin, which is at first yellow, adopts a sooty hue in the progress of the disease, and the patient generally dies about the third day with violent atrabilious discharges upwards and downwards.'[32] A theory existed at this time that there was an intimate connection between scurvy and 'putrid fevers' (the name applied at the time to what was afterwards called yellow fever) and therefore the favoured treatment was by giving sweet water, fresh provisions, and a liberal use of vegetable acids such as limes, lemons, bananas, oranges and other fruits. Kempthorne says that the immunity to yellow fever observed amongst some of the Spaniards was ascribed to their fondness for sirops.

Let us describe in general terms the cause and the distribution of yellow fever. It is conveyed by the stegomyia mosquito which is found chiefly in the vicinity of towns, unlike the anopheles mosquito the carrier of malaria which breeds in swamps and marshes; the stegomyia breeds in such places as the old tins and flower pots and similar receptacles in house yards; in barrels used for water storage and in cisterns. The disease can only be transmitted in a temperature of 70°F. and above, and the mosquito is rarely found at an altitude of over 2,000 feet. The endemic area covers the West Indies, Central America and the west coast of Africa. The victim contracts fever some five days after being bitten by a mosquito which has become infected from a previous sufferer of the disease.

On the 5th May the fleet sailed away to Jamaica and the grim tragedy of Carthagena was over. But the agony of the troops was not yet finished. The same mosquito was just as prevalent in Jamaica, and within a month of arrival 1,100 more had perished, and for the next three weeks the death rate continued at 100 a week; the strength of the British troops fell to 1,400 and the American to 1,300 men.

It was next decided to make an attempt on Santiago de Cuba, but after the troops landed, the operations came to nothing because of the difficulties of the terrain and further recriminations between Vernon and Wentworth. The troops lay idle in their camps from the end of August until November, all the time sickening and dying, so that by October 1741 there were 566 sick in camp out of a strength of 2,669, and the strongest regiment numbered only 237, and the weakest 99. By December there were less than 300 of the rank and file fit for duty. Of the officers no fewer than 218 had died of disease.

Once more it was decided to abandon the operations and the troops were re-embarked and returned to Jamaica. But the final curtain on this tragedy had not yet fallen. Yellow fever continued to rage unchecked and 250 of the men left in hospital when Wentworth went to Cuba died in a single fortnight. The 8 regiments in the force were reduced to 4. Then in February 1742 three thousand reinforcements arrived including three new regiments of Foot, but once again they sickened and died at the rate of fifteen men a day. At length after further delay the troops embarked for the third time in March 1742 to attempt the capture of Porto Bello a port on the mainland of Central America. Owing to inclement weather the voyage lasted nineteen days, and at the end of these nineteen days the 6th Foot alone had thrown 98 corpses overboard and of the whole force nearly 1,000 were sick or dead. Again the enterprise was abandoned and again the survivors returned to Jamaica only to discover that 500 of their comrades left in hospital died in their absence. Many more were destined to follow them to the hospital and the grave, for by the end of July there were 800 sick; in August, 150 of these had perished, and by the middle of October 300 more had joined their comrades in death. The 6th Foot had only 18 men left and of the Americans few more than 300 remained. Between the 8th March and the 18th May 1742 thirty-three regimental officers died.[33] Of the force which had sailed from Spithead under Cathcart, confident in their ability to conquer the Spaniards, nine out of every ten had perished from disease and there was nothing to report but failure and death. Kempthorne quotes a return covering the period 26th October 1740 and 26th February 1742 showing the deaths amongst officers were 284 and among other ranks 10,000.[34] So ended this disastrous campaign, and the tragedy is that this tale of destruction will be retold many times in the years to come.

REFERENCES

[1] Q. Anne C.8.
[2] N.C.O's paid 1¾d., and privates 1d. a week.

3 Clode.

4 Mates to some colonial garrisons such as Minorca and Gibraltar received commissions.

5 D'Arcy Power. *Craft of Surgery.*

6 Marshall, *A Historical Sketch of Military Punishment.* Muniment Room R.A.M. College.

7 Gore. *Our Services under the Crown*, p. 100. Balliere Tindall & Cox, London (1879).

8 Johnston. *Roll of Commissioned Officers in the Medical Services of the British Army.* Introduction p. xxiv. Aberdeen University Press.

9 *Marlborough Despatches*, vol. 1, p. 321.

10 Gask. *Essays on the History of Military Medicine*, p. 110, quoted from Hare's Journal. Butterworth, London (1950).

11 Hare's Journal, p. 110.

12 Gask. *Essays on the History of Military Medicine*, p. 113. Butterworth, London (1950).

13 Marlborough to Harley, *P.R.O., S.P.* 87/2.

14 Quoted by Gore. *Our Services under the Crown*, p. 75. Ballière Tindall & Cox, London (1879).

15 Howell. Journal *R.A.M.C.*, vol. XI, p. 533.

16 Adams. *Memorable Battles*, p. 290. Griffith and Farran London, (1879).

17 The daily pay of these officers was:

Director and Purveyor 25s. including the pay of two clerks.

Physicians 15s.
Surgeon 10s.
Apothecary 5s.
Hospital mate 5s.

18 Col. Treas. Papers 18. November 1710.

19 Fortescue. *History of the British Army*, chapter XI, p. 560 quoting Deane. Macmillan, London (1910).

20 P.R.O., W.O. 4/4, p. 286. The Horse Guards was the Commander-in-Chief's headquarters in Whitehall.

21 P.R.O., S.P. Dom., (12th March 1711), vol. XIX, p. 21.

22 P.R.O. 30/89.

23 Fortescue. *History of the British Army*, book VI, chapter XI, p. 561. Macmillan, London (1910).

24 P.R.O. S.P. Dom., vol. XVI, p. 92.

25 Dodd. *History of Gibraltar.* John Murray, London (1781).

26 Lloyd and Coulter. *Medicine and the Navy*, vol. III, p. 298. Livingstone, Edinburgh (1961).

27 A story that a wicked Spaniard had lopped off Captain Jenkin's ear.

28 Fortescue. *History of the British Army*, book VII, chapter III, p. 61. Macmillan, London (1910).

29 Kempthorne. Journal. *R.A.M.C.*, vol. XLIV, p. 275.

30 Authentic papers relating to the Expedition against Carthagena, p. 39.

31 Smollett. *Miscellaneous Works*, Edinburgh (1806) chapter IV, pp. 445–469.

32 Kempthorne. 'The Expedition to Carthagena', Journal *R.A.M.C.*, vol. LXIV, p. 272.

33 *Gentleman's Magazine*, 1742.

34 Kempthorne. Journal, *R.A.M.C.*, vol. LXIV, p. 277.

Chapter 4

WAR OF AUSTRIAN SUCCESSION

It was the death of the Emperor Charles VI which led to all Europe being kindled into a blaze of war in 1742. He had died in 1740 leaving his daughter, Maria Theresa, Queen of Hungary, as sole heiress of his dominions. Her principal rival was the Elector of Bavaria, and France, only too willing to wreak her old hostility upon Austria, actively supported his claim, while England with Hanover and Holland, backed Maria Theresa. Frederick of Prussia, later to be named the Great, was greedy to make what profit he could out of the helpless House of Hapsburg, and suddenly and swiftly invaded Silesia and defeated the Austrians in 1741. This called the whole of Europe to arms.

The strength of the British army amounted to 62,000 men, and in June 1742 some 16,000 Horse and Foot embarked from Flanders under the Earl of Stair. Here they were joined by an equal number of Hanoverians as well as an Austrian army of some 14,000 men.

The control of the medical service was in the hands of Dr. Charles Peters the Physician General who had taken up the post in 1739, and Mr. John Pawlett the Surgeon General who had been appointed two years earlier in 1737. Under their direction the hospital staff officers who were ordered overseas were Mr. Ellis who was made Director of Hospitals, 1 physician, 1 surgeon, 1 apothecary, 4 hospital mates, 2 apothecaries mates and 1 matron; a small enough staff indeed for the sick and wounded of a campaign, and one which it was found necessary to increase, so that we find them augmented a few months later by 1 additional physician, surgeon, and apothecary, 4 more hospital mates and 2 apothecaries mates; in addition to these hospital officers a special appointment of surgeon to the Commander-in-Chief was made.[1] As the war went on further officers were called for, and before its termination in 1748 4 different Directors had successively served in Flanders, and the number of physicians had risen to 8, the surgeons to 9, and the apothecaries to 3.

Ellis took with him the equipment for a general hospital of 600 beds which was opened in Ghent with Dr. Sandilands as physician. This provided hospital beds for less than 4 per cent of the force, but the regimental hospitals carried equipment for forty patients and this represented an additional 5 per cent bed cover for each battalion.[2] The regimental surgeons were encouraged to look after their ordinary sick while in garrison or in winter quarters and it was only on the march or during active operations that cases were transferred to a general hospital.

At this stage a remarkable medical officer appeared on the scene who was destined to establish a reputation which placed him among the most famous clinicians and administrators in the service. Dr. John Pringle who had been joint professor of moral philosophy in Edinburgh received a commission in 1742 as private physician to the Commander-in-Chief the Earl of Stair. Although totally ignorant of military medical routine he displayed such conspicuous ability in mastering the details of medical organization that two years later he was given the high sounding title of Physician General to His Majesty's Forces Overseas, a post he was to occupy with distinction and credit.

After arriving in Flanders in June the troops lay idle for the remainder of 1742. Although initially their health was excellent, some of the quarters occupied were low lying and damp, and intermittent fever and bowel diseases made their appearance from August onwards, especially in Bruges. Before long an average of 70 men were sick in each infantry regiment and 40 in each cavalry regiment, figures which amounted to 11 per cent of the strength; but one unit in the worst quarters of Bruges had 18 per cent of its men in hospital. This autumnal intermittent fever was undoubtedly of malarial origin, but with the approach of winter, malaria died out and bronchitis, pneumonia and pluerisy made their appearance, together with 'rheumatism', and scabies. These were the diseases which could reasonably be expected in the winter months but the one which was dreaded was hospital malignant fever or typhus which happily made only a fleeting appearance. By the end of December, 442 sick had been admitted to the general hospital at Ghent and 82 had died.

In February 1743 the Allied army at length bestirred itself and marched forward into Germany, the British leaving behind some 600 sick unable to march in the general hospital at Ghent, while some smallpox cases which had occurred were isolated in an annexe at the hospital of St. Anthony. Pringle records the interesting fact that a epidemic of influenza at this time swept through the greater part of Europe and was seriously felt at Brussels, but the troops on the march were hardly affected; when they arrived at the German town of Hoechst on the banks of the river Main on the 17th May they had covered some 250 miles and had only lost some twenty men on the march. A halt was made here for some weeks, and a flying hospital was opened at the village of Nied nearby which admitted some 500 sick before the army moved to Aschaffenburg. We are already familiar with the role played

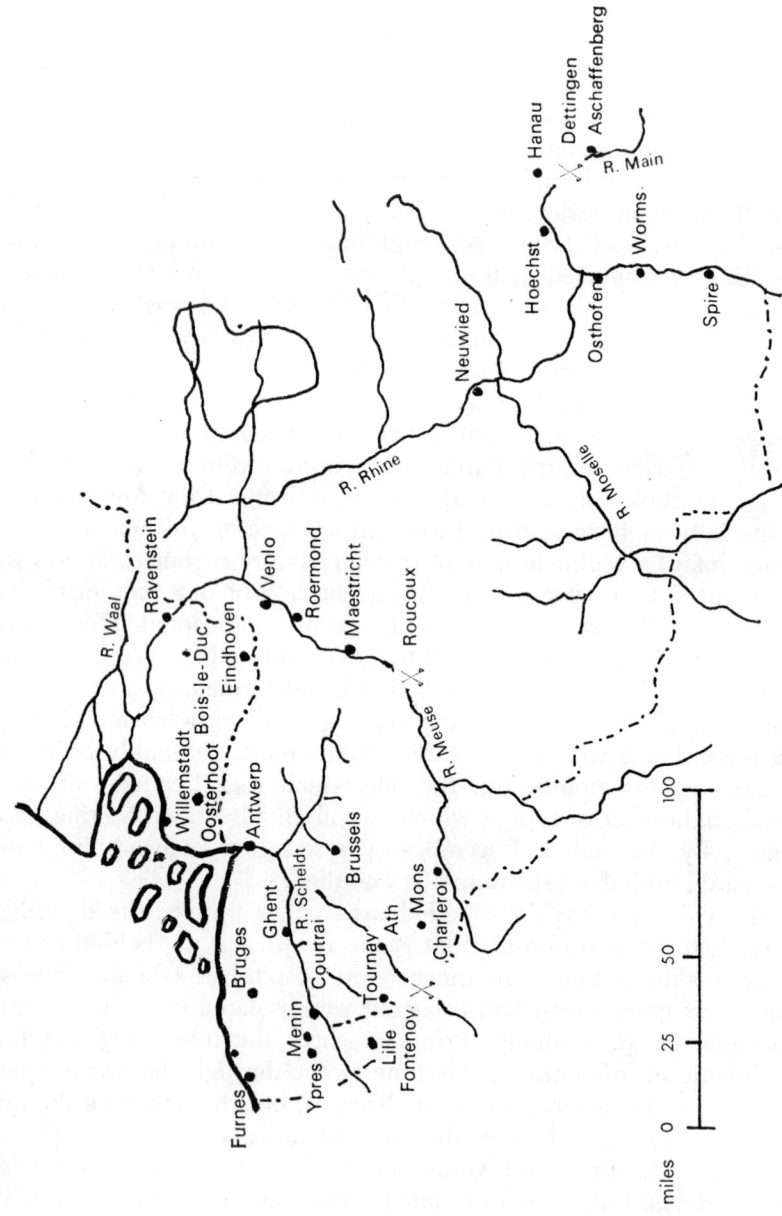

War of the Austrian Succession 1742–1748

R. Waal
Ravenstein
Bois-le-Duc
Eindhoven
Venlo
Roermond
Maestricht
Roucoux
Willemstadt
Oosterhoot
Antwerp
Brussels
Ghent
Bruges
R. Scheldt
Courtrai
Tournay
Ath
Mons
Charleroi
Menin
Ypres
Lille
Fontenoy
Furnes
R. Meuse
R. Rhine
Neuwied
R. Moselle
Hoechst
Hanau
Dettingen
Aschaffenberg
R. Main
Osthofen
Worms
Spire

miles   0   25   50   100

by the flying hospital in previous wars but we hope the reader will forgive us if we refer to it again. As its name implies it was a mobile hospital which was opened close to the regimental hospitals when they were overburdened with sick and likely to move; the medical officers came from the hospital staff establishment and the equipment from the hospital stores in Ghent. The policy was to keep cases in a flying hospital until a general hospital had moved forward to a sizeable town in the vicinity where extensive accommodation could be found in civilian hospitals, churches, or other institutions. Neither the general nor the flying hospital had any fixed establishment of beds or medical staff, and their size varied according to the requirements of the situation, but the former was generally equipped for 500–600 beds and the latter for 200–300. Moreover, the equipment did not include such bulky articles as bedsteads or hospital furniture, but rolls of bedding and ward utensils were carried. Bedsteads might be requisitioned when they were available, but for the most part patients lay on palliasses stuffed with straw, which, together with blankets, sheets and coverlets, were included in the bedding rolls. The subordinate staff for duty in the hospital and in the wards was detailed from units by order of the Commander-in-Chief. These were told to supply so many soldiers' wives as 'nurse tenders' and so many soldiers as orderlies. In addition the medical superintendent of the hospital made use of convalescent patients to fetch and carry in the wards.

On the 27th June the battle of Dettingen was fought. The French Commander-in-Chief was convinced he had trapped the Allied army, which King George II now commanded in person. After four hours of hard fighting victory was achieved by the steadiness and controlled volley firing of the British infantry and the gallantry of our cavalry, which, although outnumbered by the pick of the French cavalry, finally overcame them after a desperate struggle. But despite this the Allies were so short of supplies that they had to draw off their troops and abandon all their severely wounded on the field of battle to the French in order to reach their magazines at Hanau. This meant that a flying hospital which had been established at Aschaffenburg had also to be abandoned together with the cases under treatment.

The wounded were, however, well treated by the French, in no small measure due to an agreement made at the commencement of hostilities between the Earl of Stair and the Duc de Noailles that hospitals would be immune from attack. The cartel was signed at Frankfort on the 28th July 1743 and was entitled 'A treaty and agreement for the sick, wounded and prisoners of war of the auxiliary troops of his Most Christian Majesty and for those of the Allies'. The 37th Article laid down that 'physicians, apothecaries, directors, and other officers serving in the hospitals or armies shall not be liable to be made prisoners of war, but shall be sent back as soon as possible', while Article 41 went on to say,

'That care shall be taken of the wounded of both sides; that their medicines and food shall be paid for, and that all costs shall be returned on both sides. That it shall be allowed to send them surgeons and their servants with passports from the generals.' Finally Article 42 states, 'That the sick on both sides shall not be made prisoners; that they may remain with safety in their hospitals, where each of the belligerent and auxiliary parties shall be free to leave them a guard which shall be sent back, the same as the sick, under the passports of the generals, by the shortest way, and without being molested or stopped. So like-wise shall all commissaries, muster masters, chaplains, physicians, apothecaries, infirmarians, waiters, or other persons proper to attend the sick; who shall not be liable to be made prisoners, and shall be sent back in the same manner.' It was the Earl of Albemarle who as British representative signed this treaty which was a landmark in the treat-ment of both sick and wounded and prisoners of war, but which unfor-tunately was not always observed. On this occasion Lord Stair sent a trumpet to Marshall Noailles to acquaint him 'that his Britannic Majesty having thought proper to remove to Hanau, he had left an independent company in the field to take care of the wounded, who were strictly ordered to commit no hostilities, therefore the French might send a detachment to bury their slain; and it was hoped they would treat with humanity those who were left behind'.[3]

John Ranby attended George II on the field of battle as his personal surgeon, and from the fearless manner in which His Majesty exposed himself his services might easily have been required. But before the troops left the field his surgical instincts drove him to assist at the regimental hospitals where limbs were being amputated and wounds dressed. As the result of his experience here he proposed a scheme whereby surgeons could be of mutual assistance by several combining their regimental hospitals into one unit established some distance behind the line. 'Here,' he writes, 'let the wounded be put together under their immediate care and management. By this means they will . . . perform their duty with more exactness and dispatch.' But the difficulty of enforcing such a scheme arose from the fact that the colonels of regiments were completely autonomous in their control over their surgeons. A colonel who was difficult or uncooperative could insist on his surgeon devoting himself exclusively to the wounded of his own unit.

Surgeon Buchanan of the Horse Guards gives an account of his experiences during the fight.[4] 'It's impossible to describe the variety of wounds from cannon shot, small arms, swords and bayonets. My first intention in dressing wounds was to stop bleeding, which I did by stitching the vessels, dry dressings, bandage, etc. Having no assistant avoided amputations as much as possible, the necessity obliged me in some cases . . . The night passed amidst the groans of the dying and the complaints of those who survived them . . . Slight wounds were dressed with Balsam Traumatic. It's surprising how some people bear pain better than others . . . The like accident (compound fracture of lower leg) happened to General Campbell at Fontenoye, and during the operation (amputation) he asked an exact report of battle from his aide de camp . . . His Royal Highness the Duke of Cumberland was shot thro' the calfe of the leg with a small bullet. . . .

'Contusions from cannon balls seldom recover . . . soon spread upwards and downwards commonly attended with large emphysema over the whole body . . . Drought is the most universal complaint from all the wounded and surgeons would do better in filling their chests with proper liquors for this purpose, then stuffing them with apothecaries drugs. Shrub and water answer this intention.'[5]

'The day after the battle I was sent to the French camp in order to visit the wounded of our Army. Their surgeons went round the hospital carrying a tub of brandy and syringes with which they washed the wounds, dressing with dry lint dipt in brandy and covering with "digestive".[6] Our men say the French bleed often and cut much.'

He praises the Hanoverian medical arrangements—'their dressings are very neat drawn lint; wounds cleaned with fine spunge, soaked in warm water and brandy. Their hospital medicines are carried on a large wagon divided into many different partitions . . . any particular medicine may be easily got at, the whole easily packed and unpacked. One of their physicians visits the kitchen daily and examines the provision.'

On the night before the battle the troops were without tents and exposed to heavy rain, so that at Hanau there were soon 500 men on the sick list with diarrhoea and dysentery, and within a few weeks an epidemic broke out which affected nearly half the army. Pringle, expressing himself in the involved language which had to explain any cause of illness, ascribes this outbreak to the rain and exposure closing the sweat pores previously open and perspiring due to the heat, 'the humours became putrid and in that condition were turned upon the bowels'.[7]

The number affected made it essential to open a general hospital at Feckenheim, near Hanau to which 1,500 were admitted; and soon medical officers, nurses and hospital orderlies were victims of the epidemic as well as most of the local inhabitants. The whole outbreak was a classical example of bacillary dysentery due to flies carrying infection to food and drink. But the association of the prevalence of flies and dysentery is not altogether a modern conception, for Pringle tells us, 'There is also an old observation, that such seasons as produce most flies, caterpillars and other insects (whose increase depends so much upon heat, moisture and consequently upon corruption) have likewise been the most productive of dysenteries. Lastly, that the infection is evidently communicated by the faeces of those who are ill of the distemper.'[8]

But now worse was to follow, for the large number of patients caused the wards to be so overcrowded that typhus fever broke out, 'an inseparable attendant of foul air from crowds and animal corruption'.[9] The combination of dysentery and typhus proved deadly; of 14 hospital mates, 5 died, and all the rest contracted the disease, while the overall mortality rate was nearly 50 per cent. Those who were lucky enough to be treated in their own regimental hospital usually recovered quickly and the death rate was small, although they lacked many of the amenities of the general hospital. It was Pringle's first lesson on the danger of concentrating the sick and the advantage of dispersion, a policy he never ceased to advocate for the remainder of the war.

The Allied army made a leisurely return march commencing in August via Worms and Spire to the Netherlands to take up winter quarters. Dysentery had died out and it was now the time when the bilious, intermittent, and remittent fevers prevailed, so that 3,000 sick were left in the hospitals at Feckenheim and at Osthofen and Bechtheim near Worms. An order was then given to concentrate all sick at a hospital at Neuwied on the Rhine preparatory to their evacuation to Ghent, and in October the 800 patients remaining in Feckenheim were dispatched by river to their new destination; when it closed on the 23rd October a total of 3,386 sick and wounded had been admitted of whom 640 died, a mortality of 20 per cent. Amongst them were the usual proportion of camp followers in the form of 175 wives and 111 children, of whom 91 of the former and 53 of the latter died, in both instances a high rate in the neighbourhood of 50 per cent. The concentration of cases at Neuwied was particularly unfortunate for amongst the patients sent from Feckenheim there were typhus cases which infected the others, and on the slow and lengthy journey which was undertaken later by barge to Ghent the cramped accommodation was ideal for the spread of the disease and half the patients died on the way. Its contagious nature can be judged from the fact that out of 25 workmen at Ghent who were repairing tents which had accompanied the sick on their journey 17 died. Neuweid was closed down on the 26th November, and during less than four months it had admitted 1,467 sick, of whom 397 died, a mortality of 27 per cent.

Dysentery, fever, and typhus, the triumvirate which were the scourge of all armies in the field made an unhealthy end to the campaign, and at the close of the year one-fourth of the total strength were in hospital.

As 1743 had ended with the expulsion of the French forces from Germany it was clear that the war was now to be fought in the familiar country of the Austrian Netherlands. The year 1744 was spent by the Allies, whom the Dutch now joined, without a single major engagement, but the French enjoyed the greater success in capturing Courtrai, Menin, Yypres, and Furnes. The hospital at Ghent was open throughout the year and admitted 1,698 patients with 186 deaths, while on the 28th April a second general hospital was opened in Brussels and on 5th August another at Tournay where Dr. Wintringham and Dr. Maxwell were the physicians. By October the campaign ended and the troops went into winter quarters, the Horse at Brussels and the Foot and Dragoons at Ghent and Bruges. By December, Brussels had dealt with 1,259 cases of whom 82 had died, while Tournay when it closed on 8th November had admitted 778 with 147 deaths, a rate of 18 per cent. During the winter the medical policy was to encourage the regimental hospitals to treat their own cases as far as possible as they did in peacetime; this had the effect of decentralizing the sick and so avoiding the overcrowding which was always conducive to an outbreak of typhus.

Ellis the Director of Hospitals was succeeded during the year by Charles Garnier, brother of George Garnier the Apothecary General, but he died a few months later, and in January 1745 David Middleton a master surgeon took charge.

It was not until April 1745 that the army was stirred into activity for the new campaign. The French were engaged in the siege of Tournay when the Allies some 50,000 strong marched from Brussels under a new commander, the young Duke of Cumberland, son of George II. His army consisted of 25,000 British troops, together with Hanoverians, Austrians and Dutch.

The general orders issued each day for the advance from Brussels contain points of detail which are of medical interest from both the administrative and hygiene aspect. The projected camping area for the night was reconnoitred and marked out in advance by the quartermasters and the camp colourmen consisting of 1 sergeant and 1 man from each company; these appear to have been the billeting party and each man carried a spade or axe to construct the trench latrines in advance and act as sanitary men in the camp. The orders clearly show the strict discipline enforced, and the care of the sick on the march. A general order dated 29th April runs: 'The surgeons of ye several regiments are to carry their medicine chests and instruments upon their batt horses, which are to march at the head of each corps with their men's tents. His Royal Highness allows one waggon for ye sick of each regiment in camp; which waggon goes in the rear of ye regiment.'[10] And again on the 3rd May, 'The sick not fit to be carried forward to be sent to the hospital at Brussels by the waggons (which) return for bread. A sergeant of a brigade to be sent with them and proper certificates to be signed by an officer and surgeon to be sent with them.'[11] The evacuation of the sick and wounded by the returning daily bread waggons was the usual method of removing cases and had the advantage of being a regular service which required no special arrangement except to make the waggons report to the regiments the night before.

The Allied advance from Brussels was continued until the opposing forces met at the village of Fontenoy some 10 miles south of Tournay, where the French army held an entrenched line. Cumberland was young and impetuous. He decided on an immediate attack but despite all the courage and resolution shown by the British in particular the Allied attacks all failed and the French were left victorious at the end of the battle.

The Allied losses were terribly severe. The twenty British battalions lost 4,000 men, and the Hanoverians who fought just as nobly lost 2,000. Some regiments had 300 casualties, and the three battalions of Guards about 250 apiece. Some 600 wounded who could be carried from the field were treated in a general hospital which had been opened at Ath some 12 miles distant under Drs. Pringle and Wintringham. Here Dr. Buchanan tells us the hospital was 'the most commodious we have yet had; each room separated by a wall, and our sicke recovered well. It's a general fault in all hospitals that the apartments are too large, and containe too many sicke, by which the air is infected ... and (especially) when the house is crowded after an action. The men have much ado to keep their long hair free from vermine, and it's a custom with them to anoint their hair with ungt. mercurial instead of pomatum, and kill vermine of all sorts. Some use an ungt. of red precipitate, one pennyworth mixed with butter.'

The severely wounded who had been collected at the Chateau de Bruffoel had to be left to the mercy of the French and Marshal Saxe, the French Commander-in-Chief, sent to Allied headquarters a request for their removal; but when the Duke of Cumberland sent 105 waggons to bring them away both men and waggons were detained, and the wounded treated with such shameful severity that the Duke of Cumberland hurled a remonstrance at Saxe that 'if he intended to make war like a Turk he would learn for the future how to receive him'.[12]

There was indeed ample evidence of the harsh treatment of the wounded and the indignities medical officers were made to suffer in an article published in the *Scots Magazine*. 'We surgeons sent to take care of the wounded when carried from the field were made prisoners of war and treated in a very merciless way, for not only we, but about 1,000 more were stripped of everything valuable we had, viz. watches, swords, money and clothes, and not only so, but our very instruments were taken from us although the barbarians saw hundreds continually imploring our assistance. In this unprecedented way we remained three days, numbers dying every hour because we had nothing to dress them with, when they were flung in waggons and drove along the causeway to Lille and Valenciennes. In this jolting journey you may easily conceive the misery of the poor wretches, most with their legs, arms, etc. shattered to pieces. I assure you the impression is so strong on my mind that no time will efface the remembrance; I saw their wounds and heard their groans. At last we surgeons were allowed to pass to our regiments, and when we arrived at the camp we waited on His Royal Highness, laid before him the matter of our treatment, and presented him with a bag of chewed balls, points of swords, pieces of flint, glass, iron, etc. we had extracted from the wounds.'[13]

Furious with anger the Duke of Cumberland invoked the Cartel of Frankfort and threatened reprisals. Saxe made a conciliatory reply and assured the Duke that his surgeons were released as soon as their status was known and he undertook to return any property they might have lost in the confusion; but he added that the agreements of the Cartel of Frankfort had been previously broken by the English when they had detained Marshal Bellisle and his brother as prisoners of war and it could no longer be regarded as valid. This rejection the Duke of Cumberland chose to ignore and sent Lords Albemarle and Crawford to the French camp as commissioners under the terms of the Cartel, but the French Marshal remained obdurate.

It is pleasant to report a happier sequel. Conscious of their uncivilized behaviour even if it was done in the heat of action the French made reparation at their hospital at Lille. Voltaire says that here all wounded were treated alike and every luxury was placed at their disposal; indeed they were well nigh killed with kindness and the surgeons had to check the excessive good will of the populace. 'In a word the hospital was so well organized that wounded men preferred it to lodging in private houses'.[14]

The year turned out a bad one for the Allies. Tournay was captured by the French and this was followed in August by the loss of the important centres of Ghent and Ostend where large depots of stores were maintained. This meant that the hospital at Ath was in danger and it closed on the 25th August after treating 991 sick and wounded with a mortality rate of only 6 per cent, the lowest so far recorded. When Ghent was lost on the 10th August the main hospital fell into French hands, and Middleton, who was in the town, asked for the wounded, some of whom he considered unfit to travel, to be left on parole, but the French refused this reasonable request and despatched them by waggon the forty miles to Lille. He was however allowed to evacuate all the hospital staff officers and the equipment to Antwerp, where the hospital was re-opened with Drs. Sandilands and Lawson as the physicians. Losing Ghent hospital was a severe blow for it had done excellent work since it had opened in September 1741 and in the four years of its existence 3,274 patients had passed through its doors, with a death rate of just over 10 per cent.[15] The withdrawal to Antwerp also lengthened the line of evacuation from the forward area, and this, added to a scarcity of waggons for removing casualties, compelled many regiments to carry their cases with them. On the march, the surgeons with their medicine chests and instruments on pack horses followed the tent waggons which were at the head of the regiment, while the waggons for the sick and wounded in charge of the regimental mate brought up the rear. Ranby draws a harrowing picture of the sufferings the wounded endured, 'poor creatures . . . under the extreme misery of large lacerated wounds, bleeding arteries, or fractured limbs . . .' being moved from place to place with their units, a 'scene of terrible distress which I look upon as one of the most moving that can be presented to the human eye'.[16]

In contrast to 1745, the sick wastage in both these years was heavy; 1,500 dysentery and fever cases in 1746 filled the hospital beds, and on the conclusion of active operations in 1747 there were 4,000 men or 20 per cent of the force in hospital. There was a special reason for this last figure. Four British battalions had been stationed throughout the year in Walcheren and Zeeland, and they were decimated by malaria to such an extent that only about 100 men in each battalion were fit for duty. A naval squadron lying offshore had no cases, which, although the real reason was the absence of mosquitoes, was put down at the time to the fact that the moist and putrid air of the marshes was dissipated before it could reach them. Of the 4,000 men in hospital at the end of the year, these four battalions accounted for half. The significance of these facts must not be forgotten, for in due course history was to repeat itself, and disaster was to overwhelm those who ignored the warning.

The Allied line now ran nearly north and south through Antwerp, Brussels, and Mons, with British general hospitals at all these places; but the whole military situation was to be altered with the outbreak of the Jacobite rebellion in Scotland. Cumberland received orders to send back first a part and then the whole of his army, and in September and October 1745 the troops embarked for England, leaving about 1,000 sick behind in the hospitals at Brussels, Antwerp and Mons. The campaign had in fact been a healthy one; there had been a small outbreak of smallpox amongst recruits from England but no epidemics, and the total deaths from disease did not exceed 200. Dr. Pringle who was now Physician General went to England with Cumberland. Wintringham and Maxwell were at the hospital in Brussels, but after the troops sailed for England there was no occasion to keep it open and it closed down on the 24th November.

France quickly took advantage of the virtual evacuation of the Low Countries by the British, and both Brussels and Antwerp fell into enemy hands by June 1746 followed by Mons and Charleroi in July. Antwerp hospital closed on the 7th June after having treated 1,943 patients, of whom 209 had died, and with the loss of the Brussels hospital in the previous November and Mons in July there was no general hospital in either Flanders or Brabant.

As a result of the successful operation against the Jacobites British units began to filter back to the Continent in July, and General Ligonier disembarked with some infantry battalions at Willemstadt in Holland—the new base after the loss of Antwerp. Close by at Oosterhout was opened the new base general hospital. These regiments took part in the evenly contested battle of Roucoux in October, but by this date both Namur and Liege had been lost by the Austrians and the area of operations had shifted to the valley of the Meuse. Roucoux only caused 350 British casualties and the wounded were conveyed to a general hospital which was opened at Maestricht in July under the superintendence of Dr. Pringle who had returned from Scotland and resumed his previous post.

For the campaign of 1747 the Duke of Cumberland once more took the field at the head of 14 British battalions and 4 cavalry regiments and at the action of Lauffeld in July our troops bore the brunt of the fighting with a gallantry which extorted the admiration even of the French. The 800 casualties were carried down the Meuse in boats to Maestricht where the hospital opened in a church was so spacious and lofty that there was not a hint of overcrowding.

As the distance to Oosterhout was over 100 miles by river it was decided in June 1747 to open another hospital on the route and Venlo was chosen. At first only one apothecary and a surgeon were placed in charge but later Pringle and Wintringham both did duty here after Maestricht had closed down in November. It had been remarkably busy with over 3,000 sick and wounded admitted in five months, and with 326 deaths gave a mortality rate of some 10 per cent.

Britain after five years of war was thoroughly sick of it, and had gained no success except at the victory of Dettingen. The Dutch had proved useless allies, and the Austrians, having taken English money, had never provided the troops they had promised, and had invariably proved obstructive in active operations. When the campaign of 1748 opened, Cumberland found he had only 35,000 troops to face a French army 115,000 strong, and as war on these terms was hopeless, Britain pressed for peace. On the 30th April the Treaty of Aix la Chapelle was signed, a treaty which left matters very much as they had been before the war began.

It was November 1748 before the British army embarked at Willemstadt for England. The troops had spent the year in various camps in Holland, first at Roermond on the Meuse, where 500 sick were left in the general hospital at Cuick nearby. These were mostly malaria relapses of the regiments from Zeeland, but typhus fever occurred in some overcrowded regimental hospitals and the infection was carried to the general hospital at Ravenstein which was opened when the army moved to the Bois le Duc area; here it speedily died out as the hospital was spacious and well-ventilated, and the hospital staff officers were following Pringle's instructions in every detail. But in July and August fresh attacks of malaria developed amongst the troops in the Bois le Duc and Eindhoven areas with 2,000 in hospital. The Scots Fusiliers had 300 men struck down at one and the same time, and in the Scots Greys only 30 men escaped fever.

Under Pringle's efficient administration hospital standards had rapidly improved; strict attention was paid to ventilation, and an area of 36 square feet as a minimum for each patient was laid down. Moreover, the experience medical officers were gaining under Pringle's direction meant that dysentery and fever were being treated with greater effectiveness. Mr. Middleton, as Director of Hospitals, was the medical superintendent of a general hospital which was regarded as a model of efficiency. Each patient had the unheard of luxury of a separate bed with clean linen which was frequently changed and in each ward there were well trained female 'nurses'. These were of course our old friends the soldiers' wives, but now with several years of hospital experience behind them it is understandable that they were efficient, and infinitely preferable to the ignorant regimental orderlies provided by units. Moreover the hospital storekeepers who were often dilatory and obstructive were reported as supplying every requisition with promptness and regularity.[17]

These better methods of treatment and the more efficient administration of hospitals is plainly reflected both in the improvement in the mortality rates and the absence of typhus epidemics in the later years. In the Feckenheim Neuweid typhus episodes the mortality had been 27 per cent amongst the soldiers and as high as 50 per cent amongst the followers. From this high peak it had fallen to as low as 6 per cent in the succeeding years.

The end of the war saw the hospitals at Venlo, Cuick and Ravenstein all closing in July 1748 and evacuating their remaining sick numbering 462 to the base hospital at Oosterhout. They had admitted 1,042 cases and had 44 deaths. From Oosterhout in November the sick were embarked in hospital ships at Willemstadt, but contrary winds prevented them sailing for a month and typhus broke out on board. The infection was carried to the hospital at Ipswich where they were disembarked and 400 patients were soon under treatment; but the disease quickly abated as the wards were large and there was no overcrowding, and every man as soon as he recovered was moved from the infected wards to billets in the town. Within three months the last of the sick from overseas had been disposed of and the hospital closed in March 1749 after admitting 626 patients of whom 52 had died. As these were mainly typhus cases this mortality rate of just over 8 per cent was not excessive.

Sick and wounded admissions for the whole war totalled 32,246; of this number 2,563 died, a mortality rate of just under 8 per cent which cannot be regarded as unsatisfactory. Of the 8 physicians who served 3 died.

We conclude the account of the War of the Austrian Succession by a description of the incidence, prevention and treatment of disease based on Pringle's famous work, *Observations on the Diseases of the Army* published in 1753.[18] He was looked upon with reason as the father of military hygiene and the broad sanitary principles he laid down remain for all time.

The maladies which the troops suffered from in the winter and spring months were the so called 'inflammatory diseases', bronchitis, pleurisy, pneumonia, rheumatism and consumption. It was, however, in the summer and autumn months that the greatest incidence of sickness occurred, dysentery in the summer and fever in the autumn. Dysentery was classified as one of the 'contagious diseases' and with it were included hospital malignant (typhus) fever, smallpox and measles, the last named being by no means the mild affliction we are now accustomed to. Of fever there were three types, bilious, intermittent and remittent—the first so called by Hippocrates because of the bile which vomiting produced. Besides these so-called seasonal afflictions, both venereal and itch (scabies) were common throughout the year.

The all-embracing cause of the three great scourges was put down to 'putrid air'. Exhalations from marshes caused malarial fever, foul air from excrements and from rotting straw in tents caused dysentery; and in the case of typhus fever, although it occurred in a community habitually verminous, the true source of the infection remained unsuspected, and it was regarded as due to the foul air in hospitals overcrowded with patients suffering from putrid distempers.

The prevention of disease was therefore concerned with avoiding these pestilential vapours; areas chosen as camp sites should be on high ground away from marshes; indiscriminate fouling of the ground by troops must be penalized, and latrines covered daily with earth; a camp on fouled ground must be abandoned when an outbreak of dysentery occurs; the sick must be dispersed and free ventilation established to prevent typhus. All these were sound hygienic measures; but the enforcement of most of them depended on their execution by staff or regimental officers, and the former were too uninterested and the latter too undisciplined and ignorant to pay any attention to these doctor's fads. Under the heading of prevention too must be mentioned clothing and feeding—matters which affected the well being of the soldier. It is generally true that any improvements in the equipment and living conditions of the troops come from pressure by medical officers, for they see at first hand the effects of poor clothing and the lack of essential items reflected in the rates of sickness. In Germany, strong shoes were essential to stand up to the long distances covered by the infantry, but government policy of accepting the lowest tender meant that shoes of inferior quality were provided which quickly fell to pieces and caused great hardship. For better warmth and protection waistcoats, or undercoats as they were called, and watch cloaks for sentry duty were recommended, while a blanket per man was indispensable, even though this meant more baggage waggons to carry them.

Eating in messes meant that the soldier got better food, but even in war the custom prevailed of allowing a number of soldiers' wives and children to follow the campaign as authorized camp followers and individual messing here could not be avoided. Pringle was also a strong advocate of an issue of spirits in winter.

Every step in the prevention of typhus was so important that Pringle made new proposals to avoid concentrating large numbers in the general hospitals. His idea was to encourage regimental surgeons to treat as many as possible in the forward area, and to help them by posting a hospital mate and a nurse as an addition to the surgeons staff, and adding to their equipment. Further specialized assistance would be provided by appointing a physician to visit the regimental hospitals in a consulting capacity. Such a scheme would however be impossible during active operations owing to the need for extra waggons to carry the cases, but it might apply when troops were in winter quarters.

When by the end of each campaign there were accumulations of some thousands of sick in hospital—in 1743 there were 3,000, in 1747 about 4,000—there were so few physicians that each might have the impossible task of looking after 700 patients. But even if physicians had been appointed in adequate numbers, Pringle insists that the care and treatment of their patients would prove ineffective while the basic factors of overcrowding existed, and a mortality of 10 per cent could not be avoided. Only by dispersion of sick and ventilation in wards could better results be expected, and he remarks how difficult it was to make nurses and orderlies keep windows open. A Dr. Hales had invented a ventilator which, by a wooden tube inserted through a window to the ground outside, drew off the 'contaminated' air of the ward; but failing other measures, the 'putrid' air would be benefited by burning frankincense or juniper berries, or heating vinegar.

Now let us look at Pringle's methods of treatment. He started off by bleeding for almost every kind of disease, a remedy which was characteristic of this period of medicine. In the 'inflammatory' diseases involving the chest, such as pneumonia, pleurisy, bronchitis and even colds in the head, bleeding was described as the indispensable remedy to be performed by the regimental surgeon on the first sign of illness. Any delay might condemn the patient to drift into pneumonia or consumption, and lives might even be lost by deferring the operation or taking too little blood. Not less than 12 to 15 ounces was necessary for the first bleeding and smaller amounts for the subsequent ones. After bleeding, sweating was induced by the use of diaphoretics such as the nitrous derivatives and saline draughts, and if this did not result in cure blisters were applied. Opiates were on no account to be used. For rheumatism similar remedies are prescribed, with leeches applied to the swollen joints or rubbing in liniment; on occasion Peruvian bark might prove useful. In convalescence, wine, lemon juice, barley water or sage tea was prescribed.

For the autumnal group of fevers which lasted from July to October the sheet anchor was Peruvian bark which was given in wine to make it more palatable. But initially, bleeding, emetics such as antimony or ipecacuanha for removing bile, and purgatives were prescribed. During convalescence, fresh vegetables and spirits were recommended as tonics, but as the soldier's pay was not enough to provide wholesome food as well as spirits, Pringle recommended a free issue of spirits similar to the Navy.

Dysentery was diagnosed by frequent stools of blood-stained mucus accompanied by tenesmus. Treatment varied little from that of fever, and indeed both diseases were thought to have a common cause; the first remedy was bleeding, followed by emetics such as ipecacuanha in 5 grain doses twice or thrice daily, then frequent purging by rhubarb. Opiates were withheld until these measures had been taken because otherwise they tend to 'pen up the wind and fix the cause'. In the worst cases purgatives and astringents were combined. Rice gruel mutton broth or barley water were given but never milk unless diluted with lime water.

Malignant or typhus fever caused most of the severe cases, but attacks varied widely in their intensity, and this in Pringle's view depended on 'the virulence of the miasma or putrid ferment received into the blood depending on some internal or external source of corruption owing to exhalations from putrid animal or vegetable substances'.[19] Typhus was diagnosed from other fevers by the early tremors of the hands, delirium, petechial spots on the skin, stupor, confusion, and plucking at the bedclothes, the so called *subsultus tendinum*. In treatment, the first task was to remove the patient from the foul air of the ward; this was regarded as fundamental, but if it was impossible the freest ventilation was essential and until this was done the use of medicines gave no hope of a cure. The usual emetics and diaphoretics were prescribed with bleeding if the patient was plethoric, but if seriously ill and the pulse weak, bleeding and emetics were dangerous and opiates forbidden; reliance was then placed on diaphoretics and powerful remedies such as serpentaria or snake root, camphor, with Peruvian bark, cordials and wine as stimulants.

From Pringle's methods of treatment we turn to the account given by Surgeon Buchanan on the spread of attacks of typhus and dysentery which occurred so frequently. 'At first (after Dettingen) the distemper was moderate and occasioned by the bad air and season, afterwards communication with the sicke, and even the care taken of them spread the contagion, from whence it happened that some, neglected and abandoned, dyed thro' malignity of the disease; others received help that became fatale to all that approached them so that . . . the ears heard nothing night and day but the groans of the dying.'

The pharmacopoeia at his disposal in the regimental panniers appears to be extensive although many of the drugs mentioned are not easy to identify. For diarrhoea, ipecacuanha and opium was popular with 'Diascord in Burnt Gin every night at bedtime.'[20] For dysentery with blood in the stools Vitr. Cerat: Antimon[21] was used with marked success; for tenesmus, clysters of burnt claret with Theria: Androm.[22]

For the prevention of bowel diseases he advocated, 'warm clothing— flannel waistcoat next the skin, and socks on the feet'. 'Many men,' he says, 'attempted curing themselves by eating hard boiled eggs, old cheeses toasted, boyled milk thickened with eggs. For fever Peruvian bark was much used . . . rice gruel with cinnamon and mutton broth with rice or barley was the usual food.' For rheumatism he reports: 'Opiates were of the greatest service, especially when given in large doses with something warm; a good night's rest was always procured and sweats promoted, and seldom or never observed any bad effects from this free use of Opium, but am convinced it's the most universal medicine for soldiers.' It became a universal practice, and the pure opium is equal to any of its preparations. 'Should be kept moiste or beat up with Sap: otherwise it grows dry and hard, passing thro the body without any good effect.' This became a great favourite with the men, all asking for the little black pill, saying, *it does them a deale of good and was worth its weight in gold.*

From disease we pass to the treatment of wounds, and here Ranby gives his views. 'This work', he wrote, 'was penned in a camp' . . . and was intended 'to recommend plentiful bleeding very early in the treatment of G.S.W.'s; to advise likewise the application of light easy dressings to them, and particularly to introduce the signal use of the bark'.[23] Although bleeding was the vogue for everything, it does appear to be against all surgical principles to bleed wounded men who must already have suffered considerable blood loss. But Ranby adopted no half measures, and he describes a case of a severe wound of the leg. 'I had not omitted the necessary precaution of taking away from the arm in the field of action very little less than 20 ounces of blood'. The next morning the wounded man was carried 15 miles in a coach, and a few hours after the fatigue of the journey he bled him a second time. 'The nature of the wound considered and the quiet he enjoyed that night far exceeded my expectations. Notwithstanding which the next morning I bled him for the third time.' By this time his blood pressure must have fallen so low that a quiet night is hardly surprising. 'Repeated bleedings in the beginning', he tells us, 'draw after them many advantages. They prevent a good deal of pain and inflammation, lessen any feverish assaults, forward the digestion, and seldom fail to obviate imposthumations and a long train of complicated symptoms, that are wont otherwise to interrupt the cure, miserably harrass the poor patient, and too often endanger his life.'[24]

His penchant for bleeding is only matched by his enthusiasm for Peruvian bark, 'a medicine, which no human eloquence can deck with panegyric, proportionable to its virtues'[25]. Ranby was the originator in using bark for wounded men and in his own opinion did so with extraordinary success. In large lacerated wounds especially those made by a cannon ball where there was excruciating pain and the discharge of a 'gleety' matter which had reduced the patient to a skeleton he found that bark, given in drachm doses every three hours 'with surprising efficacy repairs the breach made in the constitution by this terrible havoc'.[26] Perhaps the explanation here is due to the tonic properties of quinine.

For the first dressing for wounds he used lint moistened with oil and a flannel bandage; this was followed at the next dressing by a bread and milk poultice mixed with oil to keep it moist, and if there was great tension a fomentation was used. Ranby was a firm believer in primary or immediate amputation. 'If a wound be of such a desperate nature . . . it would certainly be of consequence could the operation be performed on the spot, even in the field of battle.' This confirmed the practice of Wiseman in the Civil Wars who wrote: 'In the heat of fight whether it be at sea or land the chirurgeon ought to consider at the first dressing what possibility there is of preserving the wounded member; and accordingly if there is no hope of saving it to make his amputation at that instant while the patient is free from fever.' Le Dran, the most famous French military surgeon of the time also recommended primary amputation, while Bilquer, Surgeon General of the Prussian army in 1762 condemned it, and advocated secondary amputation when nature had failed to cure. This too was the opinion of one of the most famous of British surgeons—John Hunter, who was, as we shall shortly see, even now acquiring his experience at Bellisle and in Portugal.

For the actual statistics of the results of wounds only one piece of information has come to light. Dr. Macartney makes a statement that after the battle of Dettingen amongst 300 cases of amputation only 30 were completely cured.[27] Such a large number of failures would confirm the statement made by Garrison that after wars the streets of the cities were filled with mendicant cripples.[28]

Jacobite Rebellion 1745

Our history must shortly relate the campaign of 1745 undertaken against Prince Charles Edward Stuart, the Young Pretender. As early as 1743 a French fleet with Marshal Saxe and Prince Charles on board had sailed from Dunkirk but was dispersed by a storm off Dungeness. Although Prince Charles' adherents in Scotland had warned him that his success was hopeless unless he brought at least 6,000 men and 10,000 stand of arms, the Prince ignored their sound advice and determined to try his fortune. He landed on the west coast of Scotland near Moidart on the 25th July 1745, and on the 19th August raised his standard at Glenfinnan at the head of 1,600 Highlanders.

General Sir John Cope who was commanding in Scotland had some 3,000 raw recruits upon whom he could repose little trust, and after a useless march to Inverness brought his troops back to Dunbar by ship from Aberdeen. Meanwhile Prince Charles had entered Edinburgh and on the 21st October he defeated Cope at the battle of Prestonpans. His army had increased to a strength of 6,000 men and he followed up this success by capturing Carlisle in November and invading England as far south as Derby which was reached in December. Meanwhile English troops began to close in on the Jacobite army from every side. General Wade was moving down from the north, the Duke of Cumberland had 8,000 men at Lichfield, and a large force of militia stiffened by battalions of the Guards was concentrated for the defence of London.

The troops which had been pulled out of Flanders had been landed, some in the south of England and others at Newcastle, Holy Island, and Berwick. Because of long sailing delays due to contrary winds the inevitable scourge of typhus appeared on board, and this, added to many relapses of malaria, caused so much sickness that a general hospital had to be opened when the troops disembarked at Newcastle. The contagion of typhus spread to the medical officers, nurses and orderlies working in the wards, and 3 local practitioners who had volunteered their services and 4 of their medical apprentices died, while on Holy Island 40 soldiers died out of 97 patients, and 50 of the local inhabitants shared the same fate. Dr. Pringle had accompanied the Duke from Flanders and was made Physician General to the Force with headquarters at Lichfield. Here a workhouse was taken over as a general hospital, and here again typhus made its appearance, with the usual winter affections of pneumonia and bronchitis for which Pringle tells us bleeding became the most popular remedy, and the local doctors were instructed to carry this out repeatedly.

By now the hostility of the population and the lack of support which he received convinced Prince Charles that he could not continue his advance with success, and the retreat to Scotland was commenced with the intention to join a body of French troops which had landed at Montrose. Cumberland followed the Jacobite army to Carlisle but was then recalled to the south of England with most of his infantry to guard the southern coast in case of a French invasion. All the sick *en route* to Carlisle to the number of 600 to 700 were left to the care of local practitioners who looked after them it is said with every care and attention, although some forty of their patients died.

General Hawley who had succeeded Wade as Commander-in-Chief in Scotland suffered a reverse against the Jacobites at Falkirk Muir, when many of his men, from superstitious terror of the Highlanders, behaved disgracefully and ran away. Cumberland was recalled, and advancing via Edinburgh, Perth and Montrose reached Aberdeen in March 1746. He had left some 300 sick behind him on the line of march, all of whom were lodged in halls and private houses and attended by local practitioners, while in Aberdeen the hospital and other large houses were utilized. Under Pringle's supervision this good accommodation and free ventilation kept typhus in check, and when the army advanced towards Inverness some 400 sick chiefly suffering from winter chest affections were left behind.

On the 16th April 1746 the battle of Culloden was fought and the Jacobites crushed, suffering some 1,000 casualties and 500 prisoners. Cumberland's forces lost only 300 killed and wounded, and the wounded were conveyed to Inverness where two malt barns were converted into a general hospital. Here most of them were found to be suffering from cuts with the broad sword, an uncommon type of battle wound but one which was found to heal well, as the cuts were wide in proportion to the depth, and there was no hidden sepsis. As Pringle described it: 'there were no contusions or eschars as in gunshot wounds to obstruct a good digestion'.[29] For the Jacobite prisoners in the jails however, conditions were far less pleasant and their regimental surgeons complained that their instruments were taken away and they were unable to dress their cases; there were even assertions that many wounded were put to death on the field of battle.[30]

Pringle had the sick kept in separate houses, and the regimental surgeons were ordered to retain all but their worst cases in order to avoid overcrowding, and preserve his policy of dispersion against any outbreak of typhus. In a town which was now crammed with troops and prisoners and where smallpox and measles had recently attacked the civil inhabitants Pringle apprehended the worst, but by his orders the jails were cleaned every day, dead bodies were removed at once, prisoners were sent aboard a prison ship, and these measures fully succeeded. But typhus was in fact introduced by a regiment which brought with them thirty-six English deserters who had acquired it when in jail, and were being sent to Inverness for court martial. At least 6 officers and 120 men were struck down, and this otherwise small outbreak is mentioned for a special reason, for it gave Pringle the clue which confirmed his theory that jail and hospital malignant fever were synonymous.

When the troops marched off to Fort Augustus some 600 sick besides the wounded were left in hospital in Inverness, and at Fort William another 300 to 400 suffering from 'agues and the bloody flux' were evacuated back to the general hospital after ¡Pringle tells us they had undergone large and repeated bleedings.

The final figures for the campaign show that between February and August 1746 there were 2,000 admissions to hospital out of a force of 12,000 or 16·6 per cent and nearly 300 deaths, the majority of them due to typhus.

Cumberland's inhumanity in hunting down the fugitives, burning the villages and destroying their crops, earned for him the name of the 'butcher', and although this blot is indelible it must be remembered 'that at a time of extreme national peril the Duke lifted the army in a few weeks from the lowest depth which it has ever touched of demoralization and disgrace to its old height of confidence and respect'.[31]

REFERENCES

[1] The daily rates of pay were as follows:

Director of Hospitals and payment of one clerk	25s. 0d.
Physician	20s. 0d.
Surgeon	10s. 0d.
Apothecary	10s. 0d.
Hospital mate	5s. 0d.
Apothecaries' mate	5s. 0d.
Matron	2s. 6d.
The total daily pay of hospital staff officers amounted to	£8 17s. 6d.

[2] The strength of a battalion was 813.

[3] Howell. Journal, R.A.M.C., vol. XXII, p. 330.

[4] Extracts from Dr. Buchanan's Journal presented to Muniment Room, R.A.M.C. by Major A. J. Dickinson by permission of Baroness de Ros. This is an illuminating account of the daily duty of the regimental surgeon to the Royal Horse Guards.

[5] Shrub was made of the fruit of orange or lemon with sugar and rum.

[6] Digestive ointment (New Dispensatory 1770), yellow basilicon, black basilicon, balsam turpentine, used as a styptic.

[7] Pringle. Observations on the Diseases of the Army, p. 20. Wilson and Durham, London (1753).

[8] Pringle. Observations on the Diseases of the Army, p. 226. Wilson and Durham, London (1753).

[9] Pringle. Observations on the Diseases of the Army, p. 22. Wilson and Durham, London (1753).

[10] Howell. Journal. R.A.M.C., vol. XXII, p. 456.

[11] Howell. Journal. R.A.M.C., vol. XXII, p. 451.

[12] Kempthorne. Journal. R.A.M.C., July 1938, p. 60.

[13] Scots Magazine, July 1745.

[14] Voltaire. Siecle de Louis XIV, chapter XVI, p. 215.

[15] This number does not include the figures for 1744 which are not available.

[16] Ranby. *The method of treating gun shot wounds*, pp. 32–33. Knapton, London (1744).
[17] Gordon. *Army Surgeons and their works*, p. 26. Lewis, London (1870).
[18] It was translated into French, German and Italian.
[19] Pringle. *Observations on the Disease of the Army*, p. 280. Wilson and Durham, London (1753).
[20] Diascordium (London Pharmacopoeia 1618) contained herbs such as germander, gums, opium, seeds, pepper and honey with conserve of roses and wine. Used as a tonic and restorative.
[21] A powder made from glass of antimony and yellow wax.
[22] Theriacum Andromachus. London Pharmacopoeia (1618) lists 62 ingredients including opium, powdered seeds, barks, roots, gums, and viper's fat.
[23] Ranby. *The method of treating gun shot wounds*, pp. 2–4. Knapton, London (1744)
[24] Ranby. *The method of treating gun shot wounds*, p. 21. Knapton, London (1744).
[25] Ranby. *The method of treating gun shot wounds*, p. 36. Knapton, London (1744).
[26] Ranby. *The method of treating gun shot wounds*, p. 38. Knapton, London (1744).
[27] Macartney Lectures 1833.
[28] Garrison. *Notes on the History of Military Medicine*, p. 128. Washington (1922).
[29] Pringle. *Observations on the Diseases of the Army*, p. 45. Wilson and Durham, London (1753).
[30] Maclachlan. *William Augustus Duke of Cumberland*, p. 24. Henry S. King and Co., London (1876).
[31] Fortescue, *History of the British Army*, book VII, chapter VI, p. 148. Macmillan, London (1910).

Chapter 5

SEVEN YEARS WAR

In the latter part of the eighteenth century which covers the reign of George II and George III the campaigns of major importance were the conquest of North America between 1755 and 1760, the Seven Years War in 1756, the American War of Independence in 1775, and the commencement of the wars against Revolutionary France in 1793. These campaigns will be described in due course and we are concerned here with events in Britain and the affairs of the separate Irish establishment up to the date of the formation of the Army Medical Board in 1793.

A major change in adminstration was effected in 1756 with the creation of the post of Inspector of Regimental Infirmaries. The title makes the duties self-evident, namely to inspect the regimental hospitals; to ensure that the professional standards of the regimental surgeons were maintained; to see that the medicine money was correctly used for the purchase of drugs, and that an adequate diet was provided for the patients from the hospital stoppages. Unlike his contemporaries, the Physician General and Surgeon General, the Inspector was a regular officer with a full time task and with headquarters at the Horse Guards. Similar appointments were created on the staff of overseas expeditions both on the Continent and in America.

In control of the medical service during this period were:

Physician Generals

Sir Edward Wilmot	1746
Sir Clifton Wintringham	1786
Sir Lucas Pepys	1794

Surgeon Generals

David Middleton	1748
Robert Adair	1786
John Hunter	1790
John Gunning	1793
Thomas Keate	1798

Inspectors of Regimental Infirmaries
Robert Adair	1756
John Hunter	1790
Thomas Keate	1793
John Rush	1798

Apothecary General
George Garnier	1736

Of the Physician Generals, Wilmot held office for the long period of forty years and died at the age of 93. He was followed by Wintringham, already 76 years old when he succeeded. Like his predecessor, age seemed to be no bar to his appointment. Unlike Wilmot, however, Wintringham had a good deal of active service experience to his credit, having been first appointed physician to the forces in Germany in 1743 during the war of the Austrian Succession. After going on half pay he was restored to full pay in 1756 for home employment, and was then made Director General of Hospitals and Chief Physician to Albemarle's expedition to the West Indies in 1762. For some years before his death he was incapacitated from the more active duties of his office by age and illness and was nothing but a cipher when the Revolutionary War against France broke out in 1793. In spite of this there was no question of his resignation and he was made a member of the Medical Board created in that year, until early in 1794 at the age of 84 death removed him from the scene. He was replaced on the Board by Sir Lucas Pepys who was a distinguished physician, but had no army experience.

Turning to the Surgeon Generals, Middleton also continued in office for the long period of thirty-eight years, but again was too old latterly to perform active duty and the onus of work fell on the Inspector of Regimental Infirmaries. This was Robert Adair, who first joined the service as a staff surgeon in March 1742 during the war of the Austrian Succession; in 1748 he had gone on half pay but was recalled from civilian practice to full pay in 1756 and made Chief Surgeon to the Forces in Britain and Inspector of Regimental Infirmaries, a post which he held for the next thirty years. Adair soon became Surgeon General in all but name, and it was Adair who corresponded with the various commanders and principal medical officers, who detailed reinforcements and ordered periodical supplies of hospital equipment and medicines. It was Adair too who nominated all surgeons and mates, and direct commissions in regiments were granted to such doctors as had enough money, interest, or patronage to obtain them. His rate of pay at 30s. a day was a high one and contrasts with that of the Physician and Surgeon General which was still only 20s., but the full time nature of his appointment explains the difference. When Adair succeeded Middleton as Surgeon General in 1786 he appears to have combined this duty with that of Inspector, as also did John Hunter when he followed Adair in 1790. This combination of duties was possible while Britain was at peace. It is interesting to record that Adair married in 1759 Lady Caroline Keppel, daughter of the Earl of Albemarle, and was the hero of the well known song 'Robin Adair' which was composed by his wife.

In Britain the peacetime system of billeting the troops in ale houses and in private dwellings was most unsatisfactory; there was no check on the men's health or cleanliness except on parade, and there was no corporate messing. The soldier's pay was only 6d. a day of which half was spent on food and drink and they often augmented this by doing odd jobs about the town with a pot of beer as a reward. In billets they had to feed and cook for themselves, with the result that their diet was often so little varied that they lived solely on bread and cheese while the rest of their money went on drink. The only way to solve the billeting problem was to build barracks, and this had been first started as far back as 1739, but as late as 1762 there were only two permanent army barracks in the country, one at Chatham and one at Hilsea. Brocklesby condemned both of them on medical grounds, for having been built of salt bricks these attracted humidity, drainage was lacking, and the ventilation poor. He was convinced they 'bred disease and swept off men like a perpetual pestilence'.

Under the Duke of Cumberland, who showed himself a good administrator, the discipline of the army was improving and a new and better stamp of officer was emerging. The soldier's equipment and clothing was gradually being improved; a goat skin bag or knapsack was issued, and in 1751 the standards, colours, and clothing were for the first time regulated. Medical officers began to wear the clothing of the regiment to which they belonged. Recruits were ordered to undergo a phsyical examination and in the Impress Act of 1745 rupture first appears as a disqualifying disability.[1] Garrison however states there was no regular medical examination until 1790.[2]

On the medical side the regimental surgeons' pay remained precisely the same at 4s. a day, and the mates at 2s. 6d., rates which had been in existence since the foundation of the Standing Army nearly 100 years before; the only exceptions were the surgeons to the Household Troops who drew 6s. a day. But the stoppages from pay were many and varied, and included deductions for poundage, for the medical agent who granted pay, and for warrants.

The regimental surgeon was responsible for the hire of a building to accommodate the regimental hospital, and for the supply of medicines. To do this he received money from two distinct sources. To pay for the hire of a building an order was published in 1768 authorizing the sum of £30 a year to each regiment for the contingent expenses to hospitals; this was also to include the pay of a nurse. The Secretary of State for War when addressing C.O's of regiments in this connection said, 'That as the allowance was sufficiently ample to bear any expense that can properly occur for the relief of the sick, and being considered an essential service to the regiments, His Majesty had no doubt of the colonels careful application of it to that service agreeably to the most gracious attention'.

Secondly on the Government dictum that the army must pay for itself the money to provide medicines was raised by stoppages from the soldiers' pay, 1d. a month from each private and 1¾d. from each N.C.O. If the establishment of Foot is taken as being 800 N.C.O.'s and men, the sum amounted to about £44 in a year. The medicines were then purchased through the Apothecary General, the type of drugs and the quantities supplied being entirely dependent on the surgeon's discretion. Any money unexpended at the end of the year would go into the medical officer's pocket, so it was a temptation for the unscrupulous to deal in nothing but cheap medicines. This applied particularly to Peruvian bark, for the cheap variety which was much less efficacious could be purchased for only half the price of the best quality. Moreover a dishonest surgeon would often make soldiers pay for items of treatment which were not included in the pharmacopeia and so deprive the sick of their just benefits; such common remedies as bread and milk for poultices, flannel or oil for rheumatic complaints, oatmeal and stale beer as dressings for ulcers were often placed to the soldiers' account and he naturally objected to this further inroad into his meagre pay. It was not until a recognized list of drugs was published in a Formulary in the 1760's that a certain amount of control could be exercised to stop these dishonest practices, while the creation of the post of Inspector of Regimental Infirmaries helped this officer on his annual inspection to check such abuses.

Most of the houses hired as regimental hospitals provided very poor accommodation and some were merely wretched hovels. This was not the surgeons' fault because the sum of 12s. a week could provide nothing better, and although it was the surgeon's duty to reconnoitre the area a day or two in advance this was seldom done. Brocklesby's picture of the average hospital makes distressing reading. 'Most commonly the habitation hired for an infirmary has for some time been unoccupied, with the walls all damp, the boarded floors half rotten, and the roof in several places open above . . . I have indeed seen such a cottage stuffed with 40, 50, or 60, nay with 70 or 80 poor soldiers all lying heel to head, so closely confined together with their own stinking cloathes, foul linen, etc., that it was enough to suffocate the patients as well as others who were obliged to approach them.' Brocklesby also quotes Pringle's remarks 'that air corrupted by putrefaction is of all other causes of sickness the most fatal and least understood . . . and ripens all distempers into a putrid or malignant nature'; and again 'that among the chief causes of sickness and death in an army the reader will little expect that I should rank what is intended for its health and preservation the hospitals themselves'.[3] Often there was lack of warmth or fire. The sick attendants were soldiers changed every twenty-four hours, and a 'nurse' to do the cooking and washing was chosen from one of the soldiers' wives and paid 6d. a day. The hospital was self supporting in the way of extras for the sick, which were bought by the hospital sergeant in the local market out of the stoppages of 2s. 6d. a week which were levied from each patient. This had to provide the milk, eggs, vegetables, chickens and fish which their illnesses required, while the basic ration of bread and meat was drawn by the Company to which the sick soldier belonged and sent to the ward. Regulations now began to appear for administering the hospital and these are the rules first laid down by Mr. Gordon, a regimental surgeon, at Winchester in 1762.

(a) A hospital sergeant will be appointed to preserve order and regularity.

(b) The pay sergeant to pay the hospital sergeant every day the subsistence money for the sick, and settled by the latter weekly with the regimental surgeon, and by the surgeon with the paymaster.

(c) Two regimental orderlies to be provided to attend the sick.

(d) No man to be excused parade etc. unless reported to the surgeon, and every man found sick in quarters subsequently to be punished.

(e) Every man to bring his knapsack to hospital containing his necessaries.

(f) A sentry to be posted at the hospital to prevent unauthorized visitors bringing in strong liquor.

Further detailed regulations for the conduct of a regimental infirmary about this time are given in an appendix.[4]

Brocklesby and Monro were the two outstanding military physicians and ardent reformers, and published works on both medicine and hygiene in 1764. Brocklesby's suggested reforms ranged over every aspect of the service. He wanted to improve the quality of the regimental surgeons by the offer of pay up to £250 a year. This would provide young gentlemen duly qualified, of a good education and liberal turn of mind who would carry enough weight to alter the prevailing custom which took little account of professional ability but depended upon some influential regimental colonel choosing some 'raw youth just emancipated from half his apprenticeship'.[5]

Brocklesby affirmed that the great preponderence of medical cases both in peace and war required doctors who were skilled in physic rather than surgery, consequently the rule that surgeons should be examined at the College of Surgeons with the Surgeon General present was wrong and should be replaced by an examination carried out by a censor of the College of Physicians, attended by a physician acquainted with army practice. Brocklesby forgot that operating ability in a regimental surgeon was essential for war, and the army would forgive the surgeon who failed to cure a medical case but not one who was incompetent to amputate a limb in battle.

His views on man management were probably the first ever to be expressed. 'The well being of the men and the preservation of their health ought to be a constant serious business and in increasing care of their officers as well as the physicians.[6] This presented an entirely new conception of the regimental officers' duties but one which was not to be accepted in the army until many years had elapsed.

We have already seen that in every general hospital it was a combatant officer and not a medical officer who controlled discipline and order in the wards, as medical officers had no executive power and were unable to arrest or punish any wrong doer. Brocklesby appreciated the consequent lack of medical control which led to confusion and hampered treatment and wished to remedy it by investing the medical officer in charge with executive power, 'as he alone must be the most competent judge of all physical (medical) matters under him on the spot, or why he should not be invested with a power from the Commander-in-Chief or other sufficient authority to establish a well preconcerted plan for the hospital he has the care of'.[7] The hospitals, he says, at the commencement of a war were formed too much upon temporary shifts and never on preconcerted measures so as to give the suffering soldier contentment or satisfaction. 'It is well known that numbers of brave men are annually lost in hospitals for want of order and proper subordination among the physical (medical) officers, and that the most able and active men, unless they have a military character, cannot prevent a total relaxation of that regularity which should be observed as well here as in the field among the soldiers and gentlemen of the profession.'[8]

All this was sound common sense, but the Horse Guards would never accept the idea that a doctor could be trained as an administrator; he was only capable in their view of the professional care of his patients. The medical officers themselves were partly to blame, for the intense jealousy between the physicians and surgeons always led to friction and argument when one attempted to exercise control over the other. This was in large measure due to the fact that the physicians who were regarded as senior were generally recently commissioned civilians without army experience, whereas the staff surgeons and apothecaries were regular officers with long service and experience behind them.

Brocklesby's treatment of disease was in conformity with that of Pringle and Monro. In his opinion typhus fever caused eight times as many deaths as those killed in action; nothing he said, was more conducive to recovery 'than a continued attention to nurses, cleanliness, frequent shifting of foul linen, bedding, and invariably a free and almost uninterrupted current of fresh air by treating the patients in tents'.[9]

Passing to other changes in medical adminstration certain items of interest must be mentioned which took place before the formation of the Army Medical Board in 1793. On the outbreak of the Seven Years War in 1756 a medical board was set up to control the proper conduct of the medical arrangements while engaged in hostilities. This will be referred to in due course. Another important event was the establishment of the first general hospitals in Britain which were opened from 1781 onwards at the ports where troops embarked and where invalids from overseas were landed.

In 1761 the first authorized list of drugs which would be supplied by government was published in the form of a Dispensatory or Formulary which was supplied to all medical officers to guide them when submitting their lists. Any items outside this list would have to be paid for by the medical officers of regiments out of their yearly medicine money.

It was in 1783 that the time-honoured custom of buying and selling regimental medical commissions was abolished, but before this occurred there was some confusion in the orders published for their guidance. At first surgeons were forbidden to sell their commissions on retirement even though they had been purchased; then it was decided that this was a harsh rule and to get over the loss in income which the surgeon would suffer an ensign's commission in the regiment could be sold and the money handed to the surgeon; when the surgeon actually held a double commission this combatant commission could be sold;[10] finally in 1784 it was decided that those officers who had bought their commissions would be allowed to sell.[11] The banning of the purchase of commissions stopped the direct entry of doctors as regimental surgeons, and they were now forced to begin their army career as regimental mates and undergo a period of probation before a King's commission was granted. In point of fact this regulation was never strictly enforced, and the practice of purchase continued unofficially for many years, as may be witnessed ten years later when in 1793 the name of Dr. James McGrigor appears as purchasing a commission as surgeon in the 88th Foot—The Connaught Rangers; these candidates then received a direct King's commission with the tacit approval of the Surgeon General.

A further noteworthy advance came in 1783 when new regulations were brought into force which abolished for ever the iniquitous order which deprived the soldier of pay to provide the medicine money for the unit. A sum of £70 a year was now paid by government to surgeons whose regimental companies were fifty men or under, with proportionally larger sums in regiments of greater strength. This policy was in fact a mixed blessing to some of the more unscrupulous surgeons. It simplified the regimental administration, but it also did away with the temptation of pocketing some of the medicine money by purchasing cheap drugs, or by unjustly making further inroads on the soldiers' pocket by making them pay for the forms of treatment not in the accepted Formulary which they said the medicine money did not provide for. However open to condemnation such practices were it must be remembered that peculation was rampant in all classes of the army. So the surgeons with their miserly pay of 4s. a day lost a source of income however illicit, and thirteen years were to elapse before in the Royal Warrant of 1796 medical officers' pay was improved. It is easy to condemn medical officers for their lack of morality but there were many unfair financial hardships which they had to endure mainly owing to lack of definite orders. In 1782 a surgeon asked to be reimbursed £22 which he had had to pay for treatment of twelve sick men left behind at Plymouth when the regiment sailed; Adair replied that regimental surgeons frequently incurred expenses of this kind and there were no funds to meet it but their medicine allowance. Although he acknowledged the case was a hard one it was a kind which every surgeon was liable to meet and there was no precedent for any relief. Such an example of Treasury parsimony may well explain the reason why surgeons were driven to underhand transactions to put a few pounds in their pockets, and this dishonesty was not confined to the medical service. The colonels of regiments were responsible for clothing their units, but how often this was neglected is evident from a letter written from Dominica by General Hamilton to the Secretary at War in July 1795. 'The mortality of the soldiers on these islands in many instances may be attributed to the neglect of the medical tribe in the hospitals and the criminal inattention of officers of different ranks, who have left soldiers without second shirt, or shoes, and uniform in tatters, nine months pay due, clothing five years in arrears. The evil originates in the condemnable avarice and neglect of colonels, agents and master tailors.'[12]

One of the most notable advances of this period was the great increase in literary activity by many medical officers in describing the symptoms and treatment of the diseases which were encountered especially in the tropics. Brocklesby, Monro, Cleghorn, Hunter, Jackson, and others produced contributions of great value which covered not only diseases but the organization of the medical services.

We must now refer to the affairs of the Irish Establishment. The year 1784 was noteworthy, for this marked the establishment by Royal Charter of the College of Surgeons in Ireland, one of its chief duties being the provision of a sufficient number of properly educated surgeons for the army. Four years later in 1788 the Kings Royal Military Infirmary was completed in Dublin at a cost of £9,000, the first military hospital for the care of soldiers built in that country, and much superior to the few small general hospitals so far constructed in England. The Physician General and the Surgeon General were appointed Commissioners, and to ensure that full use was made of it, positive orders were given that all sick suffering with acute diseases were to be sent for admission within twenty-four hours of being taken ill.

Medical officers' pay was even less than in England, regimental surgeons drawing only 3s. and mates 2s. a day; but the regimental hospital expenses and the medicine money allowances were then on a more generous scale. Formerly the contingent allowances for hospital hiring expenses was £30 a year as in England, raised by stoppages of one day's pay from each officer, N.C.O. and man. For the hire of hospital buildings it is true only £20 was now allowed, but in addition to this sum £30 was provided for nurse hire and bedding. Medicine money came to the comparatively large sum of £125 a year based on 12 guineas for each company of sixty men and upwards; if the regiment consisted of less than 500 men it was reduced to £75 a year; all medicines were bought from local chemists by the surgeon.

In 1784 most barracks and hospitals attached to them had been allowed to fall into decay by the Irish Parliament who were not enamoured of a military force. Since the days of William III this was still rated at 12,000 men.

To control the medical arrangements a Medical Board on the English model was set up on the 1st June 1795 consisting of the two joint Physicians General, the Surgeon General, and the surgeon of the Kings Infirmary, Mr. George Renny, now made Director of Hospitals, and previously a regimental surgeon of the regular forces. The Medical Board decided that the unsettled state of the country during these years of the Revolutionary wars against France made it necessary to establish general hospitals for the first time and enlist a staff of medical officers. These hospitals, each of 100 beds, and housed in wooden huts, were erected in the four major encampments which had been established throughout the country; allotted to each was a staff comprising physician, surgeon, apothecary, purveyor, hospital mate, and nurses. In addition one physician was permanently stationed at Cork during the war where a general hospital was opened in 1790. To recruit these medical staff officers it was found necessary to offer rates of pay which would recompense them for the loss of their professional prospects, and physicians received 20s., and surgeons 10s. 3d. a day, both being entitled to half pay; apothecaries and purveyors were paid 10s. a day, and mates 7s. 6d., but the last not entitled to half pay. Both the physician and surgeon were to visit the regimental hospitals within the encampments daily to supervise treatment and assist in diagnosis.

while as Director of Hospitals Mr. Renny had the authority to visit all camps and hospitals in the country. Allowances for medicines were also authorized by government varying from 20 to 40 guineas a year according to the strength of the troops in camp.

The Board drew up rules and regulations for regimental surgeons and mates and introduced a system of accurate medical reports which included a list of the prevailing diseases, a system which proved so informative that the Duke of York ordered their adoption in England and a copy was sent to the King for his information. In all its actions the Board showed a progressive outlook which showed it was in advance of what was happening in England.

The banning of double commissions in Ireland was not enforced until June 1797 but in fact, as in England, it was only loosely applied. The point of substance about these double commissions was that a junior medical officer who held one might in certain circumstances in virtue of his combatant rank exercise command over his more senior medical officer who did not buy one, and in active operations the regimental hospital might be left to shift for itself with the medical officer engaged with the enemy.

It is reported that during one of the engagements in the East Indies one such officer who was both surgeon and captain in his regiment had led his unit out of action, and as the only senior surviving officer, commanded it on its return to England.

North America 1755–1760

Hostilities and rivalry between the British and French in Canada and America had been going on ever since the early seventeenth century, but by the Treaty of Breda in 1667 French dominion over Canada was established. Meanwhile the first English emigrant had founded New England in 1621, which was destined to swallow up New France. In 1664 the Dutch settlements at New Amsterdam were captured and renamed New York, and after the Treaty of Breda the position was that the French held the key to Canada at Quebec, and the British the key to New England at New York.

The French aim was to cut off the British North American colonies from any expansion west of the line of the Ohio river, and they built a chain of forts from the Canadian border at Crown Point through Niagara and Lake Erie along the Alleghany and Ohio rivers. In 1755 a dispute arose as to whether French troops were not occupying British territory, and the result was an expedition under General Braddock in an attempt to capture Fort Duquesne at the junction of these two rivers. Braddock's force of two regular British regiments, American Provincials and Indians, was totally defeated at the action of the Monanghela river chiefly because their commander insisted on adopting the tactics of European warfare. Of 1,373 men engaged only 459 came off unharmed, largely thanks to an American officer by the name of George Washington after Braddock himself had been slain. Then there was an attack on Nova Scotia which succeeded, but others on Crown Point and Niagara failed.

In the following year, 1756, Lord Loudon was sent out to command, with two British regiments, but the only result was the capture of Fort Oswego, an important trading post on Lake Ontario. With Loudon came as physician Dr. Richard Huck, a great friend, who had been surgeon to Loudon's Scottish Regiment in the 1745 rebellion, and was renowned as a gay and learned wit. Mr. James Napier was Director of Hospitals and Chief Surgeon, and the hospital staff officers under him apart from Huck numbered 4 surgeons, 3 apothecaries, 12 surgeons mates and 10 hospital mates. These were distributed between the general hospitals at New York, Albany and the distant port of Halifax, and there was also a flying hospital in touch with the troops in front of Albany. These hospitals were well equipped with what are called 'lock' beds, with bolsters, blankets, and sheets, and the usual hospital utensils. The wives of soldiers in the proportion of 1 to every 25 patients were employed in the wards as nurses to prepare food, wash linen, and keep the patients clean and comfortable.

Napier appointed a hospital board composed of the senior staff medical officers which laid down hospital regulations, and had the power of dismissing unsatisfactory mates and subordinate staff, and reporting to the Commander-in-Chief the name of any commissioned medical officer who proved negligent.

Loudon's forces were so scattered that Napier wanted to disperse his staff surgeons from the general hospitals to help the regimental hospitals in the field, but fortunately this suggestion was not adopted, as events proved that the maintenance of general hospitals to deal with the sick and wounded at fixed centres was a more realistic policy.

Although exact figures are not available it appears that a sickness rate of 7 or 8 per cent was common, with an average of some 40 to 45 men in each of the regimental hospitals, and 15 to 20 of each unit more seriously ill in the general hospitals, while the annual losses by death, desertion and discharge were 15 per cent for troops in New York and twice that amount for troops in Nova Scotia.

The diseases which brought men into hospital included fluxes or enteritis, a considerable incidence of venereal complaints,[13] fever, scurvy and smallpox. Scurvy was prevented as far as possible by the issue of spruce beer, and at some stations one half of the meat ration was exchanged for fresh vegetables; but many of the worst sufferers were sent to New Jersey where the vegetable supplies were more plentiful.

After the outbreak of the Seven Years War in 1756 when Pitt became

Prime Minister a more comprehensive and concerted plan was made for the operations in North America; Loudon was recalled and General James Abercromby appointed to New York in his place. A force of 11,000 men under Lord Amherst was now assembled at Portsmouth and a fleet comprising in all 157 sail left our shores to attack the French citadel of Louisburg on Cape Breton Island. In the face of enemy fire a landing was made from open boats under an officer of the name of James Wolfe, and after a siege of some six weeks, the fortress surrendered in July 1758. Our losses had not exceeded 500 killed and wounded while capturing nearly 6,000 of the enemy. Amherst with five battalions then sailed for New York. Meanwhile Abercromby was given the task of pushing northwards from New York by way of the Hudson river and Lake Champlain with a force of some 7,000 regular and 9,000 Provincial troops with the object of capturing Fort Ticonderoga. Abercromby chose to make a direct frontal attack upon the French position and was repulsed with heavy loss. Of the seven British battalions engaged no fewer than 1,600 had fallen and of the Provincial troops 334; the 42nd Foot (Black Watch) alone lost close on 500 officers and men.

After Abercromby's failure General Amherst took over command of the renewed operations in 1759 with 11,500 men, including 6 British battalions and 5,000 Provincials. A vast flotilla of river craft set forth on Lake George in four columns—the hospitals at the rear of the administrative and baggage column. This time the French abandoned Ticonderoga without a fight and fell back to the northern outlet of Lake Champlain, where, as they had four armed vessels on the lake, Amherst was brought to a standstill and the operations ended for the year. Nevertheless, the news of Amherst's advance to Crown Point caused great alarm in Quebec and steps were taken to reinforce Montreal.

Napier as Director had 32 hospital staff officers under him including 22 hospital mates, and in addition he had 12 apothecaries' mates to act as dispensers. Albany was the chief hospital centre for the forward area although it lay 100 miles behind Amherst's headquarters at Crown Point, and the evacuation of sick and wounded from the regimental hospitals to Albany, and from Albany to New York, was carried out entirely by boats on the lakes and rivers. The general hospital at New York had only 150 beds, but when Napier came down from Albany to visit it in November 1759 there were 531 in hospital including 292 wounded, and part of the troops barracks had to be taken over as additional accommodation.

It is pleasing to record that the relations between Amherst and Napier were of the friendliest, and like all capable administrators Amherst kept his Director well informed of all his projected operations. It has not always been so; too often principal medical officers have been left in the dark in such matters by their Commanders, not so often by intention as through sheer thoughtlessness. Napier we find writing many letters to Amherst, sometimes wishing him health, safety and success in his operations, and he does not hestitate to show his loyalty to the Crown when he writes as a postscript 'Long live great George our King.'[14]

We must now follow General Wolfe's fortunes in the expedition planned to capture Quebec. Wolfe had been selected for the enterprise by Pitt and perhaps a short description of a man famous for his skill and daring is not inappropriate—'A shock of red hair tied in a queue, and a tall lank ungainly figure added neither grace nor beauty to his appearance; but within that unhandsome frame lay a passionate attachment to the British soldier and an indominable spirit against difficulty and danger.'[15]

With 10 battalions divided into 3 brigades, making a total strength of 8,500 men, Wolfe in June 1759 sailed for the St. Lawrence river, and after much skilful seamanship on the part of the Royal Navy necessitated by the shoals in the river, anchored a few miles below Quebec on the 26th of June. The first attack made on the eastern side of the city was defeated by the overwhelming French fire and caused a loss of 500 men.

Hospitals had been established on the Isle of Orleans which lay in midstream, and at Point Levis on the southern shore. It was to these hospitals the casualties were brought, but the wounded who fell close to the French defences had to be left on the field only to be mercilessly scalped and murdered by the Redskins.

Wolfe was in a dilemma on the next steps to be taken but then several vessels of the fleet sailed by night to an anchorage above Quebec, successfully running the gauntlet of the enemy batteries and covered by the fire of British guns erected on the southern shore. This success directed Wolfe's attention to an attack on the city from above. More and more ships braved the passage of the batteries; troops were landed from them and laid waste the country inland thus effectively cutting off the food supply of the French garrison of some 13,000 men. By August, Wolfe's force had lost 800 killed and wounded, but was weakened more seriously by fever and scurvy. Troops on the eastern side were now withdrawn and marched along the southern bank of the river to the position where the ships of the fleet were assembled. Then for several days Wolfe kept the French in uncertainty by pretending to threaten various possible landing places, but at last on the pitch dark night of the 13th September nearly 2,000 men in open boats approached by stealth a cove now known as Wolfe's Cove and started scaling the 200 foot cliff by a narrow path. By sunrise some 4,500 had scaled the cliff and were drawn up on the plains of Abraham. Montcalm, the French Commander, at once accepted battle with his 5,000 troops at hand, and marched his men upon the British line which shattered them with one decisive volley. Wolfe at once gave the order to advance and the British line strode forward with bayonet and claymore to complete the French rout. Both commanders were slain—Wolfe with a bullet through his lungs, and Montcalm mortally wounded by a shot through the body. The French hospital, full of sick and wounded, which was situated over a half a mile from the town was captured, and the whole French army streamed away in disorderly flight up the St. Lawrence river. Our losses were trifling amounting to 58 officers and men killed and 572 wounded. For the wounded who were brought into Quebec an Augustinian convent provided splendid accommodation. Here each officer had a room to himself and the men had clean comfortable beds in well aired wards.

During the succeeding winter our troops in Quebec suffered severely from bad quarters, bad food and insufficient clothing and fuel. Frostbite attacked both sentries and men gathering fuel, and before Christmas 150 men were affected. Then scurvy added to their miseries. There were of course nothing but salted provisions available and soon hardly a man was wholly free from the disease; by the middle of April there were only 3,000 fit for duty and 700 bodies were awaiting burial when the thaw would come.

Moreover the French were not yet beaten, and in an attempt to recapture Quebec the bloody battle of Sainte Foy was fought on the 28th April 1760, when the 3,000 British troops attacked a superior French force and were defeated with over 1,000 casualties. Unable to carry off the severely wounded these had to be left on the field and were cruelly neglected by the French; less than thirty were removed to hospital and the remainder were abandoned to the savagery of their Redskin allies, who proceeded to scalp and massacre them.

Brigadier Murray, the Commander, was now hard put to it to defend the city with his remaining 'half starved skeletons'[16] and even the sick were set to work making cartridges and sand bags. The loss of Quebec was averted by the arrival of a British naval squadron on the 9th May after the ice had broken, and the French Commander realizing his chance had gone, withdrew his forces, leaving all his sick and wounded behind.

Amherst now completed the conquest of Canada by advancing from three directions on Montreal. Murray with 2,000 men from Quebec advanced up the St. Lawrence and encamped just below Montreal on the 24th August; Brigadier Howland with 3,400 men including two regular battalions, Provincials and Indians, drove back the French from the northern end of Lake Champlain to the banks of the St. Lawrence. Amherst himself with 11,000 men including 8 British battalions, 4,500 Provincials and 700 Indians advanced from Lake Ontario. The three forces met under the gates of Montreal on the 5th September, a major triumph in co-ordinated action.

These widely dispersed expeditions necessitated an extended distribution of medical resources. For Amherst's column moving down the St. Lawrence there was a hospital at Fort Ontario which in August had 305 patients; nearer the front there were other hospitals at Oswegatchie, and at Fort Oswego, where there were some cases of smallpox under treatment. But on the whole the troops were fit and healthy. For the central line of advance the general hospital at Albany received the bulk of the cases and had between 80 and 100 patients under treatment between May and July 1760. But as the advance continued what was probably a flying hospital was opened successively at Crown Point, then at Fort Edward, and finally at Fort George, with all movements and evacuation of patients depending on river transport. At New York the general hospital was now far from the scene of operations and had only thirty-two patients in its wards in July 1760.

The end of the war was now in sight. The French forces had been demoralized by ill fortune and defeat, and so many had deserted that only 2,500 men remained at Montreal to oppose 17,000 British and Provincials. On the 8th September the capitulation was signed and half a continent passed into the hands of Great Britain. Amherst's fame has been lost in the renown attached to Wolfe, but it was he who conquered Canada, and Fortescue fittingly describes him as the greatest military administrator between the death of Marlborough and the rise of Wellington.

We must complete the story of the North American scene, and it must be realized that in addition to the hospitals for the operations against Canada there were small hospitals in the colonial provinces at Philadelphia, Bedford, and Pittsburgh; while mention must also be made of those at Halifax and Louisburg. Between December 1758 and March 1761 the hospital expenses for the pay of officers, nurses, subordinate staff and medicines obtained locally amounted to £17,407, or about £620 a month and Napier who appeared to be responsible was sending frequent letters to Amherst asking for funds. The local purchase of medicines was allowed to supplement the supplies sent out regularly from home at half yearly intervals.

We have already mentioned that the sick rate in the years 1756–1757 appeared to be 7 or 8 per cent, and there is nothing to indicate that the succeeding years were different except for the devastating effects of scurvy in Quebec. At the end of the war there were no fewer than 2,500 invalids awaiting embarkation at Quebec, the majority unfit from rheumatism and old age, which points to their long service in the ranks. Scurvy, fever, dysentery and smallpox were the diseases which caused the heaviest wastage and leg ulcers were very common. With regard to treatment, Peruvian bark was of course the stand by in all types of fever, and dysentery was treated by giving 4 to 5 grains of tartar emetic and 2 ounces of manna in a pint of water; 3 to 4 ounces of this mixture were administered every half hour until vomiting and purging occurred, and this treatment was repeated as the symptoms required for three or four days.

It was an agreed policy for troops who were sickly and convalescents who were recovering from illness to come from the West Indies to America to recover their health, and in 1762 we find preparations being made to receive many from Albemarle's expedition to Havana. To explain this point we must say something about this operation and its disastrous record of ill health. It was in February 1762 that Lord Albemarle had been chosen to lead an expedition to Havana, the modern Cuba, for war had been declared against Spain, and this was one of the major prizes to be seized. Sailing from England to Barbados, his force was augmented by what he termed 'the remains of a very fine army'[17] much reduced by sickness, and this addition brought his strength up to 11,000 men. Arriving in sight of Havana City on the 6th June the army was landed, and the British siege batteries which opened fire on the Spanish forts had with the help of the fleet silenced the enemy guns by the 15th July. But the forts defended themselves obstinately, and soon Albemarle had only half his troops fit for duty for yellow fever, malaria and dysentery had decimated the ranks.

Luckily he had an extensive hospital staff to support him. Dr. Wintringham was Chief Physician and Director General coming direct from his duties in Germany, and with him came 3 other physicians; as surgeons he had Mr. Landep, chief surgeon and deputy director, a master surgeon, and 4 other surgeons; there were also 5 apothecaries, 1 apothecary and purveyor, and no fewer than 42 hospital mates. With the regimental surgeons and their mates there must have been something approaching 100 medical officers with this army of 11,000, which meant one medical officer to every 110 men of the force. It was not long before every M.O. was needed, for as early as the end of June, 1598 sick or nearly 15 per cent of the strength had been admitted to hospital and 194 were dead; one regiment alone had 154 men in hospital, and 21 deaths.

On the 27th July, 3,000 reinforcements arrived from America, and after one of the forts had been stormed and another silenced the town capitulated and the Spaniards were granted the honours of war, for with his army melting away from disease Albemarle was thankful to obtain possession of the town on any terms. He had hoped that rest and better quarters after the siege ended might restore the health of the army but on the contrary sickness increased. It was the height of the yellow fever season and this deadly disease swept away the men so fast that there were 5,000 soldiers and 3,000 seamen sick at one time. Less than 800 had been killed or wounded in the siege but by the 18th October over 5,000 men[18] or 35 per cent of the strength of the force had been buried and one brigade of four battalions could only muster twenty men fit for duty. The naval physician Dr. Lind[19] who served with the fleet quotes a dejected letter from an officer, 'I think myself extremely happy in being among the number of the living, considering the deplorable condition we are now in. You will hardly believe me when I tell you that I have only 33 of my company alive out of 100 which I landed. The other regiments have lost in proportion. We are now very sickly when out of seventeen battalions here we cannot muster 600 men fit for duty. The appearance of the country is most beautiful. Yet a man's life in it is extremely uncertain as many are in health one morning and dead before the next.'

Lind says there was a prejudice against the liberal use of bark because it was apt to produce dropsy and jaundice, and James' Powder which had recently come into vogue was the most popular febrifuge. Lind attacked its use because he did not know its ingredients and was suspicious of its inflated reputation; in his opinion a wine glass of infusion of bark would have saved hundreds of lives.[20] This was certainly true for malarial fever which no doubt caused much of the illness, but the doctors did not suspect that the jaundice was due to yellow fever and not the use of bark.

Anxious above all to put a stop to this terrible waste of life Albemarle hastily arranged for as many of his troops as possible to be shipped off to America, and Amherst directed Napier to arrange extensive accommodation for the sick. Accordingly between £1,200 and £1,400 was spent in equipping hospitals at Trenton and Burlington in the state of New Jersey and at Philadelphia, and enlisting locally hospital mates and subordinate staff. But for some unspecified reason the hospitals were never used, although amongst the sick who arrived there were 198 deaths in a single month. Concerned with the unnecessary expense of equipping these hospitals, Amherst told Napier to dispose of the equipment with strict injunctions that he was not to reveal the facts to anyone.[21] His plans had been made in good faith, but he felt that criticism might be directed against him on the grounds of waste of money.

By 1763 the North American area had settled down to a peace establishment, and the number of medical officers reduced to twenty. At New York where there was a small nucleus of regular troops and the general hospital was staffed by 1 physician, 2 surgeons, 2 apothecaries and 5 hospital mates, while there were small hospital staffs distributed over a wide area, at Quebec, at Montreal, at Nova Scotia, Albany, Detroit and Pittsburgh. These last three served the numerous frontier posts and forts reaching from Canada to the Ohio which were now manned by the 60th Foot, or as they were called the Royal American Regiment, a corps composed in great measure of foreigners.

The war with Spain was not only concerned with the attack on

Havana but with scattered enterprises against other Spanish possessions as far afield as the Phillipines, where Manila was captured by
troops from India. Florida also lay open to attack, but this territory
was exchanged for the unwanted possession of Havana in the peace
treaty which ended the war, and we read of Mr. Mallet, a surgeon of
whom we shall hear again, being sent off to Mobile in Louisiana a
notoriously unhealthy station, with the task of establishing a hospital
there.

The wide range of foreign garrisons now included Minorca, Gibralter,
Bermuda, the Bahamas, St. Vincent, Dominica, Tobago, Grenada
and the Grenadines, Jamaica, New York, Halifax, Quebec, and Mobile.
Yet the whole force allotted for the protection of these possessions
did not exceed 15,000 men.

Seven Years War 1756–1763

On the Continent there was only an interval of eight years after
the Treaty of Aix la Chapelle before Britain was again embroiled in a
major conflict, for the Seven Years War broke out in 1756 and lasted
until 1763. The cause of the quarrel was the attempt by a league made
up of France, Austria, Saxony, Russia, and Sweden, to crush the
rising power of Frederick the Great and partition Prussia. William
Pitt was now Prime Minister and proclaimed Britain's support for
Frederick, whom he looked upon as the champion of the liberties of
Europe and the pillar of the Protestant faith.

War was formally declared in January 1756 and France struck the
first blow in June by the capture of Minorca which fell after a gallant
resistance of seventy days when many of the sick and wounded came
out of hospital to aid the defence. The army estimates for 1756 had only
authorized an establishment of 51,000 men, but in 1757 this was raised
to 100,000, although this included the Irish Establishment. Pitt introduced a new and daring experiment in the creation of Highland regiments, and the instructions laid down that recruits were 'to be none but
able bodied men, free from rupture and every other distemper and
impurity that may render them unfit for duty, not under 17 or above
40, five feet four inches and above'.[22]

The direction of the medical service was now in the hands of Sir
Edward Wilmot the Physician General, and David Middleton the
Surgeon General. Wilmot, apart from selecting physicians for the
general hospitals, also appears to have exercised some control through
the physicians over the apothecaries, and presided over the examination
of candidates for appointment as hospital mates. On the clinical side
he acted as consultant and adviser on the general lines of treatment
to be adopted for medical diseases and the introduction of any new
drugs, together with the inspection of medicines supplied by the Apothe-

cary General, whose bills were passed for payment by both the Physician General and the Surgeon General. Middleton, the Surgeon General, who, as we know had seen much active service in the War of the Austrian Succession, had all the medical arrangements for the expedition in his hands.

It was under the instigation of the Duke of Cumberland—then Commander-in-Chief—Lord Barrington being Secretary at War, that two important steps were taken to improve the feeble and ineffective attempts made in previous campaigns for the control and organization of the medical services. The underlying cause of confusion and inefficiency was the recurring fact that the physicians who superintended the general hospitals were selected from civil life and had no conception of military organization and administration. At the same time they regarded themselves as so superior in education and in status to the surgeons that they would allow no interference with their prerogative no matter how ignorant they might be of their duties. The hospital surgeons on the other hand were frequently though not always regular officers with much army experience, but any attempt they might make to advise the physicians was jealously rejected. This unfortunate attitude meant that at the commencement of any campaign the general hospitals were abominably run and their administration chaotic. It was only after the physicians had gained war experience that matters improved, and it must be accepted that in this respect the best of them became capable administrators.

The Commander-in-Chief saw the weakness of this system, and in order to bring in the experience of regular officers Lord Barrington Secretary at War was as we have already noted directed to set up a Board. 'A Board was established consisting of physicians of the hospitals . . . the Surgeon General, the principal surgeon and purveyor[23] to the hospitals, who had it given them in charge conjointly to digest certain rules for regulating all hospital matters, in order that this part of the medical service (including medicines, hospital stores, and other provisions for the sick) might be carried into execution with ability, regularity and despatch.'[24] This Board had no powers of patronage, and its activities were confined to hospital matters in the theatre of war, but after the war terminated the Inspector of Regimental Infirmaries gradually absorbed its functions.

Although specific orders issued by the Board for the running of hospitals cannot be quoted, the information available from extracts of General Orders implies that they existed, and although epidemics of disease overcrowded the hospitals, the chaotic conditions of former wars seem conspicuous by their absence. This was perhaps because no epidemic occurred during the first year, and hospitals were able to settle into an established routine under their physicians. Also there is no doubt that the experience and advice of such men as Pringle was turned to good account, and for all these reasons the general conditions afforded the sick showed a great advance on what had gone before.

A further important step in administrative control was the appointment of a Director of Hospitals who was to live at the Commander-in-Chief's headquarters and supervise all the hospitals from that centre instead of trying to conduct his operations from the rear areas. This meant that the principal medical officer would receive early information of the Commander's intentions so that he could make the necessary medical arrangements in advance. There is evidence too that the regimental hospitals came under his control for tactical purposes. Conferences were held with the regimental surgeons and plans made which included their location in time of battle or on reaching camp, although this could only be done with the full agreement of the commanding officer. It was essential if the flying hospital was to be used to the best advantage to know the location of the regimental hospitals and this could only be done by a previously agreed plan.

The shortage of waggon transport for the sick and wounded had always been a major obstacle to their quick removal to hospital and their early treatment. This was now to be improved with the establishment of an army waggon train and by contractors supplying waggons to hospitals. Each regimental hospital was to have two waggons, one for carrying sick with the unit and one for equipment, while the two medical and surgical panniers were carried on a bat horse. The generally accepted method of evacuating sick from units to the rear was by means of the bread waggons which delivered bread daily to the different regiments. Instructions on these lines were set out in detail in General Orders issued daily by the Commander, and there is no doubt that the care of the sick and their transport received the fullest attention.

Flying hospitals had proved successful in the War of the Austrian Succession, and acted as an essential link between the regimental and the general hospitals, relieving the former of their cases when they were constantly on the move or in action, and either holding and treating them, or evacuating them in turn to the general hospitals further in the rear. Dr. Monro a physician who joined the army in 1760 tells us that to be effective they should carry between 200 to 400 sets of bedding, tents and equipment, with spare waggons to convey cases to the general hospitals.

Although the war had broken out in 1756 it was not until 1758.[25] that British troops to the number of some 8,000 were first dispatched to the continent under the command of the Duke of Marlborough. He came under the leadership of Prince Ferdinand of Brunswick as General-in-Chief, whose role was in the main a defensive one. His orders were to protect King Frederick of Prussia's western flank against France while Frederick fought the combined powers of Austria, Saxony and Russia to the south and east. The areas of Western Germany over which our troops marched and fought for the next five years were the provinces of Westphalia, Hesse, and Hanover, with our main base at the port of Emden. Marlborough joined Ferdinand's forces at Coesfeld in August and here a general hospital was opened. Each regiment was ordered to send one 'careful' woman to help in the wards, while any woman appointed by the C.O. who refused to go

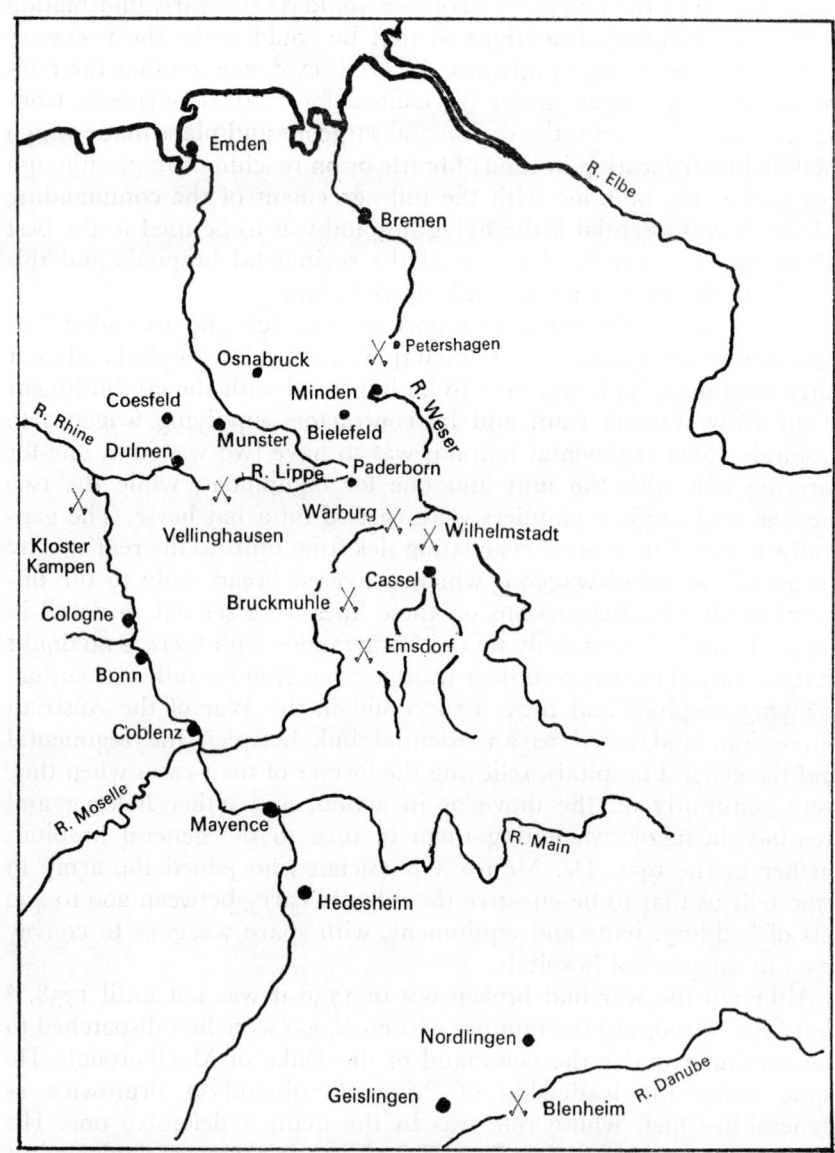

Marlborough's Blenheim Campaign 1704
Seven Years War 1756–62

would be drummed out of the regiment.[26] These women were the wives of soldiers who followed the drum and were the so called hospital 'nurses'.

The hospital board now constituted was composed of Dr. Wintringham the senior physician who became Physician General to the Forces in Germany, Mr. Young the chief surgeon, and Mr. Cathcart the head purveyor who was soon made Director of Hospitals. Wintringham had served in Flanders in the War of the Austrian Succession and was so well liked by the Duke of Cumberland that he became his personal physician at Headquarters and attended him in his final illness. We will meet him later as Physician General at the Horse Guards. Cathcart being a purveyor as well as director could not live at Headquarters but carried out his dual role from the general hospital. Mr. Burlton a surgeon of the hospital staff was made local Inspector of Regimental Infirmaries and was to succeed Cathcart as Director of Hospitals in 1761.

In September 1758 British Headquarters were at Dulmen southwest of Munster, and the regimental hospitals were being opened up. A conference of all regimental surgeons was called to meet Wintringham and Burlton on the 27th September, and a General Order states: 'The regimental surgeons are to provide regimental hospitals according to the plan laid down by Dr. Wintringham and these are to be inspected from time to time by Dr. Wintringham and Mr. Burlton who will report their state to the Duke of Marlborough.'[27] It was clear the members of the medical board were doing their duty effectively and their control was extending to the regimental surgeons, a point of particular interest as the commanding officers were always jealous of any interference with their own hospitals. While troops were on the march, sick were ordered to the hospital waggon in the rear of the column 'if the carriages of their particular regiment cannot carry them',[28] and a flying hospital which was organized to follow any movement was at Chateau D'Empte in September, at Soest on the 21st October, and at Warendorp on the 29th.

The troops were already suffering from bowel troubles and in the interests of hygiene precautions were taken that the bread waggons commonly used for evacuation of sick to the flying hospital at Chateau D'Empte should not be used by those suffering from the flux, but if this was unavoidable sufficient straw to cover the waggon floors was to be provided and this was to be burnt on arrival at the hospital. More commonly the waggons allotted to carry sick to hospital were parked with the artillery train, and were sent out on demand and returned again on arrival back in camp. Nurses and orderlies from the different regiments had to be found, and an order issued on the 17th September reads 'A nurse from each regiment of cavalry and infantry to be sent immediately to the flying hospital at D'Empte.'[29]

When troops went into winter quarters in the Munster area, a general hospital was opened in the town and to ensure that the regimental surgeons were neither negligent nor idle, every sick man admitted to this hospital had to have a pass signed by a field officer. Soon there were teething troubles; in December the returns and accounts were in such confusion that Mr. Cathcart as purveyor was ordered to unravel them with the assistance of one sergeant from each company which had men sick in hospital; and this was followed by instructions that the field officer of the day in the garrison was to visit the 'Grand Hospital' at Munster daily, and attended by a surgeon and a mate was to inspect every ward to redress any just complaints made by patients and to examine the order books. A weekly return of sick was made to the Commander-in-Chief, Lord George Sackville, who had succeeded on the death of the Duke of Marlborough.

By April 1759 Ferdinand's army was stirring from winter quarters, and each regiment marched off with two waggons for the sick and the regimental hospital stores, as well as two waggons for the regimental blankets. There was a great deal of marching and counter marching of opposing forces in the early months of this year much of it to the advantage of the French. The fortress of Munster was besieged by the enemy, Cassel was lost, and Ferdinand's forces much inferior in numbers were compelled to withdraw, so that the French were able to seize Minden and the crossings over the river Weser. It was here that British troops were in action for the first time. On the 1st August 1759 the battle of Minden was fought when 45,000 troops under Ferdinand opposed and defeated 60,000 French. Although there were only six British regiments of the Line engaged, they distinguished themselves and contributed powerfully to the Allied victory. Minden Day is celebrated by the regiments which took part by wearing roses on their head-dress, the flowers which they plucked in their victorious advance.

There were numerous farms and villages close to the battlefield in which the regimental surgeons could establish their hospitals, and when opportunity offered they were instructed to combine, so that medical officers could assist each other with their operations. After the fight was over the wounded were carried back by the drummers of each regiment to have their wounds dressed and their shattered limbs amputated. With 1,000 casualties to treat, the six regimental surgeons and their mates must have had their hands more than full, even although their surgery was of the crudest kind, but a flying hospital had been brought forward to Petershagen 25 miles away, to which the most severely wounded were sent, and here they received more effective treatment by skilled surgeons.

Because of French pressure there were no general hospitals in front of Minden, but Ferdinand had earlier occupied the free city of Bremen, and here the main general hospital had been established, the river

Weser presenting the best possible facilities for evacuation from the battlefield area by barge and boat.

The victory of Minden and the resulting retreat of the French army led to the capture of Cassel and Warburg, and the Allies in turn besieged Munster; but when Ferdinand was forced to send 12,000 men to reinforce Frederick who had suffered a disastrous defeat at the hands of the Russians, further aggression had to be suspended, and both armies retired into winter quarters in much the same areas as they had previously occupied.

Those units who could not be accommodated in villages and farms were compelled to live in tents, and during the winter months these were thatched for protection and warmth, hurdles were constructed as shelters, and deep pits dug and covered over with straw. During active operations blankets were only provided on the scale of two per tent, carried with the unit on pack horses or in waggons and wrapped in oil cloth, but in winter quarters one was issued to every man. Each regiment contracted with a butcher who accompanied the unit and was obliged to provide live sheep and oxen sold at a fixed price and paid for by stoppages from the men's pay. The midday dinner of 1 lb. of boiled meat with potatoes, root vegetables and greens made an excellent and nourishing meal; while for breakfast and supper there was gruel or porridge made from rice or oatmeal, with 1 lb. of bread as the day's ration.

It was May before the campaign of 1760 was opened, and in the meantime the British had been reinforced by additional infantry and cavalry regiments, bringing the force up to a total of over 20,000 men. At the victories of Emsdorf and Warburg, British troops played a notable part, but as the total wounded amounted to some hundreds only these battles call for no special mention. After the fight at Warburg, which took place on the 21st July, a severe epidemic of diarrhoea and dysentery broke out. The battlefield area on which the troops camped was covered with the carcasses of dead horses, fouled by human excrement, and many of the dead were only partially buried. The swarms of flies which were generated under these noisome conditions caused widespread bowel infections, and the nearest general hospital at Paderborn became grossly overcrowded and sick were dispatched to the other hospitals at Osnabruck, Bielefeld and Nutzungen. But the total beds in these hospitals only amounted to 800, and this number was quite insufficient to cope with the size of the epidemic. Inevitably, typhus fever appeared and swept through the wards at Paderborn, spread to the local villages and devastated both soldiers, hospital staffs, and civilians.

Ferdinand being a bold and audacious leader attempted a winter campaign in Hesse but was defeated in the battle of Kloster Kampen and after failing to take Cassel and losing a flying hospital and its staff at Alsdorf, went into winter quarters at Warburg. All through the winter and spring typhus cases were being continually admitted from all the regimental hospitals and the nine month period between July 1760 and May 1761 was the most unhealthy of the whole war. Dr. Monro who had recently arrived from England at Paderborn as medical superintendent was soon striving desperately to avoid overcrowding, and could only keep his 400 beds from being swamped by continually discharging convalescents to billets in the surrounding villages. To the epidemics of dysentery and typhus were added the usual 'inflammatory' diseases of winter origin caused by exposure—bronchitis, pneumonia and rheumatism. On the 1st April 1761 returns show that there were no fewer than 3,024 sick in the general hospitals at Paderborn, Osnabruck, Bielefeld and Bremen and 515 sick with their units, a sick rate of 18 per cent. Moreover as there was a reported mortality of 30 per cent—(in May 1761 there were 309 deaths)—something like 1,000 soldiers must have lost their lives. Some doubt exists about the accuracy of these figures, for General Conway of the Q.M.G. Staff at Headquarters reported dreadful confusion in the hospital statistics over a period of two years. He had therefore in October 1760 appointed Captain Douglas, an officer 'much afflicted with the gout', to take charge of all hospital returns and the arrangements for accommodating and exercising convalescents. Now Mr. Cathcart was once more summoned to put some degree of accuracy into the work of the hospital clerks. Conway declares he had no criticism of the medical care and treatment, and there is little doubt that the physicians such as Wintringham and Monro were of high professional status and the hospital wards were run with increasing efficiency as the physicians acquired the details of administration.

At Bremen the wards were equipped with bedsteads or cradles, and each patient was allotted 36 square feet of floor space in the large wards and 42 to 60 square feet in the smaller ones; palliasses with straw were preferred, as mattresses were difficult to clean; bed linen was issued twice a week; cleanliness was considered so important that walls were first scraped and then washed with soap and water followed by warm vinegar; ward floors were sprinkled with vinegar daily and then fumigated with the smoke of wetted gunpowder, then aired and dried before the sick were admitted. No less attention was paid to the patients themselves; every man on arrival was washed or bathed, and given a clean shirt;[30] face and hands were washed daily and feet occasionally; patients shaved twice weekly.

Separate wards were provided for medical and surgical cases, and dysenteries and putrid fevers were nursed apart and given ample floor space; dysentery wards had their own latrines which at Bremen opened directly into the river Weser, a system which was considered highly commendable and ingenious. Windows were opened morning and evening, and ventilation in wards was increased by removing panes in windows and cutting apertures in doors controlled by slats.

The dieting of hospital patients was a refinement which was just beginning, and could only be really effective when the salt meat of the ration could be replaced by fresh meat from local sources. When this was not possible the feeding of dysentery cases on salt provisions had proved disastrous because of their irritating effects upon the bowel. Happily the availablity of fresh meat in Germany for all troops naturally extended to the hospital patients, and it was a matter of common sense to introduce different diets for the various types of disease. Monro was one of the first to do so, and diet scales and diet boards were introduced for every patient.

	Breakfast	Dinner	Supper
Full diet	One pint of water or rice gruel*	One pound of boiled fresh meat	As for breakfast
Middle diet	One pint of water or rice gruel*	One pint of broth ½ lb. boiled meat	As for breakfast
Low diet	One pint of water or rice gruel*	One pint of broth or ½ pint of panada, with 2 spoonsful of wine and ¼ oz. sugar.	As for breakfast

To each diet 1lb. of bread was added.

* Water gruel was really porridge and made of 3–4 ozs. of oatmeal, salt, with or without a little sweet oil, and two spoonsful of wine. Rice gruel was 2 ozs. rice, some flour, salt and sugar.

For drink—3 pints of barley water and rice water, to each pint of which was added 2 spoonsful of brandy and ¼ oz. of sugar. Extras consisted of additional wine, brandy, milk or water gruel, or other articles ordered by the medical officer, and paid for by the purveyor out of the hospital stoppages which amounted to 7¼d. a day.

The Allies had suffered so terribly from hardship and exposure during the unfortunate winter expedition to Hesse that out of 8 British battalions there were only 700 effectives fit to take the field, and it was necessary to allow the army two months' rest. But the excellent work the hospital service performed in saving sick wastage can be judged from the fact that between April and June 1761 nearly 4,500 convalescents rejoined their units, and as a result Ferdinand in the latter month was able to make up his depleted British regiments, although the Allies could only muster 93,000 men against a French army of 160,000.

It would be out of place to follow the manoeuvring between the rival forces which characterized the campaign of 1761, which was fought in the area of the river Lippe between Paderborn and Munster. The only battle worthy of mention was the defeat of the French at Vellinghausen in July when 12 British infantry and 6 cavalry regiments suffered some 450 casualties. For this campaign the Paderborn hospital was too exposed to enemy attack, and it was closed in April after the 300 sick remaining had been evacuated to Osnabruck and Bremen. Monro went on to Osnabruck as superintendent, but transferred the hospital to Bielefeld in June.

When the convention to make hospitals neutral in the War of the Austrian Succession was agreed to the general hospitals were free to be located wherever necessity required. But the chivalry which characterized war between British and French forces did not extend to the Seven Years War when France fought Prussia. That hospitals could now be exposed to capture resulted in constant changes of location which caused a disastrous breakdown in evacuation of the wounded and the sick, and the regimental surgeons were compelled to trail their cases around for one, two, three and even more weeks before they could be evacuated. This caused great hardship because it involved long slow journeys in country carts and waggons over execrable roads. The lack of treatment and the exposure involved in these journeys often led to a mortality of 30 per cent. But apart from these difficulties in evacuation there was an epidemic in the summer of 1761 of autumnal fever probably malarial in origin which had helped to pack the hospital wards with 1,200 sick.

Besides autumnal fever there were also a few small outbreaks of typhus at Osnabruck and Munster, but the prompt measures taken of immediately giving each patient greater floor space and ample ventilation of the wards had killed any epidemic. However, the potential danger was ever present amongst a soldiery habitually vermin infested. That Monro appreciated the danger of acquiring typhus from personal contact is revealed by the precautions which he took in visiting patients, and this applied to smallpox cases as well. A waxed linen coat he said should be worn on visiting typhus or smallpox wards, to be discarded on quitting the wards, and the hands washed. A dose of bark should be taken, and small rolls of lint dipped in camphorated spirits should be put up the nostrils, and a vessel with warm camphorated vinegar should be held near the patient. While taking the pulse of a patient the doctor should not breathe.

Smallpox made its appearance at Osnabruck but died out when the cases were promptly isolated. Protection by inoculation or variolation as it was called with the human variety of smallpox was being practised at this time, as Jenner's method of vaccination with cowpox did not come into existence until 1796. It had been introduced from Turkey by Lady Mary Wortley Montagu in the early part of the eighteenth century. Although the inoculation method was sometimes dangerous and uncertain in its effects it was widely practised though never compulsory in the army. Soldiers undergoing it were prepared for some days beforehand by purges and light diet, and after the scabs had dried, by further purges and mercury; a popular idea was to keep the victim in 'cool air', and some doctors even advocated exposure to severe frost. Be that as it may there are records of 100 cases being inoculated with only one fatality, and as an added precaution it is possible that the inoculated material was taken only from those victims who were suffering from the mildest attacks.

Cholera was reported for the first time at Munster in July and August. As none of the patients died the diagnosis may be open to question, but Monro was an accurate observer, and the cases may indeed have been of European cholera, which must be distinguished from the Asiatic variety. At Bremen there was an outbreak of influenza in April which affected civilians more than the troops, and there were cases of true scurvy characterized by the spongy foetid gums, the livid blotches on the skin and the leg ulcers. This was due to a diet of nothing but salt meat and salt herrings without any root or fresh vegetables, which were so expensive that the soldiers could not afford to buy them.

After further fighting which did not seriously involve British troops the campaign of 1761 ended in November, and the Allies' winter quarters once again extended from Munster along the line of the river Lippe to Hedensheim. The year 1762 covered the last campaign of the war. Two battles must be mentioned, both fought in the vicinity of Cassel, but in neither were the British casualties of great account; at Wilhelmstadt in June the French were beaten with a loss to our troops of 450 men, while the stubbornly fought final action of the war at Bruckmuhle cost some 250 killed and wounded. After Cassel had been captured by the Allies in November, Lord Bute the Prime Minister decided that the war must end. In 1763 peace was finally concluded.

By the terms of the Treaty of Paris the French lost all India except Pondicherry and Chandernagore; they also lost French America, Canada, Tobago, Dominica, St. Vincent and Senegal.

From the world of battle and politics we must turn to medicine. Dysentery, fever, and typhus were as always the cause of the greatest wastage; typhus due in contemporary opinion to the putrid exhalations in overcrowded wards, dysentery from obstructed perspiration, and fever from marshy miasmas. Their forms of treatment differed but little from those adopted ten years before.

In acute dysentery, salts were now replacing rhubarb as a purge, with starch and opium enemas for tenesmus. Some doctors gave opium throughout, but the consensus of opinion was in favour of purges being administered for twelve to fourteen days, followed then by opiates for relieving pain and procuring rest. The great majority of patients recovered from these acute attacks but some drifted into chronic dysentery which was very hard to cure. Many patients died from its effects. For these cases a bland nourishing diet[31] was prescribed with astringent medicines and opiates, including Dover's Powder, but many appeared to do better without any medicines at all. Relapses, which were caused by errors of diet and catching a chill, were frequent. For fevers the new remedy James' Powder was used, consisting it was now revealed of a mixture of antimony, mercury, sal ammoniac and spirits of nitre. This was a diaphoretic in small doses, but an emetic and purge in larger doses, while it could be dangerous and deadly if given too frequently. Monro claims it had no specific effect on fevers, and makes the libellous suggestion that Dr. James gave it to put money into his own pocket,[32] for James himself always relied on Peruvian bark to effect a cure. He also used a mild powder which included antimony and powdered crab's eyes, and this quaint remedy is also mentioned by Monro as sometimes being given with bark in the treatment of malaria. This last remedy had gained such an universal approval that it was now used in the treatment of wounds and of small-pox.

Medical officers now had the advantage of the *Dispensatory*, a booklet which gave a list of drugs authorized in 1761 by the physician, surgeon and apothecary generals. The governing factor was to provide only drugs which would keep, and had not to be used fresh, so we find 56 principal prescriptions followed in an appendix by a further 94. We have such items as Roman philonium for dysentery and Lenitive electory for gonorrhoea, but crab's eyes are not among them. Perhaps these had to be used fresh!

In none of the wars of this century do any official reports appear to exist which describe the activities of the medical service and it is from Dr. Donald Monro that we learn the administrative lessons of the war in Germany which he published in his *Observations on the means of preserving the health of soldiers*. He was a member of the famous Monro family who were professors of anatomy at Edinburgh, and his father had served as a surgeon in the army of William III and lent his help to the wounded after the battle of Preston Pans. He took his M.D. at Edinburgh in 1753 at the age of 26, and the L.R.C.P. London in 1758 when he was on the staff of St. George's Hospital. Monro suggested strengthening the medical arrangements in the forward area in several ways, in addition to the flying hospital he wanted a hospital with 200 to 400 sets of bedding, with tents and equipment to move with army headquarters and to reinforce the regimental hospitals in the event of an action until the flying hospital could arrive; to supplement this there should be additional staff surgeons chosen for their operating ability attached to brigade headquarters to perform early surgery at brigade level; these surgeons should be provided with instruments and dressings carried on horseback so they could rapidly move to where the casualties required their attention.

As medical officers possessed no executive powers of discipline over the subordinate hospital staff this duty was as we know performed by a military officer. He was responsible for order and cleanliness in the wards, listened to any complaints of patients, saw that the convalescents were exercised, and inspected the hospital returns made out by the purveyor. An important duty was the punishment of offences committed by the nurses and subordinate staff, and nurses guilty of great neglect of duty, drunkenness, or stealing the effects of the dead, were put in the guard room, court-martialled and confined, whipped or otherwise punished. This lack of executive command meant that the Director of Hospitals was unable to order the movement of hospitals except through military channels, a method which inevitably entailed delay.

This dual medical and military control could never be satisfactory and medical officers were already pressing for full authority over their own hospitals. Monro saw the disadvantages and wanted the physician attached to the Commander-in-Chief to be made the Director of Hospitals, and in his own right issue orders which had to be obeyed without hesitation. To do this he wanted medical officers given a form of military rank, but over a 100 years were to pass before mere doctors were judged to have the capacity to control their own affairs. Monro was supported in his opinions by Dr. Brocklesby who condemned the interpolation of military officers into the hospital wards. Brocklesby was physician to a force under Lord Moira which made a landing at St. Malo in Northern France, and was afterwards stationed in the Isle of Wight where he gained the experience which he published in his book *Oeconomical and Medical Observations tending to the improvement of military hospitals and the cure of camp diseases.*

Mr. Burlton had now succeeded Mr. Cathcart as Director of Hospitals and also continued his duties as Inspector of Regimental Infirmaries. His task to provide a reasonable standard of nursing in general hospitals was bedevilled by the ignorance and unwillingness of the soldiers detailed for hospital duties. The only members of the hospital staff who had seen previous service were the apothecaries, a sprinkling of the surgeons promoted from regimental duty and the hospital mates, but even some of these were often civilians hastily enlisted for the war. Under these circumstances the apothecary was often a key man and apart from the care of the drugs and the dispensing was given many administrative tasks to perform. He was responsible for the nurses and orderlies doing their medical duty, he had to examine diets and rations, supervise the prescriptions made up by the hospital mates, and visit the hospital morning and evening. Further, he was ordered to live near the hospital to assist at once in case of emergency. The hospital mates carried out the bleeding of patients and the dressing of wounds and ulcers, and they attended ward rounds with the physician or surgeon, and received the admissions. There was an orderly mate who slept at the hospital and by the C-in-C's instruction was provided with 'a joint of meat, roasted or boiled for dinner and a bottle of wine' so that 'they might not absent themselves from their duty'.[33]

As in the case of Cathcart, there was a tendency at this time for a Director of Hospitals to combine his own speciality with that of purveyor, but Monro condemns this dual role in no uncertain terms. 'The directing and purveying branches,' he says, 'ought never to be entrusted to the same person, as the temptation to accumulate wealth has at all times . . . given rise to the grossest abuses which have been a great detriment to the service as well as to the poor wounded and sick soldiers, and has occasioned the loss of many lives.'[34] The Director should have nothing to do with accounts and contracts for as he has the ear of the C.-in-C. he can prevent any subordinate making complaints of abuses. Further he advocates the purveying and contracting branch being entirely separate from the medical, a policy which as we shall see was to be adopted in the future.

Both Monro and Brocklesby reiterated the proposals on hygiene previously stressed by Pringle; dispersion of cases of itch, measles, and smallpox in separate wards or preferably in separate houses with separate nurses; better ventilation, cleanliness, conservancy in camps; strict attention to latrines, moving camp sites when ground was fouled, etc. But attention to drinking water was a new measure. The adoption of crude filtration by sand with the aid of one barrel let into another was a measure still mentioned in text books on the subject, and if no other means was possible water was to be boiled, and vinegar or cream of tartar added to it.

All the measures described reveal the improvements which characterized the Seven Years War, and it is evident that the medical service which according to Monro dealt with 25,000 cases of sickness, came through it with an enhanced reputation.

At the end of the war the newly acquired possessions wrested from France such as Minorca, Grenada, St. Vincent, Dominica, Tobago and Senegal were all supplied with garrison surgeons who acted as local medical staff officers. In Senegal a special unit was raised known as 'A Corps of Foot serving in Africa' and there were other districts, Goree and Galam on the west coast, which were temporarily in our hands before being returned to France at the Treaty of Paris. Mr. Boon, who for three years was the garrison surgeon at Senegal, reports that of the troops sent to Galam consisting of 6 officers, a surgeon's mate, and 56 other ranks, only the mate survived. In Senegal itself between the months of December and March he had 400 patients under treatment 'prodigiously ill of tertiary (tertian) fevers which were so obstinate that he had been obliged to order bark to be taken almost as common food, and indeed,' he says, 'had it not been for this medicine we might not have had five men living on the island.'[35] The troops themselves were so conscious of its efficacy that 'mutiny amongst the troops was the alternative if the surgeon would not undertake at his own peril that bark in sufficient quantities should be sent along with each detachment'.[36] The one-time garrison surgeon at Goree stated that the price of bark in scarce times was at the rate of an ounce of gold dust for the pound.

Our history must record the capture of the island of Bellisle off the French coast in 1761, not because it was of military importance, (it was wanted as a port for the British fleet), but because it was here that John Hunter of surgical fame had his first and only experience of treating gun shot wounds of recent origin.

Hunter had come to London from Scotland at the age of 20 primarily to help his brother William in his studies on anatomy, but this was soon to give place to a growing attention to surgery. He entered St. George's Hospital as a surgeon's pupil in 1754 and was house surgeon there in 1756. At the same time he began to teach anatomy in William Hunter's school and was appointed one of the Masters of Anatomy of the Surgeon's Corporation. By the time he was 32 these years of hard work had affected his health, and after an attack of pneumonia he decided to join the army. By his brother's influence with Adair who had recently been made the Inspector of Regimental Infirmaries, Hunter obtained a commission in 1760 as a surgeon on the hospital staff. Already in collaboration with his brother he had done much original work, including the study of the placental circulation, the lymphatic system, and the nature of pus, and it may well be that apart from being beneficial to his health, joining the army gave him the opportunity he sought of studying the effects of gun shot wounds. Thus we find him present at Bellisle where in April 1761 an assault was made by a force numbering some 8,000 men, which after two months of fighting proved successful.

The total casualties were some 700 killed and wounded. In a general hospital opened at Palais under the Director, Mr. Young, Hunter gained his first experience in the study of coagulation of the blood and the inflammation and the repair of tissues in recent gun shot wounds. In due course he made a valuable contribution to the literature of surgery based on these cases in his book *The Blood, Inflammation and Gun Shot Wounds*. The occupation of Bellisle was followed by a great deal of sickness due to 'a severe fever and flux', one of the cures for which 'clarified butter given two spoonfuls at a time, twice or thrice a day, is an infallible cure for the bloody flux'.[37]

Then in 1762 war broke out with Spain, and on the pretext of Portuguese friendship with England Portugal was invaded and the country overrun as far as the river Douro. A force under the command of Lord Loudon of nearly 7,000 men was dispatched to Lisbon arriving in May and June 1762, and four regiments from Bellisle were included. Hunter had been longing to go to Portugal but feared his name would not be included and he would be left behind kicking his heels doing routine hospital duties in Bellisle. 'I hear,' he wrote to his brother William, 'that Dr. Blyth is to go to Portugal. I suppose Mr. Young goes as Surgeon General. God help the hospital when directed by such two.'[38] But eventually his orders came and he arrived in Lisbon about the 16th July; with him there were others of the medical staff—an apothecary, 5 mates, the matron and 4 nurses. In his methodical way he gives a list of the invalids left behind in Bellisle, their age and infirmities, which includes blindness, paralysis, consumption and rheumatism,[39] a list which would certainly exclude them from any form of active service.

No fighting occurred in this short campaign in Portugal and its interest for us lies in the medical arrangements, which are depicted in more detail than other more important campaigns have been able to provide. For the first time we come across a previously prepared hospital plan based on an estimated sick rate. This was the work of Mr. Fordyce, surgeon to the Third Foot Guards, and why he carried out a task which should have been the responsibility of the Surgeon General is not clear. Here is his plan. 'For 6,000 men in eight regiments, and supposing each regiment to have 100 sick. First for bedding: one hundred palliasses . . . to be filled with straw . . . if the hospital is fixed and not a field or flying hospital there must be 100 bedsteads with boarded bottoms of strong work.'[40] Fordyce tells us that the sick seldom exceed 100 men in a regiment unless they lie encamped on the same ground for any length of time and this gives the average sick rate as something over 13 per cent. In fact the sick rate in Lisbon in June 1762 was 13·6 per cent and in July 14·2 per cent. Doubtless, the danger of an increase in sickness was due to the deteriorating sanitary conditions with fly breeding possibilities, and this fact was fully appreciated in Jamaica some twenty years later, when it was found that troops could occupy camping grounds for indefinite periods if the closest attention was paid to sanitation. A further point of interest is the establishment of the general hospital, details of which have been recorded. Here we find that the subordinate staff were largely composed of women who sailed with the hospital from England and this is so unusual that we have thought fit to record the fact. On this occasion only two men are borne on the establishment, one as quartermaster and one as store-keeper. There are 28 women, including a matron paid 2s. 6d. a day, 2 head nurses at 1s. a day, and 18 nurses at 6d. a day. The matron and the head nurses must obviously have had some previous training, but those nurses who were paid at rates lower than the washerwomen were probably soldiers' wives. Fordyce estimated 800 sick of the force of

6,000 required hospitalization and as the 8 regimental hospitals were equipped for 40 beds apiece this would leave 480 in the general hospital. With 20 nurses employed on the wards this would give them 24 patients apiece to look after, a number which would be a reasonable standard at the time.

Mr. Young was Director, with 2 physicians, 3 surgeons including Hunter, 2 apothecaries and 16 hospital mates,[42] and he opened his general hospital in Lisbon in July 'with great difficulty and confusion'[43] for it was housed in four separate buildings with a total capacity of 496 beds. As so frequently happened when general hospitals first opened with an inexperienced staff there was a complete lack of order and discipline in the wards. A Standing Order by the D.A.G. had to be issued to curb the misbehaviour of the patients, 'it having been reported to General Townsend that there is not that discipline at the hospital which can enable those that have the care of it, to do as much for the recovery of the men as he could wish'.[44] Accordingly, a hospital guard under an officer was to be made responsible that order was observed, and that fatigue parties would be provided to carry water, bury the dead, and generally assist the nurses in work which was too heavy for them. Refractory and disobedient patients were to be confined on bread and water as long as the medical officer directed and if necessary placed in the black hole or in irons. The guard was to visit 'the tippling houses' in the neighbourhood to prevent any men drinking and quarrelling with the inhabitants.

Lord Loudon's force was now pushed forward to an area some 100 miles east of Lisbon stretching from the Serra da Estrella in the north to Portallegre in the south. The regimental hospitals served their own units, and to keep in touch with them on this extended front five small flying hospitals were organized at Tancos, St. Domingo, Montalvao, Vendas Noves and Apalhao. Each was in charge of a hospital mate and visited from time to time by a more senior member of the hospital staff. Ox or mule waggons brought the sick from these flying hospitals to an embarking point on the Tagus at Abrantes or Punhete, and thence it was a six to eight hour journey by boat to Santarem, where a second general hospital was opened in a good site in a Jesuit College with a capacity of 250 beds. By the end of the month it was overcrowded with 400 sick mostly fevers and dysenteries, and Young who visited it on the 28th August found many of the sick were lying on the bare ground, and both fuel and straw were difficult to obtain from the Portuguese corregidores. 'The wards,' he said, 'are as clean and their cookery as well conducted as it can be . . . and upon the whole are pretty comfortable.'[45] But the flying hospital at Tancos was bad and overcrowded with 130 patients. Hunter was sent up to report. He was feeling disgruntled. He had got it into his head that he was to be made deputy director of the hospital, (a post which in fact did not exist), for brother William in

London had been told by the Secretary at War he would get it—a piece of solicited patronage which proved to be quite false. 'They want to cheat me out of it,'[46] was Hunter's disgusted comment.

September was a sickly month and the number of patients in Santarem had increased to 694 most of them suffering from ague, fluxes, and fever. But according to Young the 'distempers' were not bad, although in the last few days twenty-five men had died, several of them brought out dead from the boats. And waggons were always hard to come by. 'I wish,' said Young, 'we had a small number to ourselves with a guard over them to secure them from being pressed. Indeed, I think if a battle should happen there would be a good deal of distress.'[47] Such has been the complaint of medical officers in many a campaign.

Loudon now ordered a hospital to be opened at Abrantes, a further forty miles up the Tagus from Santarem, and equipment for 200 patients and four supernumerary mates[48] were sent from Lisbon which was nearly empty. When a vacancy occurred at Lisbon owing to Dr. Cadogan one of the physicians falling sick, Hunter, in spite of his limited experience, was bold enough to apply for the post, and on the 16th November wrote to his brother, 'I am now applying for physician. If I can get it I shall be a doctor as well as the best of you.' To obtain this coveted post with its large increase in pay the patronage of his Commander was essential, and Hunter wrote to Loudon, 'to throw myself upon your favour.' This was done behind Young's back, whose approval Hunter neither seemed to value or care about. In fact he was not popular with either Young or his brother officers whom he described as a 'damned disagreeable lot',[49] and his biographer Jesse Foot tells us, 'He had scarcely arrived at Portugal before he excited an uneasiness among the faculty . . . he turned the common intercourses of social good humour into suspicious tauntings of jealousy; he created a faction and a consequent disgust.'[50] On one heated occasion Mr. Tomkins, a fellow surgeon, became so annoyed with Hunter's behaviour that he drew his sword on him. Anyhow, Hunter was to be disappointed in his attempt to become a physician for the vacancy was filled by Dr. Richard Huck an old friend of Lord Loudon's whom the reader will remember in North America. But this experience of Hunter's was to have an important sequel, for we will find in due course that when he became Surgeon General he changed the existing policy and laid it down that a physician must have had previous service as a regimental or hospital surgeon before he could be regarded as competent.

One of Hunter's chief regrets was the loss of the additional pay which a physician's appointment brought, but his Director was luckier in this respect. In October, Young was pressing Lord Loudon to make him surgeon to the Lisbon hospital in addition to being Director, as this would bring him pay for both appointments, and when he succeeded in getting it the letter of thanks he wrote to Loudon on the 23rd

October 1762 is worth recording. 'Nothing', he says, 'can equal the satisfaction your Lordship has been pleased to give me by my new commission but the gratitude I feel towards my noble patron. I now humbly heartily thank your Lordship. This most pleasing and expressive testimony of your Lordship's approbation of my conduct came unsolicited and was never in my thoughts, now it will never be out of them.'[51]

When November came the autumnal fevers especially malaria caused a heavy sick wastage; some mates died and several others were sick, so that Loudon sent for seven additional hospital mates as well as bedding and equipment from England.[52]

Further details of the campaign need not detain us except to say there were difficulties over the supply of mules or horses for moving the medical officers and equipment of the flying hospitals. These were evacuating their patients in January and February 1763 preparatory to closing down, and it was in May that the last ships took away the invalids.

At the end of 1762 Young had a bill for £5,112 0s. 6d. to pay for the hospital purchases of bread and meat and other contingencies including over £1,000 for subsistence allowance for the hospital staff officers. This was the only emolument they received, for their pay was not allowed until the campaign was over, and then only after a complicated procedure with certificates jointly signed by the Commander of the Forces, by the Director of Hospitals, and the Paymaster General, stating the exact period the general hospitals were open and functioning, from 16th February 1762 to the 14th May 1763.

When Hunter left Lisbon after his sole experience of active service, an experience which was to serve him in good stead when over twenty years later he became Surgeon General, it is said he embarked with 'two hundred specimens of beasts, lizards and snakes'[53] many of which were doubtless to find places in his historic museum.

REFERENCES

[1] But in 1762 the requisition for medical stores made by Dr. Young, the Director of Hospitals in Portugal, included ten dozen trusses which shows that men with rupture were commonly serving.

[2] Garrison. *The History of Military Medicine*, p. 137, footnote 6. Saunders, London (1929).

[3] Brocklesby. *Oeconomical and Medical Observations*, pp. 54–55. Becket and de Hondt (1764).

[4] See Appendix A.

[5] Brocklesby. *Oeconomical and Medical Observations*, p. 45. Becket and de Hondt (1764).

[6] Brocklesby. *Oeconomical and Medical Observations*, p. 21. Becket and de Hondt (1764).

[7] Brocklesby. *Oeconomical and Medical Observations*, p. 28. Becket and de Hondt (1764).

[8] Brocklesby. *Oeconomical and Medical Observations*, p. 27. Becket and de Hondt (1764).

[9] Brocklesby. *Oeconomical and Medical Observations*, pp. 226–7. Becket and de Hondt (1764).

[10] P.R.O., W.O. 7/96, p. 8.

[11] P.R.O., W.O. 7/96, p. 126.

[12] P.R.O., W.O. 40/7.
[13] Many sufferers from venereal complaints were made to serve with their units.
[14] P.R.O., W.O. 34/64, p. 8.
[15] Fortescue. *History of the British Army*, book X, chapter III, p. 360. Macmillan, London (1910).
[16] Fortescue. *History of the British Army*, book X, chapter IV, p. 394. Macmillan, London (1910).
[17] Fortescue. *History of the British Army*, book X, chapter XI, p. 541. These were troops sent from America after the conquest of Canada for operations in the West Indies. Macmillan, London (1910).
[18] Corbett gives a figure of 4,708 deaths.
[19] Lind. *Essays on Diseases incidental to Europeans in hot climates*, p. 334. Becker and de Hondt (1771).
[20] Lloyd and Coulter. *Medicine and the Navy*, vol. III, p. 120. Livingstone, Edinburgh (1961).
[21] P.R.O., W.O. 34/64.
[22] Gore. *Our Services under the Crown*, p. 89. Ballière Tindall & Cox, London (1879).
[23] Purveyors were promoted regimental surgeons and therefore regular officers.
[24] Clode. *The Military Forces of the Crown 1869*, Appendix BB, p. 462. John Murray, London (1869).
[25] Except for a minor engagement in 1757.
[26] Historical Manuscripts Commission Report. Various Collections VIII, p. 446.
[27] Historical Manuscripts Commission Report. Various Collections VIII, p. 451.
[28] Historical Manuscripts Commission Report. Various Collections VIII, p. 451.
[29] Historical Manuscripts Commission Report. Various Collections VIII, p. 459.
[30] Monro suggests a stock of shirts should be carried in hospital stores.
[31] Sago, rice, salop, white meat with wine or brandy.
[32] Monro. *Observations on the means of preserving the health in soldiers*, p. 14. John Murray, London (1780).
[33] Monro. *Observations on the means of preserving the health in soldiers*, p. 140. John Murray, London (1780).
[34] Monro. *Observations on the means of preserving the health in soldiers*, p. 135. John Murray, London (1780).
[35] Gore. *Our Services under the Crown*, p. 97. Ballière Tindall & Cox, London (1879).
[36] Gore. *Our Services under the Crown*, p. 97. Ballière Tindall & Cox, London (1879).
[37] Howell, Journal *R.A.M.C.*, vol. XIX, p. 145.
[38] Peachey. *Memoirs of William and John Hunter*.
[39] Amongst the soldiers at Portsmouth rejected for service in Portugal there was one of 61 years of age, another of 53, and two of 50.
[40] Gask. *Essays on the History of Military Medicine*, p. 119. Butterworth, London (1950).
[42] Their daily rates of pay were: Mr. Young 25s., physician 20s., surgeons and apothecaries 10s., mates 5s.
[43] P.R.O., W.O. 1/165.
[44] Gask. *Essays on the History of Military Medicine*, p. 122. Butterworth, London (1950).
[45] Gask. *Essays on the History of Military Medicine*, p. 128. Butterworth, London (1950).
[46] Gask. *Essays on the History of Military Medicine*, p. 122. Butterworth, London (1950).
[47] Gask. *Essays on the History of Military Medicine*, p. 130. Butterworth, London (1950).
[48] Supernumerary mates were recruited locally.
[49] Foot. *Life of John Hunter*, p. 80. Becket, London (1794).
[50] Foot. *Life of John Hunter*, p. 80. Becket, London (1794).
[51] Gask. *Essays on the History of Military Medicine*, p. 128. Butterworth, London (1950).
[52] Two sets of instruments for the trepan, 2 sets amputating knives complete, 2 dozen dissecting knives, 20 dozen lancets, 6 dozen bag trusses, 4 dozen spring trusses.
[53] Howell, *John Hunter*, Journal, *R.A.M.C.*, vol. XIX, p. 145.

Chapter 6

AMERICAN WAR OF INDEPENDENCE

Following the famous Boston 'tea party' the first shots of the American War of Independence were fired at Lexington in Pennsylvania in April 1775, when a small British force dispatched from Boston to seize a quantity of American military stores at Concord was severely mauled by a superior force of American Militia. The Americans were naturally much elated by their success and before long the British troops in Boston, consisting of eleven weak battalions, were surrounded by 16,000 to 20,000 of the enemy, and held in a strict blockade. General Gage, the Commander, being so heavily outnumbered had no alternative but to await reinforcements from England, and in June 1775 seven battalions of infantry and a regiment of cavalry arrived under General Howe.

The British army everywhere numbered only 33,000 men and recruits were so difficult to obtain that officers were loathe to part with their old soldiers as long as they could crawl. Even when the establishment was raised to 55,000 men, this increase was far too small for the reconquest of America, and the history of the American War is bedevilled by the chronic shortage of troops and their transportation by ship over a distance of 3,000 miles.

The American plan was to attack and drive the British out of Boston, but at the battle of Bunker's Hill fought on the 17th June 1775 they were heavily defeated. The British losses were severe and a temporary hospital was opened in a wooden building at Charlestown which was soon extended to include the town's workhouse, the almshouse, and every empty warehouse in the place as some 800 wounded poured in. At the general hospital opened at Boston just across the water there was a staff of only 2 surgeons and 8 hospital mates under Dr. Blagden a physician, with 1 purveyor and 2 apothecaries, and the hospital staff must have been desperately busy dressing the wounded and amputating limbs. Additional help in the wards was obtained by detailing 2 soldiers' wives from every unit to act as nurses, and 2 N.C.O's and 18 men reported daily as hospital orderlies.

Hospital equipment had been arriving from England, more than 5,000 palliasses, 1,250 blankets, over 8,000 sheets, 2,500 coverlets and bed rugs, with ward utensils of every description. One item which deserves attention was the blood porringers for blood letting which was an essential part of the treatment for both wounds and disease. All this equipment together with hospital rations and other necessaries had been carefully divided amongst different transports as a measure of safety, so that if any ship was sunk only a fraction would be lost.

The effect of the skirmish at Lexington made itself felt throughout the American colonies, and in September 1775 General Washington set on foot a daring enterprise for the conquest of Canada from a base at Fort Ticonderoga, which the Americans had surprised and captured with its small garrison. The 3,500 American troops threw back the small British forces in their advance and in view of this threat Montreal had to be evacuated. But they were finally defeated at Quebec in December and Canada was saved.

Our troops in Boston spent the winter of 1775 hemmed in by much superior enemy forces and soon outbreaks of scurvy and smallpox were causing between 10 and 30 deaths every day. With only rations of salt pork and dried peas to eat with an occasional diet of fish, scurvy was unavoidable. Smallpox, although it affected the British to some extent never appeared in epidemic form as it did in the American army; most of our soldiers had either suffered from it before enlistment or were already protected by the current practice of inoculation. The Colonists had no such immunity. Blagden and his hospital staff earned Gage's approbation during the trials of the siege and the Secretary at War expressed his approval when he wrote in March 1776, 'I am glad to find you are so well satisfied with the care and attention of the gentlemen in the Medical Department.'[1]

General Howe now arrived to assume command. Boston was evacuated after an American attack, and he sailed with his whole force to Halifax in Nova Scotia. Here a new plan was evolved of attacking Washington's army along the line of the Hudson river in New Jersey, and in June 1776 Howe landed at Staten Island near New York with a force of 25,000 men. After a successful engagement at Brooklyn, when the Americans were defeated with a loss to the British of some 400 officers and men, the way to New York lay open, and the city was captured on the 15th September. Unfortunately, the army then remained motionless for a month, but then advancing northwards on the east bank of the Hudson River it again defeated Washington's force at White Plains on the 28th October. The American army through desertion was fast dwindling in numbers so Howe was able to push his advance to the Delaware River some 50 miles to the west, where the campaign for the year 1776 ended.

In these operations around New York we have the personal experiences of Dr. Forster to present a picture of his duties as a staff surgeon to what is called His Majesty's Detached Hospital which was probably another name for what has been previously described as a flying hospital. At the action of Brooklyn on Long Island in August 1776 Forster was on duty with 2 other surgeons and 6 hospital mates. Not only was treatment provided for the wounded in his hospital but individual surgeons were dispatched on horseback with pockets full of bandages to wherever the fighting was most severe. The slightly wounded went straight back to a hospital ship lying off the Island, while the severe cases were operated on and retained until they were fit to move.

At the capture of New York on the 15th September Forster was well forward behind the regimental surgeons and set up a dressing station in a barn until the flying hospital arrived. Having laboured strenuously all day and disposed of their casualties to the general hospital just opened in the city, the medical officers Forster tells us 'opened our canteens, spent a jolly evening' (with the feeling of work well done) 'rolled ourselves up in our cloaks, and slept as sound till daylight the next morning as if we had been in the best house in Europe'.[2]

On occasion he got into trouble for being too venturesome. At the fight at Bloomingdale on the 16th September 'I dressed the wounded and had them put into barns and stables till I could establish a proper hospital'[3] and on the following day he set about this by cleaning out three empty houses, and laying down bedding so that very shortly 'I had nurses, stewards, orderly men, and in short as complete a hospital as if I had been a month about it.'[4] But it was so near the enemy that the hospital was soon under shell fire and he was compelled to ask for infantry to protect it and a frigate to stand by at sea. Eventually he was compelled to abandon the hospital site in the middle of the night clad only in a shirt. 'The laugh', he grudgingly admits 'is against me.'[5]

With Howe's advance to White Plains he sailed up the East River in the hospital ship *The Peace and Plenty* and after the action on the 25th October had 143 wounded to treat on board and take back to New York. Then an incident occurs which is typical of the reverse side of any war; for men to keep sane and balanced in time of conflict the mental stresses and physical dangers of the battlefields must at times be set aside for pleasures which are often simple ones, but by contrast to the horrors which have preceded them are wonderfully gratifying. We read 'of a comfortable house shared with the colonel and other officers—a small room—a good fire—a grilled fowl and sausages—a bottle of port and excellent porter completed a comfortable repast— jolly and hearty ones we have had but this was comfortable—we had table cloths, ate off plates, and had glasses for our wine, and breakfast with good soft bread, new butter, cream and tea'.[6]

The drain of troops for the American war made it imperative to raise the army establishment again, and this was increased to 89,000 in 1777, including 24,000 foreign troops, mainly Hessians. But after the troops left for the protection of the British Isles and the Mediterranean stations there were only 57,000 for the prosecution of the war as well as staffing the colonial garrisons. America could be recovered only by an overwhelming force, and the numbers available were plainly inadequate.

The main base for general hospitals was now at New York and before long there were seven of these scattered in buildings throughout the town. They were known respectively as the General, College, Vauxhall, Brick Meeting, Ranelaugh, Poor House, and Quaker Meeting hospitals with a total of 3,000 beds, of which the College Hospital was the largest with over 1,000 beds. Naturally there was an increased medical staff and there were now 5 physicians, 3 purveyors, 8 surgeons, 8 apothecaries and 60 hospital mates. Of these the highest paid were the purveyors[7] at 25s. a day, no doubt with the idea of discouraging peculation by providing good pay; physicians received 20s., surgeons and apothecaries 10s., and hospital mates 5s. a day. The purveyor's task was to provide accommodation, supply equipment, beds, bedding, fire and light, and 'good wholesome food'. The subordinate staff of clerks, stewards, storekeepers and cooks were often locally enlisted, while orderlies from regiments and soldiers' wives attended the patients in the wards.

It was obviously necessary to co-ordinate the work of these hospitals by appointing some administrative head, and in 1776 Howe informed the Secretary at War that he wished to select for this post Mr. Mallett, whom we last met at Mobile fifteen years before and who now held the dual commission of surgeon and purveyor. To supervise the treatment in the regimental hospitals Dr. Morris was made Inspector of Regimental Infirmaries.

In these wartime general hospitals the essential need for smooth administration was to co-ordinate the work of physician and surgeon and define their responsibilities, so as to avoid the 'confusion and disagreement' which so often arose between them. Mr. Adair the Inspector of Regimental Infirmaries at the War Office who controlled the overseas medical arrangements fully appreciated these problems and laid down hospital regulations to make the position clear. 'The physician and chief surgeon are the principal officers of the hospital, and the physician has the chief administrative control and responsibility to visit the sick, prescribe diet and medicines, see sick are in well ventilated wards, and assign duty to other physicians, apothecaries and mates. He can suspend any doctor from duty until the Hospital Board sits.' This Board composed of a physician, a master surgeon and a purveyor, was set up to exercise disciplinary powers, and could dismiss mates, nurses and hospital servants, but could only report commissioned medical officers to the C.-in-C. for his final decision. The reader will notice that there is no mention of a physician giving orders to a surgeon, but regulations contained a paragraph which said that operations could only be performed with the consent of both physician and surgeon. This was done to ensure that a surgeon was not free to exercise his skill or the lack of it on the patient until the diagnostic ability of a physician had agreed with the treatment. It is not clear whether this regulation applied to men wounded in battle and as a proportion of amputations were done at regimental hospitals level it would in any case have been impossible to implement. In spite of this attempt to create good relations between the branches of the profession Adair reported in 1782 that the harmony of the hospitals had suffered by disputes concerning precedence between the physicians and surgeons and the whole corps thereby rendered contemptible.

Howe's plan was now to capture the capital, Philadelphia, but his forces, strung out on the Delaware River, suffered a reverse when Washington, whose army had been increased to 6,000 men, out-manoeuvred General Cornwallis, and by a bold and skilful action in January 1777 drove his troops back to Princeton. The spirits of the revolutionary party revived and recruits flocked to join, not omitting however to keep their certificates of loyalty to King George safely in their pockets. The farmers cared little about the quarrel but a great deal about their farms, and were quite ready to swear allegiance to anyone for the sake of peace. Howe realized that his enemies were ready to swarm upon him from every side at the first sign of a British reverse, and the loss of nearly all New Jersey meant that apart from the capture of New York the whole operation required to be done again. This campaign had been based on the promised help of the loyalists, but these, as events proved, never fulfilled his expectations.

Our history must now trace the events of the war in the northern part of the state of New York which bordered on Canada. In 1776 eight battalions had arrived as reinforcements in the St. Lawrence River, and together with some 4,300 Hessians the strength of this force amounted to some 13,000 men. Driving back the Americans with heavy loss from Three Rivers, a town on the St. Lawrence between Quebec and Montreal, General Carleton advanced some 100 miles to the southern end of Lake Champlain, which meant the Americans were driven completely out of Canada. The dense woods and mountains, the rough tracks, and the long lines of communication made progress slow, so that it was not until October that the British were able to resume the attack. But the Americans slipped away in retreat and escaped capture, and then, instead of advancing to take Fort Ticonderoga which was only 15 miles away, Carleton, against the advice of his officers, refused to do so. This proved a serious error because it disheartened the loyalists of whom there were many round the town of Albany some 70 miles to the south. The coming of winter ended the operations for the year.

Medical arrangements in Canada were under the control of Dr. Knox, Inspector of Hospitals at Montreal, and Dr. Kennedy who held the appointment of Inspector of Regimental Infirmaries at Quebec. General hospitals were situated at the bases at Montreal, Quebec, and later at Three Rivers, with small hospitals at St. John's, south of Montreal, at Oswego on Lake Ontario, and at Sorel on the St. Lawrence. At Montreal the staff comprised 3 surgeons, 2 apothecaries, a purveyor, 20 mates and 5 temporary mates.[8]

During Carleton's advance Dr. Kennedy accompanied him as chief medical officer. Owing to the long line of communications a flying hospital was formed to act as a link between the regimental hospitals and the general hospitals at the base. First established at St. John's south of Montreal, it moved forward behind the advancing troops, and when Lake Champlain was cleared of American vessels it was established at Crown Point. Kennedy found it necessary to issue dietetic instructions to prevent outbreaks of scurvy, but in general the troops enjoyed excellent health.

It was far otherwise with the Americans. The whole of their operations were broken up by an epidemic of smallpox and their hospitals were ill-supplied to deal with the outbreak. The disease had begun when their small force was in front of Montreal in 1775 and as the men were highly susceptible and unprotected by inoculation it spread with fearsome rapidity. During an early stage of the retreat from Canada Dr. Sullivan had written in ominous terms: 'The raging of the smallpox,' he says, 'deprives us of whole regiments in the course of a few days. Of the remaining regiments, from 50 to 60 in each are taken down in a day, and we have nothing to give them but salt pork, flour, and the poisonous water of the lake.'[9] In June and July 1776 Crown Point was a lazar house. Dr. Lind reported 1,800 men sick with smallpox at one time, with a total of 3,300 unfit to bear arms and with scarcely any medicines to treat them with, and on the 4th July John Adams wrote: 'Our army at Crown Point is an object of wretchedness enough to fill a human mind with horror—displaced, defeated, discontented, dis-spirited, diseased, naked, undisciplined, eaten up with vermin, no clothes, no beds, no medicines, no victuals but salt pork and flour.'[10] Driven to desperation the troops took to inoculating themselves with pus from the dried scabs.

Undoubtedly the Lake area proved most unhealthy in the summer and early autumn causing fever and ague which must have been malaria, and at Ticonderoga in September 1776 men were dying daily in the American camp without a scrap of medicine to treat them. 'It would make a heart of stone melt to hear the moans and see the distress of the sick and dying.'[11] That the American hospitals were ill-equipped there is no denying, but it must be remembered that the whole army medical service had to be built up from scratch at the beginning of the war and it was to be many months before they came to be properly organized.

At the opening of the campaign in 1777, General Burgoyne, who had arrived from England to assume command, now had at his disposal some 7,000 regular troops, 2,000 Canadian levies and a large body of Indians. By skilful manoeuvring, Burgoyne made the Americans abandon Fort Ticonderoga and pursued their retreating army, fighting rearguard actions, all the way down the upper waters of the Hudson River. By the middle of September he was at Saratoga but his troops were soon beset with extreme difficulties of supply and baggage because of the rough state of the forest roads and the destruction of the bridges, and he did not dare to advance further.

For this campaign Dr. Knox controlled the medical arrangements on the spot by going forward with General Burgoyne's staff, and detailed 1 physician, 2 surgeons, 2 apothecaries and 14 hospital mates as hospital staff. These were instructed to rendezvous at Montreal preparatory to joining the army on the 20th June at Cumberland Point at the northern end of Lake Champlain. The general hospital at Montreal admitted all sick from the regiments before their departure and a medical store depot was located between Montreal and Lake Champlain. Owing to its success in the previous campaign a flying hospital was again formed and equipped with 300 sets of bedding, with a further 300 sets in reserve; all its personnel and stores were to be taken forward along the waterways in covered boats; it was to receive sick and wounded from the regimental hospitals as they moved forward, treat and return to duty those who recovered, and evacuate by boat to Montreal those who required further treatment. There the staff included 1 physician, 1 surgeon, 1 apothecary and 8 hospital mates. On the 3rd July the flying hospital was at Three Mile Point, but by the 10th of the month Ticonderoga had been captured and a general hospital of 230 beds was opened a few miles away at Fort Independence to which the sick and wounded were sent by boat. Fever and dysentery were both common complaints and the former was so prevalent that Knox reported that not 1 man in 50 escaped, and he himself went down with it and had to return to Montreal. As treatment by Peruvian bark was highly successful this tends to confirm a malarial origin. As usual in all these campaigns soldiers' wives shared the hardships of active service and two from each battalion were ordered to help in the hospital wards, and ten men from Provincial units were brought in to act as storekeepers and orderlies. In spite of the acute shortage of provisions, Burgoyne, who was anxious to contribute everything in his power for the comfort of the wounded, directed $\frac{1}{2}$ lb. of fresh meat daily to be added to the existing ration. Fatigue parties were detailed to attend to sanitation.

By the middle of September the general hospital was some 60 miles behind the troops and orders were issued to move forward to Saratoga as soon as carts could be provided, while the regimental surgeons were summoned to a conference with the hospital surgeon to settle details of evacuation from the regimental hospitals.

In the face of outnumbering American forces Burgoyne's position was soon critical. As the result of casualties and the necessity to garrison Fort Ticonderoga he had only some 5,000 men fit for active operations, but because instructions from the War Office were imperative, he continued to press on southwards to join forces with Howe in New York. On the 19th September he won the battle of Bemis, but at the cost of 500 killed and wounded or a third of the force engaged.

While these operations were taking place General Clinton was advancing northwards from New York with a force of 3,000 men to join up with Burgoyne, and by a brilliant action on the 6th October 1777 he stormed and captured Fort Montgomery on the Hudson River. Splendid as it was, this success was too distant (nearly 150 miles) to have any pronounced effect upon Burgoyne's desperate position. In this dilemma he determined to make a last violent effort to overcome the enemy, but after the hard fought battle of Bemis Heights he was forced to retreat to Saratoga on the 8th October abandoning some 460 sick and wounded to the enemy. Burgoyne wrote feelingly to General Horatio Gates the enemy commander: 'Sir, the state of my hospital makes it more advisable to leave the wounded and sick officers whom you will find in my last camp than to transport them with the army. I recommend them to the protection which I felt I should show to an enemy in the same case.'[12] Dr. MacNamara Hayes who was in charge of this tented hospital carried the white flag, and Gates immediately responded and showed his humanity by providing a guard to protect the patients from his Redskin savages.

At Saratoga Burgoyne was soon surrounded by some 18,000 of the enemy, and he was in a critical situation as he had barely 3,500 men left of the original force of 7,000. It was in a house above the heights of Saratoga that the hospital was situated but this was quite inadequate to deal with the 598 sick and wounded in camp, and all the regimental hospitals were full. Thinking it was Burgoyne's headquarters the enemy threw some shells into the house, and the wives of officers and soldiers who were helping to tend the sick and wounded had to take refuge in the cellars. With only a muddy spring of water to supply them the patients were soon tortured by thirst until a plucky soldier's wife went down to draw water from the river. She was not fired upon, and the gratitude of all was expressed it is said in a reward of 20 guineas.

But the end was at hand for on the 17th October 1777 Burgoyne had no alternative but to surrender. Heading the medical staff captured was Dr. MacNamara Hayes with 7 British and 7 German surgeons and 8 hospital and regimental mates. When in due course the medical officers and the sick and wounded were evacuated to Albany the total of over 1,000 British prisoners who were now under treatment caused overcrowding which was distressing. Under their captured medical officers the best was done for them, although medicines and dressings were short and many of the wounded were found to have wounds crawling with maggots. The standard of treatment provided by the German surgeons was not regarded favourably by the American doctors and Dr. Thatcher wrote, 'I have been present at some of the capital operations and remarked that the English surgeons performed with skill and dexerity, but the Germans with a few exceptions do no credit to their profession. Some of them are the most uncouth and clumsy operators I ever witnessed and appear to be destitute of all sympathy and tenderness toward the suffering patient.'[13]

Dr. Hayes remained in charge of the sick and wounded prisoners at Albany from October 1777 to June 1778 when he was exchanged, and the last return from the hospital which he superintended shows that in this period of nine months 477 had been admitted, 341 discharged, 76 had died and 417 were remaining. To strike a lighter note, the immortal tune of *Yankee Doodle* was said to have been composed here by Dr. Shuckburgh, a surgeon in the hospital.

Our history must now return to events in the neighbourhood of New York where earlier in 1777 General Howe had made plans for the capture of Philadelphia. As the American army lay athwart his objective he decided to use the Navy's command of the sea to make a landing in Chesapeake Bay, some 300 miles to the south of New York. With 14,000 troops he arrived here late in August, and dividing his force into two columns with two British brigades in each column, he advanced some 30 miles and defeated Washington at the battle of Brandywine early in September with a loss of 577 killed and wounded. The American losses were nearly twice as heavy and 400 prisoners were taken.

The casualties after the battle were evacuated in waggons to a flying hospital which had been set up at Wilmington. Here too the Hessian wounded were treated until their own general hospital had come forward. Under Dr. Schoeff, their Director, they had always provided their own medical staff for their hospitals, as well as their own transport. Dr. Benjamin Rush (who was later to write an account of his experiences) and three American surgeons were allowed to come across to our lines and treat their own serious cases who were left scattered in houses after the battle and unable to be moved in their retreat; all were later returned on parole.

We have seen that Mr. Mallett, who had now served in America continuously for twenty-two years, had been recommended as director of the New York hospitals by General Howe. But with the more extensive operations against Philadelphia, Lord Barrington, the Secretary at War, informed Howe that the considerable number of general hospitals already in existence and projected, required a director more senior in rank, and proposed sending out Mr. Napier who the reader will recollect had served with zeal and ability in the previous war against the French. But after Napier had been honoured by the receipt of a knighthood his appointment was countermanded, and the post having subsequently been offered and refused by Mr. Adair the Inspector of Regimental Infirmaries at home, the choice fell on Dr. Nooth who was then serving as a physician on the hospital staff at New York and had been commissioned at the outbreak of war. This was promptly followed by ineffective protests from Mallett who was a regular officer, and from Dr. Kennedy in Canada, both of whom had been passed over.

Nooth had now seventy-three hospital staff officers under his command,[14] and a proportion of these including Nooth himself had sailed with Howe from New York and had provided the staff of both the flying and general hospital at Brandywine. Transport for these hospitals was always provided on an allotted scale, and for a general hospital twelve waggons were allowed.

Philadelphia was occupied on the 25th September 1777. A fortnight later Washington attempted a surprise attack on Germantown, some 10 miles to the north of Philadelphia, but was beaten off at the cost of over 500 British casualties while that of the Americans again exceeded 1,000 in killed, wounded and prisoners. A local resident tells us he saw a hospital being improvised in a stable, where the surgeons were beginning to arrange long tables made of doors on which to lay the wounded, friends and foes alike, for amputation.[15] Here it is pleasant to recall that in all the many instances in the war when wounded prisoners were under treatment the opposing medical forces were invited to collaborate in a manner which transcended the bitterness of the struggle. This attitude not only benefited both sides by providing additional medical assistance when it was most needed, but it emphasized the feeling that the medical profession, especially when they spoke the same language, had a fraternal aim in doing their utmost for friend and foe alike, a feeling that was to come to fruition under the aegis of the Red Cross 100 years later. Here after the fight at Germantown the British surgeons were assisted by surgeons from the neighbouring Medical College of Philadelphia, while those of the American wounded who were evacuated with their own troops were treated in an American hospital at Bethlehem where 750 were crammed into accommodation fit for only 250. It is little wonder typhus raged in the wards and in one regiment which had 40 men in hospital only 3 came out alive.

After further skirmishing between the rival forces, Howe withdrew to winter quarters in Philadelphia, and thereupon threw up his command. He had previously written to Lord George Germaine, the Minister at Whitehall, requesting 10,000 additional reinforcements in an attempt to conclude the war in the coming campaign of 1778; Germaine had refused, and Howe consequently resigned. He was ignorant of the disaster at Saratoga which had happened five days previously.

Dr. Nooth took up his headquarters in Philadelphia with Dr. Morris the Inspector of Regimental Infirmaries, and here our troops remained from September 1777 until June 1778. The hospitals were able to settle down to static conditions, and by December had 1,000 sick in their wards. Nooth appeared to exercise little effective control, for instead of taking action himself he complained to Adair of the excessive consumption of wine by patients and strangely enough of the excessive use of vegetables. One hospital had acquired a 12 acre garden, but this, he said, would not be large enough if the present 'rage' for vegetables continued. There was also trouble with hospital stoppages; soldiers were charged 5d. a day but the purveyors were allowing sailors, women and children and refugees to be treated free instead of paying their regulation charge of 4d. a day. Moreover Adair complained of the excessive number of hospital mates and hospital servants employed, and agreed with Nooth that the consumption of 3 pipes of wine[16] every week was much too high. When instructed by Adair to supervise the Hessian Hospital and provide their medicines Nooth did it with an ill grace complaining that his 'paltry' commission did not warrant the extra work involved, especially to check their accounts which he said were very irregular; the bill for medicines for 1776 and 1777 amounted to £9,200 and in one item of £656 stated to be supplied by an apothecary, the individual in question denied he had ever provided the medicines specified.

General Clinton who succeeded Howe was now ordered by Whitehall to abandon Philadelphia and concentrate his 15,000 troops on New York, some 70 miles distant. As he set off in June 1778 his march was interrupted by an American attack which was beaten off with the loss of 358 officers and men, of whom no fewer than 60 fell dead from sunstroke owing to the overpowering heat of the day.[17]

The disaster of Saratoga decided the French Government to support the cause of the revolting colonies, and a French fleet bringing 4,000 troops arrived at the mouth of the Delaware river in July 1778. This was a welcome addition to Washington's resources, and introduced a new element which he had foreseen was vital to his success. The new French and American forces lost no time in launching an abortive attack on Rhode Island which ended in recriminations between the new allies. On the British side the loss of sea supremacy which war with

France meant might bring disaster to our plans, and it was imperative to readjust them to meet this threat.

Our forces were widely scattered over the globe; in India, in the West Indies, in Gibraltar and Minorca, while in America itself there were troops at New York, on the Delaware, in Florida, Quebec, Halifax, and on the Great Lakes. Forty thousand men were required for the reconquest of America, and at a time when every British garrison needed reinforcement, this was out of the question.

It was Lord George Germaine who, at the request of the Governors of the Southern American States now directed a new sphere of operations by ordering an expedition to Georgia. The old argument was used of the number of loyalists who would assist British arms, and Germaine was not yet cured of this reliance upon the loyal section of the American population. Accordingly, a force of 3,000 men including four Provincial regiments of American loyalists was sent from New York and landed at Savannah in Georgia in December 1778. There were in fact some twenty-three regiments of American loyalists which fought with the British forces, and all these had regimental surgeons and mates of American origin. Savannah was captured following a short fight, and soon afterwards the expedition was joined by a body of troops under General Prevost who had brought them from Florida, and who now took command. An advance was made up the Savannah river to Augusta and by February 1779 the State of Georgia was in British hands. With this force to Georgia went Dr. MacNamara Hayes whom we last saw a prisoner at Saratoga, and who in accordance with custom had with other medical officers been exchanged with American medical personnel; with him he had 1 surgeon, 2 apothecaries and a number of hospital mates with the equipment for a general hospital which was established in Savannah.

An attempt to capture Charleston had to be abandoned from lack of troops and the presence of superior American forces; and then in September 1779 a French fleet suddenly appeared off the mouth of the Savannah river and the combined American and French forces proceeded to lay siege to the town. The British forces amounted to some 3,700 men of whom some 1,500 were sick, but after they had gallantly repulsed a fierce enemy assault in October with a loss to the enemy of 900 men, the attack was not resumed, and the siege ended with angry reproaches between the Americans and French.

With so many sick both the regimental hospitals and the general hospital were desperately busy. Georgia in the summer had a shade temperature of between 90° and 103° F., and the soldiers clad in their scarlet tunics were badly affected by the heat, while malaria and dysentery were rife. Adair had dispatched ample supplies of bedding and ward utensils from England and an item worthy of note was the provision of 300 mosquito nets.[18]

Meanwhile, since the end of 1778 General Clinton, except for fighting the minor action of Penobscot, had remained practically impotent at New York awaiting reinforcements from England. They came in August 1779, but instead of nearly 6,000 men expected, only 3,400 arrived, and they brought with them typhus fever which spread amongst the troops so rapidly that within six weeks 6,000 men were in hospital in New York.[19] Luckily Dr. Nooth with 58 hospital staff officers at his disposal including 4 physicians was well off for medical officers, but finding beds and equipment for such an epidemic strained his resources to the utmost, although supplies had been arriving from England at regular intervals. In March 1778 came 217 bales of bedding, hospital utensils of all kinds, provisions, 20 hospital and 30 surgeons' tents, 36 chests of medical stores, followed by additional quantities later in the year. Then in March 1779 further extensive supplies arrived.[20] The tentage was often needed for hospital use, for although buildings were taken over wherever they were available the country was in particular areas so sparsely populated that tents often provided the only form of shelter. The unexpected typhus epidemic had resulted in a shortage of medicines, and it was necessary to appropriate the West Indian supplies which came through New York, a step which as we shall see caused much suffering to a force of 5,000 troops which by Germaine's order had been dispatched to that area under General Grant.

Still wedded to the foolish plan of over-running the Southern States, Germaine now sent instructions to Clinton to undertake once again the capture of Charleston and at the end of December 1779 he sailed from New York with a force of 7,600 men. By thus dividing his army in two he had insufficient men for both enterprises, for one army was needed for the defence of New York, and one for operations against Charleston. Owing to stormy weather and the loss of some of his transports it was not until the end of January 1780 that he landed opposite the town, which was defended by 7,000 American troops behind strong entrenchments and redoubts. After a brilliant engagement when three regular regiments of American cavalry were signally defeated, he had completely invested the city by April and it capitulated on the 9th May, with insignificant losses to the besiegers and the capture of some 6,600 Americans, including the headquarters of the Hospital Department of their Southern Army and seventeen of their medical officers. As there were considerable numbers of sick in both armies suffering from fever and diarrhoea this additional medical aid was doubly welcome to staff the general hospital opened in the town. Nine medical officers including a physician had come with Clinton from New York and Dr. MacNamara Hayes who had joined Cornwallis with fourteen of his hospital staff from Georgia was now placed in charge with the pretentious title of Physician General and Inspector General.

After his resounding success Clinton was compelled to return with part of his army to New York, for he learnt that another French fleet bringing reinforcements was crossing the Atlantic and he wished to be ready to meet it. Cornwallis was left to complete the occupation of North and South Carolina, but his force was soon pitifully small, numbering only some 2,000 men fit for duty with 800 sick. In spite of these handicaps he insisted on fighting the battle of Camden in August 1780 when he defeated the Americans, losing 324 killed and wounded but killing and wounding over 1,000 of the enemy and capturing 1,000 prisoners. Hayes was present at this fight and had brought with him the staff for a flying hospital which he organized to operate with the force, but dressing the wounded was not their only task for August was a notoriously unhealthy month and a week after the battle Cornwallis wrote, 'Our sickness is great and truly alarming. Dr. Hayes and almost all the hospital surgeons are laid up.'[21] It was therefore no wonder that Dr. Williamson, an American who was given permission to visit his wounded compatriots, found they had been neglected for as long as ten days; some 250 of them, including many dangerously wounded, were found in houses without straw or covering of any kind; there were hardly any medicines and not an ounce of lint or tow, nor a single bandage.

Indeed, the climate of the Carolinas in summer was so hot and steamy that active operations were usually suspended. 'To keep troops,' wrote Cornwallis 'within one hundred miles of the coast between June and October is to risk them being rendered useless for some time . . . if not entirely lost.'[22] Dr. Jackson who was surgeon to Fraser's Highlanders had two-thirds of his regiment sick with ague within a period of nine days and he had to evacuate 220 of them to a general hospital which it had been found necessary to open at George-town, some 50 miles up the coast. Of this number 100 went by boat down the river, the other 120 in open waggons, although this entailed exposure to the scorching heat of the sun and drenching rain. But this exhausting journey did at least end in their safe arrival, while the boat party were all captured and carried off to North Carolina.

It was probably owing to Hayes initiative that we meet for the first time a new medical appointment described as Field Inspector. His duties were both sanitary adviser in the forward area and co-ordinator of evacuation by river and road from the regimental hospitals.

In spite of the heat and his losses from disease Cornwallis pushed on towards North Carolina and reached Charlottetown in September, but he was continually harassed by some 3,000 American backwoods-men who were well trained and expert in guerilla tactics, and many of his own small force were local militia who proved most untrustworthy and deserted whenever occasion offered. Then his whole plan of campaign was wrecked when one of his columns was defeated in October at King's Mountain[23] by much superior forces, and beset with scarcity of food and sickness caused by exposure and incessant rain he was forced to retreat to Winnsborough in South Carolina to conclude his operations for 1780 and to await reinforcements.

By August 1780 there were 92 hospital staff officers under the Superintendent General's direction, half of them in New York and the remainder scattered amongst the general and flying hospitals in the Southern States or with the garrisons as far south as Florida.[24]

Much hospital equipment arrived in April and August 1780, and in August 1781. Medicines were supplied in blocks or 'divisions' each containing quantities sufficient for 5,000 men for specified periods, and bedding was sent in sets each containing palliasses, bolsters, sheets, blankets and coverlets. In addition to ward furniture and utensils, surgical instruments and dressings, there was a particular item of eight machines for impregnating water with fresh air.[25]

Early in 1781 after reinforcements including the Guards Brigade had arrived, Cornwallis resumed his advance northwards with some 4,000 men. General Tarleton one of his commanders was heavily defeated at the engagement of Cowpens in January and lost 800 men killed, wounded and prisoners, very few of his force escaping. It was here that Dr. Robert Jackson distinguished himself while saving the life of his General, when his brave conduct so struck the American Commander that he was returned with the wounded when they were exchanged, without an exchange being demanded in his own case. Jackson was a remarkable character. He had arrived at New York from Jamaica in 1778 attracted by the prospect of active service, and enlisted as a volunteer in Fraser's Highlanders. Being a medical man, his Colonel gave him a temporary appointment as surgeon's mate, which would not, he said, prove a bar to his taking a combatant commission if he preferred it. Essentially a man of action, Jackson ultimately decided to devote all his energies to the profession in which he was trained, a decision which was to prove in due course of immense benefit to the service.

After Tarleton's defeat Cornwallis tried to entrap the American forces and penetrated deep into North Carolina, where on the 15th March he fought the bloody battle of Guildford and won a resounding victory over an enemy who outnumbered him by two to one. The Americans fought stubbornly and the British losses were 532 killed and wounded, more than a quarter of those engaged. The wounded of both armies were collected by the British but this took time as the ground to be covered was extensive; there were no tents or houses to shelter the cases; the night was dark and there was heavy rain; fifty died before morning.

Although a brilliant feat of arms it was no real victory for the troops were terribly reduced in numbers, had undergone great hardship and fatigue and were starving from lack of provisions. Cornwallis had no choice but to accept the inevitable and retreated the 150 miles to Wilmington, compelled owing to lack of waggons to leave his wounded under a flag of truce to the care of the local inhabitants at a Quaker Meeting House, with many assurances that he would speedily return. But worse was to follow. Throughout this time there had been practically no communication between Cornwallis and Clinton in New York and both were soon working at cross purposes. Clinton imagined that Cornwallis after the victory of Guildford had completed the conquest of the Carolinas, and the former wished to withdraw some troops which he had sent to the Chesapeake area; Cornwallis on the other hand had now decided to abandon the operations in the Carolinas, and to Clinton's utter astonishment embarked without orders on a march of some 200 miles to Virginia where he joined Clinton's forces on the Chesapeake and established himself at Yorktown. In the meantime the detached garrisons in South Carolina were one by one overcome by the enemy and many loyal Americans were abandoned.

Clinton was gravely upset by Cornwallis' tactics, but he did not order him to return to Charleston, and Cornwallis, after some skirmishing and contradictory orders from both Clinton and Germaine remained inactive at Yorktown. Here he was soon surrounded by a crushing superiority in numbers of Americans and their French allies, for a French fleet had arrived in overwhelming strength with twenty-eight ships of the line. The defences of the town were by no means contemptible but after heavy bombardment the outer defences were abandoned, and on the 14th October, after three attacks had been repulsed, two redoubts were lost which made the position almost hopeless. It was here again that Dr. Jackson's name comes to notice for his devotion to the wounded while exposed to heavy enemy fire. 'Our gallant friend,' said Sir Thomas Saumarez, 'declared he was fully determined to remain with us to the last . . . Dr. Jackson was ever greatly esteemed by all who had the good fortune of knowing his amiable qualities and very extraordinary talents.'[26]

As soon as Clinton heard of Cornwallis' predicament he hurriedly set sail from New York with 5,000 troops and 26 ships of the line, but on the 19th October 1781, Cornwallis, with hardly a gun left able to fire, with 500 casualties on his hands and over 1,500 disabled by sickness, capitulated. Clinton arrived five days too late, and sick at heart was forced to sail back to New York. This blow was perhaps the heaviest that has ever fallen on the British army and to all intents it put an end to the war. Charleston alone remained in British hands, but after much desultory fighting in South Carolina it was evacuated in December 1782, when the American War of Independence finally ended. The number who surrendered at Yorktown including hospital staff and non-combatants was 6,618 of whom 1,545 or over 23 per cent were in hospital; there were 16 hospital staff officers captured including 3 surgeons, 2 purveyors, and 10 hospital mates; while added to this number there were the regimental surgeons and mates and the German medical officers.

It was now the turn of the British to complain of the lack of treatment, and according to Duncan, the American army marched away and left the sick and wounded to fend for themselves, although every assistance had previously been promised. The sick got no proper hospital supplies and many of the slight cases wandered about the country and would have been badly off except for their own officers' help; those unfit to move were concentrated at Gloucester Point on the York River where they were under the care of their own surgeons.

Although there are no comprehensive medical records for the sick rates for the whole period of the war the figures for the year 1781 are available. These show that in June the rate was 10 per cent and in September in a strength of 37,876 there were 4,997 sick or 13 per cent. For the different areas where operations were taking place the rates varied between 12 and 28 per cent the latter figure relating to Georgia with its unhealthy climate.

	Strength	Number of sick	Percentage
New York	14,991	1,780	12
Virginia	8,018	1,545	19
South Carolina	8,852	1,045	12
Georgia	984	272	28

Within the non-operational areas of the North American command the rates varied between 5 per cent in Nova Scotia and East Florida, 7 per cent in West Florida and 12 per cent in Rhode Island.

Colonel Duncan of the United States Medical Corps has given his views on the morbidity rates in his book *Medical Men in the American Revolution*. His opinion is that the British army suffered less from sickness than the American forces because the camp discipline was better, many of the soldiers were veterans and inured to active service conditions, and the hospitals were better managed and supplied. Another American, Dr. Benjamin Rush reported that neither typhus nor smallpox affected the British to any appreciable extent and Dr. Schoeff the Director of the Hessian Medical Service agreed with this view.

Duncan's estimates in fact made out the American army as twice as sickly as the British.

> British   100   per thousand per year
> American   200   per thousand per year
> German   62·5 per thousand per year

As the average strength of the British forces was 39,196 this rate would give the total numbers of sick as 23,520 for the period of six years.

The deaths for the six years 1775–1780 amounted to 6,107 which gives an average rate of 1,018 per year or 2.6 per cent.

Deaths in North America:

	American colonies	Canada including Burgoyne's force
1775	781	
1776	869	200
1777	1202	301
1778	1311	178
1779	1154	50
1780	No return	61
	5317	790

6,107

Turning now to the German (Hessian) figure the records show that 29,687 came to America and the total deaths were 7,774, of which 1,800 were killed in battle, and 5,974 died from disease, an average over six years of 996 or 3·4 per cent. Dr. Schoeff, the Director, said that they lost many men from dysentery in the summer and autumn after their arrival in 1776, and in the winter months from chest troubles. But recently 'the surgeons', he said, 'had scarcely anything to do throughout the whole winter'.[27] This is borne out by the figures for New York where out of 8,000 Hessian troops there were only 250 in hospital.

There is little doubt that the endurance of the troops was severely tried during operations in the Southern States. Not only was their strength sapped by attacks of malaria and dysentery but the long distances they marched clad in scarlet tunics and burdened with equipment when the temperature stood at times at over 90° F. was the cause of much heat exhaustion. Supplies too were often short and hunger added to the hardships which bore heavily on their health.

One of the greatest tragedies in the American Army was the amount of disease which was contracted in the general hospitals. These institutions proved veritable death traps. It was not the bullets of the enemy but the filthy straw of the pallets or the very instruments of the surgeons that were the carriers of death; many a man going to hospital with a mild affliction caught smallpox or typhus and died miserably. But according to Jackson the American hospitals were not the only ones at fault when he complained that 'The miseries of sickness measured with the miseries of general hospitals were of small account.'[28] In the specific treatment of wounds we have found nothing to add to the description by Ranby thirty years before in his book on gun shot wounds with its bleedings and dressings of lint. Dr. Thatcher praised the skill of the surgeons after Saratoga. But these remarks probably referred to the general hospital surgeons for in later years Surgeon General Keate had no good word to say of the skill of the regimental surgeons in America and gave his opinion that 'regimental surgery was in a very defective state, the surgeons having been either appointed by purchase or taken from the mates who had been recommended by the colonels of regiments without any proof of their medical qualifications'. Duncan estimates the number of wounded as 5,000 based on the number of wounded officers which is known to have been 395, but this appears to be a low figure if a proportion of 1 officer to 25 other ranks is taken.

It is only Jackson's book that gives us any information on the treatment of the sick. The remedies chiefly used for fever included of course Peruvian bark, which was combined with many other drugs, acid of vitriol, alum zinc, tinctures of aloes and myrrh, powder of charcoal, rhubarb, calomel, camphor and blisters. Bleeding was resorted to in all illnesses and blood porringers were necessary items of all medical stores. Jackson also practised some novel methods of treatment which he had found beneficial during his own attacks of fever in Carolina. These may be called the cold water cure and the open air cure or what he called 'gestation' in the open air. The first included cold applications to the head and body in fever, cold baths and douches and drinking large amounts of cold water. Gestation in the open air he discovered accidentally himself when suffering from fever. After being driven round in an open carriage he felt much better and the fever then left him. This was probably fortuitous and coincided with the fall of temperature which occurs in malaria. Be that as it may it remained in Jackson's view a sound adjunct to treatment by drugs, and fever-stricken patients were dragged from their beds and jolted over rough roads, whether they liked it or not. On occasion this violent method of treatment became a military necessity to prevent the sick falling into enemy hands, and Jackson quotes the occasion when 120 men of Fraser's Highlanders were sent to Camden in open waggons. When they started all were diagnosed as obscure bilious remittent fever but after three days of this rough treatment and exposure to scorching sun and heavy rain the 'obscure' fever had resolved itself into definite ague which responded to bark. In the treatment of dysentery, purges and emetics such as antimony and ipecacuanha were employed; but cold water also had its uses in the form of cold compresses to the abdomen (provided, as Jackson said, there was no inflammation of the underlying organs), and by cold water injections into the rectum. With these scanty references to treatment we must leave the subject but we shall have something to say about Jackson's methods of diagnosis and treatment on a future occasion.

One of the severest criticisms made by the Americans was the harsh treatment of prisoners. Most of them were incarcerated in prison ships and the inevitable overcrowding and confinement spread disease with dreadful effect; of 2,000 prisoners confined in this way after the capture of Charleston, 800 had died from smallpox and typhus within thirteen months. At New York too complaints were continually made of the barbarity with which the prisoners were treated; starved and ill clothed, crowded into jails and prison ships, 1,700 were said to have perished in three weeks,[29] and smallpox spread to the civil population and killed hundreds, so that as many as possible left the city to undergo inoculation.

Naturally, these allegations of neglect were refuted, and Dr. MacNamara Hayes reporting on the ships at Charleston said they were not crowded and perfectly sanitary, with no reason to expect infection or disorders; he did however admit that they were a great eyesore but regretted 'there was no help for it—it must be done'.[30] The fact that epidemics did occur goes to show that either the lessons relative to overcrowding so ably demonstrated by Pringle and Monro on the Continent had been forgotten, or that as Hayes said it was under the circumstances impossible to adopt them.

One of the problems which worried Adair and the Secretary at War at Whitehall was what they considered the extravagant use of medicines. Under war conditions in America it was found that the medicine money was not enough to purchase medicines locally and provide for the surgeon's other expenses. It was therefore decided that medicines should be drawn through apothecaries at the general hospitals, but this resulted in the regimental surgeons taking advantage of their release from financial control and making extravagant demands. Moreover this allowed the surgeons to put the whole of the medicine money in their own pockets and Adair thought they should be controlled and only allowed to retain half. He also blamed the senior officers of the hospital for not exercising more judgement and control. The Secretary at War agreeing that the consumption of medicines was unreasonably high published his view on the 6th February 1781 that 'To correct these abuses it has been in contemplation to give an order that the regimental surgeons abroad should supply their respective regiments with medicines to the full amount of the stoppages made on their account from the pay of each soldier, but in consideration of the increased expenses of living to the surgeons employed on Foreign Service it is now intended that only half of these stoppages should be applied for that purpose. Each surgeon is to send annually a list of medicines he is accustomed to use in his own practice to the amount of one half of the medicine money; this list is to be sent to the Agent, who will deliver it to Apothecaries Hall, and that upon acquainting the Inspector General he has done so, it will be the Inspector's care that the full amount be sent to the regiment, but if he does not, one half of his medicine money will be stopped and paid to the Apothecary General who will account to the public for what he receives. As this may frequently be insufficient, what is further necessary will be supplied by the hospital stores but under control of the Superintendent General.' When Dr. Nooth heard of this complicated procedure he proposed a simpler and more sensible solution. He advised dispatching from home a supply of medicines based on the strength of the regiment, and if any surgeon found this insufficient he would make demands on the general hospital, where a hospital board would give its views on the necessity of each case; if the demand was found to be exorbitant, deductions would be made from the surgeon's pay with the assistance of the Apothecary General.[31]

These problems of control arose from the Government's dictum that the army must pay for itself, a rule which led to a vastly complicated system of finance which as far as the Medical Department was concerned included the payment of hospital stoppages in time of war. The clerical labour involved in this was immense, as units were continually changing location, and unless prompt payment and careful supervision was exercised the purveyors found great difficulty in maintaining accounts. At Philadelphia it was discovered the hospitals were owed the sum of £22,000, partly from units which had left the country and had to be traced. Moreover it sometimes encouraged dishonesty, and an instance occurred where a clerk had received £271 in stoppages while the purveyor was absent, and promptly deserted to the enemy!

Although the custom of a medical officer holding a combatant commission was winked at mainly because it was a pretext to increase the surgeon's wretched pay, this was not intended to include other double commissions. When it was discovered that Mr. Mallett the chief surgeon in New York was holding a commission both as surgeon and as purveyor and drawing the pay of both, the Secretary at War put his foot down. Owing no doubt to Mallett's continuous absence of twenty-two years in this distant sphere this anomaly had so far escaped the notice of the War Office. As a purveyor drew pay of 25s. a day and a surgeon only 10s., Mallett naturally chose to keep his purveyor's commission, but he complained that this new rule personally affected his honour as a surgeon, and defended his action by asserting that Mr. Napier before him had held a similar double commission.

Then a medical scandal arose when Mr. Jefferies, a surgeon, was refused leave to go home on urgent private affairs. He promptly resigned and sold his commission to Mr. Loring, a hospital mate, for the sum of £600. Adair was horrified when he heard of it and said that such a thing had never occurred before, although Jefferies quoted a previous case in Havana which the War Office denied. The Secretary at War at once put a stop to such transactions on the grounds that the sale of commissions between doctors might lead to a medical man entering the service who would be unfit to look after the health of the troops. Most of the regimental surgeons being of indifferent professional ability the Medical Board refused to advance them to the position of physician and only occasionally to that of hospital surgeon, although from their knowledge of drugs it was conceded that they could be appointed as apothecary; but as this was a limited avenue of promotion the regimental surgeons had little cause for satisfaction. Not so the hospital mates, who in 1781 were rewarded by an increase of pay from 5s. to 7s. 6d. a day provided they showed zeal and ability; at the same time the Secretary at War said mates of poor standard were to be discharged and future ones made to pass an examination. As mates only held warrants and not commissions, they could be discharged at any time without compensation as they did not qualify for half pay.

Although fighting had ended in 1782 British troops remained in the country until peace was signed in 1783. There were then general hospitals at New York and Boston, with hospital staff detachments at St. Augustine in Florida, in South Carolina, at Providence in Rhode Island, and at Halifax, Newfoundland, and Bermuda. In 1782 Mr. Lorimer was made Inspector of Regimental Infirmaries in place of Dr. Morris with pay of 20s. a day. This was a step in promotion which encouraged the regular officers, for Lorimer had been a regimental and garrison surgeon for twenty years, seventeen of them spent in West Florida. The accepted policy was to allow these garrison surgeons, who after all had little prospect of promotion, to settle down in one station for the greater part of their service, and Mr. Catherwood at St. Augustine in Florida was another who preferred to spend nearly twenty years in this remote location. No doubt happy to be independent of too much official control, he found this at times tiresome when equipment and medicines failed to arrive, and for bedding he was forced to use spruce branches and palliasses filled with leaves, and provide medicines out of his own pocket. But he was not averse to making a few guineas when the opportunity offered, and he astonished Adair by sending in a bill for 63 guineas for inoculating thirty-six men against smallpox. Not only, said Adair, was this double what it would cost at home where the charge was a guinea for each recruit but the inclusion of 4 gallons of rum and a equal quantity of brandy was a pure waste of money when the correct treatment after inoculation was water gruel and bread pudding!

It was in June 1783 that the hospitals finally closed down and the surplus equipment was either sent to hospitals in Canada or was disposed of locally. In Canada the general hospitals at Three Rivers and Montreal remained, with an additional one at St. John's, Newfoundland. But as there had been no operations since Burgoyne's surrender at Saratoga in September 1778 there were fewer than 100 in hospital, most of them suffering from fever and the effects of scurvy. The general hospital of 130 beds at Quebec had been closed in 1781; previously in the Augustinian convent, it had been moved in 1778 to a new site because serious trouble had arisen over the nuns attempts to proselytise the Protestant patients, attempts which are described in more vivid language by the medical officer in charge 'it has been said I believe with truth that the nuns of the Hotel Dieu have killed some of our sick by tampering with them about their conversion when in a state of great weakness of body and mind'.[32]

Hospital diets laid down by Dr. Knox the Inspector of Hospitals in Canada can be regarded as typical of all hospitals in North America.

Full diet;	Breakfast	Rice, gruel or water gruel, sugar and butter.
	Dinner	1 lb. fresh meat and vegetables.
	Supper	2 oz. butter or cheese.
Half diet:	Dinner	Broth and pudding $\frac{1}{2}$ lb. fresh meat four times a week.
	Breakfast and Supper	As for full diet.
Low diet:	Breakfast and Supper	Rice or water gruel, milk porridge, sago or salop.
	Dinner	Broth and pudding.

To these diets was added 1 lb. bread and 3 pints spruce beer in summer and a quart in winter; wine, vinegar etc. as prescribed. Rice water was given as a common drink in enteritis, and barley water in fever.

Supplementing the general hospitals there were small detachments with a hospital mate at Detroit; at St. John, south of Montreal; on Lake Champlain; at Oswego, Niagara, and Coteau de Les. Some of these mates had been locally enlisted for temporary service, and that their conduct was not altogether what it should be can be gathered from the following account of James Connor who was placed under arrest at Niagara on the 21st August 1783. The charge made against him was 'For having gone on board H.M.S. *Seneca* at 3 o'clock in the morning on Sunday 17th August (having no business whatever there) and obliging Captain Bouchette, the commander of said ship to get out of his bed at that unreasonable hour when he was under sailing orders, to get him grog; for having insulted, beat, and abused the said Captain Bouchette, forcing him to quit his own ship and seek shelter on board the *Limnade*, for following him on board the *Limnade* and attacking him again there, also following him out of the *Limnade* to the wharf when he was going to his boat to complain of the violent treatment he had met with, and afterwards presenting him with pistols to fight on board the *Limnade*; and for stopping three of H.M. Ships four days idle at Niagara, breaking his arrest when put on board the *Mohawk* to go to Canada, quitting said ship on the 20th and coming on shore where he now is.' It is difficult to believe that after this wild drunken spree Connor was not instantly dismissed.

There were other enemies to fight besides America and France for in 1779 Spain and 1781 Holland had been added to the list. But first we must record the events which occurred in the West Indies during the American War if only to emphasize the lethal effects of the climate, effects which had already taught bitter lessons in the past and were to prove of deadly import in the years which lay ahead.

In 1778 General Grant sailed from New York for the West Indies with a force of 5,600 men, at the very time when every soldier was required for the conquest of North America. The French in the West Indies had already struck first and taken Dominica, but Grant after arriving at Barbados, sailed for St. Lucia within twenty-four hours and captured it. Although it was the winter and the healthy season of the year sickness soon began to take its toll. On leaving New York his sick rate had been 11 per cent, by February 1779 it had risen to 15 per cent, and by April to 24 per cent with 1,350 men in hospital and 100 deaths within the month. Grant wrote to Lord George Germaine on the 5th April, 'Without bark we should not have a man fit for duty in three months, but the hospital at New York would not give us so much as I looked for.'[33] As we know the authorized West Indies supplies of medicine had been misappropriated by Dr. Nooth at New York when the disastrous typhus epidemic had overcrowded every hospital in the place. Now the soldiers here were to pay the price in lives.

In June 1779 the French scored another success when they wrested from us the island of St. Vincent. Grenada then fell in July, and under these threats Grant redistributed his troops to safeguard our other possessions at St. Kitts and Antigua, with three battalions 1,600 strong left to garrison St. Lucia, while two further battalions had to be detailed to man the fleet, which owing to sickness and deaths was desperately short of seamen.

St. Lucia now became the chief hospital centre of the Windward Islands with a general hospital staffed by a physician, a surgeon, an apothecary, a deputy purveyor and 5 hospital mates. At Barbados the Inspector of Hospitals made his headquarters, and garrison hospitals under the charge of surgeons and mates were located here and at St. Kitts, Antigua and Tobago. As soon as Germaine realized the medicine shortage, 1,200 lbs. of bark was dispatched to the Windward and Leeward Islands in June 1779, and 600 lbs. to Jamaica, followed in November by a further 800 lbs. This ample supply brought relief to the sufferers from malaria, but much of the sickness was due to yellow fever and this disease was not affected by quinine. In St. Lucia by September there were 1,137 men fit for duty and 510 sick, a sick rate of over 30 per cent; on the 29th October the number fit for duty had dropped to 933, with 500 sick, and by the 30th December 1779 it was only 685, with 576 on the sick list, a rate of over 45 per cent; the remainder were dead. The other islands showed similar figures.

General Vaughan arrived from England to take command the following year and immediately asked for more medicines, pointing out that some medical officers had criticized the unsuitability of many of the drugs dispatched. Adair promptly asked Dr. Young the physician at St. Lucia to send a list of his essential requirements, but when he included the drug serpentaria in his list for the treatment of yellow fever Adair sent him a supply, but pointed out that it cost 9 guineas a pound. Every drug however proved useless. In the three months of June, July and August 1780 600 men died in St. Lucia alone, and between the 1st March and the 30th October there were 1,556 deaths. A reinforcement of 8 hospital mates had to be hurriedly dispatched from England to reinforce the 14 already on the island. But following a severe hurricane in October the same year which did immense damage and caused much loss of life the island became much healthier, a result due probably to the wholesale destruction by the storm of the mosquitoes and their breeding places.

Over the years the appalling loss of lives continued and a War Office return of January 1781 shows that between 1774 and 1780 3,895 soldiers were buried in island graves.

1774	—	59	
1775	—	121	
1776	—	86	
1777	—	303	
1778	—	236	
1779	—	1,054	Strength in 1779—7,130
1780	—	2,036	
		3,895	

In Jamaica conditions were almost as bad. In August 1780 out of a strength of some 2,300 men 780 were sick and 100 dead, and the mortality increased so alarmingly that between the 1st August and the 31st October 1,100 men died out of the seven and a half battalions in the country, and half of the remaining 3,000 were sick.

It is a sad reflection on the policy of government in general and the War Office in particular that over the centuries the lives of men have been considered of small account, and money spent on preserving the health of soldiers or constructing hospitals bears no comparison to the sums expended on military equipment, on transport, or on the appurt-enances of war. Such health factors were universally applicable but the authorities were blind to them, for the hidden economics which the preservation of the lives of soldiers led to were not so apparent. So the bones of countless numbers of British soldiers are scattered through-out the world, lives which might have been preserved if rules for the preservation of health had not been ignored by the commanders of armies or by Ministers in Whitehall.

A medical officer who was to make a name for his work in Jamaica was Dr. John Hunter[34] who as physician was in charge of the medical arrangements in the island. He reasoned correctly that much of the sickness was due to the unhealthy location of the barracks which were built on low ground near the coast. But in spite of the utmost pressure which Dalling the Governor and Hunter could bring to bear on White-hall, the Government on the grounds of expense strenuously opposed the construction of barracks at a higher site. Dalling wrote angrily to the Minister expressing his disgust and disappointment. 'Considered only as an article of commerce,' he said, 'these 1,100 men have cost £22,000, a sum which if laid out above ground might have saved half their lives.'[35] Once again it was the oft repeated story of the lives of soldiers being sacrificed to parsimony and neglect in Whitehall.

It would have been thought that with thousands of sick, provision of a general hospital was desirable if not essential, but Hunter con-demned such a proposal both on the grounds of expense and as being inimical to the best interests of the patients. No doubt he was influenced by the unfortunate experience of the recent American war when general hospitals had obtained such an unemiable reputation. This was because they were invariably overcrowded, and it never appears to have occurred to medical officers that a hospital extensive enough to avoid overcrowding would have been the best place for dealing with large numbers of sick by concentrating the available resources instead of dispersing them. Probably the fact was that convenient buildings large enough to accommodate large numbers without overcrowding could not be found, and therefore dispersion under the regimental hospital system was the best practical answer. This then was the policy now adopted under Hunter's advice and as it saved expense it was assured of War Office approval. The capacity of the regimental hosp-itals was increased by providing extra equipment and additional help was detailed from the hospital staff officers; a physician was sent on a tour to visit and advise on treatment; a purveyor to supervise the stores; a surgeon and four hospital mates to attend the additional number of patients. At the same time 108 bales of bedding and 137 bales of stores were sent out from England to deal with the extra numbers, an amount which should have been ten times as large.

Adair became so impressed with Hunter's ability that he had his pay increased from 20s. a day to 30s. a piece of patronage which may seem highly irregular but was excused on the grounds of the extra work involved in his visits as consultant to all the regimental hospitals. To make it appear less conspicuous the purveyor's pay was at the same time raised to 20s. a day for undertaking *his* added responsibilities. Adair was careful however not to publicize the fact, and warned Hunter it 'must be kept within your own breast'.

In his book *Observations on the Diseases of the Army in Jamaica* Hunter quotes figures of the fearful losses suffered *annually* between 1779 and 1783, deaths and invaliding being reckoned together. In his careful analysis he tells us that in the 1st Battalion of the 40th Foot two-fifths of the whole were lost in one year; in the 79th Foot four-ninths; in the 88th about one-third; in the 85th one-half; in the 92nd eleven twenty-fifths; in the 93rd nine-elevenths; in the 94th six-sevenths. On his reckoning the most severely hit regiments were wiped out in two years or less, the others within three years.

Hunter studied the combination of circumstances that was calculated to give rise to such a terrible loss of life and his rules for preserving health were sound and efficacious. Had they been adopted who can say how many lives might have been saved, even although the anopheles and stegomyia mosquitoes were the unsuspected carriers of malaria and yellow fever respectively. Troops, he said, must be well disciplined, and should arrive in the winter months to give them time to become seasoned before the rains begin; camping areas should be either on dry sandy shores or on high ground in the hills; negroes should be employed to do fatigues; soldiers must eat in messes and not cook individually; parades should be held in the early morning and never in the evening. During epidemics of yellow fever on board ship the only remedy was to remove the men to a temperate climate; and science has shown the effectiveness of this step depends on the fall in temperature, as yellow fever can only be transmitted at a minimum temperature of 70°F. He observed, as many other medical officers had before him, that the ground floors of houses were more unhealthy than the upper storeys; this again was because of the greater infestation of those lower rooms by disease carrying mosquitoes. But the excellent advice contained in these proposals suffered the fate which so often rendered them ineffective; some, such as the location of barracks were rejected on the grounds of expense; others were ignored as doctors' fads; while the hazards and exigencies of war rendered others impracticable.

Not only was Hunter observant but he was scientifically sound in some of his theories and deductions. Experiments, he said, made upon mixtures of small proportions of decaying animal matter kept moist and in a certain temperature might throw some light on the subject of disease; the different kinds of elastic vapour arising from such mixture should be carefully examined and the various kinds of 'mucores' that come upon their surface and the *insects that breed in them* should be noted. Hunter little knew how near he was to the truth, and what is more, his hygiene proposals bear the modern look, for he said that troops might remain on the same camping ground for a long time without injury to health 'if care were taken from the beginning to bury at a good depth all excrementious matter, and to have proper receptacles underground for the water used in cooking, and also all remains of victuals'.

Yellow fever defied all the variations in treatment which were tried—bleeding, emetics, purges, stimulants. The mortality varied in the different epidemics between 5 and 75 per cent, but was commonly in the region of 50–60 per cent. Malaria of course responded quickly to the use of Peruvian bark to which arsenic was sometimes added, while dysentery was then commonly treated by a combination of opium and ipecacuanha in the well established remedy of Dover's powder.

One of Hunter's important discoveries was the cause of 'dry belly ache' or *Colica Pictonum*, which he traced to the lead derived from the pipes through which rum passed in the process of distillation. Having detected the nature of the complaint and its cause the remedy consisted of substituting another metal for the lead tubing in the distilling apparatus; and this indeed had in 1723 been laid down by Public Act.[36]

From the consideration of these medical problems we must make a short reference to military activities, and refer briefly to the expedition against the Spanish and Dutch possessions in the West Indies and in Central America.

A force of 1,400 troops was sent from Jamaica on a futile expedition to the Spanish province of Nicaragua which ended in such a disastrous toll of human lives that only 320 men came back alive. The Governor of Jamaica was responsible for the station of Pensacola in Florida, which had a medical staff of 1 surgeon and 6 hospital mates; also for Mobile in Mississipi where British troops now risked attack by Spain. Mobile was in fact captured by the Spaniards in 1780. The Dutch possessions of St. Eustatius, Demerara and Essequibo were captured but lost again to the French, and they were poised for an attack on Jamaica when they were thwarted by the great victory of Admiral Rodney at the naval battle of the Saints. Jamaica was saved.

The end of the American war in 1783 was followed in the same year by the conclusion of peace with France, Spain, and Holland. By 1784 the garrisons had all been reduced and the medical staff on the other side of the Atlantic was cut down to a handful of regimental, garrison surgeons, and mates, scattered in stations between Quebec in the north through Nova Scotia and Newfoundland to Jamaica and the Windward and Leeward Islands in the South.

Concurrently, the Government reduced the size of the army, a policy which was consecrated by precedent. Scores of medical staff officers were delegated to half pay and we learn in January 1784 that many gentlemen were 'in a situation next to starving'. Ten years were to elapse before their services were again required.

REFERENCES

[1] P.R.O., W.O. 4/275.

[2] *Forster Diary*, p. 105. Essame. *Military Review*. Vol 42 No 5, Fort Leavenworth, Kansas (1962).

[3] *Forster Diary*, p. 105. Essame. *Military Review*. Vol 42 No 5, Fort Leavenworth, Kansas (1962).

[4] *Forster Diary*, p. 105. Essame. *Military Review*. Vol 42 No 5, Fort Leavenworth, Kansas (1962).

[5] *Forster Diary*, p. 105. Essame. *Military Review*. Vol 42 No 5, Fort Leavenworth, Kansas (1962).

[6] *Forster Diary*, p. 133. Essame. *Military Review*. Vol 42 No 5, Fort Leavenworth, Kansas (1962).

[7] Purveyors were medical officers.

[8] These temporary mates were enlisted locally.

[9] Trevelyan. *The American Revolution*, p. 222. Longman Green, London (1905).

[10] Duncan. *Medical Men in the American Revolution*, p. 100. Pennsylvania Medical Field Service School (1931).

[11] Duncan. *Medical Men in the American Revolution*, p. 102. Pennsylvania Medical Field Service School (1931).

[12] Duncan. *Medical Men in the American Revolution*, p. 254. Pennsylvania Medical Field Service School (1931).

[13] Duncan. *Medical Men in the American Revolution*, p. 257. Pennsylvania Medical Field Service School (1931).

[14] Three physicians, 1 chief surgeon and purveyor, 7 surgeons, 1 apothecary and deputy purveyor, 3 apothecaries, 58 hospital mates.

[15] Duncan. *Medical Men in the American Revolution*, p. 216. Pennsylvania Medical Field Service School (1931).

[16] A pipe of wine was 105 to 138 imperial gallons according to the kind of wine.

[17] Fortescue. *History of the British Army*, book XI, chapter XII, p. 254. Macmillan, London (1910).

[18] Palliasses, bolsters, coverlets 600 of each, sheets 900, blankets 1,200, wooden bowls, spoons, knives, forks 600 of each, close stools 50, bed pans 30, chamber pots 300, urinals 50, blood porringers 36, hospital tents 12, provisions, stationery, mosquito nets 300.

[19] Fortescue. *History of the British Army*, book XI, chapter XIV, p. 285. Duncan suggests this may have been an epidemic of influenza. Macmillan, London (1910).

[20] Bedding—1,800 coverlets, 3,600 blankets, 3,600 sheets, 1,000 palliasses, 800 mattresses. Wooden ware—2,500 bowls, 4,000 spoons, 1,000 trenchers, 500 platters, 600 brooms. Pewter ware—50 bed pans, 600 chamber pots, 100 urinals, 100 close stool pans, 50 wash basins, 100 blood porringers. Kitchen ware—tools, provisions, stationery.

[21] Duncan. *Medical Men in the American Revolution*, p. 320. Cornwallis to Clinton. Pennsylvania Medical Field Service School (1931).

[22] Duncan. *Medical Men in the Americal Revolution*, p. 312. Cornwallis to Clinton. Pennsylvania Medical Field Service School (1931).

[23] Two surgeons were killed and one captured.

[24] *New York*. Dr. Nooth, Superintendent General; Dr. Morris, Inspector of Regimental Infirmaries; Mr. Mallett, master surgeon and purveyor; 1 physician, 5 surgeons, 3 apothecaries, 38 hospital mates.

South Carolina, Charleston and Georgetown. Dr. MacNamara Hayes, Physician General and Inspector General; 2 surgeons, 2 apothecaries, 1 deputy purveyor, 12 hospital mates.

On operations with General Cornwallis—Mr. Alexander Grant, Field Inspector and surgeon 1 physician, 1 surgeon, 6 hospital mates.

Georgia. One apothecary, 6 hospital mates.

Florida. St. Augustine. One surgeon, 2 hospital mates.

Pensacola. One surgeon, 6 hospital mates.

On detachment to regiments or prisoners—Six hospital mates.

[25] This may have been soda water.

[26] Gore. *Our Services under the Crown*, p. 120. Ballière Tindall & Cox, London (1879).

[27] Duncan. *Medical Men in the American Revolution*, p. 374. Pennsylvania Medical Field Service School (1931).

[28] Jackson. *An Outline of the History of Fever*, p. 392. Mundell and Son, Edinburgh (1798).

[29] Duncan. *Medical Men in the American Revolution*, p. 152. Pennsylvania Medical Field Service School (1931).

[30] Duncan. *Medical Men in the American Revolution*, p. 320. Pennsylvania Medical Field Service School (1931).

[31] Dr. Nooth to Mr. Adair 6th July 1781.

[32] P.R.O., W.O. 28/6.

[33] P.R.O., C.O. 5/173.

[34] Not to be confused with his famous surgical namesake.

[35] Fortescue. *History of the British Army*, book XI, chapter XVII, p. 341. Macmillan, London 1910).

[36] Act 10, George I, C.2.

Chapter 7

ARMY MEDICAL BOARD

The last we saw of John Hunter was at the termination of his experiences in Portugal in 1763 when he retired on half pay. Now over twenty years later he is to make his re-appearance on the medical stage and in a position of importance. When Adair succeeded Middleton as Surgeon General in 1786 he was over 70 years of age and it soon became evident that younger blood was needed to carry the administrative burden. Therefore in the same year 1786 a deputy surgeon general was officially appointed, and the choice fell on Hunter who at 58 years of age was recalled from half pay. Although this half pay was only 5s. a day it had proved a desirable addition to his income, and he had continued to draw it for over twenty years. Hunter was at this time at the height of his civilian career. He had been made a Fellow of the Royal Society in 1768, Surgeon to St. George's Hospital the following year, and in 1776 Surgeon Extraordinary to the King. When his life of scientific investigation and unremitting toil is taken into account it is strange that he should have accepted the extra duties which his new task involved, although he could hardly refuse while continuing to draw half pay. Apart from this he was no doubt glad to earn the extra 10s. a day, for as a good Scot he was always mindful of the 'bawbees'. Moreover in 1786 Britain was at peace, and his duties were not arduous, for there were only 133 regular medical officers in the service.

There is some uncertainty about the date of Hunter's appointment, for although most authorities give 1786 as the year of his becoming deputy surgeon general there is evidence that he was engaged in medical affairs as early as 1781[1] when he was living in Leicester Square, and in 1782 he was already engaged in making plans to change the methods of army promotion. From his previous service in Portugal Hunter was convinced that the experience the regimental surgeons gained in the treatment of medical diseases in all climates and in all parts of the world fitted them to become physicians and more than compensated for their lack of academic medical qualifications. The reader may remember the application he had himself submitted in Portugal to be made a physician on similar grounds. When in 1790 he became Surgeon

General after Adair's death he was in a position to enforce his policy. There is also some confusion over the date when Hunter succeeded Adair as Surgeon General. Everard Home in his *Life of Hunter* gives it as 1792; Joseph Adams says 1789[2], but the official records show that Robert Adair died on the 16th March 1790 and Hunter was appointed Surgeon General on the 17th March 1790,[3] and combined this appointment with that of Inspector of Regimental Infirmaries.

The main task he set himself was to improve the professional standard of the regimental surgeons which had been adversely reported on in the American War. Hunter himself had remarked, 'It is hardly necessary for a regimental surgeon to practice in the army anything of surgery,'[4] and Adair had also formed the same opinion. He started with the regimental mates. It had been customary for colonels of regiments to promote their own mates to vacancies as regimental surgeons in their own unit, but Hunter stopped this and insisted on keeping their selection under his personal control. This led to many clashes with commanding officers but he refused to be intimidated or alter his policy. 'No man,' he wrote to the Secretary at War, 'but a professional man is judge of professional merit, and even few of them.'[5] His next step was to promote regimental mates into hospital mates, for he decided that a period of hospital service would broaden their experience; only after recommendation by the physicians and surgeons of hospitals would they then be eligible for appointment as regimental surgeons.

Further, as his chief aim was to create capable hospital surgeons he wished to select the best of the regimental surgeons who showed aptitude and ability but discard the older long service men who had little opportunity for surgery while serving in the isolated conditions of regimental life. 'I think the little practice the generality of regimental surgeons have done does not qualify them to be hospital surgeons.'[6] But as he considered that many regimental surgeons would make better physicians than operating surgeons he was ready to promote them in that class as well as appointing them apothecaries and purveyors. All these steps indicated his passionate desire to recognise talent in promotion rather than patronage, and by this he hoped to attract good potential surgeons to enter as regimental mates. As a further encouragement he created in hospitals the new rank of staff surgeon.

The Secretary at War gave his blessing to this policy and all the regular medical officers were delighted with the improved chances of seniority and higher pay. Complaints were made by commanding officers to Lord Amherst the Commander-in-Chief at the Horse Guards but Hunter stood his ground, for as he said, 'Since the above plan has been adopted and most religiously exercised on my part the Physical (Medical) Gentlemen of the Army have looked to me as their protector.'[7]

Next, he took steps to widen recruitment, for up to 1788 candidates were admitted only by appearing before the Surgeon General in London; this was now extended to Dublin, and in special cases to Edinburgh.

One may ask where the training of regimental mates as hospital mates was to take place? The answer is that the establishment of general hospitals at home had at last been forced on an unwilling Treasury by public opinion which had been scandalized by the hardships suffered by the invalids arriving at the ports from America. To pay medical staff officers at home was an expense which so far had been strenuously resisted, but by 1781 there were general hospitals at Portsmouth for 60 patients, at Chatham for the same number, and at Carisbrooke in the Isle of Wight; while in 1782 Adair was pressing for one at Plymouth of 100 beds. It was not only at the ports that complaints arose, for Hunter raised the question of invalids arriving from New Brunswick and Halifax who were quartered in public houses round Chelsea, who were in want of comfort and good nursing, and free to drink spirits which Hunter says, 'will make disorders incurable and desperate'.[8] He asked the Commissioners of Chelsea Hospital to provide shelter for them. Providing medical staff officers for general hospitals presented no difficulty for there were 178 who had served in the American campaign on half pay,[9] amongst them 15 physicians and 59 surgeons.

An account of the life and prospects of the regimental medical officer is given by Dr. Robert Hamilton in his *Duties of a Regimental Surgeon* published in 1787. It is not an encouraging one. The pay of surgeons at 4s. a day or £73 a year was so poor that no doctor, unless he was attracted by the adventure and comradeship of a soldier's life would think of taking up a commission when he could make four times that amount in civil life, and it is not surprising that in general only candidates of poor quality came forward. The mode of entry was either by purchase of a regimental surgeon's commission or as a regimental mate without purchase. For a commission by purchase a candidate was required to be a university graduate or at least a Licentiate of the College of Surgeons and he had also to pass a form of army examination at the college in the presence of the Surgeon General who possessed no great power of patronage. A few well qualified men who could not afford to purchase a commission at the cost of some hundreds of pounds entered as regimental mates.

The majority of surgeons spent their whole army career with their regiments, and were happy to do so because the regimental feeling was extremely strong and they preferred a carefree life; on the other hand there was in peacetime practically no choice, for the opportunities for promotion were extremely limited. A few were offered appointments as garrison surgeons which gave them slightly increased pay and a permanent station which might prove an inducement if they were married. As the Empire grew the opportunity to take up such posts became more numerous, ranging from the West Indies to the Mediterranean garrisons, and from Canada to West Africa. It was, however, in time of war that much wider avenues of promotion presented themselves, for general and flying hospitals were then created and appointments as surgeons, apothecaries, and purveyors on the staff became available to the more efficient regimental surgeons.

There was, however, a major disadvantage which faced the holder of any appointment on the staff of a general hospital for at the end of hostilities these hospitals were disbanded and the staff relegated to half pay. By this policy the more efficient medical officers were lost to the service in peacetime and were forced to take up private practice to maintain themselves until the outbreak of a fresh war made a recall to the colours possible.

Hamilton then refers to the regimental mates. We have already pointed out that with their shabby rate of pay, 2s. 6d. a day, they were inevitably of poor quality even in peacetime, but when war broke out and the strength of the army increased, the necessity for additional mates was so demanding that they were accepted after the briefest training under a country apothecary without ever having been to a medical school or heard a single lecture. So desperate was the need that the case of a private soldier can be quoted who, after assisting the surgeon to 'spread plasters' in the capacity of orderly man was appointed regimental mate. 'Diligence,' wrote Hamilton, 'and a mind turned to enquiry and observation may in a great measure supply the place of education, but when both are wanting the consequences are obvious.'[10] Such a scandalous state of affairs was bound to occur until more pay could be wrung from a hard-fisted Treasury, and at last in 1763 the Government was forced to give way and the rate increased to 3s. 6d. a day. Even with this addition a regimental mate, at the end of a year would have been able to save less than £5 to spend on himself, as the following table shows:

Mate's pay at 3s. 6d. a day		£63 17s. 6d. a year
Subsistence issued at 3s. a day	£54 15s. 0d.	
Poundage stopped by Government at 1s. in the £	£3 3s. 10½d.	
Chelsea Hospital, one day's pay	3s. 6d.	
Warrants and contingencies—two days' pay	7s. 0d.	
Agency fees 2d. in the £	10s. 7½d.	£58 19s. 6d.
Remainder of pay		£4 18s. 0d.

The mate performed most of the hospital duties, the surgeon paying only occasional visits, while he never failed to get an admonition from the Surgeon General to 'beware of expense in medicines'.

To conduct the affairs of the regimental hospital an infirmary board of three captains sat once a month to examine the state of the hospital and report to the commanding officer. The surgeon had to lay a statement of expenses and other matters relating to it before the board for their inspection. When the regiment was in barracks a subaltern visited the hospital daily between 10 and 12 noon to make his report to the commanding officer of the number of patients and how they were attended. The surgeon or his mate had to attend morning and evening roll-calls at all times when the regiment was under arms, and had to be present at all punishments to judge if the deliquent's life was in danger, so that no punishment might endanger life or limb. One order to note which is in direct contrast to modern army ideas, says that any man presuming to cut off his hair, except thought necessary for medical reasons, shall be confined for disobedience! In fact it was not until the Peninsular War that the soldier was permitted to remove his queue.

In peacetime the opportunities for promotion depended on vacancies amongst the regimental and garrison surgeons, and these were so infrequent that a mate might serve in this rank for as long as twenty years. Moreover, only holding warrant rank meant that he could be dismissed at will, for he was not entitled to half pay; further, he could be flogged or sent to the regimental prison in the same way as a private soldier. But when war broke out his chance of promotion greatly improved with the formation of new regiments which required surgeons, or with the prospect of becoming a hospital mate on the staff of a general hospital. The steps in promotion which were then open were: regimental mate, hospital mate, regimental surgeon, apothecary, purveyor and even surgeon to a hospital. The last named might be selected from a wide range of possible candidates: apothecaries, regimental surgeons, hospital mates, or direct from civil life. The reader will note that physicians do not appear in the promotion ladder because they were an *imperium in imperio* and maintained their exclusiveness.

The policy of keeping regiments in individual stations had the effect of isolating surgeons from their medical colleagues, and they had no opportunity to interchange ideas. Combined with the inducements of sport which always pervaded regimental life this isolation tended to make surgeons rusty and out of date in their knowledge of recent advances. It is true they were encouraged to discuss their cases with local practitioners and to borrow their medical books, while Hamilton is insistent that they should carry about with them their own library of some thirty books for 'without an almost daily application to them his practice must be mere quackery and his views confined'.[11] A list of these is given in an appendix[12], but amongst the more important are Lynd on scurvy, Pringle and Monro on soldiers' diseases, Simmons and Hunter on venereal disease, and the works on operative surgery. Such a list may seem extensive for a regimental medical officer, but it must be remembered that he was both physician and surgeon and for the most part the sick lived and died in their own hospitals.

During the summer months regiments were often encamped together for exercises and it was then that surgeons were able to meet their brother officers for an interchange of ideas. On these occasions a combined regimental hospital would be established and a physician sometimes appointed to assist with more specialized treatment.

Hamilton who was writing about conditions some twenty years after Brocklesby, describes the regimental hospital in less depressing terms. Accommodation for twenty-five patients was the common provision, ten beds being set apart for single patients who were seriously ill, the remainder for double occupancy; this was often a compulsory measure due to the difficulty of finding a house with space enough for separate beds. Mattresses of flock or straw, sheets and bolsters were provided but hospital furniture was scanty and Hamilton says he never saw a bed pan in use until he had one made of tin. Sometimes it was impossible to find a civilian willing to let his house as a hospital for 10s. a week, and the surgeon had to visit the sick in their billet which was often a cold dark foul garret with such difficulties in treatment and attendance that the chances of cure were certainly retarded.

Let us now consider the treatment of the commoner diseases. Fever cases generally were treated with Peruvian bark (quinine) and Fowler's solution which contained arsenic. For typhus fever many remedies were prescribed; opium was a popular drug, up to 80 drops of the tincture combined with wine, or from 9 to 13 grains of the powder. Lung tuberculosis was common and often fatal, and made worse, says Hamilton, by the purgings, bleedings, and low diet which sent thousands to their graves. Operations were rarely performed except for accidents such as fractures. Leg ulcers were a common disability, often caused by the gaiters which the soldiers wore and sometimes aggravated by the men themselves when they wanted to malinger. Venereal disease was common and mercury carried to the point of salivation was the sheet anchor for syphilis. Medical electricity was just coming into vogue and the Galvanic battery recently discovered was used for the treatment of eye cases, chronic rheumatism, and hemiplegia, more it would appear with enthusiasm for a new method of treatment than with any scientific reason.

Turning to the prevention of disease we find that the first glimmerings of hygiene were beginning to be applied after the writings of Pringle and Brocklesby, while Dr. Miller wrote: 'Success in war depends upon preserving military force in health and vigour. Disarmed by sickness the most intrepid warrior becomes a prey of the most pusillanimous adversary. Fleets and armies moulder away by diseases.' Although a good C.O. might sometimes listen to his surgeon's advice in attempting to preserve his men's health, the medical officer's low status (junior in rank to the youngest ensign) meant that his word carried little weight and his preaching was usually in vain.

Hunter during his period in office was much concerned with military operations in the West Indies. Like his namesake the physician he was totally opposed to opening general hospitals which he was convinced were fatal to the sick, and preferred regimental hospitals supervised and inspected by the island garrison surgeons every three months. Although the expenses of regimental hospitals in peacetime were expected to be paid out of hospital stoppages, a free hand was given to the Governor to provide extra articles of diet required on indent by the garrison surgeon and their cost written off as expenses. A further indulgence was allowed for medicines in those islands where there was a high incidence of disease or epidemics of yellow fever. Items such as cantharides, calomel, jalap, rhubarb, ipecacuanha, and vitriolic acid were sent out free from England at six monthly intervals. Dr. James' powder too had such a great reputation and was such a high price that twelve dozen powders were sent to units in the West Indies for trial in 1789.[13] The hospital allowance for which £30 a year was allowed in Britain varied between £20 and £40 in countries abroad according to conditions and prices.

With the outbreak of the French Revolutionary War in 1793 which will be dealt with in the succeeding chapter heavy responsibilities devolved on the Surgeon General to make medical arrangements for the expeditionary force which was dispatched to Flanders in that year. As Wintringham was incapable owing to his poor state of health, Hunter had all the work to do, but unhappily he had little chance to show his capabilities for on the 16th October 1793 he died from what appears from the evidence available to be coronary thrombosis. For some years he had been a victim of angina pectoris which was made worse by any form of excitement or mental worry. As he himself declared 'his life was in the hands of any rascal who chose to annoy or tease him'.[14] One day while he was attending at St. George's Hospital he suddenly dropped dead. The post mortem examination confirmed that the coronary arteries were calcified.

Hunter's scientific achievements need not be emphasized here as they are sufficiently well known to merit universal acclaim. But during his short period of three years in the highest army medical office he brought a new vision on medical problems and quickly perceived that the unchanging routine of regimental service was inimical to the advancement of clinical medicine and surgery. His instructions to broaden medical officers' experience by giving hospital training before promotion was distinctly beneficial to the efficiency of the service.

Dr. Robert Jackson described Hunter as 'a man of an original mind and considerable discernment, but too little acquainted with military operations in the field to foresee everything that was likely to occur in military service and provide on all occasions . . . the best means of remedy'. This is probably an accurate assessment of his work as Surgeon General when faced with wartime responsibilities, for his service experience was limited by the short period he spent at Bellisle and in Portugal.

As a writer from the military angle his treatise on *The Blood, Inflammation and Gun Shot Wounds* which was published a year after his death was a masterly work. Billroth the German surgeon called it the cornerstone of modern English and German surgery. In it Hunter condemned what he called 'meddlesome surgery' and his advice was to leave well alone, especially in the case of abdominal wounds; the finger, he said, was the best instrument for exploration, while bullets in a non-vital area should be left alone. For the same reason he was against the immediate amputation of limbs in all cases and was the first to advocate excision of joints as an alternative to removing the whole limb. Owing to this he has been represented as preferring secondary to primary amputation, a principle which was regarded with disfavour by subsequent surgeons. With his genius for scientific observation he appreciated the damage caused by the velocity of bullets. Moreover, he was the first to investigate the problems of surgical pathology. This fact was aptly referred to by MacCormac when he said Hunter elevated surgery to a science.

Our history now comes to the period of the French Revolutionary Wars and the rise of Napoleon; a time of almost continuous warfare which spanned a period of twenty-two years from 1793 to 1815. This conflict ranged over many continents and many countries and involved not only France but Holland, Spain and North and South America.

The month of October 1793 was an important landmark in the history of the medical service for under orders of the Secretary for War the direction of affairs following the death of Mr. Hunter was now invested in a Board of three members, which exercised control from 1793 until 1809. When they took office the members were Sir Clifton Wintringham, Mr. Gunning, and Mr. Keate, and in this chapter we follow the fortunes of the Board from its inception until it ceased to exist.

Sir Clifton Wintringham, already a sick man, died only a few months later in January 1794 and was succeeded by Sir Lucas Pepys. Pepys had studied medicine at Edinburgh and Oxford when in 1774 he had taken his degree of M.D., and in keeping with the policy of choosing an eminent civilian he was Physician in Ordinary to the King. In 1804 while holding the appointment of Physician General he was made President of the Royal College of Physicians. His high professional

attainments were regarded as outweighing his lack of military knowledge for he had no previous experience of army medicine or administration. Mr. Gunning, also a civilian, was nominated Surgeon General,
and held the appointment of surgeon to St. George's Hospital and
Master of the Surgeon's Company. Thomas Keate, the only officer
who had had regular service was made Inspector of Regimental Infirmaries. He had been regimental surgeon to the Foot Guards in 1778, and
was surgeon to the Royal Hospital at Chelsea; he at least had some
knowledge of army procedure.

In accordance with the established custom these appointments were
only part time ones and the members continued to pursue their civilian
vocations. When the Board came into being they were given no specific
instructions by the Secretary for War as to how they should proceed,
and for the first few years the members acted in unison.

With many campaigns being fought simultaneously in Europe, in
the Mediterranean, and the East and West Indies, it might have been
thought that the members would have been overwhelmed by their
army duties. Nothing could be further from the truth. Their official
office hours lasted from twelve noon until two o'clock daily, when as
Mr. Keate observed, they were *generally* at their desks, although
officers complained they could never be found, and there is evidence
that a great deal of their army work was done from their private
residences, the rest of their time being devoted to their private practices.
For these few hours of military duty the members drew pay at the rate
of £2 a day, and with the addition of their lucrative civil appointments
they were handsomely remunerated. Mr. Keate was made surgeon to
the Queen and the Prince of Wales; as surgeon to the Royal Hospital
Chelsea, he drew £100 a year; for operating sessions at the York Military Hospital in Chelsea he was paid the generous sum of £700 a year in
peace, and £900 a year in war. He was in addition Inspector of the
National Cow-pox Establishment, surgeon to St. George's Hospital
and examiner to the College of Surgeons. Together, his official emoluments came to over £1,800 a year apart from what he earned in private
practice. There is little wonder he could spare only two hours a day for
army duties.

At the Medical Department headquarters at Upper Brook Street
and later at Berkeley Street there was an office hardly worth the name.
One hundred pounds a year and an allowance of 10s. a day was the
total sum allowed to cover the office expenses, and it was not until
1796 that a niggardly Treasury was persuaded to allow an establishment of three clerks, one of whom acted as Secretary to the Board.
Under such straitened conditions it is a wonder that the Department was
able to function effectively at all, but if their duties are examined in
detail certain points emerge. In the first place the Board could not
interfere in the purely administrative side of the regimental hospitals

which were under the colonels of the regiments, and were run by them as they wished. The regimental surgeon and his assistant were essentially regimental officers, being by right servants of the colonel according to the old regimental system. The Inspector of Regimental Infirmaries whose duty it was to make periodical inspections of these establishments was primarily concerned with the professional standards of treatment, the adequacy of the diet, and the quality of medicines supplied.

For overseas expeditions the Board had extensive responsibilities mainly devoted to three objectives. These were the provision of general hospitals and their equipment, the selection of the medical staff officers to serve in them, and the free supply of medicines and surgical instruments. The provision of the subordinate medical staff such as ward masters, stewards, and attendants, was not their concern as they were all supplied under local arrangements. The basic allotment for planning was a physician for every 2,000 soldiers in the force, a staff surgeon for every 1,000, and a hospital mate for every 160, but this number would be varied according to the destination of the expedition and the amount of sickness expected.

Hospital equipment was provided in conjunction with the purveyors department which was now directed by a Purveyor-in-Chief, and this included the bedding, the ward furniture, and all the paraphernalia needed from tents to cooking pots. Medicines, dressings, and surgical instruments were received from the Apothecary General who controlled the supplies from civil firms, and it was the task of the Board to dispatch the quantities required calculated on the strength of the force and the duration of the campaign'

Although the Board had collective responsibility for these decisions the arrangements for overseas expeditions were the particular concern of the Surgeon General. But once the expedition had left these shores its principal medical officer took complete control. The delays of communication caused by sailing ships and the distances involved made this essential, and the Board could do little or nothing to influence policy or treatment. Indeed, it is clear that the inspector generals of these expeditions looked upon themselves as completely autonomous even to the extent of promoting their own officers when vacancies occurred from death or invaliding. Instances occurred when, having sent out additional physicians or staff surgeons because they were convinced the need existed, the Board found they were sent home again because the inspector general wanted to promote some of his own officers who had proved their ability. Although they did not recognize this power the Board was sometimes forced to accept it, and the independence exercised by the principal medical officer meant that their responsibilities were limited to the dispatch of medical officer reinforcements and the supply of medicines and hospital stores.

All these factors limited the duties of the Board in its initial stages but as the exigencies of war developed so the medical requirements multiplied, and to these duties were added increased responsibilities on the home front. The creation of general hospitals at the chief ports of embarkation, the medical preparations for the militia, and the opening of depots of hospital equipment and medical stores throughout the country owing to the risk of invasion absorbed much time and energy. From every point of view it should have been apparent to Ministers that part time members working limited hours and with totally inadequate office staff would have great difficulty in exercising the required degree of administrative control which would meet the requirements of a nation at war.

In common with the rest of the army the Medical Board was faced with a recruiting problem. Even with the increase of regimental mates' pay to 3s. 6d. a day it was, owing to the numbers required in time of war, difficult to obtain mates of an acceptable standard. As the demand increased with the expansion of the army the Board was forced to accept more and more men without proper qualifications. The sole training of many of these so called doctors consisted of a few years or even months as assistants to some country apothecary or walking the hospital wards. They possessed neither degrees nor diplomas nor even certificates of attendance. Dr. Maclean asks, 'if it be true that a certain Mr. Williams is now actually a hospital mate doing duty with the army whose age scarcely exceeds seventeen years, and whose apprenticeship was of the duration of four months?' To such low standards was the Board forced, and even so, one expedition to the West Indies sailed with only one-third of the mates required.

When the new rank of staff surgeon came into being Surgeon General Hunter's policy was to promote the most capable regimental surgeons to these posts in order of seniority tempered with ability. But after his death the new Board introduced a policy of selection, and staff surgeons were chosen for their operating skill, not only from the regimental surgeons, but from hospital mates, medical officers from the militia, and direct from civil life. Efforts were made with success to get keen young doctors who would enlist as hospital mates and receive quick promotion to staff surgeon's rank. These hospital mates were paid 7s. 6d. a day, a rate which made it even harder to enlist good regimental mates.

By long established custom, physicians were regarded as a superior class for they were better educated and better qualified than the average surgeon and drew twice the rate of pay. During his period as Surgeon General we have seen that Hunter's policy had been to nominate physicians both from the more experienced and better qualified apothecaries or regimental surgeons, and from civil life. But when Sir Lucas Pepys became Physician General he was determined to raise the standard of medicine in the army and would accept only physicians with the highest qualifications. He refused promotion to any officer unless he was a graduate of Oxford or Cambridge and a licentiate, member, or fellow of the College of Physicians of London. Although he acknowledged that the advancement to the post of physician would be an incentive to the morale of the regular officers, the appointment of anyone less well qualified would be, he said, at the sacrifice of soldiers' lives and could not be justified. This extreme arbitrary rule meant that the university graduate from Scotland and Ireland and in point of fact nearly every regular officer was excluded from a physician's appointment at a time when, owing to the expansion of the service the opportunities for promotion had never been so favourable. The practical effect was to limit these appointments almost exclusively to newly qualified physicians from civil life and as the rank of physician carried with it seniority above that of staff surgeon as well as double the rate of pay, the regular officers were soon seething with discontent when these young doctors without a scrap of army experience were placed over their heads. Entirely ignorant of the treatment of tropical diseases, these young physicians were made medical superintendents of the general hospitals and gave orders to the surgeons, who by virtue of their foreign service were years ahead in experience. The resulting breakdown in hospital administration will be subsequently seen. Pepys' folly in adhering to this strict standard is illustrated by the case of a Dr. Wright, a fellow of the College of Physicians of Edinburgh who had served for seventeen years in the army, mostly in the West Indies, before taking up private practice in Jamaica. Dr. Wright applied for the post of physician, but was refused unless he became a fellow of the College of Physicians of London. He expressed his willingness to sit the examination, but the expedition he was due to join sailed for the West Indies before it could be held. In this particular case, however, Pepys was overruled by the personal intervention of the commander of the expedition, and Dr. Wright duly sailed with the force as its physician. This power vested in local commanders to override the rules of the Medical Board was a source of concern to the members, and they appealed against it with success to the Commander-in-Chief at the Horse Guards. However, the necessity to mollify the feelings of the regular officers could not be ignored, and Pepys was persuaded later to modify his policy and to accept as physicians medical officers who possessed the degree of M.D. of universities other than Oxford and Cambridge, although this may have presented a risk if the following statement made by the Board can be believed. 'It is well known,' they said, 'that from many of the Scotch universities a degree may be sent for by the stage coach on paying eleven pounds.'[15]

The syllabus of training for a licentiate of the College of Physicians of London was a residence of two years at Oxford or Cambridge, and taking a degree after passing three examinations conducted in

Latin in the subjects of anatomy and physiology, pathology, and thera-
peutics. Their 'Knowledge of Principles,' wrote Dr. Bancroft, himself
one of Pepys' nominees, 'inevitably made them superior to the surgeons
who were often of obscure origin, sons of millers or bakers who trust
in curing diseases without licence. They have neither the knowledge,
habits, nor manners of members of a learned profession, and many
assume the title of doctor without any justification.' The flaw in Pepys'
policy was the fact that these young physicians knew nothing of service
conditions and Dr. Jackson contended that every medical officer must
enter the service as a mate, and gain regimental experience; 'the only
station where a correct knowledge of the physician's duty can be
acquired'. Bancroft rejected this argument and said that there was
nothing special in the diseases met with in army hospitals, and any well
educated man could quickly learn the special peculiarities of soldiers'
diseases. All the bad blood which was generated by this controversy
involved only a score of officers, for the number of physicians in the
army never exceeded that number during this period, so that by far
the greatest number of medical cases were treated by surgeons anyway.
However, this step to improve professional standards was the first
incentive for regular officers to acquire higher qualifications, and
ultimately it proved beneficial, for in the course of time officers elected
to go on half pay in order to obtain them.

The increase in army strength and the growth of the medical organization which followed made it necessary to create additional administrative posts. In overseas expeditions the administrative officer was the
inspector general of hospitals, but with extensive operations in areas
like the West Indies it became essential to exercise control by assistant
inspectors who would superintend the regimental, garrison, and general
hospitals. At home too, they were needed at the headquarters of the
military districts which had been formed to command the large numbers
of Militia and Volunteer units which existed throughout the country.
The institution of the rank of assistant inspector in 1795, with seniority
below that of physician, was an important step in overcoming the block
in promotion which had angered the surgeons and went some way to
appease their ruffled feelings.

In 1798 Gunning died, Keate was made Surgeon General, and the
appointment of Inspector of Regimental Infirmaries or Hospitals as
it was now called, was given to Mr. John Rush. Service with the
Guards seemed to be the chief criterion for selection to the Board, for
Rush had been surgeon to the Horse Grenadier Guards in 1782 before
being sent as apothecary to North America.

The opportunity was now taken to alter the duties of the Board,
because for members who spent such a short time at headquarters
working together it was found more convenient and less exacting
to allow them to work independently, and a Royal Warrant of the

12th March 1798 stated, 'the Physician General, the Surgeon General, and the Inspector of Regimental Infirmaries shall each have his distinct province of business and of recommendation, and be each made openly and solely responsible for his own acts'.

As the senior member, the Physician General's most important duty became the appointment of physicians, but he also inspected the medicines supplied by the Apothecary General and checked the bills in conjunction with the Surgeon General. The Surgeon General now appointed the staff surgeons and the regimental and assistant surgeons[16] and continued to control the arrangements for all overseas expeditions so that the major portion of the work fell on his shoulders.

Under his designation of Inspector of Regimental Hospitals Mr. Rush was allowed to nominate the apothecaries, the purveyors and the hospital mates. This was quite irrelevant to the scope of his appointment and was simply to give him a share of the patronage which each member insisted upon regarding as an indication of his prestige.

This division of responsibility suited the members of the Board but in other respects it proved unrealistic. The Physician General having appointed the physicians had no further control over them for this was the prerogative of the Surgeon General by virtue of his authority for the general hospitals in which they served. The Surgeon General having selected the whole category of surgeons only controlled the staff surgeons, for the regimental surgeons and assistant surgeons were under the Inspector of Regimental Hospitals. And finally, the Inspector of Regimental Hospitals who selected the apothecaries, purveyors and hospital mates, had no further say in their future for they came under the Surgeon General. No procedure could be more calculated to cause confusion than this curious mixture of duties.

Mr. Rush died in 1801 and was succeeded by a man who was ultimately to prove a disruptive element in the Board. Like Rush and Keate before him, Francis Knight had been regimental surgeon to the Guards, and like his predecessors had never held senior rank in the Department. His only claim to fame was his reputation of having the best administered regimental hospital in the Brigade. This extraordinary choice of men without administrative experience can only be accounted for by the fact that the higher appointments were chosen from a clique who had the ear of the Commander-in-Chief because of their service in the Guards. Ability and experience were sacrified to nepotism.

Knight joined the Board with his new title of Inspector of Army Hospitals, a significant change, because it brought under one authority not only the regimental but the general hospitals at home which had until then been controlled by the Surgeon General. Knight opposed his colleagues' policy and considered that service in the junior ranks was essential before promotion to physician or staff surgeon. Moreover, under the Royal Warrant of 22nd May 1804 he succeeded in creating a further avenue of promotion for the regular officers by replacing assistant inspectors by the new administrative rank of deputy inspector[17] which would be senior to that of physician, and as these posts were reserved for officers of previous service and experience this displeased the physicians brought in from civil life, who found themselves compelled to take orders from officers whom they regarded as professionally inferior.

Knight then revised the administration of the regimental hospitals, but soon showed that he was more concerned with their economy than their professional standards. The surgeons found that they had to devote their time more to keeping accounts and feeding patients on low priced foods such as oatmeal than on their medical duties. Highly professional men like Pepys and Keate disagreed with Knight's methods. 'There is little novelty,' said the latter, 'in the mere attempt to reduce the expenses of hospitals—various expedients have been adopted at different times with more or less success, but every one must be founded upon depriving the sick of those comforts which the most able and honest practitioners have usually deemed proper for them, and in employing remedies which cost nothing, such as bleeding, water, salts, etc. a species of economy which has, I believe, always proved ultimately very expensive by the consequent loss of lives.'

The differences between the members of the Board made co-operation difficult. Knight was blamed for being too ambitious, and Pepys and Keate resented what they considered his determination to exercise more than his due share in the control of the Department. The most serious split came over the question of general hospitals. Pepys and Keate considered them essential, Knight did not, and by virtue of his new authority as Inspector of Army Hospitals took it upon himself to close the general hospitals at Gosport, Plymouth and Deal between the years 1802 and 1806. This was a foolish and unwarranted step which nearly brought disaster upon the Department, for when in 1809 some 4,000 sick riddled with typhus arrived at Portsmouth from Spain there was no accommodation except in the local regimental hospitals and these, of course, were quite unable to cope with such numbers. In due course it was McGrigor who as Inspector of the South West District averted a scandal by his firm and decisive action. McGrigor deserved the approbation which Knight expressed for getting him out of this awkward predicament—one of his own choosing.

Pepys and Keate argued convincingly against closing the general hospitals. How could the regimental hospitals, they said, small and poorly equipped as they undoubtedly were, provide proper accommodation for thousands of cases? They expressed their concern to the Commander-in-Chief stressing 'the calamities which must ensue if the system of regimental hospitals on foreign service was to be persevered in to supersede the use of general hospitals'. But although the use of regimental hospitals to replace general hospitals had been tried in the West Indies and received Treasury support, Knight was only concerned with defending his policy of the closure of the hospitals at home. Having procured a copy of Pepys and Keate's letter, he anticipated any criticism of the Portsmouth incident by convening a board of Generals who backed him up by saying 'that so far from having found any pretence for imputing blame or neglect on any part of the Medical Department charged with the duty of providing for their reception and treatment, we cannot but express our satisfaction not unmixed with surprise that so large a number of sick could have been so well provided for.' With this powerful support Knight won the day, and Pepys and Keate gave in, protesting, however, that 'Knight's ambitious views, implacable temper and over-bearing disposition have been the cause of all trouble and the destruction of the Board.'

Knight now felt secure enough to take a further step, and in turn condemned his colleagues saying he could no longer act in a public capacity with them. 'My best exertions are paralysed—the ground shakes under me. I dare not risk responsibility with authority so questionable.'

The quarrels grew in intensity and bitterness. Pepys said that ever since Knight's appointment in 1801 collaboration had decreased and efficiency had suffered, and he made an appeal for the Board to revert to the policy adopted between 1793 and 1798 when control was exercised by all three members conjointly and the pay was equal. Keate supported him strongly, and wrote on the 4th August 1809 a long series of complaints against Knight, accusing him as the cause of disharmony and hostility because he failed to get the post of Inspector of Regimental Infirmaries in Keate's place on the death of Surgeon General Hunter. He accused him of creating the newly made posts of deputy inspector because he wanted to procure the patronage of nomination to these posts for himself and secure the direction and control of the Department although he was the junior member. He attacked him for his parsimony in running the regimental hospitals and saving money from stoppages against the soldiers' interest.

The personal animosity; the struggle for power amongst the members of the Board; and the discontent amongst medical officers at what they considered unfair methods of promotion and selection were bad enough; but all these signs of discord and unpopularity were brought to a climax by the medical disasters which befell the Walcheren expedition to Holland in 1809. When the Physician General and the Surgeon General both refused to visit the hospitals in Holland to see things for themselves this was the final nail in the Board's coffin, and the Secretary at War wrote to the Treasury, 'The disunion which exists among the principal members of the Army Medical Board is productive of very serious inconvenience to the public Service.'[18]

In the following year the Government decided to appoint a Commission of Military Inquiry to investigate the whole field of appointments, duties, emoluments, and allegations of waste and inefficiency in the control of expenditure. This decision was undoubtedly influenced by the volume of criticism expressed by officers such as Dr. Charles Maclean who in his pamphlet *An analytical view of the A.M.D.*, accused the members of the Board with lack of public integrity, unnecessary extravagance, promotion by favouritism, patronage, speculation, and indirectly, (caused by their inefficiency) of the sacrifice of some thousands of soldiers' lives each year.

It was soon obvious that the main object of the Commission was to seek every excuse to reduce expenditure rather than promote efficiency. The policy of divided responsibility adopted by the Board from 1798 onwards was condemned, not only on account of the fact that it was anomalous for each member to possess the power of appointments to a category of medical officers over whom he would later exercise no authority, but it led to unnecessary increases in establishment by creating higher ranking appointments resulting in extravagant expenditure. If the Board had acted together they would have checked each other's activities. Commissioners questioned the need for general hospitals at home because they considered the regimental hospitals were capable of dealing with the sick; they conveniently ignored the problem of dealing with the thousands of patients and invalids who poured in from the overseas expeditions. It was of course possible to deal with such emergencies as the arrival of the cases from Spain by opening temporary hospitals, but these *ad hoc* arrangements were the negation of efficiency. But when it was found that it cost 17d. a day to maintain a patient in a general hospital and only 10d. a day in a regimental hospital, this was enough to convince the Commissioners that general hospitals were unnecessary. This decision received added support when it was found that the stoppages of 9d. a day exacted from the patients in the regimental hospitals showed a surplus of £8,528 between the years 1802 and 1806. They shut their eyes to the fact that Knight's drive to produce economy in these hospitals meant that the patients were receiving inferior and inadequate food and were deprived of good quality medicines.

Knight however had a powerful supporter in Deputy Inspector James McGrigor who, giving evidence before the Commissioners, praised his remedy of the abuses which previously existed. 'It is well known and indeed universally acknowledged by the great body of medical officers . . . that these reforms originated in the judicious and unwearied exertions of the present Inspector General of Hospitals. By these improvements the service has been benefited, immense retrenchments have been made, the effective strength of the army has been increased, and by a more liberal remuneration being offered, men of superior talents and education have been induced to enter the Medical Department.'

But the most powerful indictment brought against the Board was the accusation of wastage and extravagance in the provision of medicines and surgical instruments. The cost of these was undoubtedly heavy. Between 1795 and 1806, a period of twelve years, the money spent on medicines amounted to over £800,000, including over £70,000 for instruments. Medicines were purchased from civil firms by the Apothecary General who was paid 10s. a day plus a profit of 10 per cent, but this percentage was increased when payment of bills by the Government was delayed. Civil supplies were delivered to the Army Elaboratory in Bury Street from where they were distributed after they had been inspected and passed by the Physician General; but it was found that when they were dispatched they were not checked by a medical officer, and no receipts were obtained; moreover the prices paid were at times considered excessive, and the Board was blamed for not exercising more control; 'the Physician General to whom this branch of the Department seems more peculiarly to belong takes no part in it', and they 'have reason for thinking there had been great inattention to the assortment of the medicines sent abroad'.

With regard to the £70,000 spent on instruments the stocks were held to be excessive. At the main depot of army medical stores at Portchester there were found to be 1,100 capital[19] cases of instruments and 1,300 sets of pocket instruments, and McGrigor who was ordered to investigate said there were sufficient instruments to supply all the armies of Europe for a century. The Surgeon General explained that capital cases of instruments were issued when the danger of invasion had been present, and these had to be replaced in the depots for further eventualities, while when replacement sets were sent overseas before the damaged ones were returned, duplicate sets had to be kept in reserve. The Commission considered that as the regimental surgeons had to buy their own instruments it was only to supply instruments for the wasteful and unnecessary general hospital system that so much money had been spent and they saw no reason why staff surgeons should not buy their own instruments in the same way.

Owing to the danger of invasion in 1803 Keate had been ordered by the Horse Guards to make the necessary medical arrangements and he established a number of temporary general hospitals and reserve depots of medical stores in the eastern and south-eastern counties. He provided the hospitals with a small basic establishment of medical officers and the minimum of equipment in readiness for expansion if necessary, but as the invasion threat never materialized they never received a single patient. The Commissioners now blamed him for maintaining such hospitals and took the easy line of condemning the quantity of medical stores as excessive. 'We cannot omit to observe,' they said, 'that the continuance of these expensive establishments seems to have been unknown at the War Office.' This remark was quite untrue.

The total annual budget for the Medical Department came to nearly a quarter of a million pounds a year, but owing to the various headings under which money was issued for the different services the whole cost was not obviously apparent to the Government. This amount was made up of £45,000 for the pay of the hospital staff officers, £79,000 for the subordinate ranks in general hospitals, £67,000 for medicines and surgical instruments and some £50,000 for purveyors stores.

The well founded system of the payment of officers through the Army Agent was then attacked. This had been the practice for nearly twenty years, and the cost had risen from £150 in 1792 to £670 in 1807. In this last year the payments amounted to £85,000 for 319 medical officers of the hospital staff (apart from the regimental establishment) with a further £16,902 for officers on half pay, a total sum of £103,009.

The proceedings of the Commissioners' investigations was published in their Fifth Report in 1808. They found that the members of the Board had shown a lack of proper control; irregularities in promotion had occurred; new and unnecessary appointments had been made; extravagance and waste in stores had been allowed; and general hospitals had been opened unnecessarily. Their recommendations covered all these points; economy was to be the watchword; general hospitals at home were to be abolished; the Agent's office closed; purveyors were to be downgraded to the rank of stewards; the half pay list was to be resorted to before making new appointments, and officers drawing half pay who were found to be ineffective were to be discharged from the service; reserve stocks of medicines and stores were to be run down before further items were purchased, and checks of expenditure introduced. It was obvious, the Commissioners said, that the personal antagonisms between the members had affected their efficiency and lowered their influence over the control of the Department and in the eyes of the officers; consequently the only solution was to dissolve the Board.

And so, after sixteen years, the control of the Department passed into new hands. No one was sorry to see the old Board disappear, for the members had never been popular. Promotion by seniority had given place to promotion by selection, and this policy in the hands of members who were disliked and mistrusted was dangerous. The time honoured qualities for promotion—industry, education and talents—were replaced by partiality and favouritism. Complaints were made that inspectors were selected from regimental surgeons instead of staff surgeons, and junior officers were promoted out of their turn. Mr. Keate was accused of preferring the young doctors from St. George's Hospital and it was rumoured the fees went partly into his pocket! The suppression of all lists of seniority made it impossible for officers, particularly those on foreign service, to know to what extent their rights might have been disregarded. Dr. Maclean quoted one such case of favouritism of the nephew of the Surgeon General who was promoted inspector of hospitals; originally a purveyor, he had never gone through the regular steps of promotion and had never been out of the United Kingdom; as a contrast, he mentions the case of a hospital mate who had spent thirty years in the service, the greater part abroad, who had never received promotion. But the standard of mates was often so poor that promotion by seniority alone was not always advisable. 'It has happened,' wrote Dr. Bancroft, 'that very deficient persons who could scarcely write even a single line of English correctly have had the health of considerable armies entrusted to them.'

Bribery too was not unknown. The secretary to the Board was dismissed for accepting fees from candidates who had been appointed to vacancies and Mr. Knight, shortly after his appointment in 1801, said, 'In future, any officer presuming to offer bribes at this office would incur the displeasure of the Medical Board!' This 'displeasure' may have been an answer to a libellous suggestion made by Dr. Maclean, that each inspector promoted must have made gifts to Mr. Knight to make it worth his while! Maclean states that 95 per cent of the establishment had not been promoted in due order. Officers who dared to report on these matters were, Maclean says, dismissed the service or placed on half pay. Adverse criticisms were said to have been lost in a fire which destroyed many of the Departmental records in 1803.

All these disruptive practices were now to be put right; promotion from surgeon to staff surgeon was to be strictly by seniority, and from staff surgeon to deputy inspector after seven years on full pay.

The Apothecary General with his profit making privilege was to be abolished and in his place a medical officer as inspector of medicines was to be appointed with pay of £600 a year. The Army Elaboratory was to supply not only the Army but the Navy and the Ordnance Medical Department as well, a first attempt at inter-service co-ordination.

With the emphasis on economy, staff surgeons were to be made to buy their own surgical instruments in the same way as regimental surgeons, and as the price of a capital case of instruments was nearly £20 this would save the Government a great deal of money.

The new Board was to consist of a chairman receiving £1,200 a year, and two members, both principal inspectors in rank, drawing £1,000 a year, with a secretary and cashier in receipt of £600. All were to be selected from senior regular medical officers with knowledge and experience. Part time civilians indulging in private practice were to be swept away for ever. When the dissolution occurred the members were not dismissed without monetary compensation and Pepys, Keate, and Knight, were all retired on an allowance of £1 5s. 4d. a day, a sum which they contested was quite inadequate after their long service. Keate showed his lack of patriotism by complaining that he was poorer by several thousand pounds because his public duties interfered with his private practice. It was only given to Knight, who had been the chief disruptive element, to make a successful appeal and receive an additional sum in virtue of his holding the appointment of Comptroller of Accounts.

Although Pepys on the whole cuts a poor figure in these inquiries we feel this cannot be said of Keate, who, when he was Surgeon General, carried out most of his duties with ability and success. The bulk of the blame fell on his shoulders, for although the provision of temporary hospitals and depots of stores against the risk of invasion were measures which one might expect would have had the Commissioner's approval, when invasion did not occur it was easy to condemn them as wasteful and unnecessary. Keate defended himself vigorously against his critics,[20] to 'rescue my character from their unwarranted imputations'[21] and made out a strong case quoting chapter and verse which his opponents would have been hard put to repudiate. But they were never called upon to do so. They had already given evidence against him under oath and refused to indulge in any controversial arguments.

Keate concludes his defence in these words: 'I have carefully reviewed and considered my past conduct and have found nothing to occasion sensations of shame in any but my accusers, or afford ground to impeach my integrity or my honour. For fifteen years I have endeavoured to discharge beneficially for the Public the laborious, difficult, and very numerous duties imposed upon me, in which a greater or more embarrassing variety of military operations have occurred than at any period in the history of the country.' In spite therefore of the Commissioner's condemnation of his conduct we cannot but feel for him a measure of respect.

The history of the Medical Board which controlled the Department between the years 1793 and 1809 and its ultimate fate has been described. It is necessary here to relate the problems which the Board had to deal with at home.

One of the first of these was to make arrangements for the treatment of the sick and wounded from the overseas expeditions which in previous wars had been dealt with by the regimental hospitals. The conflict which spanned the years of the Napoleonic wars against France and later against Holland and Spain, was on such a scale that general hospitals became essential to cope with the numbers which poured in from overseas.

A start had been made during the American War of Independence in 1781 to provide hospitals at Portsmouth and Chatham on a small scale and the time had come to expand them. Accordingly, at ports from which expeditions set sail and casualties and invalids from abroad disembarked permanent general hospitals were established. The first was completed at Gosport near Portsmouth in 1796 and this was followed by one at Deal in 1797. Both were built of brick or stone, with ceilings 15 feet high, windows on both sides, and upper sashes which opened to give improved ventilation. The internal facilities for the sick were greatly improved; every patient was allotted his own bed, fever cases and fluxes were to have separate wards, and smallpox and measles patients isolated; cleanliness and ventilation were given special attention, and daily fumigation with vitriolic (sulphuric) acid and nitre brought into use.

At the important port of Southampton a temporary general hospital was established in a granary of several storeys, low roofed, and badly ventilated. One regimental surgeon described it as a hot bed of contagion where there was a 30 per cent mortality amongst typhus cases compared with one of 15 per cent amongst those treated in his own regimental hospital. These complaints against the higher mortality in general hospitals became common, and was blamed on the overcrowding and the poor standard of nursing. This certainly applied to Southampton where just before the hospital closed down in June 1796 there were 1,262 patients who were transferred to the new hospital at Gosport.

Plymouth was another port where a general hospital was badly needed, but it was only after years of slow negotiation that a sail cloth factory was purchased for £7,200 in January 1795 which provided accommodation for 1,000 sick[22]. This type of converted accommodation could never be satisfactory and this was confirmed by Dr. Jerome Fitzpatrick who during a visit found the hospital in a bad state of repair with broken windows and patients in some wards lying on the floor.

It is necessary here to explain Dr. Fitzpatrick's appearance at Plymouth. He was an Irish doctor who had been Inspector of Jails and Asylums in Dublin, and was noted for his humanitarian ideas and reforms. In some way his name came to the notice of Henry Dundas who was Pitt's Minister for the conduct of the war, and Fitzpatrick was appointed to a new post, Inspector General of Health and Transports. His terms of reference included the inspection of transports, barracks, and hospitals, and as his reports were made direct to the War Office he was in no way under the authority of the Medical Department. During his visit to Plymouth he found many sick in the transports which were due to sail for the West Indies, and as he found the hospital unsuitable and overcrowded, two transports were converted as temporary hospitals, and he engaged civilian apothecaries to look after the sick. Dr. Boone, the physician in charge of the Plymouth hospital objected strongly to Fitzpatrick's interference, but Fitzpatrick retorted by sending in a damaging report to Dundas on the state of neglect in the hospital where, he said, there was a scarcity of medicines, medical comforts, and wine. Furthermore, on his own authority he orderd repairs to the hospital wards and requisitioned a building as a convalescent hospital of 400 beds, where patients on discharge from the general hospital were exercised, their garments fumigated, and themselves reclothed. Boone now complained to the Medical Board about Fitzpatrick's intervention, and Mr. Keate the Inspector of Regimental Infirmaries came down to investigate, rejected Fitzpatrick's criticisms, condemned his unauthorised interference, and as a counterblast fell back on the safe Government objection that his expenditure on wine and alcohol amongst convalescents had been excessive; apart from costing £750 in a single month it had provoked amongst the convalescents a state of 'riot and disorder'. After this dispute had died down strong pressure was brought on the War Office to build a permanent hospital, but it took a further three years of effort before it was completed.

The next hospital to be opened was the York Hospital in Chelsea, opened on the site of the Star and Garter Inn. To start with it received the severely wounded cases from Flanders who were sent here to be under the Surgeon General's personal care, but it increased in size and importance over the years until in 1799 it was capable of accommodating 500 patients. Added to this list there was the Depot Hospital at the Army Recruiting Centre, first at Chatham and later at Newport in the Isle of Wight, and finally the hospital for the Foreign Legion at Eling near Southampton.

The military commandants of these hospitals were retired officers who acted under the orders of a director who resided at York Hospital. An order issued in October 1797[23] defined their duties. They were made responsible for order and discipline, which was to be enforced by frequent visits to the wards at uncertain hours; cleanliness and ventilation were to be supervised, and they were to see that proper attention was given to the sick by the regimental orderlies, that medicines were regularly administered and hospital rules obeyed. Further duties included the exercising of convalescents, and the posting of sentries and guards. They were to receive from the medical superintendent of the hospital a daily report on the state of the sick. From the range of these duties and responsibilities it will be appreciated that many aspects of administration were entirely in their hands and medical officers had little chance of showing their initiative or ability; while as none of the commandants had previous experience of their tasks, their reputation for efficiency was not of a high order, and many medical officers complained. The disasters which later overcame the general hospitals in Flanders was largely the responsibility of the military commandants. But it must be emphasized that in every case it was the Medical Department which received the blame.

The continual change of medical officers in hospitals due to postings overseas led Mr. Knight to appoint a permanent 'Principal Medical Officer' with additional pay of 5s. a day who would not be posted abroad and would supervise the internal hospital administration. This was a sound idea, but the physicians who were always extremely jealous of their status objected strongly, and at times refused to acknowledge them. Dr. Gordon even went further and wrote to the Surgeon General on the 23rd January 1804: 'I find an inferior officer is to direct or command me under the pompous denomination of principal medical officer. It is full time this farce was concluded, this mockery of justice was done away with.' Dr. Gordon however paid for this indiscretion by being court martialled and reprimanded, and the Medical Board subsequently succeeded in getting him dismissed the service.

The numbers under treatment in these general hospitals varied between 300 and 1,000, and the figures below show the distribution and staff during a period in the year 1800.

		Medical Officers	Female Attendants
Depot Hospital at Chatham	391	—	—
Deal	130	14	31
Gosport	286	16	45
Plymouth	56	9	19
York Hospital	199	27	—

As an example which would apply to them all the details of the staff of the Gosport hospital and their rates of pay about this time are given in the footnote.[24]

We have already seen the provision of general hospitals was by no means universally acclaimed by all medical officers. The ignorance and inefficiency of the military commandants and the mistrust of the physicians at any attempt to diminish their professional status were only two of the many problems which brought the general hospitals into disfavour, and fierce arguments on the merits and demerits of regimental versus general hospitals split the Department. All were agreed that the latter were essential in overseas campaigns, but they had different views on their necessity at home. Many senior officers, Knight, McGrigor, and Jackson amongst them favoured their abolition; Pepys, Keate and Bancroft wished to retain them. Those who condemned them based their arguments on such factors as the higher mortality rates, the greater expense, the lack of training and bad discipline of the orderlies who were drawn from different units, the temptation amongst patients to malinger when treated by strange medical officers, and the long delay before their return to duty. In the regimental hospitals the opposite applied, there were no military commandants to interfere, and the orderlies were better trained and imbued with the regimental spirit; each patient's characteristics were so well known that malingering was rare. Those who supported the general hospitals argued that they provided a higher standard of treatment by virtue of the professional qualifications of the physicians and staff surgeons; better food and wine for the chronic sick; while the mortality rate was bound to be higher and the expense greater because the patients were more severely ill. Both were wrong, for the real cause of the higher mortality depended on factors unknown at the time. Typhus fever from which the majority of the patients suffered was spread by the body louse from one patient to another by close contact in overcrowded wards, while the presence of hospital gangrene amongst surgical patients was due to bacterial contamination by septic instruments and infected dressings carried from case to case.

McGrigor described general hospitals as having 'the most destructive consequences to the sick soldier and greater expenditure and waste of every kind'. Another experienced officer, Deputy Inspector William Fergusson, said the 'general hospitals are needed for active operations and not required as a permanent institution for the care of the sick. Even under these circumstances these hospitals will always prove a great though necessary evil, destructive of the effective strength of armies, for diseases are difficult of cure wherever a large body of sick is aggregated together; new conditions are certainly generated, and discipline is imperfectly preserved because the dread of immediate military punishment is removed. The soldier too often becomes infected with vicious and malingering habits when no longer in the presence of his officers and under the eye of his corps, for the villains and malingerers are always found to skulk in general hospitals.

In all armies therefore the sick should never under any circumstances except those of active service, be sent to general hospitals while their regiments are present. To do otherwise must wound the professional feelings, and operate as a proclamation of idleness and freedom from responsibility of the medical officer of the regiment deprive the sick soldier of his home, and prove hurtful by the loss of time or change of treatment which transfer to the hands of strangers implies.

Instead of collecting the sick of an army into one spot it ought to be a rule to separate them as far as possible. This prevents undue accumulation of human effluvia from bodies in a state of disease, and accelerates recovery by ensuring ventilation, discipline, repose and attendance.'[25]

Jackson was a passionate believer in the superiority of the regimental hospital when he wrote, 'Good soldiers are generally unwilling to go to general hospitals and good surgeons are unwilling to separate good soldiers from their comrades.'[26]

These powerful arguments were endorsed by many officers, and when Knight finally decided to close the general hospitals at home on the grounds of economy he had many supporters. Plymouth, Gosport and Deal were all shut down between 1802 and 1806 leaving only York hospital and the Depot Hospital now established at Newport in the Isle of Wight. The former was retained because as well as a hospital it was fast becoming a headquarters to which medical officers were posted on first commissioning for instruction in army duties.

But the closure of the home hospitals undoubtedly lowered the standards of medical treatment, and hospital mates lost the teaching facilities provided by the physicians and staff surgeons, while Bancroft who advocated their retention was so contemptuous of regimental hospitals that he regarded them as unworthy of serious attention: 'Men cannot excel in everything,' he says, 'and he who is great in such little things will I am persuaded generally be little in those which are great.'[27]

A scheme was then evolved for cutting down the expense of general hospitals overseas by administering them on what was known as the regimental plan. This meant running them with fewer staff, abolishing either the purveyor or apothecary but employing two staff surgeons instead of one. Robert Jackson had in fact already been at work on similar lines at home. In 1801 he had been appointed as medical superintendent of the Depot Hospital for the Recruiting Centre at Newport and also held this position when it was previously at Chatham. With his passion for economy many original ideas in adminstration were introduced. The purveyor was dispensed with; the office staff was reduced to one clerk; the patients were moved into successive wards as their condition improved so that those in each ward were all on either low diet, half diet, or full diet; porridge was served for breakfast and supper, and the meat ration reduced. In all hospitals orderlies on the scale of 1 per 10 patients was the rule but for convalescents on full diet Jackson allowed only 1 orderly for 40, and in all there were 16 attendants, a reduction of some 50 per cent. But to each ward of two beds for serious cases one female nurse was allotted. The hospital was equipped with painted iron beds; palliasses and bolsters were filled with straw; there were linen sheets, two or three blankets, and a rug for each bed; flock mattresses were provided for special cases. Patient's clothing was a linen shirt, a woollen night cap, a gown, and slippers, and when allowed up, pantaloons and his own shoes and stockings were added.

His G.O.C. was so impressed by Jackson's measures of economy that the scheme was submitted to the War Office for their consideration. But the Medical Board, grasping at any opportunity to denounce Jackson, would have none of it, and attacked him on two counts: first for depriving the patients of their full ration, and secondly they said his hospital showed an unprecedented number of deaths, frequent relapses, and a debilitated state of the patients, and instead of being economical his form of adminstration caused a serious loss of men and this meant a greater expenditure. This report was made without any member of the Medical Board ever having visited the hospital. Jackson 'denied the second charge, but a board of senior physicians were ordered to inspect the hospital, and Sir John McNamara Hayes, Dr. Hunter, Dr. Weir and Dr. Pinckard arrived. Their report on the whole was favourable except that full diet should be increased to the normal 1 lb. of bread, 1lb. of meat, and one quart of beer daily. They did not blame the relapses or the mortality to this cause but said these were due to the sick being young recruits often of poor constitution, the overcrowding, when there were often some 400 sick in the 200 authorized beds, and the severe nature of the diseases.

A Dr. Maclurin had written a letter blaming Jackson for excessive blood letting, but the inspectors could not substantiate this and ended their report by saying, 'We feel ourselves called upon in justice to say that Dr. Jackson appeared to us as zealous, diligent, and a meritorious servant of the public and full of humanity in the discharge of his duty.'[28] This exculpated Jackson from any form of malpractice but the Medical Board was determined to condemn him. He could not in fairness be dismissed, but two physicians were appointed for duty in the hospital and he was forbidden to treat cases and left solely as the administrative head. This did not suit his proud spirit and he tendered his resignation in January 1802. It was accepted, and he retired on half pay.

But the scheme for running general hospitals on the regimental plan was adopted in 1807 and welcomed by the Treasury because it enabled the whole cost of the hospitals to be defrayed from the hospital stoppages.

Knight's absurd decision to close the general hospitals placed an impossible burden on the regimental officers and their hospitals, for they were now compelled to accommodate not only their own sick but the wounded and invalids arriving from overseas. In September 1808 there were no fewer than 5,861 patients in the regimental hospitals including 987 wounded; after the Walcheren expedition the numbers went up to 7,139, and one regimental hospital was dealing with 337 patients and another 220. To provide acceptable standards of treatment for such numbers must have been impossible when the regimental surgeons were not noted for their professional skill. Then a fresh crisis arose early in 1809 when thousands of typhus cases poured into Portsmouth from Spain after the retreat to Corunna and there was no hospital to put them in.

We have seen previously how both the Physician General and Surgeon General protested violently against Knight's high handed action, but the independent authority which each member of the Board now enjoyed in his own department allowed the Inspector of Hospitals to ignore their opposition. The Board in fact was a Board no longer.

In addition to these permanent hospitals, temporary general hospitals were opened as occasion demanded either to deal with casualties from overseas or as a precautionary measure against the danger of invasion. The influx of over 1,000 sick from Holland and Germany after the end of the Flanders campaign in 1795 was met by opening temporary hospitals at Colchester and Harwich, and these were again brought into use after the campaign of the Helder in 1799. In 1803 the fear of invasion led the War Office to issue orders for temporary hospitals to be opened at Chatham, at Dunmow in Essex for 500 beds, at Bury St. Edmunds in Suffolk for 300, and at Edinburgh for the same number. Each had a basic establishment of one staff surgeon or apothecary, hospital mate, matron, steward and wardmaster. When the invasion scare had subsided they were all closed down between 1804 and 1806 without having received a patient. For the same reason twelve depots of hospital stores and medicines sufficient to treat over 7,000 casualties were formed at selected points, the largest one at Portchester near Portsmouth. It has already been described how the Surgeon General was unfairly accused of extravagance in retaining these hospitals and depots by the Commissioners of investigation into the activities of the Medical Board when he was in fact complying with War Office orders.

The risk of introducing yellow fever into the country by invalids from the West Indies was regarded as serious, and a strict quarantine lasting three weeks was therefore imposed in May 1796 on all transports arriving from that quarter. Not until the Medical Board had informed the Horse Guards could the restriction be lifted, when the transports were fumigated and cleansed with quicklime.

We must now turn to the problems which affected the regimental medical establishment. The regimental surgeon was still the keystone of the service. He often served with his regiment throughout his whole army career, was proud to be identified with it in every way, and sometimes refused often with good reason all offers of further promotion. Above all it was a life of good fellowship and good sport which suited many of the less professionally minded, for there was little incentive or opportunity for the surgeon to keep his medical knowledge up to date except by friendly contact with civilian doctors in garrison towns. McGrigor described him as a man who 'reads less and less every day, makes his hospital duty as light as he can, stops but a short time with his patients, and is in haste to join his brother officers in their plans of amusement'.

Under the stern test of war the poor quality of many of the regimental surgeons and mates after ten years of peace was soon revealed and the Medical Board undertook an examination of their capabilities by an investigation into their medical qualifications, the hospitals and clinics they had attended, and their records of experience. That many of the regimental mates were deplorably ignorant cannot be denied, but this was due to the poor pay of 3s. 6d. a day, a rate no self-respecting doctor would accept unless he was dedicated to a military career. To provide even a minimum of medical care the Board was compelled to accept unqualified mates who were no more than dressers, and even so, by March 1794 there was a deficiency of seventy regimental mates, and the Board pointed out the seriousness of the position to the Secretary at War. These deficiences however only affected the regiments ordered to serve in the West Indies where the risks to health from yellow fever were so great that few volunteers were forthcoming, and the Board, who usually allowed mates to select the regiments in which they chose to serve, was now compelled to nominate them, a policy which angered the C.O.'s who were accustomed to select their own.

There was a further reason for the shortage. On the outbreak of war the need for hospital mates to staff the general hospitals being formed for overseas became a matter of urgency, and as their pay was 7s. 6d. a day, many regimental mates naturally transferred as hospital mates and there consequently arose an acute shortage in regiments. The Medical Board became extremely alarmed pointing out to the War Office that the low pay and status of regimental mates was the cause.[29] The only concession the Secretary at War would allow was to give the Board the power to refuse the enlistment of mates whose professional knowledge was regarded as unsatisfactory, which was no concession at all, and to promote regimental mates to the rank of surgeon as vacancies occurred.[30] Three years afterwards these paltry concessions had brought no improvement in recruitment and the crisis was not resolved until under the Royal Warrant of the 30th November 1796 pay for both regimental surgeons and mates, the former unchanged for nearly 150 years was at last substantially improved. Cavalry surgeons were given an increase from 6s. to 12s. a day, and surgeons to regiments of Foot from 4s. to 10s. a day. For the purpose of allowances and quarters surgeons were now to rank as captains, and after twenty years service they were granted half pay of 5s. a day. The designation of 'mate' which had originated in the Navy and had never been regarded with favour was now abolished, and they were to become assistant surgeons with pay at 5s. a day, raised to 7s. 6d. both on active and on foreign service. What was of equal importance was the removal for ever of the stigma of warrant officer's rank by the grant of King's commissions, and their status was raised to the rank of subaltern for quarters and allowances. There were separate arrangements for the Foot Guards; the 3 senior surgeons were paid 15s. a day, and subordinate to them there was 1 battalion surgeon and 3 assistant surgeons to each of the three regiments of Guards, and there were also improvements in their status. None of course were entitled to exercise their military rank.[31] Stoppages from pay of officers under the name of arrears were also abolished.

This warrant took effect from the 25th December 1796, and had an immediate response so that by 1799 most of the vacancies had been filled, and in some regiments one, and in others two assistant surgeons had been appointed. In September 1803 an additional assistant surgeon was allowed for regiments of 500 men and upwards. It still remained the prerogative of colonels of regiments to have assistant surgeons of their own choice, and although this practice was thoroughly disapproved of by the Board, the Commander-in-Chief refused to undermine the colonels' authority in this respect, but compromised by accepting Surgeon General Hunter's rule that candidates must also be acceptable to the Medical Board. But with these improvements in pay and status higher professional standards were demanded, and all regimental surgeons now had to pass an examination before promotion. In addition to the new privilege of being able to retire on pension, regular officers now had the right to go on half pay whenever they desired, even during a war period, except that medical staff officers were debarred if this meant that fresh appointments had to be made.

Common foresight might have assumed that the pay of medical staff officers would be improved concurrently with the regimental officers but nothing of the sort occurred, and it soon became difficult to induce regimental surgeons to take up appointments as staff surgeons, as financially they were worse off. Surgeon General Keate showed up the impossible position produced by this niggardly approach by the Treasury and wrote strongly to the Secretary at War on the 4th June 1799.[32] How, he asked, could good staff surgeons be attracted when their total pay per annum was £147 5s. 2d. (the sum remaining after the various deductions out of their gross pay of £182 10s.[33]), for this amount was now inferior to the pay received by the regimental surgeons, and staff surgeons who came from regiments were now asking to revert. He emphasized that regimental surgeons were not proficient in the 'science of medicine' which could only be obtained at an university, and to provide operating surgeons of experience candidates were needed who had spent five to seven years working in hospital wards. The drudgery involved in this was much greater than that undergone by most regimental surgeons, whose experience was usually that of a country apprenticeship followed by three to twelve months in London wards. There were, he said, only seven really competent surgeons in the whole army, and five of these were appointed directly from civil life. To attract the enlistment of surgeons with more experience, he asked the Secretary at War to pay staff surgeons 12s. a day regularly every three months, and proposed a higher rank of surgeon major at 15s. a day. The latter would not be permitted to become physicians but staff surgeons would have this right. These were sound and rational proposals but they were all rejected outright by the Secretary at War.[34]

Following the Peace of Amiens in 1802 there came about an immediate reduction of forces both in Britain and in Ireland. Many medical staff officers serving at home were placed on half pay and only three phys·icians and a handful of garrison surgeons and mates were retained for duty in the general hospitals; but even with these reductions there were still 600 medical officers on full pay, the great majority being on the regimental establishment.[35] Such a sudden change from war to peace disrupted the whole prospect of a settled army career for the medical staff officers, and explains why many regimental surgeons refused advancement. Promotion as a medical staff officer meant that half pay was always just around the corner. However, only two years were to elapse before war broke out again in 1803, when in spite of recalling officers from half pay a shortage again made itself felt. In an attempt to overcome this recurring deficiency several steps were taken by the Board. Grievances which affected recruitment were removed; one was the allotment of prize money which had never been granted but was now permitted after a table of comparative rank for medical *vis-a-vis* combatant officers had been worked out; also there were improvements in the standard of quarters, and better pensions for widows.[36] The much disliked West Indian service was made more attractive by increasing the outfit allowance from 10 to 20 guineas, and making two years service to count as three.

The disparity between the pay of regimental surgeons and the medical staff officers could not be maintained with any sense of fairness or justice and after a memorial setting out their grievances had been submitted by the staff surgeons in 1802, two years later increases of pay were granted by the Royal Warrant of the 22nd May 1804. The hardly hit staff surgeons were now to get 15s. a day (half pay 6s.) which was more than Keate had originally asked for; deputy inspectors 25s. a day and 30s. after twenty years' service, and inspectors of hospitals 40s. a day; both with half pay at 50 per cent of these rates. Hospital mates now also received King's commissions and were paid 6s. 6d. a day at home and 7s. 6d. abroad;[37] apothecaries and district surgeons 10s. Physicians and purveyors were considered adequately paid and received no increases. Not only were these overdue increases granted to medical staff officers, but regimental medical officers were to benefit further, and were now advanced to 11s. 4d., with 14s. after seven years' service as such or ten years completed service, and 18s. 10d. after twenty years; half pay was 6s. a day; at thirty years' service they had the unqualified right of retiring on pension; assistant surgeons were also advanced to 7s. 6d. a day. No officer was entitled to half pay unless he had served for five years at home or for three years abroad. Then in 1805 was first instituted the policy of medical cadetships.[38] Government consented to pay for the education of medical students provided they engaged for service in the army, and special steps were taken to include training in operative surgery at the Westminster Hospital. Then the Irish Medical Board was asked to help recruitment by placing notices in Dublin University and this applied also to Edinburgh. Within a year these combined measures had taken effect, and by 1806 when the danger of invasion was acute the strength of the medical staff officers in Britain had risen to 138.

These welcome improvements in pay were reflected in the Irish Establishment and its composition and the daily rates of pay are given below:

Two joint Physician Generals	10s. a day each
Surgeon General	20s. a day
Director General of Hospitals	50s. a day
Deputy Inspectors (4)	25s. a day each
	plus horse money of 7s. 6d. a day and lodging money of £1 2s. 9d. a week.
Staff Surgeons (4)	15s. a day each
	plus horse money of 5s. a day and lodging money of 15s. a week.
Apothecaries (4)	10s. a day each
Purveyors (4)	10s. a day each
Deputy Purveyors (4)	5s. a day each
Hospital mates (30)	7s. 6d. a day each
Total expenditure	£17,478 16s. 4d. a year

Shortly afterwards in the same year important new regulations were introduced for the grant of commissions. Sir Lucas Pepys' strict rules in the case of physicians which had caused so much controversy and bitterness were now modified, and although a degree of Oxford or Cambridge, or a membership of the College of Physicians of London was desirable, it was not now regarded as indispensable. Graduates of an university in Great Britain or Ireland were now eligible, but only if they were found fully qualified in other respects after examination by a board comprising the Physician General and two army physicians. Assistant surgeons of regiments were to be chosen from the hospital mates and the regimental surgeons from the assistant surgeons, and promotion depended on length of service and merit. Before promotion, mates were now required to pass an examination before a court of examiners at Surgeons Hall, and had to undergo a medical examination by the heads of the Department; if serving abroad they had to appear before a local board of medical staff officers. Selection of staff was to be made primarily from those on the half pay list. Apothecaries were now to be downgraded and chosen not as before from the senior regimental surgeons as a step in promotion but from the assistant surgeons and hospital mates. On the other hand purveyors were selected from staff or regimental officers who were drawing at least 10s. to 12s. a day. Although double commissions were prohibited as far as the regular officers were concerned this was not the case in the Militia where it continued to be normal practice. The following titles which were borne by senior officers were now discontinued—field inspector, assistant inspector, deputy inspector-general, inspector general, and superintendent general.

On Easter Sunday, 15th April 1797 the whole country was alarmed by the mutiny of the fleets at Spithead and the Nore. Some army units became disaffected during the crisis, and on the 25th May the Government showed its concern by granting the pay increases for the army which had been pressed on the Treasury for years. The soldier was now to draw the proverbial 1s. a day.

This increase in the soldier's pay was followed by improved living conditions in which the regimental hospitals participated when an extensive barrack building programme was introduced in 1797. The barrack room ceilings were to be 12 feet high, ventilated by sliding boards; each man was to have a bed to himself and no double berths or tiers were allowed. Troops were not allowed access to their sleeping quarters by day, and the mess room was also used as a sitting room. The kitchens, wash houses, and privies were detached. Regimental hospitals were to be accommodated within the barracks and equipment provided from the barrack department, while an important innovation was the provision at last of transport for the hospital—a cart for equipment, and a waggon to convey the sick.

From the year 1796 the Government had agreed to provide medicines both at home and overseas through the Apothecary General, and the iniquitous medicine stoppages which had plagued the soldier for so many years and had incidentally often benefited the surgeon was at last stopped. 'Ordained,' the order runs, 'that surgeons should be regularly paid and all perquisites abolished. Medicines and hospitals to be paid by Government.'

It has already been shown in a previous chapter that the cost of medicines for the period of twelve years between 1793 and 1806 amounted to the large sum of £800,000 and this meant that the Apothecary General who was allowed a 10 per cent profit had amassed a very considerable fortune. The Treasury now stepped in and did their utmost to cancel this arrangement, but Mr. Garnier who held the appointment refused to be deprived of it, and with his patent of office securely in his pocket rejected the Treasury offer to pay an annuity of £2,500 a year to his wife in return for its cancellation. It was not until 1810 that the appointment of Apothecary General was done away with by Act of Parliament and a medical officer appointed to control the supply of medicines at a salary of £600 a year.

The Medical Board followed this in 1798 by new *Regulations to regimental surgeons for the better management of the sick*. This included a more extensive range of medicines, but the half yearly indent for them had to enclose an affidavit by the regimental surgeon before a magistrate that none of the medicines had to his knowledge been converted to private purposes, while if drugs not in the Formulary were prescribed he was bluntly told he must pay for them himself.

The rise of pay for the soldiery to 1s. a day inevitably caused an increase in hospital stoppages, and these were now assessed first at 9d. and then at 10d. a day. This however did not mean that the diet in hospital was more substantial or varied. The principal reason for its introduction was to prevent the soldier accumulating money while in hospital which he would immediately spend on dissipation when he was discharged. A weekly account of expenditure of the regimental hospital of the 31st Regiment in 1810 shows that only two types of diet were supplied, High and Low. Patients on Low diet had to exist on bread, tea and soup, with perhaps one egg a week. That there was a surplus of 16s. at the end of the week from the hospital stoppages shows what a low standard of feeding resulted from Knight's policy, and bears out the critical remarks of the Surgeon General that the patients' comfort was being sacrified to economy.[39]

In general hospitals the diet scale was more ambitious and divided into Full, Half, Low and Milk with extras in the shape of mutton, fish and other items which the medical officer considered necessary.[40]

Maclean condemned the whole system of hospital stoppages as iniquitous. It resulted, he said, in soldiers with families to support out of their pay refusing to be admitted to hospital unless absolute necessity compelled them to, and by then perhaps it was too late to effect a cure. Or again on discharge from hospital to convalescence with his unit a man might find his pay wholly exhausted and have no money to buy the comforts necessary for his convalescence. 'This,' says Maclean 'is a punishment for being sick which is wrong, and the whole upkeep of the regimental hospitals should be borne by the public.' But the Government's firm policy was that the army must pay for itself, 'Sufficient funds,' the regulation said, 'should be established for the support of the sick without any additional charge to the Government'.

It was in fact due to the enlightened and progressive outlook of the Duke of York that the soldiers' lot improved, for the Commander-in-Chief took a keen interest in their health and well being, and supported the efforts constantly being made by medical officers to better living conditions and hygiene. This was plainly the task of the regimental officers, but by their laziness and ignorance they were too often neglectful of any attempts at good man management. The Duke was the first

C.-in-C. to ask for monthly sick returns showing the hospital state both at home and overseas, and although these returns are incomplete they give an approximate indication of the general state of army health. During a period of five months in 1797 there were an average each month of 3,396 sick in the regimental and general hospitals at home, and with a strength estimated at 60,000 this gives a sick rate of 5·6 per cent per month.

The Medical Board poured out a spate of orders. On the 31st March 1800 new regulations for general hospitals were published and in 1806 for regimental hospitals. The latter were now defined as 'subject to the general superintendence and control of the Inspector of Regimental Hospitals', who was authorized to point out to the commanding officers of regiments any faults found and remedies required. Thus was the C.O.'s exclusive control materially diminished. This was followed by an order in August 1809 directing that surpluses and deficiencies in the hospital stoppages or contingent account were to be dealt with in future by the agent for the Medical Department and no longer by the regimental paymaster.[41] Regimental medical officers were reminded too that as their practices included far more medical than surgical cases it was essential that they should have a complete knowledge of pharmacy and that they would not be recommended for promotion by the Medical Board unless they could prove this on examination.[42]

All these activities of the Board necessitated an expansion in personnel and extra accommodation in Berkeley Street. A Comptroller of Hospital Accounts was appointed and three assistants became necessary where before there had been none. The increase is clearly shown in the following table:

	1799	1806
Physician General	£730 0s. 0d.	£730 0s. 0d.
Surgeon General	£730 0s. 0d.	£730 0s. 0d.
*Inspector of Hospitals	£730 0s. 0d.	£730 0s. 0d.
Comptroller of Hospital accounts	—	£730 0s. 0d.
Three assistants	—	£1,435 0s. 0d.
Agent and Treasurer	£669 6s. 3d.	—
Treasurer	—	£670 0s. 0d.
Contingent Expenses	£556 5s. 0d.	£2,423 3s. 3¾d.
	£3,415 11s. 3d.	£7,448 3s. 3¾d.

* The Inspector of Hospitals also received for expenses £100 a year and 10s. a day.

In June 1807 the Secretary at War gave instructions that no regimental personnel would in future be employed in general hospitals as orderlies but that these would be supplied from the Veterans battalions who were men of low medical category from age and disability. There is however no evidence that this measure ever took effect in the Peninsular War now shortly to commence.

Ordnance Medical Department

It was in 1727 that medical officers for artillery were first appointed, but the rise in importance of both the artillery and the engineer arms under the Master General of the Ordnance now led to the creation of a separate medical department, controlled by its own surgeon general. 'The Medical Establishment for the Military Department of the Ordnance', as it was named, came into existence on the 1st May 1797 and was regularized by Royal Warrant on the 1st September 1801. Dr. John Rollo, the first holder of the appointment of Surgeon General had eighteen years service with the Royal Artillery. From its inception the new Department acquired a good name, and as there was considerable competition to join, a relatively high standard of entry could be imposed and permanent commissions were granted only to those who had passed the College of Surgeons examination and could produce certificates of good moral character. On administrative grounds a separate Department for the number of medical officers on the establishment seems unjustified, for they only amounted to 30 in 1806, and not until 1814 did they reach the maximum of 103.

The Surgeon General had his headquarters at Woolwich and unlike the members of the Army Medical Board he was solely employed in the administration of his department. There was also an Inspector General of Hospitals and Deputy Inspector General, Sir John MacNamara Hayes,[43] whose duties were to inspect the Ordnance Hospitals throughout the United Kingdom. In 1804 Rollo became both Surgeon General and Inspector of Hospitals with remuneration of £3 a day, and in 1806 the total cost of the establishment was £12,457 a year.

Between 1801 and 1814 there were four additional Royal Warrants authorising alterations in establishment and pay, and in 1813 the 'Ordnance Medical Department', as it was now named, appeared in the Army List for the first time. Both Rollo and Sir John Hayes died in 1809, and Mr. John Webb[44] who succeeded, assumed the title in 1813 of Director General. The status and titles which were accorded to the senior medical officers controlling such a small service could only have resulted from considerable pressure exerted by the Master General of the Ordnance and after all the Royal Horse Artillery were the right of the line.[45]

At the Royal Artillery headquarters established at Woolwich a new hospital was built which possessed many original features, and was considered, with justification, the best in the Kingdom. Each of its three floors were divided into small wards holding 5 to 6 patients apiece in accordance with the recently introduced idea of segregating different diseases to avoid the risk of 'contagion'. Modern schemes of ventilation were installed by removing a portion of the bottom sash of each window pane and substituting a glass frame fastened by hinges, which allowed it to be tilted to form an angle and direct a current of air towards the ceiling. This is still an approved method. Other innovations included a vapour bath, showers, and portable water closets. In accordance with the current idea there was a separate convalescent hospital to avoid patients on discharge going straight back to barrack life.

Rollo was justifiably proud of his hospital. 'The want of proper accommodation,' he said, 'deranges and disgusts, as it produces very serious and extensive defects in the minds of soldiers by damping the spirit of enterprise and exertion and may have some share in inducing desertion.' Words which are as true now as when they were uttered. There were two resident surgeons who were paid at the high rate of £1 a day, and instead of the usual regimental orderlies, nursing was carried out by a staff of female nurses under a matron who also did the duties of quartermaster. The food was good and more varied than other army hospitals, with five different types of diet, and roasts and stews substituted for the eternal boiled meat, while in marked contrast to Knight's policy of economy which restricted the spending of any surplus money from hospital stoppages, any favourable balance was expended on poultry, fish, fruit and beer. As the soldier was now paid 1s a day and stoppages were 9d. a day, he was, while in hospital saving money, and Rollo thought this might induce him to feign disease; on the other hand a married man's family suffered hardship while he was in hospital, so that he was as far as possible treated in quarters.

Surgeon General Rollo's control of his department indicates that he was an able and popular administrator who possessed the confidence and exacted the co-operation of the officers of the Regiment in a happy relationship which has always been a feature of the Royal Regiment of Artillery with its reputation for good man management. He was, too, well known as a writer on military hygiene, on elephantiasis, dysentery and diabetes,[46] and his views on the prevention of ill health merit attention, as indicating the lines of current opinion. Four causes of disease were named, (a) intemperance, (b) exposure, (c) marsh vapour, and (d) contagion.

(a) That intemperance was the foremost cause is a reflection on the hard drinking habits of the time. Often the soldier started the day with a glass of spirits which destroyed the appetite, and the remedy for this was to provide a breakfast at an early hour of gruel or porridge, beer, rice milk, milk and bread, or chocolate. A common breakfast amongst regiments in the West Indies was a glassful of rum with a slice of salt boiled pork, and the thirst which this engendered not infrequently led to spirits being repeated during the forenoon.

(b) Exposure to heat or to cold, with or without moisture, resulted in changes of the external temperature which affected the lungs causing inflammation, or the abdomen leading to bowel diseases. If the wet and exposure were severe this might bring on cholera, rheumatism, or consumption, and the most effective measure of prevention was the issue of flannel shirts.

(c) The well established cause of 'marsh vapour' induced fever and dysentery. It could be avoided by camping $\frac{1}{2}$ to 1 mile away from marshes, or by draining them, or by wood fires to which was added a mixture of manganese and sulphuric acid which acted as we now know by repelling mosquitoes.

(d) Disease due to 'contagion' could occur only from uncleanliness and lack of ventilation, and included smallpox, measles, whooping cough, scarlet fever, plague and typhus. Current opinion considered the last named could be spontaneously produced from want of cleanliness, poor food, depression of mind, and stagnation of air, while the remedy against smallpox was compulsory vaccination which was now being widely practised.

Amongst surgical cases the danger of infection spreading from open suppurating wounds or compound fractures was recognized, and in these cases clothing was fumigated and patients were isolated, even to the extent of posting sentries on the wards.

It was during the Peninsular War that the first general hospital used exclusively for artillery and engineer units was opened at Lisbon in 1811 with a staff of 18 medical officers under the charge of Dr. Kearsley, who also inspected the battery hospitals which were established in the army area. Senior Ordnance medical officers were now appointed to various commands overseas, and in 1812 the holder of the appointment in the Leeward Islands had his headquarters at the Ordnance Hospital established at Barbados.

During the Waterloo campaign Dr. Wittman who was then Assistant Director General was attached to the headquarters staff in Belgium and charged with the local administration of the battery hospitals although these had to conform to the general orders of the Army Inspector of Hospitals. Mutual assistance between the two branches occurred to the extent of admitting sick and wounded from all branches of the service while the provision of medical stores which up to 1815 had been carried out through A.M.D., was now taken over by Ordnance. In the post Waterloo period when much pressure was brought to reduce army expenditure it was surprising that the Department managed to maintain its independent role notwithstanding that almost every year Parliament discussed the necessity for its existence. It only survived by the forcible arguments of the Master General of Ordnance that its abolition would cause great inconvenience and loss of morale. In the larger stations such as Chatham, Woolwich, and Plymouth separate Ordnance hospitals existed and when this could not be justified separate wards were set aside in regimental or garrison hospitals for the sick of artillery and engineer units. This also applied to India.

There were only 28 officers serving in the Department in 1822, 38 in 1841, and 47 in 1850, and inevitably the chances of promotion for medical officers in such a small service were desperately slow. Many of the medical officers were old and too infirm to carry out their duties with any degree of efficiency. They were very unwilling to retire before they got a step in promotion, while if amalgamated with the Army Medical Department they would serve under officers junior to them in years of service owing to promotion in A.M.D. being so much quicker.

That a separate department with such limited responsibility should have existed, however desirable for *esprit de corps*, appears unnecessarily complicated, but after much discussion the War Office decided to retain the Department until the post of Director General held by Sir John Webb (he had fifty-five years service) became vacant, and after his death in 1853 the Ordnance Medical Department ceased to exist and was absorbed by the Army Medical Department. Henceforward, separate battery hospitals continued to exist until the re-organization of the Department in 1873 abolished regimental hospitals.

REFERENCES

[1] P.R.O., W.O. 7/96.

[2] Adams. *Memoirs of the Life and Doctrine of the Late John Hunter*, p. 108. Callow, and Hunter, London (1818).

[3] P.R.O., W.O. 7/97.

[4] Gore. *Our Services under the Crown*, p. 105. Ballière Tindall & Cox, London (1879).

[5] P.R.O., W.O. 7/97, p. 66.

[6] P.R.O., W.O. 7/96.

[7] P.R.O., W.O. 7/97.

[8] P.R.O., W.O. 7/96, p. 194.

[9] The rates of half pay were: physicians 10s. a day, surgeons and apothecaries 5s. a day, regimental surgeons 3s. a day.

[10] Hamilton. *Duties of a Regimental Surgeon*, p. 100. J. Johnson, London (1787).

[11] Hamilton. *Duties of a Regimental Surgeon*, p. 306. J. Johnson, London (1787).

[12] See Appendix A.

[13] P.R.O., W.O. 7/96.

[14] *Dictionary of National Biography*, p. 290.

[15] P.R.O., W.O. 7/103 d. 11th May 1796.

[16] Regimental mates were renamed assistant surgeons in 1796.

[17] *Fifth Report Commission of Military Enquiry 1808*, p. 158. Act 45, George III, Cap 47.

[18] P.R.O., W.O. 4/408.

[19] This was the official term given to the case containing the surgical instruments.

[20] His chief critics were Dr. Borland, Dr. Jackson, Dr. McGrigor and Mr. Young.

[21] Keate. *Observations on Fifth Report*, p. 157. J. Hatchard, London (1808).

[22] P.R.O., W.O. 40/7.

[23] P.R.O., W.O. 3/31.

[24] Military superintendent 15s.; staff surgeon as P.M.O. 20s.; physician 20s.; staff surgeon 15s.; apothecary 10s.; deputy purveyor 10s.; resident mate 7s. 6d.; hospital mates each 6s. 6d.; purveyors clerk 3s.; matron 2s. 6d.; head nurse 1s.; nurses each 1s.; steward 2s.;

surgery man 1s. 1½d.; wardmaster 1s. 1½d.; porter 1s.; orderlies each 1s. (if soldiers 3d.). Officers were allowed furnished quarters, coals and candles.

[25] Fergusson. *Notes and Recollections of a Professional Life*, p. 59–60. Longman Brown Green and Longman, London (1846).

[26] Jackson. (1808). *Remarks on the constitution of the Medical Department of the British Army*, p. 114. Cadell and Davies, London (1803).

[27] Bancroft. *Commissioners of Military Enquiry*. Fifth Report, p. 81.

[28] Jackson. *Remarks on the constitution of the Medical Department of the British Army*, p. 170. Cadell and Davies, London (1803).

[29] P.R.O., W.O./1/896.

[30] P.R.O., W.O./1/896.

[31] *A Treatise on Military Finance, etc.* London 1804, p. viii.

[32] P.R.O., W.O. 40/12. Paper No. 18.

[33] This refers to basic pay of 10s. a day and takes no account of allowances.

[34] P.R.O., W.O. 40/7.

[35] There were 36 cavalry regiments, 144 regiments of Foot, 9 West India regiments, and some miscellaneous units.

[36] Widow's pension for physician and purveyors was £30 a year, for surgeons, staff surgeons and apothecaries £26 a year.

[37] Temporary hospital mates were not given commissions.

[38] P.R.O., W.O. 4/402.

[39] See Appendix B.

[40] See Appendix C.

[41] P.R.O. W.O. 4/282.

[42] Horse Guards. 30th January 1804.

[43] He was created a Baronet in 1797.

[44] Afterwards Sir John Webb.

[45] This meant they were the senior corps in the Army.

[46] He proposed a meat diet for diabetics.

Chapter 8

FRENCH REVOLUTIONARY WARS I (1793–1798)

On the 7th February 1793 France declared war on Britain and Holland, and the Prime Minister, William Pitt, approached Austria and Prussia to unite in concerted action. Our foreign policy had always been based upon the independence of Holland and the free navigation of the Scheldt, for its occupation by a powerful foe was a threat to Britain which could not be tolerated.

The country had been at peace for ten years and was in no condition ready for a Continental war; both the Navy and Army had been neglected, and Ministers had practically reduced the two services to the strength of one. Our commitments overseas had already drained most of our military strength, and there were only some 15,000 regular troops in the country. Moreover, recruiting had been neglected and units were well below strength. Of 87 battalions in the Army, there were no fewer than 19 in the West Indies providing security against a general rising of the coloured population; there were 9 battalions in India, and 28 understrength battalions besides the Guards and cavalry for the defence of the country. Energetic measures were taken to attract recruits by offering bounties and lowering medical standards, but many of those enlisted were old men or boys, and even after a modicum of training were totally unfit for service. Laws were passed increasing the strength of the militia, and for drafting militiamen into the regular forces. This was followed by an Act for a compulsory levy of men to be drafted into the militia, and then asking them to volunteer for the regular army for service overseas. These steps failed to produce the number of regular recruits required and because of this the disgraceful policy was introduced of offering commissions for payment provided recruits were brought in, and unscrupulous young adventurers without a scrap of military knowledge were made officers overnight. As Fortescue says, 'The folly of ten years was not to be made good by the belated wisdom of a day.'[1]

Pitt, however, in spite of these difficulties promised an army of 40,000 men composed of British, Hanoverians and Hessians. But it was one thing for him to promise an army and another thing to produce it. However, several battalions of Guards amounting in all to some 2,500 men were hurriedly embarked for Holland, and with Hanoverian and Hessian troops hired by English gold they joined the Dutch and Austrian armies with the object of protecting the Austrian Netherlands which was threatened by the French revolutionary armies. Our polyglot forces were commanded by the 28 year old Duke of York, the son of George III, who had received his training under Frederick the Great.

As we have already indicated Sir Clifton Wintringham the Physician General, and John Hunter, who held the dual appointment of Surgeon General and Inspector of Regimental Infirmaries, were in control at the War Office. But Sir Clifton was too incapacitated by ill health to take an active part, and the task of organizing the medical arrangements fell upon Hunter. These took the usual steps of organizing general hospitals to accompany the force overseas, the selection of medical staff, and the provision of equipment and medicines.

To staff the hospitals he could either call on serving officers or those who had been on half pay for the ten years since the termination of the last war. He selected what he thought were the best from both sources.

To distinguish the surgeons appointed to the general hospitals from the regimental surgeons he created the title of staff surgeon, and these were chosen for their operating ability from the regimental surgeons, the apothecaries and the purveyors. In accordance with his accustomed policy they were appointed by seniority but he was still selective in his choice; this earned him the warm approval of his officers, but as we shall see in due course it was not entirely successful.

The Guards went overseas with their regimental hospitals, each equipped for forty patients. Hospital cots made of wooden frames with canvas bottoms were carried for the more severe cases on the scale of 2 for every 100 men in the regiment, and the other beds were simply wooden boards. Palliasses, sheets, pillow cases, blankets and ward equipment were provided, with close stools, bed pans, and urinals, cooking and feeding utensils, and medical comforts[2] such as oatmeal, sugar, sago, etc. A field chest contained a comprehensive list of some 120 different drugs and dressings. Stretchers were issued before embarkation, but the regimental establishment included no stretcher bearers. When a man was hit he made his own way to the regimental hospital set up beyond the range of cannon fire in a building or in a tent; if badly wounded he lay where he fell until the end of the battle or was helped to safety by his comrades. When the fight was over the wounded were dressed and any immediate amputations performed by the regimental surgeon and his mate assisted by the regimental orderlies.

The carriage of the bulky hospital equipment was always a problem on active service and as no army transport service existed,[3] reliance had to be placed on carts and waggons provided by the regiment from

local sources. Later in the campaign when the Minister for War came
to realize the need, a separate Waggon Corps was instituted, a need
which should have been apparent at the start.

The 10,000 Hanoverians in the force proved to be good troops, and
had a medical service larger in numbers and better equipped than the
British, for there were 7 regimental surgeons and 56 regimental mates,
or 1 mate to every 178 men. In addition there was a numerous hospital
staff of 1 superintending physician and 1 staff surgeon, 2 hospital
physicians, 1 hospital surgeon and 14 surgeons, 4 purveyors and 60
attendants and nurses. And moreover they were self-contained for
transport with fourteen waggons for the general hospital equipment.
A medical contingent of 14 medical staff officers came with the
8,000 Hessian troops, the senior doctors distinguished by the high
sounding titles of Physician General and Surgeon General, while more
impressive still was the four-horsed coach in which the Physician
General rode to war.

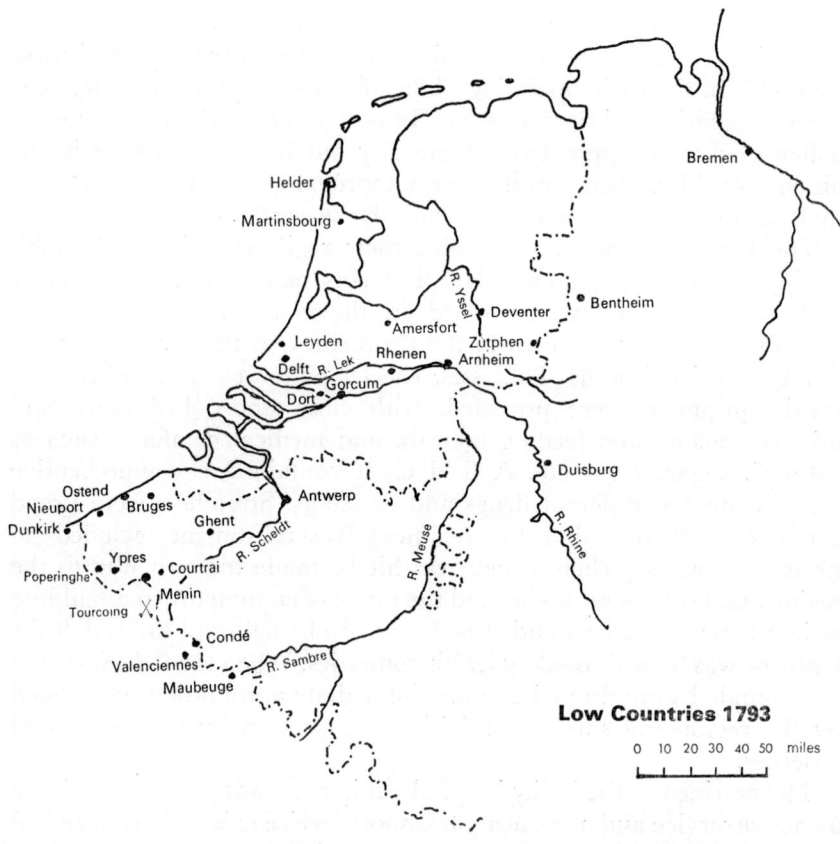

Low Countries 1793

0 10 20 30 40 50 miles

On the 1st May 1793 the Allied Army numbering some 100,000 men under Prince Coburg, the Austrian Commander-in-Chief, made a slow and deliberate advance in a huge arc which stretched from Mauberge to Ostend, spending two months in the reduction of the French fortresses of Condé and Valenciennes where the British forces were engaged and suffered some minor casualties.

Bruges was selected as the site for the chief general hospital for our troops with a smaller one at the base at Ostend, and to staff these, 2 physicians, 2 staff surgeons, 2 apothecaries, 2 purveyors, and 14 hospital mates with the necessary equipment were sent over. In order to make their duties clear Hunter drew up seven rules of conduct for the medical staff, which he hoped would settle any argument or jealousy between rival claims of physicians and surgeons.

(1) Every part of the management of sick in the General Hospitals is to be governed by the physicians except the strictly surgical procedures.

(2) The physician and surgeon is answerable for the treatment of the patients under his charge, and if more than one doctor is involved in attendance on the patient the Rules of Practice will apply.

(3) Apothecaries will have the charge of medicines and will act for the surgeons if required.

(4) Hospital mates will attend the cases both medical and surgical as mutually arranged.

(5) If there is any detachment of forces being made, the physician will nominate the necessary staff without regarding seniority or other distinction.

(6) The purveyor will give stores to the physician and surgeon as required and will engage the subordinate staff consisting of clerk, storekeepers, stewards, cooks and nurses. His accounts will be rendered every three months.

(7) The stoppages will be deducted at the rate of 4d. a day and paid once in three months.

In spite of Hunter's instructions it was not long before the inherent jealousy between these two branches of the profession made itself conspicuous by squabbles over the running of the wards and the responsibility each should bear. Perhaps this was inevitable without a senior officer to take overall control, and on the 27th July the Surgeon General appointed Dr. Hugh Kennedy to act as Inspector General to the Duke of York. Kennedy, the reader may remember, had served previously as a physician to the forces in North America, and was recalled from half pay to take up the appointment; currently he was physician to St. Bartholomew's Hospital.

The Allied plan of campaign under Austrian leadership continued its slow and deliberate advance on an extended front, but now King George put in a claim for the capture of Dunkirk, and the Duke of York with his British forces which now comprised the Guards brigade, Abercromby's brigade, and some cavalry regiments, together with his German troops, broke away from the Austrians and moved north through Ypres, Poperinghe and Nieuport. Brushes with the enemy caused some 600 casualties, but by the end of August some 22,000 troops were entrenched around Dunkirk.

Events were soon going badly for the Allied armies. The French struck at the long extended Allied line which was weak at every point. A covering force of Hanoverians between Dunkirk and Nieuport was overwhelmed, and the Duke of York, threatened with encirclement, was forced to raise the siege and to retire hastily towards Ostend, abandoning guns and stores.

Sick wastage had been heavy at Dunkirk and before, because incessant marches and fighting, swampy encampments and bad drinking water had caused outbreaks of both dysentery and fever. Fortescue reported that this operation cost the Allies nearly 10,000 men. The general hospital at Bruges was quickly in difficulties for over 1,000 sick arrived without warning before accommodation could be found for them. Ostend too was soon full as it only held some 200 patients and the overflow was sent to Bruges only to be sent back again. To relieve the pressure on Bruges another general hospital was opened nearer the front at Menin, and additional hospital staff dispatched from England.

Complaints about the ineffectual treatment of the wounded were now reaching the Surgeon General's ears and anxious also to know how the general hospital system was working, Hunter sent out his brother-in-law Mr. Everard Home, on a visit. Home, however, at once ran into difficulties with Kennedy who insisted that as Inspector of Hospitals to the Commander-in-Chief he was entirely independent and would not allow interference. He intended, he said, to communicate his reports direct to the Minister, and to demand medicines direct from the Apothecary General. Home was, however, allowed to visit the general hospitals where he found nothing radically wrong in the forms of treatment, nor had any of the sick and wounded officers any criticisms to make, but he made certain suggestions for improving working conditions and conducting surgical operations. On the administrative side however there was a great deal to criticise. Some of the faults were not medical in origin but hinged largely on the lack of transport for casualties, and the hardship caused to the sick by the long journey from the regimental to the general hospitals in slow jolting country waggons. But he still found a good deal of confusion caused by the shortage of hospital accommodation, and lack of co-operation between physicians and surgeons. He had moreover to use restrained language in making suggestions, to avoid anything which might be interpreted as orders to upset Kennedy's absurd prerogative of independence. The complaints about the care of the wounded arose because of the complete absence of facilities for treating casualties in the area between the regimental hospitals and the general hospitals in the rear. To cover this gap he now proposed the revival of the 'flying hospital' to act as a link and serve as a centre to which the regimental hospitals could evacuate their casualties. With two staff surgeons in charge it would be a self-contained unit carrying its equipment and tentage in six waggons; the former would include boards for beds, bedding, ward, and kitchen equipment, medical comforts, instruments, dressings and medicines.[4] The Duke of York at once gave his agreement to the proposal.

Ostend was the port from which invalids were embarked for England, and Home now offered to arrange transport and go home with them, but he was snubbed by Kennedy on the grounds of interference. 'It showed me,' Home remarks, 'that my stay on the Continent would not materially improve the service.'[5]

Henry Dundas, the Minister for Home Affairs who had been made responsible for operations, now recalled to England some battalions for service elsewhere and this reduction in the Duke's strength was followed by a further French advance. After defeating the Austrians at Wattignies, a thrust was made towards Nieuport and Ypres, which threatened the British base at Ostend. The hospitals at Bruges and Menin which held 1,474 sick had to be moved back to Ghent for safety. This represented a 20 per cent sick rate which was distressing. As always in campaigns, fever and dysentery were the major causes, although the term dysentery was applied to all cases of enteritis; while fever included malaria, typhus, and typhoid. The Hanoverians and Hessians suffered equally, with a 20 to 25 per cent sick rate at their hospital at Tournai, which meant a further 2,000 cases under treatment there.

Both armies shortly afterwards went into winter quarters, engulfed in the Flanders mud, with the Allied front on the French frontier. The campaign for 1793 had achieved little more than turning the French out of the Austrian Netherlands, but it had proved an arduous year for the troops due to the constant alerts and the endless marching and counter marching which the tactics employed by the old school of the Austrian high command demanded.

Towards the end of the year, as we have already indicated, the control of the medical service had changed hands by the death of Hunter followed by the institution of the Medical Board with its three members.

It was not long before the Board changed Hunter's policy of promotion by seniority asserting that he had relied too much on length of service instead of ability in the selection of the medical staff officers. This applied especially to the staff surgeons whose lack of operating skill had come in for a good deal of adverse criticism. On the 23rd November 1793 the Board addressed a letter to the Secretary at War explaining their motive. 'They found themselves,' they said, 'under the necessity of deviating from lately established custom of . . . choosing through a regular gradation and motives of length of service and seniority only . . . because these surgeons had lost their skill and (were) only fit for retirement.'[6] 'Our policy,' they affirmed, 'is to make physicians of gentlemen bred to physick, and hospital surgeons of men bred to surgery.'[7] In theory nothing could be more sensible or straight forward than this declaration but in practice their change of policy was to riddle the Department with discontented officers and to prove a significant cause of their own ultimate downfall.

The Board was quickly at loggerheads with Kennedy, for in his passion for independence he had now taken upon himself to control the promotion of both regimental and staff officers, and wrote on the 28th November from Army headquarters at Tournai, 'As I hold myself responsible for the abilities of those whom I think worthy to recommend to H.R.H. for promotion I am sedulous in my selection. H.R.H. has given me confidence in these matters and will not permit any interference.'

Alarmed by this restriction of the Board's powers, Gunning said it was 'repugnant' to the commands of His Majesty. But Kennedy proved most obstructive. Letter after letter asking for a return of the deficiencies of regimental surgeons and mates remained unanswered and the Board was finally driven to making the position known to Lord Amherst, the Commander-in-Chief at the Horse Guards. They pointed out that their policy to obtain well qualified gentlemen would only succeed if reasonable prospects of promotion as surgeons either to regiments or on the staff of general hospitals was open to them, and they were unable to offer these terms unless they knew the vacancies. To enlist doctors as hospital mates with pay of only 7s. 6d. a day and without prospects of promotion would never attract the type of men they wanted. Without Kennedy's co-operation they could not supply the correct number of physicians, staff surgeons, and hospital mates for the number of sick in the general hospitals, and they must know the whole position of the distribution of medical officers to maintain control. This was a matter of principle which would affect all expeditions overseas, for if Kennedy was allowed to exercise his personal control in opposition to the Board this policy would also be adopted by other Inspectors.

Lord Amherst had no hesitation in confirming their authority, and laid it down that only the Board could deal with the appointments of physicians, staff surgeons for hospitals and medical staff officers both at home and abroad, as well as surgeons to regiments. Dr. Kennedy would confine himself to filling vacancies temporarily.

Gunning the Surgeon General attacked Kennedy's self importance for styling himself Director of Hospitals when he was only entitled to be called Inspector, a rank which did not give him any power of recommending any individual for special appointments.

In December the newly constituted Board drew up fresh instructions for the conduct of medical staff on foreign service, with the object of stopping the bickerings and arguments between physicians and surgeons. Although the physician was still to remain in control, the surgeons were now to have an entirely free hand in treating their own surgical cases, and, obviously worried by the complaints, the Surgeon General enjoined them to treat their patients with 'tenderness and humanity'.[8] They were ordered to visit the wards once a day at least; mates were to be allowed to operate only in the presence of surgeons; and the purveyors were directed to provide all the items needed by both physicians and surgeons.

To relieve the congestion in the hospitals, Keate the Inspector of Regimental Infirmaries proposed the evacuation of as many cases as possible to England, and arranged for the naval hospital at Deal to receive them. But when he went there he found it was crowded with seamen and poorly equipped. Hammocks and cots were in use instead of bedsteads which were at once installed for the army casualties and he procured another building for the 'putrid contagious cases' who were spreading infection in the over-crowded wards. Many lives, he said, may be lost in such conditions. Being a keen and able surgeon he wanted the surgical cases under his own care in London and this brought about the creation of the York Hospital in Chelsea—a house which was formerly the Star and Garter Tavern, and was increased by building huts to accommodate a total of 200. The transports bringing the sick and wounded from Ostend would disembark the medical cases at Deal and take the surgical cases on to Deptford where they would be transferred to barges and taken up the Thames to Chelsea.

Between November 1793 and March 1794 some 30,000 recruits were enlisted for the regular army, and 13 new infantry battalions and 5 new cavalry regiments were raised. The practice of selling commissions to anyone with money, provided they brought in a certain number of recruits, made officers of many undesirable types. Some were commissioned in the immediate rank of lieutenant colonel or major and even mere youngsters were exalted in the course of a few weeks to the dignity of field officer; political interest rather than meritorious service was the road to promotion. Bounties for recruits were offered and the price of men rose to £30 a head. Even the prisons provided their quota. But of the troops raised many were untaught owing to the scarcity of officers who knew their job. With a possibility of invasion, scores of Militia and Volunteer Corps were formed. The number of regular troops provided for in the estimates for 1794 was 175,000, and with Volunteers, Militia, and foreign troops, the army strength amounted in all to a total of 265,000 men.

For the 1794 campaign in Flanders, the Duke of York, who had not shone as a military leader, was kept in command, but made subordinate to Austrian supervision. The British forces which now included four cavalry brigades had been made up to strength by young and raw recruits, but there was a deficiency of drivers and horses, guns and transport. The Hanoverian and Hessian units were far below their proper strength from sickness and losses from constant skirmishes. In all the Duke had under his command some 30,000 men. The troops of our Austrian allies were in poor condition, and the local inhabitants refused as far as they could the food, fuel, and shelter which could make conditions bearable. The strength of the Allied armies was about 120,000, while the French were reported as over 200,000 strong.

This year saw the appointment of the first Secretary for War, a step of the first administrative importance but for the fact that the holder of it was Mr. Dundas, the former Minister for Home Affairs, whom Fortescue describes as 'the very worst man that could possibly have been chosen to found the traditions of such an office'.[9]

The Medical Board had followed up Home's suggestion for a 'flying hospital' by sending out in March 1794 1,500 sets of bedding, 5 hospital tents, 100 cots, 50 stretchers, and ward equipment which included over 500 bed pans, close stools and urinals, and a wide range of hospital necessities including 20 fumigating lamps; with medical comforts of oatmeal, currants, raisins and portable soup.[10] Additional reinforcements of medical staff officers, physicians, staff surgeons and 14 hospital mates were dispatched and a surgeon's mate was now provided for each cavalry regiment as the numerous engagements over wide areas of country had shown the necessity for increased medical aid.

The fighting which now developed saw the Austrians defeated at Mouscron, and the French capturing Menin and Courtrai. On the 17th May the battle of Turcoing resulted in a British defeat by a greatly outnumbering French force, after suffering nearly 1,000 casualties, while the Austrian troops close by observed a conspiracy of inaction, which embittered the relations with our troops. On the 22nd May after severe fighting the French in turn suffered a reverse at the hands of the Austrians with the loss of some 6,000 men.

Two additional infantry brigades had now arrived as reinforcements One was Lord Moira's brigade which had been kept inactive in the Channel Islands while the troops sickened and died of typhus fever in overcrowded transports in Jersey. The other brigade which came from the Isle of Wight left behind 100 dead from typhus and 250 men invalided, over and above a further 500 sick whom they foolishly carried to Ostend to clutter up the already overcrowded hospital.

These reinforcements were badly required, for the Guards brigade which had been continuously in action could only muster in May 1,266 men fit for duty and 400 sick.

But now the situation in Poland drew off the attention of the Austrian Emperor who had been leading the Allied armies, and he left the front for Vienna, leaving his army dispirited and discouraged. The loss of Ypres in June caused a wave of despondency and with the defeat at Fleurus in the same month the Austrians retired on Brussels. The British were forced to evacuate Ostend and fall back towards Ghent. This meant that the general hospital at Ghent had to be closed down and on the 5th July it was moved to Antwerp. Here it only remained until the 19th July when it was again sent northwards to Rhenen between the rivers Maas and Waal. As the number of sick increased and Ostend had also been abandoned a second general hospital was opened at Gorcom on the Maas, and a third at Dort, while transport vessels were utilized at the port of Dordrecht. These repeated moves disrupted the medical arrangements; neither did the jealousy and lack of co-operation between the medical staff officers make things easier. Colonel Craig of the Adjutant General's staff wrote on the 19th July: 'It gives me very great concern to say that the department which is so essential is most extremely ill conducted. I know not to whom to attribute it and still less how to remedy it but I feel for it very much. One great cause of the mismanagement is undoubtedly the spirit of discord which reigns in the department. I declare if I had my will I would change them all from the first to the last.'[11]

This spirit of discord was abundantly evident when in June Dr. Kennedy's control of the Department was heavily criticised by some of his own officers. Their complaints became so abusive that a court of inquiry was held at Tournai by order of the Duke of York to examine into 'complaints brought against him by one physician, four staff surgeons and one apothecary'. They stated Dr. Kennedy's conduct had been 'inimical to the recovery of the sick and injurious to the professional character of the complainants, that either by ignorance or inattention to the duties of his officers he had been the cause of much injustice to the sick and wounded . . . and that in the hospital many men had materially perhaps fatally suffered for want of medicines, dressings and bedding'. Some of these shortages were undoubtedly true, but often they came about from shipping delays due to adverse winds and weather. The Medical Board could not be blamed for the want of medicines for Kennedy with his self appointed freedom from control had adopted the short sighted policy of getting his supplies direct from the Apothecary General and the responsibility was therefore his alone.

The inquiry did not resolve the disagreements, and matters became so serious that Mr. Gunning the Surgeon General went out in August 1794 to see things for himself. He found some 3,500 sick in the hospitals;

1,300 at Gorcum, 800 at Dort and 1,400 at the main hospital base at Rhenen. He gave orders at once for additional physicians and apothecaries. Meanwhile Colonel Craig had written to Dundas on the 12th August, 'the business which of all others weighs heaviest upon me and which I own I despair of ever bringing to any sort of regulation is that of the hospital. The dreadful mismanagement of it is beyond description and the remedy is beyond my ability. Every branch and every fibre of every branch draws a different way. I really doubt if there will be any other way to get any good from the Department but by tying them all up together and sending them to you to be changed for a new set.'[12]

Although these criticisms were no doubt justified, the handicaps under which Dr. West, one of the medical superintendents was forced to work is typical of them all. When the only attendants in the wards were untrained regimental orderlies or unwilling convalescent patients changing every twenty-four hours the nursing standards were deplorable. The so-called female 'nurses' were only employed to cook the medical comforts or extra diets or to act as washer women, and they were often as disorderly as the convalescents. To control these unruly elements each hospital had its military commander with disciplinary powers, but these officers were ignorant of hospital administration and moreover they were so frequently changed that their power of command lacked all continuity. It was impossible to make bricks without straw and expect well managed wards in the face of such unreasonable conditions. It was the system which was to blame.

After further manoeuvring and fighting, the Austrians in August decided they were tired of the war in Flanders and withdrew their forces eastwards beyond the Meuse. This separation of the Allied armies left the Duke of York with no alternative but to retire northwards towards Holland. Although considerable reinforcements had brought his strength to nearly 40,000 men including seven brigades of infantry his army was now in poor shape. In the retreat to Holland the discipline suffered, and the officers, many of senior rank, who had bought their way into the service, were a disgrace with their hard drinking habits and entire lack of military knowledge.

Much of the hardship suffered by the troops was due to the poor clothing and the lack of greatcoats. The system was still in force whereby the colonel of the regiment received an allowance to clothe his men, and if unscrupulous he was able to make money out of it, which in wartime was at the expense of their lives. Moreover, the materials for clothing had to be made up by the regiment itself, but it was impossible to spend three or four months in making up clothes during a campaign, and the Duke's army was left almost naked. Even the Secretary at War appealed to the public to supply shoes for the soldiers because the clothing allowance was exhausted. It does not appear to have struck him that the obvious answer was to ask the Treasury for more. An attempt to change this iniquitous and out of date system which caused so much hardship on the soldier was made in 1798, but was abandoned as the cost interposed a fatal objection. To train a recruit cost £20 and it was beginning to dawn upon the authorities that many lives were being thrown away by allowing soldiers to perish from exposure due to insufficient clothing. 'It has needed,' said Fortescue, 'many years to drive from the heads of British statesmen the idea that it is not sound economy to pay a heavy price for a man on one day and kill him within a month in order to save a few shillings.'[13]

With the British and Dutch armies left to defend Holland owing to the refusal of the Austrians to participate, it was not long before, under French pressure, the British were forced to retreat to the line of the river Maas, and then to the river Waal. The Dutch proved reluctant fighters and surrendered fortress after fortress. By November the British troops were in desperate straits, naked and many barefooted. Twenty thousand pairs of good shoes were ordered. 'We will pay for these,' said Craig, 'but let us have them over without a moment's delay.'[14] Not only were shoes deficient but greatcoats as well, one brigade had no tents, and the civil population at home subscribed together to provide flannel shirts.

All this had a disastrous effect upon the health. Dysentery and fever decimated the units, and the number of sick amongst the British troops which on the 1st September had amounted to 3,391 men or 15 per cent had risen by the end of November to 6,501 or 31 per cent, nearly a third of the force. The German troops with 2,764 sick out of a strength of 15,000 were less unhealthy with a rate of 18 per cent, and this no doubt was due to better provision in the way of clothing and footwear. To provide adequate medical arrangements for over 9,000 sick was utterly beyond the capacity of the Medical Department; the hospitals were swamped, and many of the medical officers were themselves sick, including 2 of the 4 physicians, both dangerously ill. The death rate was enormous. When a man was ordered to hospital his comrades would exclaim, 'Ah, poor fellow, we shall see thee no more for thou art under orders for the shambles!'[15]

Our Dutch allies resisted every effort at collaboration and the British Ambassador at the Hague tried for two months in vain to find places where additional hospitals could be located. The only help he could get was an offer to send 500 patients to Delft. To relieve the overcrowding, 800 of the more severe cases were sent off to England, transport vessels were used to house convalescents, and many cases were kept on the barges which were largely used on the numerous canals, for they provided a smooth journey and good shelter. On one occasion 500 sick and wounded were embarked at Arnheim under the care of a single hospital mate without sufficient straw or provisions and were brought to Rhenen where they had to be left on board because the hospital was already full. A Dutch gentlemen counted at one time the bodies of forty-two men who had perished and been thrown out on the bank. 'Meanwhile,' says Fortescue, 'the rascals who bore the name of surgeon's mate charged £40,000 for wine for the sick and, not content with robbing the State by drinking it themselves, actually plundered the helpless patients committed to their charge.'[16]

Such wholesome condemnation of the hospital mates is hard to believe and the allegation is taken from an account published by an officer of the Guards.[17] There is no mention of such a scandalous state of affairs in the reports of the Adjutant General but it is true that the Medical Board were worried about the excessive consumption of wine and considered there must be some leakage between its issue by the purveyor and its reaching the patient. Because of the hardships suffered by the sick, port wine had been authorized as a general issue for the first time, although it was also a popular form of treatment, and 38 pipes or nearly 4,000 gallons had been consumed within eighteen months which at £78 per pipe would cost approximately £3,000, less than one-tenth of Fortescue's allegations.

Hard drinking was a common failing amongst all ranks and with the lapse of discipline which characterized the retreat, instances had been reported when senior officers who had bought their commissions had been found too drunk to march off with their units. As far as the hospitals were concerned it was equally likely that it was down the throats of the hospital orderlies and the nurses that the port wine disappeared. To try and bring consumption under control the Medical Board issued orders that each medical officer must sign the particular quantity for each day's delivery and must see it mixed with medicine or nourishment before it was given to the sick, and purveyors must have the power of dismissing anyone they considered was untrustworthy.

During November and December the British forces occupied the area between the rivers Maas and Waal and it was hoped that active operations would end and that this would provide their winter quarters. The regimental hospitals which had been unable to retain cases during the retreat were now re-opened to relieve the pressure upon the general hospitals, but the accommodation in barns and outhouses without any form of heating was harsh and comfortless when the cold became intense. Added to this the men's clothing was in tatters, some were destitute of blankets, and there was a shortage of hospital bedding. The troops were housed in tents or hastily constructed huts, but straw was scarce and in the severe weather sickness increased rapidly. Forty to fifty men in every battalion were barefooted, and flannel waistcoats and drawers were badly wanted. The surgeon to the Buffs reported that 150 sick were admitted within six weeks, all with one or other forms of fever. The returns from the infantry show that on the 21st December there were 12,604 men fit for duty and 7,728 in hospital, a rate of 38 per cent. But the cavalry regiments with better footwear and no marching to do had a sick rate of only 8 per cent.

There is no information as to how the 'flying hospital' performed its function in the field but that it was a success may be inferred from the fact that both the Hanoverians and Hessians had adopted the same policy, and with these three flying hospitals now reinforcing the general hospitals there were eight in all in the following locations. British general hospitals were at Rhenen, Gorcum and Dort, and the flying hospital at Arnheim. The Hanoverian general hospital was at Leyden and the flying hospital at Bentheim, while the general hospital for the Hessians was at Duisburg and their flying hospital at Vilp.

Dr. Jerome Fitzpatrick now makes his appearance on the Flanders scene. As the following peculiarly worded phrase records, he was authorized to pay a special visit to 'make suggestions for pitching tents, forming huts or other covering for the troops in the field or in winter quarters; in the means of moving wounded or sick or sending them to England'. As he was only directly responsible for his actions to Dundas himself this anomalous role could only be expected to lead to a head-on clash with local commanders. But imbued with strong humanitarian feelings and with the power of independent action, Fitzpatrick took immediate and practical steps to remedy neglect or hardship whether suffered by the troops or the sick, Soldiers perishing from cold were taken out of the tobacco houses and barns in which they were billeted and put into the warm farmhouses occupied by officers. He constantly went in advance of the waggons carrying the sick to prepare accommodation for them, defying the cold which was so severe that some of the patients removed in open waggons during the night would be found frozen to death. He had the floors of the waggons for carrying the sick lowered to make them more comfortable, and the transports used for carrying the sick and wounded invalids to England were inspected and suggestions made for their improvement.

Fitzpatrick visited the Hanoverian general hospital then located at Arnheim and found filthy wards and poor food; 417 deaths had occurred and he says the 300 in hospital were all likely to follow their comrades to the grave. The British general hospital at Rhenen was not much better, and he castigated the medical officers for their callousness and lack of humanity. Churches, warehouses, or outhouses without any form of heating formed the accommodation and the sick were for the most part lying on straw on the floor. Both equipment and bedding were terribly short and Fitzpatrick who had been given the power of drawing funds directly on the Treasury bought blankets and supplies locally. His disregard of regulations alarmed Dr. Smith the physician in charge of the area, who was of course unable to spend money on food and blankets at the public expense; and a suggestion that all regimental surgeons should come to Rhenen and Arnheim twice a week and demand better comfort, better diet, and more medicines, appalled the medical officers by its boldness and disrespect for authority.

Fitzpatrick had a lot to criticise on the treatment of the sick which he said never varied for any disease, whether of a 'bilious, putrid or inflammatory kind'. He found numbers of men dying from dysentery, but because of the indifference displayed by the medical officers they rarely visited the wards more than once a day and, no matter how severely ill the patients were never came at night. Amidst all this disorder and neglect the accounts for hospital stoppages still had to be kept; 6d. a day was deducted for dieting in hospital, but when they were convalescent with ravenous appetites the sum deducted for the purchase of food was reduced to 4d. As Fitzpatrick put it: 'When they could eat on their recovery they had it not, either in quantity or quality.' The Commander-in-Chief at once put this right.

The advent of arctic weather suited the French because the river Waal became a solid mass of ice across which they were able to advance and our troops had to break up their winter quarters and, constantly outnumbered and attacked, were forced to make a further retreat to the line of the river Lek. All the general hospitals had to be withdrawn on the 29th December and were reopened at Amersfort and Deventer, steps which involved the gigantic task of moving some 7,000 patients in the face of an advancing enemy. This was only accomplished by the most resolute efforts under the personal exhortation of Major General Harcourt the new commander, who had succeeded the Duke of York after the latter had returned to England.

Throughout January and February constant pressure by the French army compelled a continual withdrawal to the river Yssel and beyond, and the period which followed was amongst the most tragic in the history of the army. The country north of Arnheim is at the best of times inhospitable and bare and without much shelter in the shape of houses or trees. Discipline had largely broken down and the troops of different nations fought for such scanty comforts as could be found, the waggons were plundered and the line of march disorderly. The cold increased day after day and Fortescue says 'those of the army that woke on the morning of 17th January saw about them such a sight as they never forgot. Far as the eye could reach over the whitened plains were scattered gun limbers, waggons full of baggage, stores, or sick men, sutlers carts and private carriages. Beside them lay the horses, dead, around them scores and hundreds of soldiers, dead; here a straggler who had staggered on to the bivouac and dropped to sleep in the arms of the frost; there a group of British and Germans round an empty rum cask; here forty English Guardsmen huddled together about a plundered waggon; there a pack horse with a woman lying alongside it, and a baby swaddled in rags, peeping out of the pack with the mother's milk turned to ice upon its lips; one and all stark frozen, dead.'[18]

The sick suffered terrible hardships; constantly exposed in open waggons to drifting snow and heavy falls of sleet and rain, frequently without food until the army halted, bedded in cold churches or barns on dirty straw, often with but a single blanket, they perished in hundreds: 'martyrs to a most infamous and unpardonable neglect'.[19] Under these arctic conditions frostbite added to their miseries and many suffered the loss of toes, fingers and feet; then contagious fever or typhus broke out, characterized by tremors and convulsions, bloated face, delirium and death before many days.

Up to the 20th January all sick were sent to the general hospital at Deventer, but on arrival there permission was given to impress waggons to carry the sick along with their regiments. Harcourt now considered leaving the sick behind to be looked after by the French rather than let them suffer the hardships of further movement, but it was still found possible to carry them with the retreating columns until the 11th February when some 600 of the worst cases had to be abandoned at Deventer and Zutphen with medical and combatant officers left in charge. Our Dutch allies treated the sick and wounded abominably, even refusing them nourishment, but those who were captured were well looked after by the French.

At last the retreat came to an end when at the end of February the British fell back into German territory along the line of the river Ems, and by March the army was concentrated in the vicinity of Bremen. Fortescue puts down the losses after the Lek had been crossed as amounting to about 6,000 men of which not a tithe were killed or wounded in action.

It was naturally on Dr. Kennedy that the brunt of the blame fell for the evil reputation of the hospitals and the breakdown of the medical arrangements, but in his defence it can be said that he had to contend with the worst possible conditions of over-crowding, shortage of equipment, lack of transport, and untrained orderlies. But from the following account he was also badly served by many of his medical officers. 'Such was the infamous behaviour of the medical staff that the surgeons and mates are . . . in the constant habit of robbing the sick and . . . preferring the pleasures of carousing over flagons of heady port to the drudgery of alleviating the pangs of the miserable and afflicted patients, whose hard fate placed them under the hands of such ignorant butchers . . . who scarcely knew in which hand to hold a lancet or in what manner to fix a tourniquet.'[20] Although such harsh criticism may have been exaggerated, even General Harcourt whose testimony can be relied on had no good word to say for most of the medical officers. 'Ignorance of physicians,' he wrote on the 11th

February, 'scandalous neglect of most of them, sacrifice of lives to their smallest exertion, trouble and inconvenience call for justice and help. Dr. Kennedy, Dr. Smith, and Dr. Wood the purveyor have neither ability, activity or nerves to be of the least use.'[21] The management of the hospitals, 'is disgraceful, and can never be corrected by the present Director General of Hospitals who, although good, I cannot hestitate to declare is utterly incapable'.[22]

Fitzpatrick, too, also condemned the apathy and indifference in these words—'without a zealous Director of Hospitals instigated only by the great motive of doing good, the iniquitous impolitic practices will continue'. But now Kennedy himself fell a victim to illness and died in Germany on the 28th April 1795.

Happily there were some medical officers who did not drink and neglect their patients, and amongst them was Dr. Robert Jackson whom we have seen before in America and who as Regimental Surgeon to the Buffs has been already mentioned. In defiance of the Medical Board's policy, the commander of the forces appointed Jackson as a physician at the general hospital now established at Bremen, and over the heads of the other physicians he succeeded Kennedy as Principal Medical Officer. Jackson had therefore risen from regimental surgeon to P.M.O. of the force during the period of the campaign, certainly an unprecedented promotion which emphasized the outstanding ability shown by this officer. Naturally the Medical Board was distinctly perturbed.

In the closing stage of the campaign Fitzpatrick's final duty was to inspect fourteen transports carrying some 1,200 sick and wounded from Schrevendale. He found the ships ill-suited for the purpose and filthy dirty; the food intolerable, providing only one scanty meal a day; and a shortage of all medical comforts in the shape of rice, barley, sugar, sago, wine, tea and fresh bread, all of which he proceeded to buy and supply himself. The medical officers on the transports were apathetic and 'jogged along in their own errors'. Instructions were given for the ships to be cleaned and the dark and ill ventilated corners fumigated with vinegar fumes generated in a tar kettle. In April steps were taken to send home the final batch of sick and invalids amounting to over 1,000, but as only four ships were provided the convalescents alone were embarked and the remaining 600 were accommodated in the barns and outhouses of three villages near Bremen. Jackson personally undertook the treatment of these poor wretches who were half covered with rags, incrusted with dirt, over-run with vermin, and emaciated by dysentery and typhus fever. By removing the infected rags, cutting their hair, bathing and providing clean straw and a clean blanket their appearance was transformed. Jackson who was a great believer in cleanliness had the patients bathed every day, the straw changed daily, and shirts and blankets washed. Under this regime the infection died down within three weeks, and only thirty men lost their lives before they were sent to England.

So the campaign ended in disaster to the British army, and a disaster for the Medical Department. The general hospitals had proved a colossal failure but the basic need to retain them was still clear. A combination of several factors caused the breakdown, the principal one being the inherent difficulties brought on by the Physician General's mistaken policy of insisting that civilian physicians, well qualified it is true, but without a scrap of army experience, must be appointed medical superintendents of hospitals purely on the grounds of professional superiority. As administrative efficiency was the paramount aim, the Physician General would have been well advised to forego his jealousy and allow regular officers to control the hospitals. But as this meant placing a surgeon or apothecary in the position of giving directions to a physician Pepys would have nothing to do with it. To expect recently appointed civilians to understand the complicated details of running a hospital efficiently in the midst of an active campaign was bound to fail even under the most favourable circumstances. But here there was every sort of difficulty to contend with; overcrowding from the heavy sick wastage; a shortage of equipment and of transport to carry the sick and wounded; a horde of constantly changing, undisciplined and untrained orderlies to control; and all the confusion of a fighting retreat in the face of an enemy of much greater strength. A final and important cause which must not be lost sight of is the fact that hospital discipline lay in the hands not of the medical officers but of the military commandants. There were so many changes of field officers placed in command of the hospitals that all continuity was lost and their short periods of duty precluded the possibility of them acquiring a working knowledge of hospital management and control. Lieut General Murray who was the Duke's Chief of Staff confirmed this fact when he said 'the frequent changes of military commandants never gave the hospitals a fair chance.'

Major General Harcourt appreciated these difficulties as probably no other general had before, because when a third of the army is helpless and has to be transported, the defects in the hospital system are made forcibly clear and cannot be ignored. He, in fact, put forward the first proposal for the establishment of a separate medical corps made by a general staff officer. He condemned the practice of employing only convalescent patients to do the nursing which he said made good ward management quite impossible. 'My plan,' he says, 'cannot put the Department in a worse state than it is at present.' This was to establish a permanent hospital corps, recruited from men with good qualities of 'sobriety, honesty, and assiduous attention to the sick, with implicit and punctual obedience to the medical officers'.

The proposed establishment was as follows:*

	Daily Pay
Military commandant	£1 0s. 0.
Four officers to act as paymaster, quartermasters and adjutant at 10s. each	£2 0s. 0
Four sergeant majors at 2s. 6d. each	10s. 0
Four quartermaster sergeants at 2s. 6d. each	10s. 0
Ten sergeant ward masters at 2s. each	£1 0s. 0
Twenty corporals at 1s. 6d. each	£1 10s. 0
Twenty cooks at 1s. 6d. each	£1 10s. 0
Two hundred private attendants at 1s. each	£10 0s. 0
One hundred washer women at 8d. each	£3 6s. 8
	£21 6s. 8

*The number of hospital beds this establishment was to serve is not given but might vary between 500 and 1,500 depending on the number of beds each wardmaster or attendant was made responsible for.

There was inevitably much criticism among medical officers themselves on the breakdown of the general hospital system and there were not wanting some who would have abolished them on the grounds that the mortality was greater than in the regimental hospitals, the cost of running them was excessive, and finally that by sending the sick to the general hospitals the regimental hospitals were not fully utilized and the regimental medical officers became discouraged and less active in treating their own cases. Dr. Borland emphasized this last point[23] and said that the R.M.O's were bitterly discontented because civilian physicians and staff surgeons had been brought in over their heads to command the hospitals and out of spite sent in all their cases, thus overloading them and accelerating their breakdown. Through failures of administration, malingerers and servants rioted in drunkenness, while the regimental surgeons became indolent, sulky and chagrined. The argument that civilian doctors were better educated he calls fallacious and mischievous; fallacious, if it pretends that persons properly qualified are not to be found amongst regimental surgeons, and mischievous, as thereby persons of the best education have no incentive to become surgeons.

Be this as it may the mortality in general hospitals was undoubtedly higher, not only because they dealt with the severer types of disease but because the overcrowding inevitably led to the spread of hospital gangrene amongst the wounded and of typhus amongst the sick; one observer estimated the death rate as three in five or over 60 per cent. In the regimental hospitals the sick were widely dispersed in barns and outhouses and in this way cross infection was largely avoided. Dr. Jackson who was regimental surgeon to the Buffs and avoided sending cases to the general hospitals, says he had only one death from typhus amongst 150 patients.

But neither this argument nor the complaint of excessive cost could affect the basic need for general hospitals which were essential during active operations if the regimental hospitals were to remain mobile. It only emphasized the fact that if overcrowding occurred the general hospital bed cover was based on too low a percentage. If there had been ambulance waggons to carry the slight cases while on the move, the regimental hospitals would have played a more useful role and there is evidence that they did play an effective part when the tactical situation allowed.

Similar difficulties in administering hospitals had been experienced by Pringle fifty years before at the beginning of a campaign but under less arduous tactical conditions these had in time been overcome. Kennedy from all his experience proved remarkably ineffective and never had the support of his officers, while his absurd claims to independent control antagonised and handicapped the Medical Board, who claimed that the disorders and abuses which existed were considerably exaggerated by Kennedy's obstinate refusal to supply information on the deficiencies. Moreover some of the appointments they made had aroused opposition and one staff surgeon who was sent out was rejected by the Duke of York. The Board showed its perturbation by referring the matter to the Commander-in-Chief, but with Royalty involved in the dispute Lord Amherst felt he could do nothing.

There were aftermaths of course. In June 1795 letters were received by the Medical Board making indiscriminate reflections upon the whole medical staff of the army excepting Dr. Jackson and one or two others. These censures were not always justified. One doctor whose appointment Gunning had opposed because of his drinking habits was later accepted by the Duke of York. Mr. Gunning retorted with Hunter's telling point that no medical man should be recommended to the service except by medical men. The Board requested specific charges against individuals to be made by name but no more was heard of the matter.

In their summing up the Board said that if their advice had been taken instead of Kennedy's, and they had been allowed more power to act, the disorders so justly complained of would have been remedied long before. But we cannot ignore the fact that efficiency and soldiers' lives to boot were sacrified to the Physician General's insistence on preserving the physician's prerogative to superintend the general hospitals, a task for which they had neither aptitude nor experience.

WEST INDIES

On the outbreak of the revolutionary wars against France in 1793 the operations which took place in the West Indies from that year up to 1798 had a disastrous effect on Britain's potential for war. Pitt thrust the British army into what proved to be a hornet's nest, and in the end practically destroyed it. Egged on by the demands of the French *émigrés* and the greed of the British merchants for trade and wealth the Government acceded to all the demands for more and more troops to replace the appalling losses from disease. The constant drain on the army's strength meant that there were far too few for the main struggle which aimed to overthrow the French revolutionary armies in Europe, and the effects have already been seen in the withdrawal of troops from Flanders in 1794. Fortescue calculates that in the West Indies[24] some 160,000 soldiers were lost, nearly all by yellow fever, during the operations which went on almost continuously during these six years.

The Medical Board acted with promptness and efficiency to provide an adequate medical service, but with fighting taking place in Europe, the Mediterranean, and the East and West Indies, the drain on medical officers was tremendous, and the Board was hard put to it to recruit enough regimental mates, even when forced to accept men who were unqualified and possessed only a smattering of medical knowledge. It was simply unavoidable that some of the regiments had to go overseas short of mates, and the sickness and mortality rates were so heavy that it was impossible to replace them all in time to avoid shortages. Service in the West Indies was unpopular owing to its deadly climate, and some who volunteered for service only did so on the understanding that they would not be sent there. The more senior hospital staff were given no such choice and suffered accordingly. Out of eleven physicians detailed to serve in St. Domingo, only one who had become 'seasoned' by long residence escaped yellow fever, and of the other ten, all young and recently appointed, six were dead within six months of arrival. In this connection the policy of the Physician General in appointing as physicians only licentiates or fellows of the College of Physicians of London came in for criticism from many of the regular officers, who insisted that the inexperience in tropical diseases inevitable in these young physicians who superintended the general hospitals was the direct cause of a higher mortality. Dr. Chisholm, the Inspector General of the Ordnance Medical Department in the West Indies went so far as to say, 'The absurd conduct of the Medical Board is chiefly responsible for the death of 13,000 men from yellow fever.'

Happily this criticism was confined within the Department, for in marked contrast to the deplorable record of the hospitals in Flanders not only were there no accusations of neglect but there were complimentary remarks about their efficiency. The conditions of course were totally different from war on the continent. Here war was waged in a succession of small islands where movement was circumscribed and where hospitals were static and often located in well equipped civil hospitals, or in barracks and forts, warehouses and buildings.

One of the handicaps to complete recovery after illness was residence in such an unhealthy climate, and steps were taken to send a certain number of convalescents to Halifax in Nova Scotia and to Bermuda. But it was by invaliding to England that the majority were restored to health. The evil reputation of the climate had been known since 1654 when Cromwell had sent an expedition to Hispaniola, and this experience had been repeated at the siege of Carthagena in 1741 when nearly 2,500 men fell sick within the space of a week or two. But these calamities had been forgotten or discounted fifty years later, while the compelling fact of war made it necessary that the risk should be undertaken. Yellow fever, malaria, and dysentery were all endemic, and epidemics of yellow fever were to decimate the troops, with thousands finding their graves in some remote West Indian island. The first recorded outbreak in the West Indies was in 1647 and long periods of freedom from epidemics were recorded. At St. Domingo there was no yellow fever between 1763 and 1793, and the islands of St. Kitts, St. Vincent, and Barbados 'were so healthy previous to 1793 that soldiers fresh from Europe, notwithstanding their debauched life, enjoyed good health'.[25] Between 1785 and 1792 only one officer died out of four regiments stationed in Barbados, and it was only a tragic coincidence that the pestilence reappeared in 1793 after a long interval of freedom.

Medical officers soon appreciated that it was in the coastal plain and not the mountainous interior where the chief menace to health lay, but for tactical reasons it was essential to occupy this dangerous seaboard area. The unhealthy season for fever lay between the months of May and October which coincided with the rains and as we now know the prevalence of mosquitoes, but dysentery and enteritis which were principally dependent upon transmission by flies infecting food and drink prevailed throughout the year. Fresh troops arriving during the rainy season always incurred very heavy losses, and it was repeatedly emphasized by medical officers that the winter months were most suitable for expeditions or reinforcements to arrive; but the hazards of the sea passage and the tactical situation often made this impossible. Another medical suggestion was that troops should be 'salted' by residence in Gibraltar to accustom themselves to a hot climate, while steps were taken during the voyage to prepare the troops to resist fever by bleeding, purgation and dieting.

There were other factors which affected the soldiers' resistance to disease. The uniform was thick and stifling, so that during active operations the men sweated excessively and were easily exhausted. The effects of sweating and restrictive clothing may have produced the intractable ulcers of the legs which so many men were afflicted with, and which benefited at once by a change to a temperate climate. The ration of salt beef and pork in a thirsty climate led to excessive rum drinking, a drink which was easily obtainable, and this combination was frequently the precursor of enteritis. Surgeon Donald Munro writes, 'With the idea of increasing the bodily strength, the old army custom of issuing large rations of rum was in full force. This, the most persistent and the most ineradicable of all errors was condemned by the best surgeons, and although in the American War of Independence the uselessness of rum had been proved, although in St. Domingo the immense amount of sickness showed it was producing no good result, the fatal practice was continued.'

Before the outbreak of war in 1793 the situation in the French West Indies had been disturbed. In 1791 a general uprising of the negro population had started which especially affected the island of St. Domingo, and refugees had poured into the British possessions of Jamaica, Dominica, and other islands in the Windward and Leeward groups. So nervous did the British planters become that they asked for British reinforcements, and thus it came about that before war had been declared no fewer than nineteen battalions were in or on their way to the West Indies, not for aggressive purposes, but simply for security against a general rising of the coloured population. There were therefore ample troops on the ground when war broke out, and the first steps were taken in April 1793 when Tobago was captured with trifling loss, followed a month later by St. Pierre and Miquelon. An attempt to take Martinique which followed proved a failure.

Then in June the French planters of St. Domingo implored British protection and signed a form of capitulation handing over the island to King George. It must be explained that the French held only part of the island of Haiti, or St. Domingo, the remainder being a Spanish possession. The operations in this area came under the direction of the Governor of Jamaica, and in answer to their call for help a small force of 700 British soldiers from Jamaica landed at the Mole St. Nicholas, the Gibraltar of the West Indies, and in September 1793 the French garrison of the town surrendered and swore allegiance. But the island was in a hideous state of anarchy with the coloured people and the negro slaves in rebellion and intent on massacring the white planters, while to these was added some 6,000 French revolutionary troops with 14,000 white militia. It was quickly evident that this mere handful of British troops could not hope to conquer the island without reinforcements. But only a small number could be spared from Jamaica. The initial success was, therefore not to last, for the enemy forces soon recovered from the first shock of invasion, and after many engagements against the brigands and ruffians who made up the French negro bands the position became precarious in the extreme for the various garrisons were reduced to a few hundred men by casualties and sickness. However, in May 1794 the long awaited reinforcements consisting of three infantry regiments made their appearance, and the capital town of Port au Prince was captured.

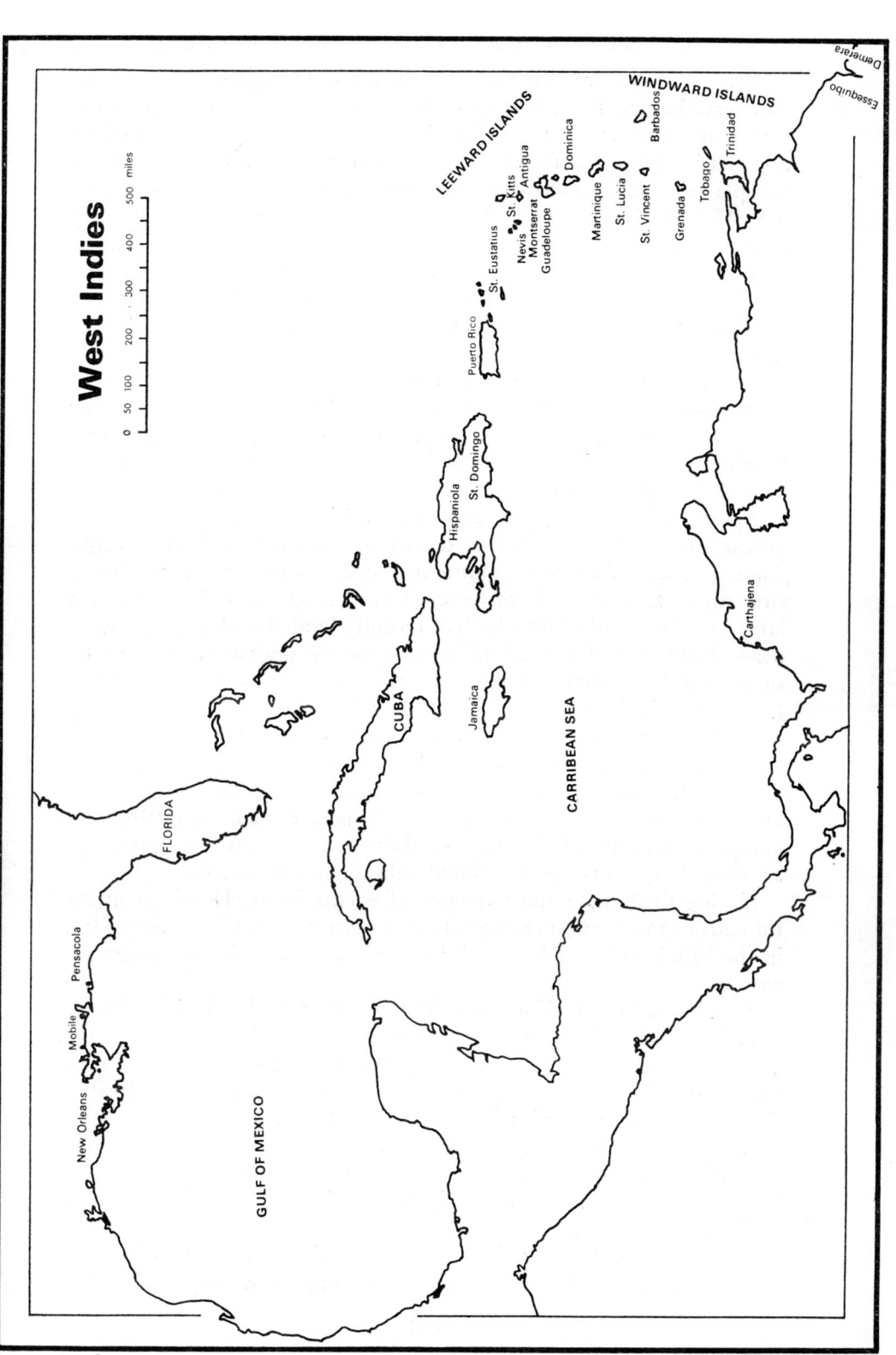

West Indies

0 50 100 200 300 400 500 miles

New Orleans
Mobile
Pensacola
FLORIDA
GULF OF MEXICO
CUBA
Jamaica
CARIBBEAN SEA
Hispaniola
St. Domingo
Puerto Rico
St. Eustatius
Nevis
St. Kitts
Montserrat
Guadeloupe
Antigua
Dominica
LEEWARD ISLANDS
Martinique
St. Lucia
St. Vincent
Barbados
WINDWARD ISLANDS
Grenada
Tobago
Trinidad
Carthajena
Demerara
Essequibo

Mr. John Weir was the senior medical officer in Jamaica where he had served since 1790, first as purveyor and then as surgeon to the forces; an officer with an established reputation of many years standing, and destined to be a future Director General of the department, he was placed in charge of the medical arrangements in St. Domingo. At both Mole St. Nicholas and Port au Prince there were French military hospitals which are described as being 'on a grand scale and when properly ordered will add much to the well being of the army'.[26] In the former there was room for 320 patients and a separate officers' hospital; while at Port au Prince 400 could be accommodated, and there was a naval hospital as well. The attention which the French gave, even in their colonies, to the construction of hospitals for the army was in marked contrast to the neglect and indifference displayed by our own Government. In these commodious buildings the regimental hospitals were speedily opened, and an urgent request was made to the War Office by the commander of our forces for hospital staff officers and equipment to open two general hospitals. But before they could arrive yellow fever had made its first deadly appearance, and on the 29th June 1794 out of the seven battalions in the island with a combined strength of 3,700 men there were 1,700 in hospital, and two months later 34 officers out of 64 who had recently landed and 729 men were dead. With such losses all offensive military operations had to be suspended, for in each of the several garrisons our troops were reduced to a few hundred men, and although they defended themselves valiantly and with success against continual enemy attacks, by the end of 1794 things were once more critical. To replace the Europeans, hopes were concentrated on raising levies of loyal negroes and some 3,000 were enlisted, but the brutal conduct of many French royalist officers and planters alienated the majority of the natives against us, and revolt arose in many areas with continual fighting and massacres.

Having dealt with the sequence of events in St. Domingo up to the end of 1794 we must retrace our steps to see what has been happening in the Windward and Leeward Islands some 800 miles to the south-east.

The first large expedition to sail for the West Indies had left Portsmouth towards the end of 1793 under the command of Lieut General Sir Charles Grey. It was made up of 7,000 men comprising nine battalions of infantry organized in three brigades, and this considerable force arrived at Barbados in January 1794. Accompanying it came Mr. Mallett, Inspector General of Hospitals, and a hospital staff of 4 physicians, 3 staff surgeons, 3 apothecaries, 1 purveyor and 18 hospital mates, with all the equipment and medical stores for establishing general hospitals.

Barbados now became the principal medical base where Mallett had his headquarters, and here a general hospital was opened and a medical store depot installed. In each of the islands of Tobago and in St. Pierre and Miquelon there were excellent civil hospitals, and these were now taken over as garrison or general hospitals. Garrison hospitals were under the charge of a garrison surgeon, who was a promoted regimental surgeon or apothecary; he had also an administrative role, and supervised the regimental hospitals in his area and rendered the weekly and monthly sick returns to the Inspector General. The general hospital had a full hospital staff of physician who acted as super-intendent, staff surgeon, apothecary, purveyor, and hospital mates. Both hospitals treated the more seriously ill cases so as to leave the regimental hospitals free for mobile operations, and the transfer of sick and wounded was generally done by sea, as speedier and more com-fortable than crossing the mountains by forest paths.

Offensive operations against the Leeward Islands were now to be undertaken, and as a result of brilliant co-operation between General Grey and Vice Admiral Sir John Jervis, Martinique was captured after severe fighting, and by May 1794 Guadeloupe and St. Lucia were also in our hands. In each of these islands general hospitals were opened; the most important being at Martinique.

In the month of June the first epidemic of yellow fever swept through the force and within a month there were 1,200 cases, a number which so overcrowded the hospitals that many had to be treated in quarters. It was not long before Grey had only 4,500 men fit for duty, and to the scourge of yellow fever was added an enemy success when parts of Guadeloupe were recaptured by a fresh landing of French troops who had evaded the British frigates in a successful passage from France. To make matters worse the growing audacity of the bands of hostile negroes in all the islands led to constant fighting amongst mountainous forest-clad country which took a severe toll of our fever-ridden troops, while the French, by promising freedom from slavery, quickly secured amongst the coloured population a formidable ally. In Guadeloupe by September there were barely 500 British troops fit for duty, 1,500 were sick, and 330 men had died in a month. The story of the garrison of Berville is typical of many. Constant French attacks were beaten off by men so weak that they could hardly stand, but finally in October the garrison was forced to surrender after losing 7 officers and 76 men killed and wounded. Thereupon, 125 ghastly figures staggered out, fitter for hospital than to be under arms, all that remained of what had once been three battalions and twenty-three companies of infantry and two companies of artillery. Fortescue says, 'The records of the British Army contain no grander example of heroism than this of the dying garrison of the camp of Berville.'[27]

In the other islands the toll of yellow fever had been equally devast-ating, and in Martinique by September the white troops fit for duty had shrunk to 600 men. To hold the islands Grey was compelled to ask for reinforcements, for by the end of 1794, of the officers who had sailed with the expedition 27 were killed or had died from wounds, and 170 had died of yellow fever or other diseases; of the men it is estimated that of the original 7,000, some 5,000 perished.

So the campaign which had started so successfully was brought to the brink of disaster by the fearful toll of lives exacted by the ravages of 'yellow jack'. It was the beginning of a story which was to be repeated over the years. Medical officers suffered death and disease no less than their comrades, and it was only by helping each other in this extremity that the hospital and the regimental officers were able to provide even a minimum of medical attention to the hundreds who crowded the hospitals. Yellow fever was not the only peril; enteritis, dysentery and venereal disease were widespread, and in the autumn months intermittent and remittent fever or malaria claimed many victims, while chronic ulcers of the legs which obstinately refused to heal were a peculiar manifestation which caused much disability.

Nor did the Navy escape; amongst the transports 46 masters and 1,100 seamen died, and Fortescue says that if the losses of the navy, the army and the merchant seamen be added together it is probably true to say that 12,000 men were buried in the West Indies in 1794. Ministers had known of the deadly effects of the climate for a hundred and forty years, 'yet they poured their troops into these pestilent islands in the expectations that thereby they would destroy the power of France, only to discover when it was too late that they had practically destroyed the British Army'.[28]

When General Grey's expedition left England the hospital equipment and medical stores had been sent out on five different transports, but the Medical Board found this method slow and uncertain and as the supply of medicines was regarded as so vital the Surgeon General persuaded the Minister to agree to the use of the packet ships which left Falmouth at regular intervals. This would ensure speed and regularity. In November 1794 the first consignment of 2 tons of supplies for Jamaica, 3 tons for St. Domingo and $4\frac{1}{2}$ tons for the Leeward Islands were dispatched, to be followed up by bulk consignments at six monthly intervals each spring and autumn.

In November, Grey had to go home worn out after repeated attacks of dysentery, and Major General Vaughan who succeeded him could muster a force of only 2,000 men fit for duty to defend eleven different islands. Guadeloupe had now been entirely lost, and although Martinique and St. Lucia still remained in our hands, the negro insurrection which was rapidly spreading everywhere created a dangerous situation. Dundas had promised thirteen more battalions, together with drafts of 3,500 men as reinforcements, and at the end of December 1794 the first three regiments arrived at Martinique. But in Vaughan's view the best chance of ultimate success lay in enlisting black levies, for while white troops died in their thousands, natives had a relative immunity from disease. He wisely set about this task without waiting for the approval of the Government.

The year which followed was to prove a disastrous one for British arms, for the negro bands assisted by the French dominated the greater part of every island. The further reinforcements which arrived in March 1795 from England consisted only of five regiments instead of the promised ten, and were recruits of poor quality.

With the example of the disastrous failure in Flanders in mind the Medical Board in April 1795 drew up fresh instructions to tighten up the administrative control. Failure had been partly due to the inexperience of hospital staffs, but the regimental hospitals had also been badly reported on and it became notorious that regimental surgery was then, as it had been during the American War, in a very defective state. The surgeons had been either appointed by purchase or taken from the regimental mates recommended by colonels of regiments; many of them were without proof of their medical qualifications or education and were unfit to perform important operations.

Now a much tighter control was to come into force. One set of instructions was issued to Commanders by the Secretary at War under the heading 'Regulations for the conduct of the medical staff on foreign service'. This laid it down that the Inspector General was to visit the sick twice a week in general hospitals and a senior medical officer either a physician or staff surgeon, to inspect every regimental hospital once a week. Medical cases were to be separated from surgical cases, and fevers from dysenteries; physicians were forbidden to instruct surgeons in the treatment of surgical cases; the stores and wine consumption were to be inspected; purveyors accounts were to be sent to the C.-in-C. every three months; sick and wounded were to pay 4d. a day stoppages.

A second set of instructions was issued direct to members of the hospital staff by the Board. This defined in strict terms the relationship between physicians and surgeons with a view to allaying the friction and jealousy caused by young physicians being given the superintendence of the hospitals. Both were asked to cooperate and act together for the harmony of the service and the surgeons were called upon to treat their surgical cases 'with tenderness and humanity'. Although many of the hospital mates were now being chosen for their surgical ability, they were forbidden to operate unless a staff surgeon was present. On the physicians was laid the responsibility for administrative control, the segregation of infectious cases and the inspectorial visits to regimental hospitals. The purveyor had the task of finding hospital accommodation with the assistance of the Q.M.G., and the provision of beds, bedding, lighting and food. As there was no establishment for the subordinate hospital staff he had to procure the clerks, stewards, storekeepers, cooks and nurses either by asking Force headquarters to detail them from regiments, or by hiring them from local civilian sources. The apothecary, in addition to having the charge of medicines, was also expected in emergency to help in the wards either as surgeon or physician.

Promotion to fill vacancies due to death, invaliding, or other causes was authorised within the command but with certain safeguards in the case of medical staff officers. Although the appointment of physicians was the sole prerogative of the Physician General, in an emergency the local C.-in-C. could nominate a medical officer to the rank of physician after examination by the Inspector General assisted by a physician on the board. Staff surgeons, apothecaries, or hospital mates could be selected from the regimental surgeons or mates after an examination before a board composed of physicians and staff surgeons. So much for the theory, but under the stress of active service conditions the meticulous regard for these orders came to be ignored or overlooked at times and the Board in London had to interfere.

During the year, desperate fighting against tremendous odds was waged in St. Lucia, Grenada and St. Vincent and after three months of continual struggle St. Lucia had to be abandoned. In Grenada and St. Vincent after hard fighting our troops managed to hold on with great difficulty, for the pestilence of yellow fever was from May onwards striking the soldiers down much faster than the enemy. Of 1,400 men who were brought away from St. Lucia before it fell, 600 were sick; at Grenada between the 7th and 23rd July, 250 men died out of a strength of 1,450, and in the Windward Islands as a whole in these sixteen days the deaths numbered 450. At Martinique in the Leeward Islands 177 men died in July, and there were 764 sick out of a strength of just over 2,000. Moreover, yellow fever demoralized the men it had not killed, and the fighting qualities of the troops was so reduced that they were easily overcome by the bands of brigands who swarmed round them in their thousands and attacked them day and night.

Inspector General Mallett himself fell sick and was invalided, and surprisingly enough, for this was contrary to the Board's policy, the appointment of his successor was left to the C.-in-C. in the West Indies. But when General Vaughan chose a young physician with only one and a half year's service the Board objected, an objection which was upheld by the King who ordered the appointment of Mr. Macdonald, a senior surgeon. Had the nomination of the young physician, Dr. Clifton, been approved there would have been uproar amongst the regular officers. By July, Vaughan himself was dead and his successor Major General Irving informed Dundas that 20,000 men would be necessary to hold the islands and that by the end of the campaign only half that number would be left. When the year 1795 terminated,

General Grey's army had largely been wiped out by disease and wounds.

The strain cast on the officers of the Medical Department by these thousands of sick has probably never been surpassed, and although there were divided ideas on whether yellow fever was contagious or not, the knowledge we now possess makes it plain that the danger in attending cases was a real one because of the risk of being bitten by infected mosquitoes. The devotion they displayed when their fellow officers were falling sick and dying was deserving of great praise. To make good some of these losses thirty-two hospital mates were sent out in October 1795 while in August no fewer than 6,000 sets of hospital bedding and other stores in proportion had been dispatched to provide for the sick, 4,000 to Martinique and 2,000 to Barbados, the islands where the principal hospitals were located.

Our history must now return to St. Domingo where by January 1795 the 3,700 British soldiers had been reduced to 1,800 of whom 700 were sick; the rest were dead. The ships of the fleet too were practically immobilized by the heavy mortality amongst the seamen, and this was serious, for it left the seas free for ships from America and other West Indian islands to pour arms and ammunition into the hands of the Republicans to allow them to continue the struggle. Fighting occurred all through 1795 with the British troops scattered in detachments over the island, principally in the coastal towns at Port au Prince, Jeremie, and Mole St. Nicholas. Reinforcements arrived from England to bring the strength up to some 3,000, but of this number 1,700 were soon sick for by June a fresh epidemic of yellow fever was sweeping the island, so that by the 1st July out of seven infantry regiments then at Port au Prince not 500 men were fit for duty. Worse was to follow, for during the height of the epidemic in August and September 900 British soldiers died, so that by the 1st October the number of troops had fallen again to 1,300 fit for duty, and 1,000 sick, and at Mole St. Nicholas in December only 300 were capable of bearing arms. This terrible shortage in man power was relieved by the raising of considerable numbers of levies from the coloured population, a policy which was to pay a handsome dividend.

On medical recommendation a scheme was now proposed to send 500 convalescents to the military hospital at Halifax in Nova Scotia, where the change to a temperate climate would promote recovery of the fever cases and the chronic leg ulcers which were a major cause of disability.

Throughout 1794 constant reinforcements of medical officers had to be dispatched from England to meet the losses by death and in- validing, but the amount of sickness amongst these arrivals had led to so rapid a wastage that in Jamaica it was only by the help of some eight hospital mates enlisted locally in February 1795 that medical care could be provided, and Mr. Weir asked the Medical Board to increase the number of regimental mates from two to three per battalion to cope with the overwhelming numbers of sick. The Board responded by sending him 32 hospital mates in October followed by a further 12 in December, while 4,000 sets of hospital bedding and stores in proportion arrived in August.

Fortescue regards the campaign of 1795 as perhaps the most discreditable that is to be found in the records of the British Army, but the conditions were so appalling it would be unjust to be too severe on regiments which were sent from one destructive campaign in Flanders, where they were decimated by typhus fever, made up to strength with raw recruits and plunged forthwith into a still more destructive campaign among the graves of thousands of their dead comrades. Even when yellow fever spared them they were worked to death under a tropical sun and tropical rain, plagued by mosquitoes and sandflies, fighting in unsuitable clothing which exhausted them, and without comforts of any kind, until the strain became insufferable and the best of them fell down, while the exhausted remnant refused to fight. There is a limit to human endurance and this was seen amongst the troops in the West Indies.

And now, persisting in their folly, the Government decided to follow up this disaster by sending out another expedition which could be certain to suffer the same fate. The command of this new force was entrusted to Lieut General Sir Ralph Abercromby, and the main body of some 18,000 men composed of twenty-four battalions of infantry organized into six brigades assembled at Portsmouth, and was destined for Barbados. At the same time a second force under Major General Whyte intended for St. Domingo was being collected at Cork. This consisted of an additional 13,000 men comprising 9 infantry battalions[29], 7 cavalry regiments, and some 4,500 foreign troops, principally Hanoverians. The recruits for the British units were mainly Irish, and the desertion, lawlessness, and drunkenness which prevailed compelled the military authorities to move them to Spike Island in Cork Harbour. During their stay here in the autumn of 1795 typhus and dysentery swept through all the units, and although a general hospital had been opened at Cork in 1790 the outbreak was so extensive that Dr. Robert Jackson who had been posted to this force as a physician describes how these cases filled every barn and outhouse on the island after the barracks and fort had already been requisitioned for the sick and the convalescents had been sent aboard transports in the harbour. By the time the fleet sailed 3,000 men had been admitted to hospital and 500 had died.

The medical arrangements for Abercromby's army were extensive.

With the Portsmouth force there sailed a group of hospital staff officers consisting of 4 physicians, 6 staff surgeons, 4 apothecaries, 30 hospital mates, 1 purveyor and 8 deputy purveyors; while in the St. Domingo group there were 7 physicians, 12 staff surgeons, 2 apothecaries and 70 hospital mates. There was a massive scale of hospital equipment to supplement the quantities already dispatched in 1795; for the Leeward and Windward Islands there were 1,200 cots with legs, 6,000 sets of bedding, 60 hospital marquees, and every item for ward and hospital use including shower baths, washing machines, filtering stoves, and fumigating lamps.[30] Then for St. Domingo there were 1,000 cots with legs, 6,000 sets of bedding, 40 hospital marquees, and the usual accompanying stores.[31] As a general reserve of bedding and equipment there were thousands of blankets, sheets, coverlets and palliasses.[32]

From these amounts it is plain the Board was determined there should be no grounds for the criticism which had been invoked by the shortages in the Flanders hospitals. Nor was this all, for there was a special supply of equipment for the Royalist forces in St. Domingo which included 1,000 sets of bedding[33], 500 cots, 10 hospital marquees, ward equipment and clothing. Medicines, too, in immense quantities were provided in scores of carefully packed barrels, bales and drums, and in order to provide ease of distribution the commoner drugs in use such as bark, opium and ipecacuanha were included in every package.

Before the troops embarked an important conference of senior medical officers was held at Portsmouth under Abercromby's orders to draw up rules for the conduct of troops during the voyage and immediately after arrival. They included Mr. Young who had been selected by the Board as Inspector General of Hospitals for this important force; he had served previously in the West Indies in 1792 and in Flanders in 1793 and proved on the whole an excellent choice. Mr. Weir from Jamaica was also present; he was now promoted to the rank of Inspector General for the St. Domingo area. The board was completed by the inclusion of Dr. Macnamara Hayes, two physicians, and Lieut Colonel Maitland of the 9th Foot, who presided.

The recommendations which follow in some detail are recorded as an assessment of the medical views of the time in preserving good health amongst troops in a tropical climate. The Board affirmed . . . that no raw and unseasoned troops should be sent, and preference should be given to men who had served abroad in places like Gibraltar; the arrival in the West Indies should be timed for November to allow troops to become acclimatised during the healthy winter months before the rains began in May, and active operations should if possible only be conducted between November and April. Natives should be employed to do the fatigues. The naval transports should be at least of 300 tons, with room to stand upright between decks; the practice of allotting one soldier for every 2 tons of ship's tonnage should be adhered to and increased if possible to 2½ tons per man; in practice this rule proved impossible as some of the ships were only 150 tons and these carried ninety-six soldiers apiece, a number which even then was in excess of the standard recommended. It is worth recording that Sir Jerome Fitzpatrick, the Inspector of Health for Transports, was at this time pressing for this basis of allotment to be scrapped and cubic space per man substituted. Every transport should be cleansed between decks with quick lime; hammocks and deck awnings provided, with bellows and wind sails to assist ventilation; no troops should be detained for long on board transports before sailing as this inevitably led to the outbreak of typhus. Good discipline, exercise, and personal cleanliness should be enforced, with a bath and clean shirt twice a week. Fumigation to be carried out between decks daily by vitriolic (sulphuric) acid and nitre in a sand bath. Fresh vegetables including potatoes were to be supplied against the risk of scurvy, with 2 pints of porter a day, while for every 100 men on board there should be a set amount of soup, pearl barley, rice and sugar for the sick.

After disembarkation the following precautions against fever should be adopted whenever possible. High ground was preferable for camps; ground floor should never be slept in;[34] tent boards should be used for camps as straw was unavailable, and the ground should be frequently changed. Men should eat in messes and not cook alone; there should be two meals a day with breakfast of coffee or cocoa and sugar, and dinner of salt meat, yams, and vegetables. No mention is made of a supper. Butter was generally rancid and was not included in the ration. Excessive rum drinking was condemned. Sea bathing was encouraged three times a week, but care was to be exercised that only five minutes was spent in the water.

The uniform consisted of a short skirted coat, loose cotton trousers and cloth gaiters to protect against bites of insects; black cloth stocks instead of leather; and watch cloaks. Each man had two flannel waistcoats which were really shirts, and flannel drawers.

Insect bites were regarded as the cause of sores and ulcers of the legs which were common and slow to heal, and for their early detection daily inspection by a N.C.O. and bi-weekly inspection by a M.O. was advised. Walking barefoot was forbidden because of the danger of jiggers which penetrated the skin.

Many of these measures recommended would be sound hygiene at any period, but the steps advocated ashore could have little effect while the peril from the disease-laden bite of the mosquito remained all unsuspected.

Dr. Macnamara Hayes was in charge of the embarkation of this force, and by medical examination had eliminated all men who were unfit, and had weeded out the aged and mere boys. The surgeons of regiments which had been broken up to provide drafts were posted as 'surgeons in second'; while for any units short of their two regimental mates, hospital mates were posted from the general hospital at Southampton. The regimental equipment was augmented and included 2 medicine chests, 2 voyage chests, 60 sets of bedding, and on Hayes' suggestion a tent was added. Staff surgeons were provided with two field chests; No. 1 contained medicines in common use,[35] while in No. 2 there were dressings and instruments which included an electric machine for treatment by electric shock.

Four so-called 'hospital ships' which carried the hospital staff officers and their equipment were just ordinary transports which Hayes says 'couldn't be worse' because of the poor accommodation and bad ventilation. But two were capacious, one was 400 tons and another 690 tons, and each carried 1,000 cots and bedding and equipment for any contagious cases which might be transferred from other ships during the voyage, and they were stocked with provisions including live sheep to supply fresh food.

So many venereal cases were embarked that three special ships for them had to be set aside so that medical officers could continue mercurial treatment during the long voyage. These were similarly supplied with fresh provisions. From the medical aspect this was the best equipped and best regulated expedition which had ever left these shores.

The start was unpropitious for when the transports set sail from Portsmouth and Cork in November 1795 they were almost overwhelmed by a terrific storm, and had to return to port. A second attempt in December encountered another storm, and eventually, instead of proceeding in convoy, many transports made their own way independently to the West Indies and the regiments arrived piecemeal at Barbados and St. Domingo from March 1796 onwards. Here the dreaded rainy season was already upon them.

Not until the end of April was Abercromby at Barbados able to assemble a sufficient force to begin his work of putting down rebellion, and with only half of the troops originally designed St. Lucia was recaptured, followed in November by the conquest of St. Vincent and Grenada, so that all the Windward Islands were once again wholly in our hands. But long before their capture had been completed the rains were in full swing and yellow fever had once again decimated the units. In St. Lucia alone during October the garrison buried 633 victims of disease, and there was hardly a regiment in the other islands which did not bury between 100 and 200. Some regiments both in St. Lucia and Grenada were reported as not having a single man fit for duty, and by November this force commanded by Brigadier General Moore, later of Corunna fame, was reduced from 4,000 strong to 1,000 fit for duty and 1,500 sick, the remaining 1,500 having died. In both the Windward and Leeward groups 3,000 British soldiers perished between the 1st April and the 1st October, and by the end of 1796 Abercromby's army had been diminished by one half.

Garrison hospitals were opened in the recaptured islands and equipped with the help of still more stores recently arrived from England,[36] but they were soon so overwhelmed with sick that thousands had to be treated in quarters. The table shows the number of patients in the hospitals and in quarters in the Windward and Leeward Islands between April and October 1796:

Month	Sick in Qtrs.	Sick in Hospital	Died	Tota
April	668	1,517	248	2,433
May	852	2,224	177	3,253
June	1,347	2,972	365	4,684
July	2,032	2,342	341	4,715
August	2,145	2,241	465	4,851
September	2,069	2,187	832	5,088
October	945	1,419	1,077	3,441
	(incomplete)	(incomplete)		

From May onwards when yellow fever became epidemic, the numbers of sick increased each month until by September the April admissions had doubled. As the strength of troops was around 16,000 this means that in the month of September, (the worst month for which all details are available) nearly one-third of the whole force was in hospital. The death rate for the seven months was 21·9 per cent, and includes all forms of disease; it was reported that the figures for yellow fever alone varied between 5 and 75 per cent of cases.

With numbers of medical officers falling victims to the epidemic Inspector General Young became desperately worried; 'St. Lucia,' he reports, 'would in my opinion require twenty mates from the dreadful sickness and mortality that prevails there, in so much that it is with difficulty I can get any to go there—the C.O's are constantly asking me for assistance; within the last twenty-four hours hospital mates Hall, Currie, Culpepper and Macauley are reported to be dead.'

His headquarters were now at Martinique, and he writes from there in October 1796 pointing out his difficulties and deploring 'the numerous sick in the regiments, amounting sometimes to 400 or 500 in each, and divided in different islands, and at an extensive chain of posts, the surgeons and mates often taken sick and dying from the fatigue of duty thereby occasioned'. On the 4th December he reports that, 'In the general hospitals throughout the several islands there are only 11 garrison mates and 33 hospital mates doing duty, (of those I have reports of death or sickness every day), which with 2 garrison and 18 hospital mates attached to regiments, constitute the effective strength of that part of the staff.'

On the 25th December 1795 in the island of Grenada a step was taken to fulfil a want which had on many occasions been put forward by medical officers and had been also proposed by Major-General Murray in Flanders. This was the formation of a separate corps to provide orderlies and other categories for duty in general hospitals which would take the place of the men supplied from regiments. The origin of this Royal Hospital Corps as it was named is obscure and its life a short one, as it lasted only from December 1795 until the 24th June 1796. The establishment of the corps was a commanding officer, an adjutant, a quartermaster, 6 sergeants, 6 corporals and 105 privates. This number was increased in April 1796 by a further seventy-five privates from the Army recruiting Depot at Chatham. Major Tinling was appointed C.O. and the adjutant was James Thornton. No records of its effectiveness and role have been discovered or the reason for its termination, but it is clear that the rank and file were used as orderlies in the general hospital in Grenada, and it is probable that it became extinct from the ravages of yellow fever.

Quite a different account of the Hospital Corps comes from the pen of Dr. William Fergusson. He places St. Domingo as the island where a Corps was formed and the commanding officer he names as Colonel Gilbert Waugh. Be this as it may the life of the Corps was equally transitory due to the utter worthlessness of the orderlies. 'Had they a man amongst them whom they were tired of flogging, and who could neither be induced to die or to desert, he was the elect for the hospital corps; or at best he might be a simpleton; not fit to stand sentry in a position of trust, or so awkward in the ranks that he could not be trusted with a ball cartridge.'[37] Drunkenness and yellow fever killed them off.

War with Holland had broken out in 1795 and a small force from Abercromby's army was dispatched to the mainland of South America to seize the Dutch colonies of Demerara, Berbice and Essequibo. A small group of medical staff officers with equipment for a general hospital sailed with the expedition and Dr. Pinckard who was present as physician has given an interesting account of the pleasant lazy life of the Dutch planters and the harsh treatment accorded to their slaves. But they were not lacking in courtesy to their British invaders, and as a doctor he was received with less hostility than the combatant officers. A general hospital was opened in a comfortable and well ventilated cotton warehouse to which the severer cases of illness were admitted from the regimental hospitals, for these from the mobile nature of the military columns which penetrated the interior were necessarily on the move. A nearby house accommodated the medical officers, and here they dined on salt beef and pork supplied by the Commissariat, supplemented by local yams and other vegetables and fruit. The staff surgeons and mates working in the hospital were at times reinforced by the regimental medical officers when the numbers of sick required it, and Pinckard himself as the physician in charge toured the regimental hospitals and supervised the treatment of the cases of yellow fever and dysentery many of whom died and many more were invalided. Bark was given as a routine in all fevers. Patients slept under mosquito curtains.

Major General Whyte's contingent of Abercromby's army had been directed to St. Domingo. Their departure from England had been delayed by storms until February and the first arrivals were in fact 2 regiments sent from Gibraltar, which were followed by 6 battalions in May 1796 bringing the strength up to 7,500 men. Although seven more regiments arrived in June the soldiers were already sickening by hundreds from yellow fever and within two months 1,300 of them were dead, so that by July this new army had shrunk to little more than 6,000 fit for duty and 2,500 sick.

Here again the strain on the medical department was overwhelming. Inspector General Weir made a report to the Board from Mole St. Nicholas where in the month of July alone 27 officers and 461 rank and file died, and the fleet, like the army, was simply paralysed by yellow fever; 'Gentlemen,' he wrote, 'I am sorry that every dispatch of mine to the Board is only a history of increasing mortality and accumulated horrors. I am under the necessity of drawing every medical man from the purveyor's line, and it is not doing them justice to make them suffer in point of emolument by giving them a more fatiguing duty—(Jackson sick, Cleghorn died yesterday, fifth day of yellow fever, Fellows sick). The whole duty of this place has fallen on Cleghorn, Lind, and myself. To attend the sick is a point of duty I thought myself exempt from, as my strength is by no means equal to that of the department of inspector.' His tale of horror was justified, for 6 of the physicians who had landed from England were dead within six months, and regimental medical officers had suffered so heavily that although 70 mates had been sent out with General Whyte's force, Mr. Wood an apothecary tells us, 'At one time the sick were absolutely in want of medical help and was obliged myself, besides the duty assigned to me of the charge and delivery of medicines, to take charge of the 56th and 67th Regiments, and also of Hospital No. 1.' In answer to Weir's urgent appeal for help the Board sent a further reinforcement of 9 mates, all they could muster.

Weir had at least no anxieties over hospital equipment for the large quantities sent from England with the expedition had arrived from March onwards, and in October 1796, the autumn supply of 28 tons of medicines had been landed. Similar amounts had been dispatched to the general hospitals in Martinique and Barbados, and 8 tons for the garrison hospitals in all the smaller islands. This was followed by further consignments in February 1797, and there were even vague references ascribed to the Inspector General that excessive amounts of medicines and equipment had been sent out and that Mr. Keate had benefited financially; but Young, when summoned before the Board in April 1799 categorically denied he had ever made such an imputation. The facts were that certain categories of medicines were more than sufficient because they were not in great demand, but the losses due to such hazards as capture by the enemy, wreckage, damage by sea water, packages going astray and theft, meant that the popular drugs such as opium, ipecacuanha, and ether, were never more than sufficient. All the islands were, however, supplied with sufficient bark for a year's consumption.

Dr. Jackson, who had arrived in St. Domingo as a physician, was now promoted Assistant Inspector under Inspector General Weir, an appointment which was only partly administrative and combined with it duties as a physician. Because of his rooted objection to general hospitals acquired in the Flanders campaign Jackson was determined to put his ideas into practice and to rely entirely upon regimental hospitals, where he was convinced that the regimental spirit which prevailed acted as a stimulus to the regimental surgeon; a better discipline was maintained with the unit's power of punishment; there was no malingering and the patient had his own comrades to nurse him. This contrasted with the undisciplined drunkards and profligates thrown out by the regiments who acted as orderlies in the general hospitals under the control of military commandants who were often inexperienced and uninterested and where patients could readily malinger.

Jackson obtained the half-hearted approval of Weir and the Medical Board to his experiment, but they covered themselves by saying that the closure of general hospitals must not be carried too far, so that if regimental hospitals had to move, the sick would not be left without care and attention. The Board's reluctance to the complete closure of general hospitals was tempered by the fact that they welcomed any chance of their curtailment on the grounds of expense. Not only did Jackson expand the use of the regimental hospitals but with that flair for reform which this remarkable man displayed he changed the system of supply. At this time the commanding officers of regiments made contracts for their regimental hospital supplies, but Jackson thought out a scheme for commuting the ration, whereby fresh meat was supplied instead of salt meat, wine replaced rum, and with the power of changing with the commissary the various items of provisions to a fixed rate of value, an immense saving to the public purse was achieved amounting it was said to £80,000 a year,[38] while the sick had every variety of fresh food which they needed.

Our narrative must now return to the islands of Guadeloupe and Martinique where there had been little fighting during 1796 and the chief enemy to be feared was not the French and the negroes but yellow fever, and again between the 30th July and the 14th November 1,549 British soldiers were sent to their graves and there were 5,731 admissions to hospital out of a strength of 13,000 men.

At this period Inspector General Young at Martinique was controlling 11 general and garrison hospitals with a total of 83 medical staff officers. In Martinique itself the principal general hospital had a staff of 16 medical officers with Dr. Pym as the medical superintendent, the author of the first clear account of yellow fever; Grenada had 10, Barbados 9, and the list below gives the detailed distribution in all the islands. To help administer these widely scattered hospitals which covered a distance of some 600 miles there were four assistant inspectors located at Martinique, St. Lucia, Grenada, and St. Vincent, but these in addition to their administrative duties were expected to help in the hospital wards either as physicians or surgeons.

Location	Inspector General of Hospitals	Assistant Inspector General	Assistant Inspectors	Physicians	Garrison Surgeons	Staff Surgeons	Apothecaries	Purveyors	Garrison Mates	Hospital Mates	Sick in Garrison and General Hospitals
Martinique	1	1	1	1	1	5	1	2	1	5	260
Barbados	–	–	–	1	1	1	1	1	3	1	30
St. Lucia	–	–	1	–	1	–	1	–	–	5	50
Grenada	–	–	1	–	1	1	1	1	3	3	21
St. Vincent	–	–	1	–	1	–	1	1	2	1	46
Dominica	–	–	–	–	1	–	–	–	1	3	96
Antigua	–	–	–	–	–	1	–	–	2	–	—
Tobago	–	–	–	–	1	–	–	–	1	–	12
St. Kitts	–	–	–	–	1	–	–	–	2	–	36
Demarara	–	–	–	–	1	–	–	1	1	3	74
Trinidad	–	–	–	–	–	1	–	–	–	4	181
Absent on leave	–	–	–	2	–	1	2				
Total	1	1	4	4	9	10	7	6	16	25	806

83

The small number of sick shown in hospital cannot be equated with the undoubtedly high incidence of sickness which constantly prevailed, unless the patients treated in the regimental hospitals and those who were sick in quarters made up the considerable difference.

At the end of this third year of war it was now beginning to dawn even upon Ministers that so costly an operation could not be further prolonged. Fortescue reckons that the army lost 25,000 men in the three years 1794, 1795, and 1796, and the fleet some 10,000. 'Official returns give the numbers of soldiers killed or dead in all quarters during 1794 as 18,600, and of soldiers discharged as unfit for further service from wounds or diseases during 1795 and 1796 as 40,600. Adding to these figures 18,000 dead during the years 1795 and 1796 and, say, 3,000 dead and discharged during 1793, we reach the total of 80,000 soldiers lost to the service, including 40,000 dead, the latter exceeding the total losses of Wellington's army from death, discharges, desertion and all causes from the beginning to the end of the Peninsular War.'[39] Yet with all this miserable waste and squandering of life England was little the better.

In January 1797 Abercromby reported to the Minister that the troops in St. Lucia and Grenada had been annihilated in spite of good hospital treatment, and such complimentary remarks on the medical arrangements was a welcome change after the accusations in Flanders. Dundas replied to Abercromby in the following terms. 'The favourable testimony you bear of the management of the military hospitals and the care of the sick is highly creditable to the Person entrusted with the direction of that Department and a source of great satisfaction to His Majesty.'[40] The 'Person' referred to was Young, and it is interesting to note that because he did not hold executive (but only equivalent) military rank he was not referred to officially as an officer but as a 'Person'. However, in whatever terms he was designated this was a feather in Young's cap, and it is all the more creditable when the strain placed upon the Department was so overwhelming. When death and disease strikes down doctors and soldiers alike, comradeship in arms makes criticism out of place. Of 6 hospital mates who had arrived in the last six months, 3 were already dead. 'From the great mortality of officers and mates that has occurred', Young writes on the 13th February, 'the number constantly sick, the promotions, etc. I am obliged to call the attention of the Board to my several letters pointing out the urgent and immediate necessity for mates being sent out. Had it not been for several young men I procured at Barbados I should have been under the most distressed circumstances.'

It was now Spain's turn to declare war in October 1796, and with the rich Spanish possessions of Trinidad lying to hand it was obvious that Dundas would order its seizure. So the campaign of 1797 opened in February with a bold landing of 4,000 of Abercromby's 9,000 remaining troops on the island of Trinidad, where the Spaniards immediately surrendered without a fight. But not content with this success, Abercromby was ordered by the irresponsible Government at home to repeat the process at Puerto Rico over 600 miles to the north-west. This was a totally different operation directed against a large island strongly held and fortified and requiring more troops than Abercromby could muster. Inevitably he was beaten off with the loss of 200 killed and wounded.

Throughout the West Indies as a whole by 1797 the resistance of the French and the negro bands was diminishing and there was comparative peace. But there was none for the medical officers, for the figures for April and May show that there were 4,639 admissions to the 23 regimental and the 11 general and garrison hospitals and 2,942 deaths, a mortality rate of over 60 per cent which is hard to believe.[41]

The sacrifice of British soldiers' lives was now to be mitigated, for at last the policy of enlisting negroes in regular battalions which had been repeatedly and foolishly rejected by Dundas at the instigation of the British planters, received official support. With the promise of liberation from slavery, recruitment proved so popular that by July 1797 there were eight battalions of the West India Regiment in being, and with the negro's comparative immunity to fever and bowel diseases these units saved the lives of hundreds of British soldiers.

At the other end of the battle line in St. Domingo the general tactical situation had also improved in 1797, but the British troops were so weakened by losses from disease that they were unable to take advantage of it. Fighting continued during that year, but was followed by an entire change of government policy, and it was decided that no further loss of lives or expense would be incurred and no further reinforcements sent to their graves. Consequently in May 1798 the British left the capital town of Port au Prince for ever. Mole St. Nicholas still remained in our hands but, following negotiations with the negro leader Toussaint L'Ouverture in October 1798, the baleful island of St. Domingo was finally evacuated and was left to be policed by colonial militia with French or Colonial officers in charge, at a cost which was not to exceed £300,000 a year. It was in fact an excellent move, for the amount of blood and treasure drained from England for its capture and its upkeep cost the lives of 7,500 British soldiers,[42] and some four million pounds sterling.

With the reduction in active operations the time had now come to cut down the medical establishments. In June, 1797, Major General Cuyler had replaced Abercromby who had returned home, and he was told by Dundas to pay serious attention to the heavy expenditure on hospitals, at the same time expressing satisfaction at the good reports on their state, in what he calls 'this interesting branch of the service'.[43] It would appear that only the appalling loss of life and the heavy wastage from invaliding had brought home to Ministers the fact that the Medical Department was at least 'interesting'. It would be many years before it would be appreciated that the Department had a great contribution to make to the winning of campaigns if their advice on hygiene and sanitation was listened to.

In Cuyler's letter of September 1797 he puts forward Young's recommendation for the reduction of hospital staff and describes him as 'the most zealous and active gentleman I have met with during my service, as he has discharged his duties of the Medical Department admirably'.[44] Perhaps the term 'gentleman' may be regarded as a more suitable expression than 'person' in official language.

Young proposed reducing by thirty the number of medical staff officers, provided certain conditions were fulfilled.[45] This included better equipment for the regimental hospitals drawn from the general hospital stores; garrison hospitals would only admit cases who could not be adequately treated in regimental hospitals and these would be inspected weekly; the medical staff of the foreign units were not to be withdrawn; and the main hospital and store base would be located at Barbados. The Minister and the Medical Board in December 1797 approved this plan in general, but wished an Inspector General and three physicians to remain, one at Barbados, one at Martinique, and a third to tour the other islands as a consultant. The hospital mates and clerks being temporarily enlisted for war could be discharged from the service whenever necessary, while the other medical staff officers would be placed on half pay. The pay of the Inspector General was also reviewed after Young had incurred the displeasure of the Board by suggesting that his pay should be increased from £2 to £3 a day; he pointed out that Inspector General Mallett under General Grey had drawn £3 a day, and this had afterwards been reduced under General Abercromby. Young won his point for he was strongly recommended by his G.-O.-C., but the Board expressed stern disapproval of such unauthorized conduct.

Medical promotions were also a controversial issue between the Board and Young, as this depended on how much power was allowed to local commanders in the matter, and Young was always running into trouble over the appointments of assistant inspectors and physicians. The Board in accordance with its settled policy would not allow civil physicians with only war service to be promoted to assistant inspector's rank with pay at either 20s. or 30s. a day for this was reserved for the regular officers. Young tended to ignore these rules in the interests of pressing local requirements when physicians and staff surgeons died or were invalided, and several promotions of this nature were approved by the Commander-in-Chief, to the annoyance of the Board, who found that their instructions on the examination of these officers were not being adhered to. Even the King did not always approve the Board's recommendations, and on several occasions had been known to reject them and promote other officers of his own choosing. Inspector General Weir in St. Domingo was also in trouble for the same reason. No doubt he was thinking of the death of the six newly arrived physicians when he wrote in December, 'The most arduous part of the service has fallen on the old officers, by the climate proving fatal to those who were never in such before.' The King approved Weir's recommendations rather than the Board's, and a purveyor and a surgeon were both promoted to assistant inspector, with the proviso that they should act also as physicians, one with pay of 30s. a day and one with 20s.

By the beginning of 1798 the bands of brigands in the Windward Islands had been thoroughly subdued or destroyed and comparative peace had returned, so that by 1799 the West Indies were practically defended by the West India Regiment and one British regiment, the 60th.

Fortescue estimates the total casualties from all causes during these campaigns including the navy, as little fewer than 100,000 men half of them dead.

It is unfortunate that no official records appear to be available of the casualties suffered by medical officers over this period, and this omission can perhaps be explained by a fire which is reported to have occurred in the Medical Board Office in 1803 when many records were destroyed.

In return for this frightful loss of life there could be shown only the British islands of Grenada and St. Vincent and the French islands of Tobago, Martinique and St. Lucia. 'For this,' says Fortescue, 'England's soldiers had been sacrified, her treasure squandered, her influence in Europe weakened, her army for six fateful years fettered, numbed and paralysed.'[46]

From operational activities we must turn to a brief description of the diseases which destroyed the British army in these fatal years. The Medical Board composed as it was of men imbued with civilian habits and ideas could not appreciate the value of a doctor such as Jackson in time of war. He was frequently unpopular with his superiors because he was outspoken, often impetuous, and inclined to be a rebel against authority. Neither was he always sound in his judgement and actions. In 1798 he brought charges against Mr. Whyte the purveyor of hospitals in St. Domingo, and at the court martial Jackson was declared to have acted throughout the whole prosecution in a 'frivolous, malicious, and groundless manner' and Mr. Whyte was most honourably acquitted.

Among medical officers there were not wanting some of a scientific turn of mind to whom we are indebted for the first accounts of certain tropical ailments. Such names as Pym[47], Bancroft, Jackson, and Nodes Dickinson are worthy of mention as successors to Hunter. Pym who was physician to the general hospital at Martinique in 1794–96 wrote the first account of yellow fever under the title of *Observations of Bolam Fever*, which was published in 1816; he estimated that in these two years 16,000 soldiers perished from the disease.

A multiplicity of theories were put forward to explain the causation, ranging from lunar influences to excessive rum drinking, and many hardened soldiers believed in the efficacy of strong drink to keep them free from both yellow fever and the marsh fevers and would smuggle rum into the hospital wards. But until the mosquito was identified as the transmitting agent of both diseases nearly 100 years later, the mystery of their origin remained unsolved. Dickinson was convinced yellow fever was a separate disease; Pym regarded it as infectious, while Jackson, who first thought it was a separate disease afterwards changed his opinion and thought all types of fever and dysentery had one overriding cause; others regarded yellow fever as a dangerous type of typhus,—typhus icteroides.

On certain aspects of malarial fever all were agreed; intermittent and remittent fever were associated with low lying coastal towns, swamps and marshes; the effect of acclimatisation was beneficial, for arrivals during the rains always suffered heavily, and fresh troops should arrive in the winter months, a recommendation which was strongly endorsed by the Medical Board but difficult to implement because of the hazards of war. Various prophylactic schemes were advocated during the voyage to prepare soldiers for their arrival in the tropics. Dickinson recommended weekly blood letting and purgation by calomel, and for six months after landing a vegetable diet, and avoidance of alcohol. Jackson advocated cleanliness by daily salt baths, airing of clothes, and active sports, scrubbing decks daily with vinegar and water, and clearing bad air between decks by explosions of gunpowder. He believed that keeping men in barracks was bad psychology and led to 'depression of mind' which was conducive to illness; and found that health improved when they were actively engaged either on patrol or on the playing field; this was contrary to the usual belief that active exercise in the tropics led to ill health.

Jackson divided fevers into seven varieties[48], but Dickinson's classification conforms to more modern thinking, (a) yellow fever, (b) marsh fever (remittent and intermittent), (c) fever with typhoid character.

The broad principles of treatment adopted for yellow fever depended on blood letting, emetics, purgatives and stimulants. A typical course was as follows: bleeding of 20 to 30 ounces; repeated doses of tartar emetic to promote vomiting; purgation by salts and calomel; frequent doses of James' (antimonial) powder, followed by further bleedings, and blisterings. In more severe cases accompanied by collapse, brandy, wine, and camphor were given as stimulants; abdominal friction with mercurial ointment; and washing frequently in cold salt water. Madeira of the first quality was the wine preferred and ample quantities were provided, for 300 pipes were sent to the Leeward Islands and 200 pipes to the St. Domingo hospitals, a total of 52,500 gallons. Some medical officers adopted mercurial treatment and pushed the drug to the point of salivation. Bark was administered in all early cases of fever but in yellow fever it was universally found of no avail. In desperate cases of yellow fever with failing pulse and all the appearances of coming dissolution heroic methods were tried; a large glass of gin with 20 grains of salt of hartshorn, a drachm of bark, 10 grains of snakeroot, and 1 grain of opium; and all repeated every two hours! But all these varied methods of treatment proved of little value and Jackson wrote despondently: 'In the sea-coast towns two-thirds at least of any given number of European soldiers will be found to perish before the expiration of the year, whether treated by French or English physicians.[49]

All cases of intermittent fever were plainly malarial in origin while many of the cases of remittent fever which occurred at a similar period of the year must also have been due to multiple infections of the malaria parasite. It was prevalent after the rainy season between the months of October and January, and Inspector General Weir wrote from St. Domingo in December 1797, 'The diseases of the season are remittent and intermittent fevers—half the garrison is on sick list. Many who were only convalescent died. I have not one relief in case of sickness at any post, Port au Prince excepted, where the greater number of sick require double assistance.'

Malaria was ascribed to 'natural causes', but medical officers never ceased to bring pressure on their commanders to avoid the low marshy areas and sea coasts where it was so prevalent. But this advice was rarely listened to and Fergusson writes, 'In the West Indies I found medical opinion equally at discount. The convenience of the engineer, the whim of the Quarter Master General or General Commanding and the profit of the contractor, seemed alone ever to be consulted. There was not a station in the command where the health of the troops seemed ever to have been thought of, or a health opinion called for.'[50]

Treatment by Peruvian bark was well established and all islands were supplied with sufficient for a year's consumption. But bark often varied in its effects for there were many types and qualities. At first yellow bark was used but this was replaced by a better form called red bark which was first taken from a Spanish prize in 1781 and analysed by Dr. Saunders of Guy's Hospital.[51] Arsenic was sometimes given in combination with bark, but bleeding, although sometimes practised in 'malignant' cases together with purging and blistering, was generally regarded with disfavour, as it caused weakness and debility. Jackson of course had his particular fad of 'agitation in pure air' and in common with many other medical officers was a great believer in cold water both internally and as cold douching. To illustrate the drastic treatment which fever cases had occasionally to undergo, a letter written by a hospital mate to the Medical Board is quoted. It is dated 6th December 1801, and it has been suggested it may have been written in malice; but it was published in an official

Blue Book, and the details appear to be correct. 'The men on admission were conducted to a wash house containing the warm and cold baths. They were instantly bled to the quantity of from 16 to 20 ounces. They were, on revival from fainting, which generally occurred, plunged into a warm bath in numbers of four to six together and confined in by blankets fastened over the machine till about suffocated. From hence they were dashed into cold baths and confined until apparently lifeless. Immediately after, a strong emetic was administered, they were carried to bed, and a dose of 8 grains of calomel and 6 grains of James' Powder given as a purge, which occasioned a train of distressing symptoms for the relief of which they were bled again and blistered from head to foot. They were bled a fourth and fifth time in the space of thirty hours, and usually lost 60 to 70 ounces of blood.'

Dysentery and diarrhoea were common diseases at all times, but worse in spring and early summer and constituted a third of all hospital cases. The universal consumption of salt meat increased bowel irritation, and although we now know that infection carried by flies to food and drink was the common cause of both the bacillary and amoebic variety of dysentery the disease was ascribed at the time to abdominal chill, or 'confined and damp air, loaded with putrid vapour'. The popular method of treatment was by enemas containing opium or sugar of lead, white vitriol, alum or corrosive sublimate, with tincture of myrrh added, followed by tonics which included angostura. Hepatitis as a sequela was understandably common after the amoebic infection and ipecacuanha was the sovereign remedy.

Pulmonary ailments, rheumatism, venereal disease and chronic ulcers of the legs were other common complaints. Dr. Dickinson reported that in the 63rd Regiment at St. Vincent there were no fewer than 200 to 300 men suffering from inveterate ulcers, and it is plain from this one instance that the trouble must have been widespread and disabling. Although their origin from injury or bites of insects was considered important enough for gaiters to be issued to protect the legs, Fergusson believed they were largely artificially produced.[52] Slow healing was probably due to excessive sweating, for as soon as the troops were taken on convalescence to Halifax or Bermuda they rapidly disappeared. These then were the diseases which led so many soldiers to their graves or sent them back as invalids.

When peace came at the end of the many years of toil and struggle, years when the strain upon the medical officers was probably greater than ever before, the Department as a whole under the able direction of men like Young, Weir, and Jackson, could look back with satisfaction upon duties well performed. Medical officers had never hesitated to sacrifice themselves for the victims of disease and many lost their lives and their health in attending their comrades in arms. Their duties may be summed up by the stirring words of Robert Jackson that devoted admirer of the British soldier who wrote: 'To be able to administer ease and comfort to a virtuous and heroic soldier affords the sublimest pleasure that the mind of man is capable of enjoying.'[53]

REFERENCES

[1] Fortescue. *History of the British Army*, book XII, chapter IV, p. 77. Macmillan, London (1910).

[2] The term 'medical comforts' is given to the extras in food and drink which were made available for patients.

[3] Transport for carriage of medical equipment was not provided until 1797.

[4] Medicines included preparations of opium and mercury, tartar emetic, rhubarb, pulv. ipecac. Glauber salts, Dover's powder, and vitrioli carne.

[5] P.R.O., W.O. 4/291, p. 122.

[6] P.R.O., W.O. 7/98.

[7] P.R.O., W.O. 7/100.

[8] P.R.O., W.O. 7/100.

[9] Fortescue. *History of the British Army*, book XV, chapter IX, p. 208. Macmillan, London (1910).

[10] This was in the form of a slab or cake which in appearance was like glue. One ounce dissolved in boiling water was said to make a quart of good soup.

[11] P.R.O., W.O. 1/169 p. 927.

[12] P.R.O., W.O. 1/169.

[13] Fortescue. *History of the British Army*, book XII, chapter XXX, p. 903. Macmillan, London (1910).

[14] P.R.O., W.O. 1/169.

[15] Fortescue. *History of the British Army*, book XII, chapter XII, p. 314. Macmillan, London (1910).

[16] Fortescue. *History of the British Army*, book XII, chapter XII, p. 314. Macmillan, London 1910).

[17] *Narrative of an Officer of the Guards*. Cadell and Davies, London (1795).

[18] Fortescue. *History of the British Army*, book XII, chapter XII, p. 320. Macmillan, London (1910).

[19] *Narrative of an Officer of the Guards*. Cadell and Davies, London (1795).

[20] *Narrative of an Officer of the Guards*, pp. 90–91. Cadell and Davies, London (1795).

[21] Harcourt to Dundas. P.R.O., W.O. 1/172.

[22] Harcourt to Dundas, P.R.O., W.O. 1/172.

[23] P.R.O., W.O. 40/22.

[24] Windward Islands—Barbados, St. Lucia, St. Vincent, Grenada.
Leeward Islands—Martinique, Guadeloupe, Montserrat, St. Kitts, Nevis, Antigua, Dominica

[25] Maclean. *Diseases of Tropical Climates*, p. 120. Macmillan, London (1886).

[26] P.R.O., W.O., 1/59, p. 211.

[27] Fortescue. *History of the British Army*, book XII, chapter XIII, p. 381. Macmillan, London (1910).

[28] Fortescue. *History of the British Army*, book XII, chapter XIV, p. 385. Macmillan, London (1910).

[29] Two battalions proceeded direct to the West Indies from Gibraltar.

[30] Bed pans 300, stool pans 120, chamber pots 1,500, urinals 360, stretchers 300, fumigating lamps 120, shower baths 6, washing machines 6, filtering stoves 12.

[31] Chamber pots 3,000, bed pans 200, stool pans 100, urinals 300, stretchers 200, shower baths 4, washing machines 4.

[32] Blankets 4,000, palliasses 4,000, sheets 12,000, coverlets 4,000, bed pans 304, stool pans 200, chamber pots 2,141, urinals 700, basins 167, blood porringers 73, plates 700, spoons 774, cots 800, cot legs 3,500, stretchers 48 and poles 96, tools, brushes, brooms, etc.

[33] Each set of bedding consisted of a palliasse, a rug, a pillow case, and three sheets.

[34] At ground level mosquitoes were more prevalent.

35 Antimony tartrate, colocynth, calomel, silver nitrate, mercury, opium, bark (pulv.cort. peruvian), pulv.ipecac; rhubarb, creta cum opio, spirit terebinth, tinct.opii, calamine, plasters, James, (antimony) powder.

36 Bedding 1,000 sets, sheets 900, blankets 830, coverlets 400, and hospital clothing. (P.R.O., W.O. 26/36).

37 Fergusson. *Recollections of a Professional Life*, p. 65. Longman, Brown, Green & Longman, London (1846).

38 Gore. *Our Service under the Crown*, p. 121. Ballière, Tindall & Cox, London (1879).

39 Fortescue. *History of the British Army*, book XXII, chapter XXIII, p. 496. Macmillan, London (1910).

40 P.R.O., W.O. 1/86.

41 The exact figures are:

Regimental Hospitals—April	admissions 1,390 and	368 deaths	
May	admissions 1,166 and	392 deaths	
General and Garrison) April	admissions 1,156 and	986 deaths	
Hospitals) May	admissions 927 and	1,196 deaths	

42 Fortescue does not accept the figure of 7,500 and says it should be doubled.

43 P.R.O., W.O. 1/86 p. 280.

44 P.R.O., W.O. 1/86 p. 280.

45 This would save the sum of £11 15s. od. a day.

46 Fortescue. *History of the British Army*, book XII, chapter XX, p. 565. Macmillan, London (1910).

47 Later Sir William Pym.

48 Bilious, yellow, remittent, nervous, continued, autumnal, putrid.

49 Jackson. *A treatise on the fevers of Jamaica*, p. 297. John Murray, London (1791).

50 Fergusson. *Notes and Recollections of a Professional Life*, p. 67. Longman, Brown, Green & Longman, London (1846).

51 Lloyd and Coulter. *Medicine and the Navy*, vol. III, p. 334. Livingstone, Edinburgh (1961).

52 Fergusson. *Notes and Recollections of a Professional Life*, p. 17. Longman, Brown, Green & Longman, London (1846).

53 Jackson. *A treatise on the fevers of Jamaica*, p. 360. John Murray, London (1791).

Chapter 9

FRENCH REVOLUTIONARY WARS II (1798–1807)

In this chapter our narrative ranges over a wide area of conflict and deals with campaigns in Holland in 1799, in Egypt in 1801, in Ceylon, and the Dutch colony of the Cape of Good Hope in South Africa. We then cross the Atlantic and describe the expeditions mounted against Monte Video and Buenos Aires in South America. On the medical side an account is given of the serious effects caused by Egyptian ophthalmia on the health and morale of the army and a reference is made to the new technique of vaccination.

After the return of the troops from Bremen in 1795 no British soldier was to set foot on the Continent for four years, for it was beyond Britain's power to provide an expeditionary force to fight the French. Pitt's policy was, therefore, based on attacking France through her overseas colonies and to employ as few British troops on the Continent as possible while paying mercenaries from Hanover and Hesse to do most of the fighting. It was in implementing this policy that thousands of troops were poured into the West Indies to moulder and die from yellow fever for the sake of a few sugar plantations.

France itself in 1795 was near anarchy, but between 1795 and 1799, Spain, Holland and Prussia had thrown in their lot with her. Conquest alone was the only antidote to her troubles, so that the French armies could live in the conquered territories by pillage and plunder. Austria and Piedmont held out with varied success as her chief enemies until Napoleon by his genius soon led to the subjugation of all Italy with its gold and its treasure. When Holland joined France the Dutch colonial possessions soon fell into Britain's power: the Cape of Good Hope was taken in September 1795, Malacca was captured by a force from India in August of the same year, the Dutch West Indies at the end of 1795, and Ceylon in 1796.

At sea the British fleet held constant watch over the French ports of Brest and Toulon, but when the Spanish and Dutch fleets were added to that of France the task of containing them proved to be almost impossible until the successive victories of Admiral Jervis over the Spanish fleet off Cape St. Vincent in June 1797, Duncan's destruction of the Dutch fleet at Camperdown in October of the same year, and Nelson's annihilation of the French fleet at the battle of the Nile in 1799, all curbed the effective power of the enemy at sea.

There were several French attempts to stir up trouble in Ireland. In 1796 an enemy fleet carrying some 1,500 troops arrived in Bantry Bay, and the country was only saved from invasion by a providential gale which drove the enemy ships back to France, and in August 1798 a Franco-Irish brigade was landed in the west of Ireland only to be surrounded and captured. These were anxious and stormy years with various revolts accompanied by the massacre of Protestants, only held at bay by maintaining a force of some 50,000 troops including 12,000 regulars and 20,000 militia for whom medical arrangements had to be made by the Irish Medical Board. The unsettled state of the country and the dispersion of the troops made it necessary to establish fourteen small general hospitals throughout the country from Belfast to Cork; the cost of maintaining these came to £10,000, with £4,000 for bedding and over £3,600 for medicines. The initial difficulty was to find surgeons for the militia regiments, as at first there was no permanency attached to these appointments until authorised by Act of Parliament passed in 1795. The Board was determined to maintain a high standard by insisting that only surgeons were appointed who had passed an examination or received a certificate from the Royal College of Surgeons in Ireland. Further, surgeons of regiments raised during the war were to be compensated by an annual pension of £36 10s. if their unit was later disbanded and they were not entitled to draw half pay. This rate it was thought 'would supersede every possible plea for the sale of the surgeon's commission', a practice we are informed 'which had prevailed to the present hour in defiance of the most positive regulations to the contrary'. Each Irish surgeon had to purchase a set of capital instruments (at an average cost of 15 guineas), and he was ordered to be responsible for the sick of all units within a radius of 10 miles. The Royal Irish Artillery had their own medical officers of the Ordnance Department under their Surgeon General.

In February 1797 some 13,000 troops were concentrated in the south of Ireland to repel any attempted French invasion, and Clonmel was chosen as the site for the general hospital with a staff of 3 physicians, 6 surgeons, 12 hospital mates, apothecary and purveyor. Twenty spring carts were specifically allotted for the carriage of sick and wounded. The credit for these ample arrangements must go to Dr. Renny the Director of Hospitals, and they drew forth the admiration of the Commander-in-Chief expressed in a letter to the Medical Board on the 23rd November 1797. Renny had a remarkable career and retired in 1847 after no less than seventy-two years on full pay, forty-nine of these as Director. This astounding record was made the occasion of a General Order issued on the 27th July 1847 expressing the Commander-in-Chief's appreciation 'to that old and meritorious officer' who had filled his position for more than half a century 'with so much advantage to the public interest'. During that long period Renny had been instrumental in bringing about outstanding improvements in the facilities for the care of the sick including the building of general hospitals; the inauguration of the medical staff with its device of a harp surmounted by a crown encircled with the words Irish Medical Staff; the preparations for the French invasion; and improvements in military prisons and substitution of separate confinement for the more degrading corporal punishment of earlier days.

Let us anticipate events here by recording that he was succeeded by Sir James Pitcairn who, on retiring in 1852, was followed by Dr., afterwards Sir Charles Maclean who was the last Director of Hospitals in Ireland. The offices of Physician General and Surgeon General ceased to exist at the same time, and the last holders of these appointments were Dr. Cheyne and Sir Philip Crampton respectively.

Over these anxious years Britain herself was often in desperate straits and Lord Malmesbury had been sent on two occasions to Paris to try and negotiate terms of peace. But the French proposals proved unacceptable. The solitary military success achieved in Europe was the brilliant capture of Minorca with its important harbour by Major General Stuart in November 1798.

At last in 1799 our fortunes began to revive for Pitt was able to form a coalition of Russia, Britain, Portugal, Turkey and the two Sicilies. Over these difficult and frustrating years Portugal had remained our only faithful ally, and the harbour at Lisbon was an important base for our ships standing guard over the Spanish naval ports on the west coast of Spain. One asset was that after the disaster of the last campaign in Flanders Britain turned her energies to building up a new army, awaiting the time when it would be employed on the Continent. With the formation of the coalition in 1799 the time to employ it had come.

Helder Expedition to Holland

The capture of Holland from the French who had driven us out in 1794 was regarded by Pitt as a keystone to his Continental strategy, and in June 1799 a treaty was signed with Russia whereby Britain engaged to provide 30,000 men and to pay for 18,000 Russian troops to attempt this enterprise. In spite of Pitt's promises, the British troops available did not amount to more than 10,000 men, and urgent steps had to be taken to find the means of raising more recruits. A ballot for the militia provided a form of compulsion for service at home, and attempts were made to convert this into a source of recruits for service abroad, so that in 1799 an Act was accordingly passed allowing militiamen to enlist in regular regiments.

For the projected invasion of the Low Countries the plan was to land on the Marsdiep isthmus near the naval base of the Helder. The medical arrangements were in the capable hands of Mr. Young, Inspector of Hospitals, recently returned from the West Indies; and a general hospital accompanied the force with a medical staff of 2 physicians, 4 staff surgeons, 3 apothecaries, 1 purveyor and 3 deputy purveyors.

The criticisms of negligence and the breakdown of administration in the general hospitals which had occurred in the Low Countries five years before had made general hospitals suspect, but General Abercromby who led the expedition admitted their necessity, although he considered the expense in running them might be heavy. To ensure success ample hospital stores of every description were embarked at Southampton, including 2,750 sets of hospital bedding and nearly 2,000 cots with folding feet, with mattresses for the serious cases, the former sufficient to provide bed cover for over 10 per cent of the force. This was the usual planning figure for campaigns, a figure which in fact had rarely proved adequate, although it does not take into account the forty beds in each of the regimental hospitals. Included in the general hospital equipment were special items such as fumigating lamps for combating infection, shower baths, and there were twenty hospital marquees for additional accommodation. The transport *Asia*, of 462 tons was fitted out with hammocks as a hospital ship, and the policy was to transfer all but the lighter cases of wounds and sickness across the North Sea to general hospitals at Deal, Harwich and Yarmouth. At Deal where there were now well-built military and naval hospitals the disembarkation facilities were adversely criticized by Dr. Jerome Fitzpatrick whom we encounter again carrying out his duties as Inspector General of Health and Transports; landing was only possible in open boats which involved great hardship on the wounded and the fracture cases, and on his recommendation Harwich was substituted and Deal used only for the sick. Both at Harwich and at Yarmouth where the Russians were treated, the hospitals were housed in halls or sheds convenient to the docks and were devoid of proper hospital facilities. To each an establishment of medical staff officers and a matron was appointed. Before embarkation a second assistant surgeon was posted to each regiment of cavalry, and a surgeon to the newly formed Royal Waggon Train which here made its first appearance in the field;[1] half of its forty waggons were earmarked for the exclusive use of the Medical Department, an innovation which heralded a welcome improvement in the transportation of sick and wounded.

Covered by a terrific bombardment by the fleet, on the 27th August 1799 a force of some 12,000 men under Abercromby made a successful landing amongst the sand dunes near the Helder, and established itself ashore. A confused struggle ensued but the invading force remained on the ground it had won. On the 10th September the French and the Dutch tried to drive the British back only to be repulsed with heavy loss, but Abercromby decided to delay further action until additional reinforcements joined him. On the 12th September two divisions of Russian troops and three more brigades of British infantry arrived, so that his force by this time numbered some 48,000 men. The Duke of York arrived to take command and on the 19th September the advance began with the Russian divisions allotted the place of honour. Rushing forward with savage yells, the Muscovites, lacking all formation or control, initially drove the French back and captured the village of Bergen. But unfortunately they had anticipated the agreed starting hour of the operation by some two hours, and there were no British troops ready to support them, so they were driven back and routed by an energetic French counter attack. On the British front the fine fighting qualities of the troops put the Dutch to flight, but battalion after battalion had to be withdrawn to rally and support the fleeing Russians, and the situation was only finally stabilized by the Guards brigade. When fighting ended the British line had been advanced from 5 to 10 miles at a cost of some 1,400 casualties, while the Russians had lost nearly 3,000.

The general hospital was opened at St. Maartinsbourg and by early September there were 1,762 British sick and wounded out of a strength of 16,806 or 10·5 per cent; on the 25th this had risen to 3,067 in a strength of 24,947 which was 12·3 per cent. The agreed plan of transferring the more severe cases to England meant that the *Asia* made successive trips to Deal, Harwich and Yarmouth. But the numbers were such that an additional hospital ship was asked for, and when this was refused, ordinary transports were utilized. At Surgeon General Keate's request, the more severely wounded were sent to Deptford and taken by barge up the Thames to York Hospital, Chelsea, where Keate acted as chief operating surgeon.

Following the destruction by the Royal Navy of a Dutch fleet at the Helder the command of the sea was safely in British hands and at this stage in the operations the Duke of York proposed an amphibious landing behind the French and Dutch lines. Admiral Dundas considered this too risky an operation, so a further frontal attack was ordered, and carried out on the 2nd October. The Russians after a successful start to the day's operations obstinately refused to press forward and, except that the village of Egmont op Zee was captured by the British, the day ended after prolonged fighting without any pronounced advantage on either side. The attack was resumed the next day without much success for the British and a defeat for the Russians.

By this time the total battle casualties since the commencement of operations had risen to the alarming total of 5,000 including 3,237 wounded; added to this, by the 14th October 2,628 British sick had been admitted to the regimental hospitals and 2,834 had been evacuated to the general hospital, a total sick wastage of 5,462 out of a strength of 25,407, which is over 21 per cent. When the dead and wounded are added to this number it is clear the army had lost a third of its strength. As far as the Russian medical arrangements are concerned the Surgeon General had sent out Deputy Inspector of Hospitals Robert Jackson to supervise their field hospitals and his task proved to be no light one for the sick rate of our Allies was even higher than the British, amounting to 24 per cent. This high incidence of sickness can almost certainly be ascribed to intermittent fever or malaria, for the autumn months were the height of the mosquito breeding season, and the Low Countries were notoriously malarious. The hospital ships were in continuous use and a further 1,500 cases were evacuated to England.

Abercromby became appalled by the thousands of casualties, by the inexperience of his young soldiers, and was baffled by problems of supply and transport. To the dismay therefore of the British rank and file, and to the astonishment of the French, the Allied army on the 7th October began to retreat, and on the 9th were back on their old lines. But at the same time the French were also in trouble, and their Commander proposed an armistice, a suggestion which was eagerly followed up by the Duke of York's staff. On the 18th October a cease fire was agreed upon on the condition that hostilities should cease and Holland should be evacuated by the 30th November. The British troops had only three days bread in hand, and there is no doubt the Allies were lucky to get away with such easy terms. When the Russians eventually reached England they astonished the people of Yarmouth by drinking the oil extracted from the street lamps.[2]

Before the final evacuation Mr. Young had warned the Medical Board that he estimated the number of hospital beds required in England would be somewhere around 5,000. The Surgeon General had taken steps to ensure this, and although accurate statistics are difficult to come by the following table shows the state of the hospitals after all the sick and wounded had arrived but do *not* show the total admissions to each hospital during the four months the expedition lasted.

Hospital	Number of patients	Total beds
Harwich	49	109
Colchester	1,300	2,500
Chelmsford	1,200	1,200
Deal	300	400
York Hospital, Chelsea	250	650
Yarmouth (Russians)	1,100	1,100
Hull	190	190
	4,389	6,149

A York Hospital return of an earlier date shows 601 admissions of the more seriously wounded who were under the personal care of the Surgeon General, while out of a figure of 2,718 admissions to all hospitals there were 186 deaths, a mortality rate of 6·8 per cent.

Young appears to have directed the medical arrangements with success, and evacuation by ship worked smoothly, a policy which prevented the overcrowding of the general hospital with its risk of hospital gangrene. At the same time the so-called hospital ship *Asia* was far from satisfactory. It was merely a transport devoid of port holes, dirty and unsuitable for patients as only one deck was available, and it was impossible to separate the different categories of sick or wounds. Surgeon General Keate in July 1800 had asked in vain that men-of-war or East Indiamen of at least 450 ton berthen should be provided with 7 feet to 8 feet depth between decks and six large port holes on each side. The hospital ships in use by the Royal Navy although better founded and equipped were never specifically built for the purpose but were slow old men-of-war reconditioned in-board, and the guns removed once their fighting days were over; they carried a full medical staff and female nurses when in port.

Fortescue says that the enterprise in spite of its failure showed that the men of the new army raw and untrained as they were fought well. So ended the expedition to the Helder.

Egypt 1801

When in 1798 the French Government decided to open the way to the conquest of the British possessions in India it sent a combined force under Napoleon to invade Egypt and this force conquered the Turks and the Mamelukes in a short campaign lasting just over three weeks. After Nelson's splendid victory and the destruction of the French fleet at the Battle of the Nile the French army was cut off from any hope of reinforcement or communication with France, although it was able to live off the country for many months. With the Mediterranean now free to British shipping, the Government decided in 1801 to remove the threat to India by destroying the French army in Egypt and the veteran Lt. General Sir Ralph Abercromby was given the command of a force of 16,000 men. To coincide with his arrival in Egypt additional troops sailed from India to participate in the campaign. The strength of the French army was estimated at 24,000 men with a force of 17,000 capable of taking the field, but their morale was low and they were longing to return to France. Moreover there was jealousy between the French generals, and Kleber their capable commander had been assassinated in May 1800.

With his constant forethought for the wellbeing of his men which characterized their Commander, Abercromby had ordered his regimental officers during the voyage to exercise every precaution to preserve their health. Embarking at Malta the expedition sailed to Marmorice Bay in Asia Minor where the troops who for the last seven months had been more or less confined on board ship were landed and exercised.

The principal medical officer at first appointed was Dr. James Franck, a physician of some distinction but without war experience and he was superseded by Inspector of Hospitals Thomas Young. This appointment shows Abercromby's influence, for Young as we know had served him well in the West Indies and at the Helder and the Commander-in-Chief had supported him in his quarrels with the Medical Board. The reader may remember that these originated from Young's insistence in the West Indies that he had the right to promote his own officers to vacancies in the medical staff, and had actually packed off to England one of the Board's nominees who had been sent out in relief. Naturally, he was distinctly *persona non grata* with Surgeon General Keate. On arrival at Marmorice Young found 1,098 sick under treatment, a sick rate approaching 12 per cent, and a clear indication that the long months spent confined on board had been detrimental to health. Included in the expedition were the medical staff, the equipment and the stores for a general hospital, while to provide further supplies of medicines and stores Surgeon General Keate had established depots at Gibraltar and Malta on which Young could draw.

Under cover of a naval bombardment an assault landing was successfully made at Aboukir near Alexandria in Egypt on the 8th March 1801. The medical arrangements for the landing were well planned, and Young directed them from his headquarters on board H.M.S. *Niger*. Sick left on board the men-of-war were to be looked after by naval surgeons, while those on the various transports were to to be transferred to one vessel and attended by assistant surgeons helped by convalescent patients acting as orderlies and nurses chosen from the soldiers' wives. For the expected casualties transports were earmarked as hospital ships, and a special division of naval boats were allocated for evacuation from the beaches. The regimental medical officers of the nine battalions in the assault scrambled ashore with their units and set up dressing stations on the beach. A medical instruction issued gives details of the allotment of medical personnel. 'A proportion of the general medical staff must be attached in the first instance to each brigade, and will be allowed such orderlies as are necessary from each brigade. Regimental surgeons are to be allowed one orderly each to carry the field case of instruments. When any wounded are brought down to the beach and a request shall be made for their being conveyed on board the hospital ships the captain of the division to whom such application shall be made is to direct some of the boats under his

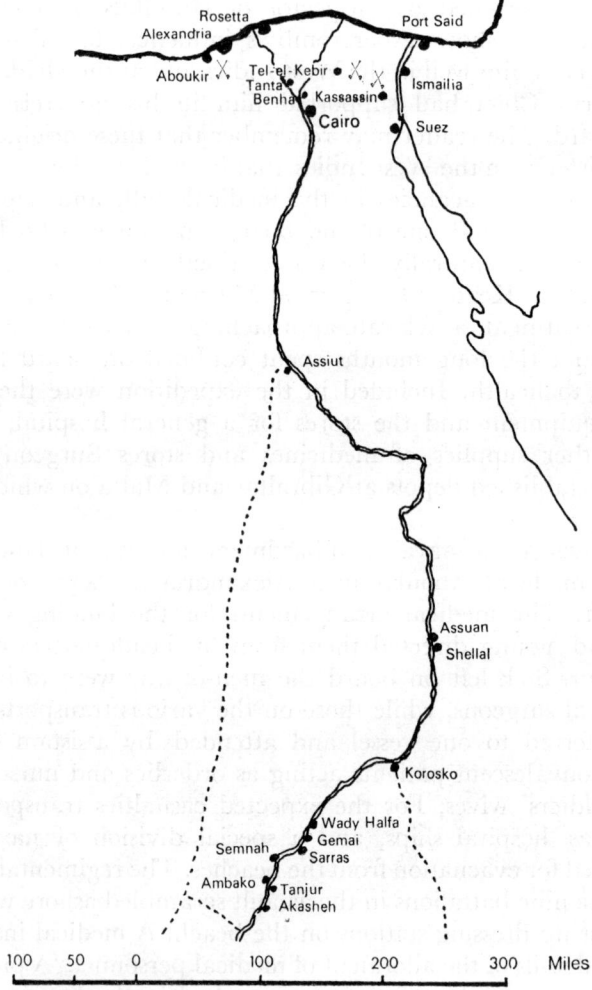

Lower Nile Valley

orders to perform this service, and, if necessary, that the flat boats shall be removed that the soldiers may be placed with convenience and ease to themselves, directing cutters and other boats to tow them. This service is particularly directed to the attention of Captain Apthorpe whose division is attached to the Medical Department. After the troops are on shore the stores belonging to the general hospital are to be landed.'[3]

By the evening, teams of staff surgeons allotted to brigades had been landed to reinforce the regimental surgeons and were to be found operating upon and dressing the wounds of the 700 casualties before sending them off to the hospital ships. Until the position could be consolidated and the general hospital equipment landed, tents were set up on the beach as temporary dressing stations. The heaviest losses were sustained by the 42nd Foot which lost 177, (including 156 wounded), and the Coldstream Guards, both caused while resisting charges by the French cavalry as they were forming on the beach. The Guards lost their surgeon George Rose. One of the chief anxieties had been the probable scarcity of drinking water, but contrary to expectations a sufficient supply was found by digging near the date palms scattered over the sandy soil, a discovery which made the troops independent of water from the fleet.

On the 13th March our troops attacked and captured the advanced part of the main enemy defensive position, but after an attempt to capture the strongly held main position was held up, the troops were partially withdrawn after a loss of nearly 1,300 men, among whom was Surgeon Egan of the Cameron Highlanders. Evacuation of the lying cases involved tremendous labour in the intense heat as there were few horses available and the sand made heavy going, but naval small craft were able to penetrate into Lake Maadieh and transfer them to the ships, while those who made their own way to the beaches were treated in the hospital tents and some palm leaf shelters which had been erected.

The heat the dust and the flies led to many bowel troubles and by the 17th March Young had some 2,400 sick on his hands while a further 1,100 had already been shipped away to Mediterranean stations. The difficulties of adequate care and attention for such a number were caused not only by the insufficient number of hospital officers to treat them, but were increased by the dispersion in the various transports used as hospital ships which were spread over 18 miles of sea. Young summoned all the medical officers and stores which could be spared from Minorca to his aid; and was already asking the Board for more supplies and for 40 well qualified hospital mates, making it clear in his peremptory manner that he could not be held responsible for the consequences if they were not provided.

The French army was now reinforced with troops sent from Cairo, and as their Commander-in-Chief was made aware that a British force from India was expected as well as a Turkish army, he determined on an immediate attack. After a fierce and prolonged struggle the enemy had to acknowledge defeat and Major General Moore later of Corunna fame said, 'I never saw men more determined to do their duty.'[4] Following the reputation they had begun to acquire at the Helder this new British army trained and disciplined under direction of its Commander-in-Chief, the Duke of York, proved itself in battle.

Our casualties amounted to over 1,400 but as no wheeled transport was available the removal of so many wounded to the general hospital on the beach was fraught with much difficulty and delay. A field hospital was therefore established in a mosque close to the battlefield, and here the staff surgeons attached to brigades supplemented the work of the regimental surgeons in their arduous task of operating upon and dressing the wounded. As the battle swayed to and fro this hospital at times came under fire, the tents were riddled with shot, and the many casualties had miraculous escapes. Victory was saddened by the death of their much beloved Commander, Abercromby. During the battle he was wounded by a bullet which became embedded in the thigh bone, but until the fight was over he refused to leave the field; he was then carried to the field hospital where it was considered too risky to amputate, and he was removed to one of the hospital ships where he died from gangrene a week later.

Treating the wounded was only a part of the heavy task which the Medical Department had to bear. At the end of March over 25 per cent of the force was in hospital with diarrhoea, dysentery, and fever, due to the bad sanitation, the swarms of flies, and the polluted drinking water. Some units had nearly 40 per cent of men off duty. The hospitals were crowded with over 3,000 cases, and there were 1,182 in the hospital ships, while Young was still shipping off the severer cases of wounds and sickness to Malta, Gibraltar and England.[5]

After a delay of six weeks to reorganize, Major General Hutchinson who had succeeded Abercromby, now had the task of defeating the French forces in Cairo, and during May advanced up the Nile Valley by slow stages with some 4,500 troops. A covering force of 6,000 men was left behind to contain the French isolated in Alexandria, and troops were pushed on to occupy Rosetta at the mouth of one of the main branches of the Nile delta. Here a general hospital was established in conditions of 'filth, mosquitoes of the most dreadful sort, vermin of every kind . . . stench intolerable, and houses almost uninhabitable'.[6]

The march up the Nile was necessarily slow for it was accomplished under conditions of great hardship in a temperature of 120° in the shade, a scarcity of water[7], clouds of dust and swarms of flies; knapsacks and tents were conveyed by boat but the single fly tents when put to use gave little protection from the sun. An account of the march has been given by Lieut Colonel Wilson: 'Certainly no troops had ever shown more resolution, patience and spirit . . . they bore every hardship without a murmur and, although four months in arrears of pay, never were guilty of the smallest excess. Frequently they were obliged to drink only water, and . . . wanting shoes, had to travel on the fiery soil and on the prickly furzes which covered the surface.' But drinking only water, although accounted a great hardship, had its good effects. 'Never indeed,' said Wilson, 'had an army before been so abstemious and consequently so well conducted.'[8] Toiling in the heat of the Egyptian sun and encumbered with their red tunics, tight breeches, gaiters and stocks, it was no wonder they fell sick. Fifty fresh cases of dysentery occurred each day, while an outbreak of bubonic plague acquired from the natives brought a new peril, added to which, fever, liver complaints and ophthalmia swelled the numbers so that a thousand more sick had to be sent down the Nile by felucca to Rosetta.

On the 7th June it was found expedient to open a further general hospital where the branches of the Nile divide, under the charge of Staff Surgeon John Webb who was given the title of Inspector of Field Hospitals. It was quickly filled with over 800 patients. By the end of May Hutchinson was 40 miles from Cairo and now joined forces with a newly arrived Turkish army; on the 21st June 1801 they appeared before the gates of Cairo where on the 27th the French unexpectedly surrendered without further resistance.

Meanwhile, the British and Indian units ordered from India under the command of Major General Baird, had, after long delays on the voyage, arrived in June at Cosseir on the Red Sea. To provide the hospital staff for this contingent Surgeon General Keate had thoughtfully dispatched via the Cape Dr. Shapter Inspector of Hospitals with a staff of 1 physician, 1 staff surgeon, 1 apothecary, 3 hospital mates and 1 purveyor's clerk, as well as hospital equipment. These reported their arrival to Dr. James McGrigor the regimental surgeon of the 88th Connaught Rangers who had been selected in India to act as the chief medical officer, an appointment which had caused some jealousy amongst the regimental surgeons of the Honourable East India Company's units when they were placed under an officer of the British service, and was duly regularized by granting McGrigor a commission in H.E.I.C. McGrigor was now superseded by Shapter, but on the representations of General Baird it was agreed McGrigor should remain as chief medical officer until the Indian contingent joined the British forces in Lower Egypt.

Before Baird's force lay the difficult task of marching across the 120 miles of desert from Cosseir to the Nile, a march which had to be carried out in the overpowering heat of June with the temperature ranging between 110° and 115°. Careful preparations were made. Movement was to take place only at night, and 2 gallons of water per man was to be carried on camels, and being brackish, the water was flavoured with vinegar. Before each march began half a pint of wine[9] and some rice water was to be issued. These sensible precautions resulted in the troops crossing the desert in fourteen days with only the loss of a drummer boy, and it was said 'never were finer men seen than those which composed this force, and no soldiers could possibly be in finer order'.[10] This was a noteworthy achievement and reflected their Indian training, but they arrived too late to take part in the fighting, and McGrigor handed over his hospital staff as a welcome reinforcement to Mr. Young's hard worked doctors.

It was not long before the reason for the Medical Board's reluctance to Young's appointment was made apparent for he showed his disregard of their orders by refusing to accept the medical staff officers whom the Board sent out in answer to his request for reinforcements. Once more he considered it was his prerogative to promote medical officers within his command, but when this included the promotion of regimental surgeons to appointments as physicians the Board found their strict control being flouted and ignored and rightly objected. But Young took so little notice of their reproof that when a physician arrived to replace a Dr. Webster who had died he ordered his return to England, because he considered the vacancy 'as coming under his patronage and to be filled by himself'. Instead, he promoted two junior officers of the hospital staff as physicians on the grounds that they had shown their competence under conditions of hardship and danger and deserved their promotion. He followed this up by demanding that all reinforcements should be of the rank of hospital mate only and no fewer than 100 of this category were asked for without delay, a number that the Surgeon General found quite unrealistic in relation to the size of the force and, moreover, quite impossible to find. However, he managed to send out twenty nine, and determined to enforce his authority he ignored Young's protests and sent assistant inspectors, staff surgeons, and three physicians, only to receive an impertinent reply that these senior officers were to be returned to England at great expense of time and money. Such high handed action was quite unjustifiable and entirely contravened the Board's sound policy that the professional standards of physicians and staff surgeons must be maintained throughout the army as a whole. In this connection the reader will remember how obdurate and independent Dr. Kennedy had proved for precisely similar reasons in Flanders.

With the surrender of the French forces in Cairo the return march to Alexandria was undertaken in company with the Turkish army and the French prisoners of war. The sick were comfortably evacuated in native feluccas, and the Inspector General's report shows that out of a strength of 4,412 in the force there were 1,922 sick. Of this number, 1,122 had been left behind at the hospitals at Rosetta and Exhove during the march up to Cairo;[11] while the remaining 800 were being dealt with in the regimental hospitals or in a hospital encampment on the Nile under the control of an assistant inspector.

The final stage in the campaign was now to take place, when, after two days' fighting, the French troops in Alexandria lost heart and capitulated on the 1st September 1801.

Reviewing the campaign we find that for the first few weeks of these operations the wastage from both sickness and wounds was so heavy that the usual provision of hospital bedding and equipment for 10 per cent of the force was quite inadequate. There were in fact by the end of March 4,501 sick and wounded under treatment or over 25 per cent. Hutchinson's troops on their march to Cairo lost 43 per cent of their effectives. After this, the falling off in the number of battle casualties, and the arrival of more staff officers from England and the welcome addition of those sent via the Cape combined to relieve Young's anxiety, although he was with the same breath complaining of their coming. By the end of the campaign he had something over forty administrative and hospital staff officers under his orders.[12] When the campaign ended the British army concentrated at Alexandria on the 13th September 1801 had 2,982 men in hospital or 16 per cent, while the total number of wounded admitted since operations started had risen to 2,998.

Amongst the various causes of disease, enteritis and dysentery held the first place, arising from the bad sanitation, the contaminated drinking water, and the swarms of flies carrying infection to food and drink. The local belief put the blame for these bowel troubles on 'checked perspiration' caused by the soldiers plunging into the Nile when their bodies were pouring out sweat, or to the damp chills at night incurred by removing breeches and gaiters and exposing the abdomen. Many of the cases of enteritis and diarrhoea were of a mild nature with recovery in a few days but true dysentery both bacillary and amoebic was also common and caused the heaviest mortality, not only from bowel ulceration but in the amoebic cases from hepatitis and liver abscess. Opium and ipecacuanha were the sovereign remedies, while flannel shirts and cloth pantaloons were advocated to prevent abdominal chills.

Bubonic plague had attacked French troops in their Syrian campaign in 1799 and it was endemic in the Eastern Mediterranean so that contact with the civil population was almost bound to lead to attacks amongst the soldiery. The immediate source of infection was put down to the arrival of a ship from Smyrna which berthed opposite the camp at Aboukir and was boarded by some of the soldiers. Between April and August 1801 there were 318 cases at Aboukir and 62 at Rosetta of whom 173 died and 207 recovered, a mortality of over 45 per cent. Strict quarantine was observed and a cordon of sentries placed round the hospital tents. As might be expected the medical officers working under strict quarantine suffered heavily, and Dr. Findlay an apothecary, Dr. Halliday of the 27th Foot and three hospital mates died. Dr. Buchan who had recently joined, volunteered his services and he and Price the deputy purveyor suffered mild attacks. Both were mentioned in General Orders for their devoted conduct under dangerous conditions. At Alexandria only one case occurred due to the stringent regulations laid down by a board of health which prevented the entry of any vessel into the harbour and moved units out of the city to an observation camp. In November 1802 a second outbreak amongst the Chasseurs Britannique was nobly dealt with by Dr. Buchan who for the second time volunteered for duty.[13]

The contagious nature of plague was recognized by all army surgeons but there were many who held that it could not be conveyed from man to man. Among the latter was Dr. White formerly a naval surgeon who was living in Rosetta. To prove his point he rubbed material from a plague bubo into the skin of his thigh, and when this had no effect, he inoculated himself with his lancet and at the second attempt he died. A pertinent observation by a French doctor showed that when a battalion affected by plague moved its quarters the disease was checked, the reason being (which was then unknown) that the rat fleas which are the transmitters of the plague bacillus were left behind.

It was March 1803 before the British troops sailed for England and during the winter of 1802 Major General Stuart who was then commanding describes his men as 'strangers to disease'![14] But on the eve of their departure a further outbreak of plague killed thirty-four men of the Regiment de Watteville, which had to be left behind. However, the sensible precaution was taken of hiring a Turkish vessel to act as a plague ship in case an outbreak occurred in any of the transports, and Mr. Blackwell a surgeon to the forces was placed in charge. Happily the voyage was free from incident, but the Medical Board at home having been warned of the danger, preventive measures were drawn up by Dr. Blane, (a well known naval surgeon), to avoid any risk of dissemination on arrival. After the British troops had returned to England the Indian contingent remained in Alexandria and Rosetta for some months, and plague broke out once more, this time in McGrigor's regiment the 88th Foot. The immediate precautions he took could not have been bettered had he known the exact cause. A pest house and an observation ward were opened, quarantine established, every patient was bathed, hair cut, clothes were baked in ovens, and fumigation with nitric acid carried out. Thirteen medical officers did duty in the pest house six of whom caught plague and three died. McGrigor himself was lucky to escape. The stringent precautions adopted prevented a more serious outbreak, while the treatment given strikes a heroic note: 2 grs. calomel and $\frac{1}{6}$ gr. opium every hour; $\frac{1}{2}$ oz. of mercurial ointment rubbed in three times a day, and ½ oz. of nitric acid by mouth during the day; immersion of feet and hands three times a day in a nitric bath.

Ophthalmia

To conclude this account an ailment must be described which may be aptly called one of the plagues of Egypt. This was ophthalmia, an affliction which was new to the army and which within a short time became one of the most distressing and widespread of army diseases. In Egypt it resulted in no fewer than 160 cases of total blindness, as well as a further 200 suffering from the loss of a single eye. The affection proved highly contagious and was regarded as a specially malignant type of inflammation which was designated 'Egyptian ophthalmia'. Dr. McGrigor referred to it as 'next to the plague in importance', and Assistant Surgeon Power of the 23rd Regiment describes it as 'one of the most dreadful diseases that has ever visited mankind'.

Egypt is well known for the prevalence of purulent ophthalmia among its civilian population due to the highly insanitary conditions in the towns and villages and the plague of flies which act as carriers of infected material. It is easy to understand that the troops living under active service conditions in the dust and sand would readily become infected, but at the time the affection was put down to the effects of the arid and burning desert, the heat and blinding glare of the sun, and once again to 'checked perspiration.'

Characterized at first by a purulent conjunctivitis, the disease in the worst cases led to a panophthalmitis, suppuration of the globe and disorganization of the eyeball. Once established in a unit it spread from man to man by personal contact or through towels or by flies and sometimes undoubtedly by the crude methods of treatment.

The prevailing opinion amongst medical officers was that soldiers with a vigorous constitution were usually attacked and therefore that the general strength of the patient must be reduced in order to lessen the severity of the inflammation. To this end venesection was performed, and anything from 20 or 30 and even up to 60 ounces of blood were withdrawn; at times this was done by opening the temporal artery. Animal food in the diet was forbidden and 'antiphlogistic' measures adopted; this meant giving drugs such as mercury in a dosage strong enough to produce salivation, and nauseating medicines like antimony. The surgical measures employed were removal of portions of the tumified conjunctiva, repeated scarification of the conjunctival vessels, and counter irritation by blistering, but as the instruments used for operation were entirely unsterilized the harm done can be well imagined. Then local applications were made of such powerful drugs as sulphate of copper, acetate of lead, and nitrate of silver.

Ophthalmia was also common amongst the French troops, but there was a notable difference between the epidemics. The famous Baron Larrey, Napoleon's chief surgeon who accompanied him to Egypt relates how after the battle of the 21st March 1801 ophthalmia broke out, caused as it was supposed by the heat of the day, the heavy fighting, the coldness of the night, and the mists from a neighbouring lake. Within two and a half months 3,000 cases were treated but not a single case of blindness occurred. This fact is so striking that the only reason appears to be the difference in the methods of treatment, for in contrast to the heroic measures adopted by British surgeons, the French avoided surgical interference and strong applications. Venesection was not performed but only superficial scarification of the skin of the temples and eyelids; no powerful drugs were applied to the eyes but only mild washes.

Even after the return of troops from Egypt ophthalmia continued to recur, and spread to units which had never been present in the campaign. It was conveyed by both English and French soldiers into almost every country in Europe, and amongst civilians too it became familiar to every medical practitioner.[15]

It will be convenient therefore to follow the course of this infection in succeeding years when it became so widespread and devastating that it became described as a menace to the future efficiency of the whole army. A few examples will suffice as illustrations. In the garrison in Malta there were 514 cases, and these were so severe that no fewer than 107 became totally blind and 102 others lost the sight of one eye; in the 2/52nd Regiment which had been newly raised in 1804 between July 1805 and July 1806 there were 733 admissions to hospital out of a strength of 691, and of these 50 became completely blind, and 40 others lost the sight of one eye; Surgeon Edmonston remarks, 'although the regiment has been removed to Maidstone, the Egyptian ophthalmia continued to rage in it to a terrible degree'[16] and this is borne out by the fact that within a period of two years there were in his regiment 1,341 cases. In the 43rd Foot there were 619 cases with 19 men quite blind and 32 suffering from the loss of an eye, while the 600 cases which occurred in the 2/12th Foot prevented the battalion being employed in the Peninsula. During the expedition to Buenos Aires in 1807 some 500 men were affected, and other similar instances can be quoted. The appalling consequences of this new plague of Egypt is apparent from the fact that in 1810 the number of soldiers on the pension list for blindness was 2,317. The spread of the disease is not always easy to explain. When once it had been established in a unit the extension was understandable as it was brought about by the uncleanly habits of soldiers infecting each other by washing in the same water and using the same towels. But it was difficult to account for its spread from one unit to another when regiments were located at a distance, and when the steps that Medical officers took to control it failed it began to be widely believed that a good deal of it was intentionally self inflicted in order to escape military service. Dr. Fergusson strongly supported this theory and called it the 'ophthalmia conspiracy'.[17] His view was that disgruntled soldiers by this means sought to escape the rigors of unlimited military service, the cruelties of flogging, the monotony of barrack life, and the restriction of furlough. Alternately he thought some worked for their discharge on medical grounds only to re-enlist and obtain a fresh recruits' bounty. Staff Surgeon Farrell completely disagreed. 'I have now,' he said, 'had under my care many thousands of ophthalmic patients and although I have used a vigilance sharpened by a bias towards that opinion, I have not as yet been able to make out clearly a case in which the soldier produced the disease in himself by improper means.'[18]

One of the steps taken to limit the spread of infection was to concentrate all cases at one centre, and an ophthalmic depot was opened at Selsea near Bognor in Sussex under the care of Dr. Vetch, Surgeon of the 52nd Regiment. This scheme would also allow treatment to be controlled by officers with the greatest experience. It had by now been recognized that Egyptian ophthalmia was accompanied by a granular condition of the inner lining of the eyelids which is now known as trachoma, and that the radical cure of the disease depended upon its eradication. Between 1806 and 1812 this depot treated upwards of 3,000 cases, and of this number there were 536 cases of impaired vision due to panophthalmitis, iritis, and corneal ulceration. Vetch's statistics show that in a period of four and a half years (17th November 1807—12th March 1812) 312 of these 536 cases were 'cured' or 58 per cent, while it appears only 20 were invalided for complete blindness, figures which show a vast improvement on the results of treatment in regimental hospitals where so many cases of complete loss of vision had occurred.

Admitted with vision impaired or lost	536
Cured of both eyes and discharged to duty	65
Cured of both eyes and discharged to Veterans Battalion	247
Invalided on account of age and other infirmities	70
Deaths by other diseases	7
Discharged with pensions for blindness being two-thirds of the total loss of thirty cases	20
Under treatment	127

By the summer of 1807, Castlereagh the Foreign Secretary had taken a hand as he was finally convinced that malingering was the root cause of the epidemic. In a letter he wrote on the 15th June to General Fox in Sicily where 263 cases had been notified he refers to this 'nefarious and abominable spread' averring that many of the men attempted to procure their discharge from the army because of a good pension. He goes on to say that in the 28th Foot alone 100 men had been proved to have infected each other and made their symptoms worse by applying irritating substances. It was largely the women in the regiments who egged on the soldiers in this dangerous practice, and after their discharge many of the men recovered their sight and some bad characters had tried the same trick more than once. Lawyers, said Castlereagh, were now making up their minds how this detestable crime could be proceeded against capitally under any law in force, and were making efforts to trace 'the abominable conspiracy'.[19]

Seriously disturbed by the wastage of manpower and the suffering caused the Commander-in-Chief in 1810 set up a Special Medical Board of eleven members comprising the most experienced civil and military physicians, surgeons, and oculists. Amongst them we find the triumvirate of Pepys, Keate and Knight, Sir Gilbert Blane the ex Naval Surgeon, and Sir Everard Home. The task the Committee undertook was to study the means of prevention and to formulate the best methods of cure, including treatment for the trachoma.

The Board's conclusions which were circulated for the guidance of all medical officers and commanding officers of regiments were as follows:

(1) *Prevention*
    (1) Separation of cases from their comrades.
    (b) Personal cleanliness. No washing in the same water but under a running tap or in a running stream.[20] Individual towels to have individual marks.
    (c) Frequent washing of bedding, clothes and towels.

(2) *Treatment*
    (a) Bleeding.
    (b) Puncture of the cornea to relieve tension and pus.
    (c) Blisters.
    (d) Irrigation with copper sulphate or liq.plumbi subacetate dil, or by fomentations.
    (e) Tonics.
    (f) Low diet.
    (g) Fresh air and exercise.

It was at this stage that the name of Dr. Adams[21] becomes prominent. He was a civilian oculist practising at Exeter and in 1809 had been attending soldiers invalided out of the service. He claimed that his treatment had restored the sight of several soldiers suffering from the granuloma stage of the disease who had been drawing pensions for blindness after their cases had been declared incurable. His claims so impressed the War Office that the Adjutant General decided to institute an extended trial of his methods, for if they proved successful there was a clear chance of reducing the large amounts paid to disabled pensioners which had now reached the considerable sum of £100,000 a year. This included soldiers invalided from the Royal Hospital at Chelsea and Kilmainham Hospital in Ireland, as well as from the Ordnance Medical Department, and officers. When the War Office proposal was put before the special Medical Board under Pepys certain objections arose, the nature of which we are not told, but they were sufficient to prevent the matter being pursued further.

Adams came to settle in London towards the latter part of 1811, when he was sent for by the Adjutant General and encouraged to repeat his methods of treatment in a fresh trial which he was assured would receive the liberal co-operation of Director General Weir. This was confirmed in a letter from the Adjutant General to Adams in the following terms:

'Sir, I have delayed replying to your note of the 2nd instant until I had an opportunity of laying the accompanying papers before the Commander-in-Chief and of stating to His Royal Highness the very satisfactory appearance of the three ophthalmic patients whom you sent to the Horse Guards. His Royal Highness commanded me to assure you that he is fully impressed with the importance of the consequences which may result from your mode of treatment; and with a view of affording an opportunity of effectually ascertaining its merit and success, has directed Mr. Weir to make an arrangement, so that you may have a sergeant and six patients placed solely and distinctly under your care for such time as you may deem requisite, and as near as possible to your residence, that you may be enabled without inconvenience to give them the necessary attendance. Care will be taken to satisfy the men that their discharges will be granted in the event of their sight being restored, that no obstruction or impediment of that nature may be in the way of your endeavour.[22] It will be proper for you to communicate with Mr. Weir as to the selection of the patients.'[23]

With these assurances in writing Adams freely communicated his methods of treatment to the Medical Department and looked forward to their full co-operation. Here he was to be disappointed, for from his first interview with the Board in 1812 he encountered their decided hostility, so much so that in December 1812 the Adjutant General wrote a peremptory and discourteous letter to the Director General asking why the Commander-in-Chief's orders had not been obeyed in a matter which so closely involved 'not only the health of individuals, but the efficiency of the Army at large'.[24] It now became obvious that Weir's procrastination arose from his reluctance to allow a purely military medical problem to be taken out of his hands by a civilian.

Tired of this continued opposition the Commander-in-Chief gave orders in 1813 that the control of the trial should no longer be the responsibility of the Medical Department but should be handed over to a committee of civilian doctors, which included the names of Sir Henry Halford, Dr. Baillie, Sir Everard Home, Mr. Cline, Mr. Astley Cooper, and Mr. Abernethy. This committee appears to have regarded Adams' treatment as promising and he was now given to understand that the Secretary of State for Home Affairs and the Secretary at War would make a combined attempt to eradicate the disease both from the army and from the civilian population.

By the time this committee's report was to hand James McGrigor had become Director General, and like Weir he was quite determined not to allow a civilian to take over a task which he felt his own officers were capable of undertaking. He went so far as to state on the 4th July that 'there now remain but a few cases (of ophthalmia) in the neighbourhood of Plymouth, and I trust this disorder will soon be eradicated from the army.'[25] From his experience in the Peninsula where the disease had been eliminated, he asserted that there were now many army doctors who were well acquainted with the methods of cure. The Secretary at War did not accept McGrigor's assertions without proof, and called for a return of all cases of ophthalmia, when it was discovered to McGrigor's discomfiture that some 550 patients had recently been treated in military hospitals, and that in fact nearly 2,500 cases had occurred in the Army of Occupation in France between the 21st November 1815 and the 20th November 1816 of whom 10 men were totally blind, and 43 had impaired vision. McGrigor therefore was compelled to acknowledge his error.

Adams had by this time proposed establishing a special hospital to which all cases should be sent, but McGrigor scouted the idea saying that they could all be dealt with at less expense in existing army establishments. Adams however won his point and he was allotted the old York Hospital at Chelsea at a cost of £2,200 a year where from 1817 onwards he treated cases from the navy, army, and artillery. Calvert the Adjutant General wrote to him on the 28th June of that year informing him that His Royal Highness the Commander-in-Chief entertained a just sense of the zeal and liberality with which he had communicated his methods of practice.

After two years' trial his results were evidently considered as entirely satisfactory, for a War Office letter of the 13th March 1819 signed by Lord Palmerston confirms that 'New and successful methods of treating disorders of the eyes especially Egyptian ophthalmia having been discovered, His Majesty's Government wishes to extend the advantage to the Chelsea and Kilmainham pensioners.'[26] These are the figures on which Lord Palmerston based his views.

Admitted	447
Cured	217
Relieved	85
Not cured	32
Remaining	48

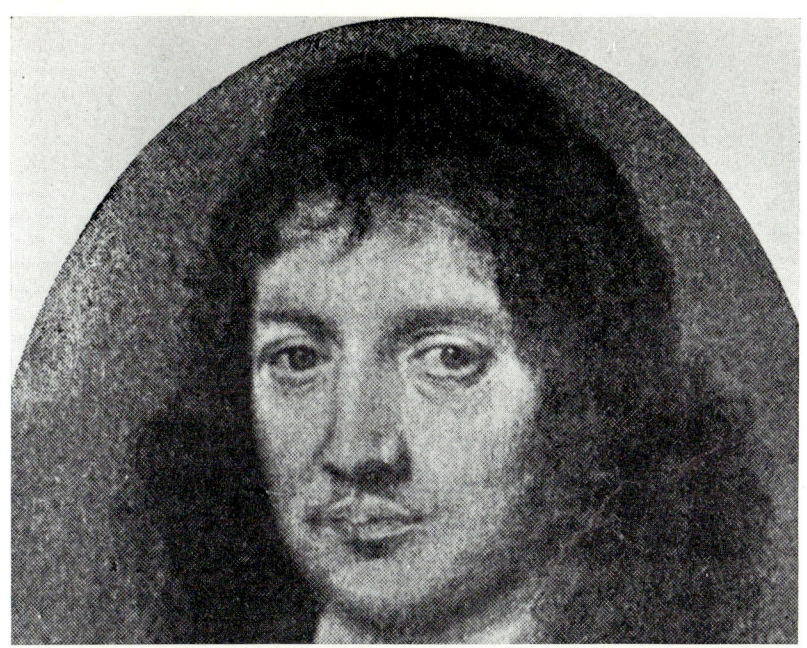

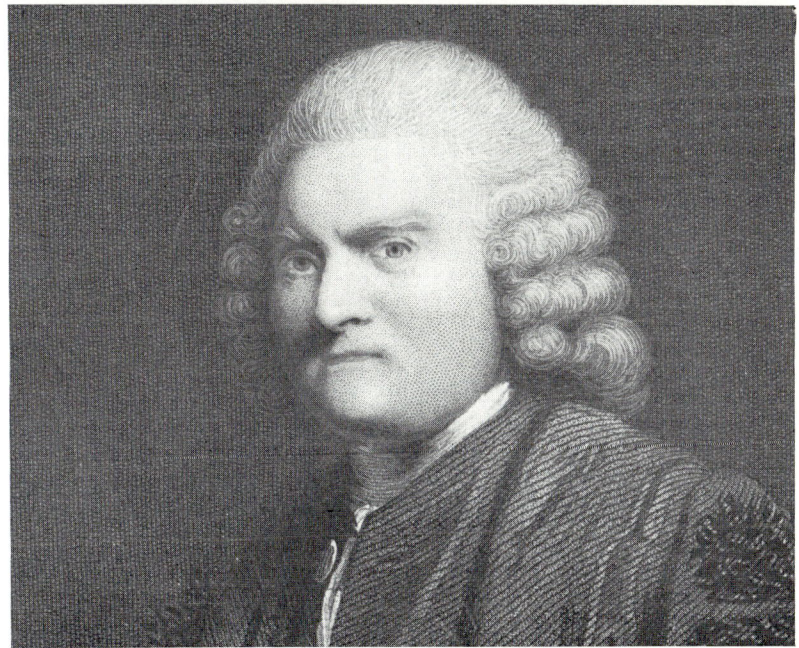

1 (*Top*) Dr. Richard Wiseman

2 (*Bottom*) Sir John Pringle

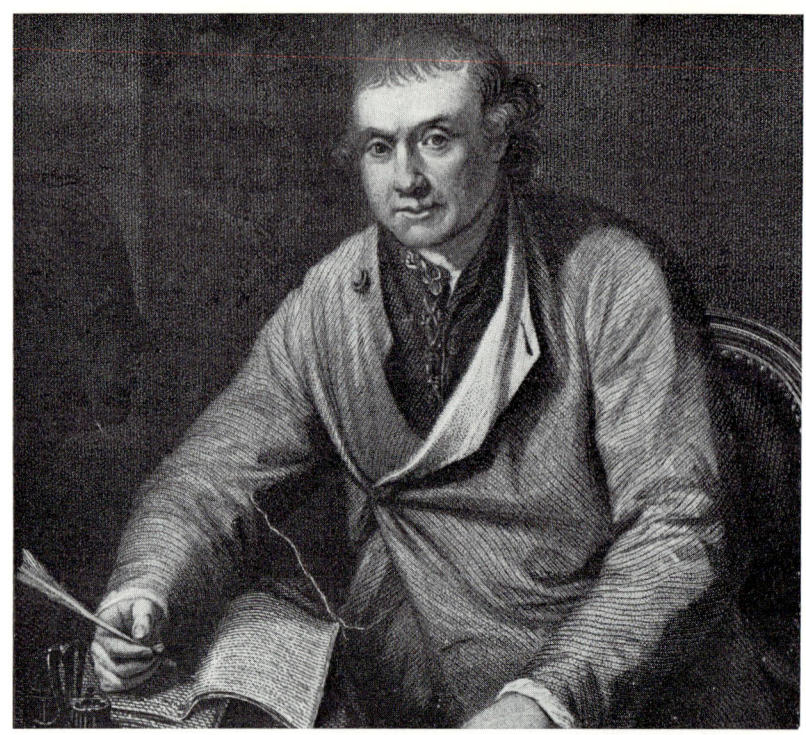

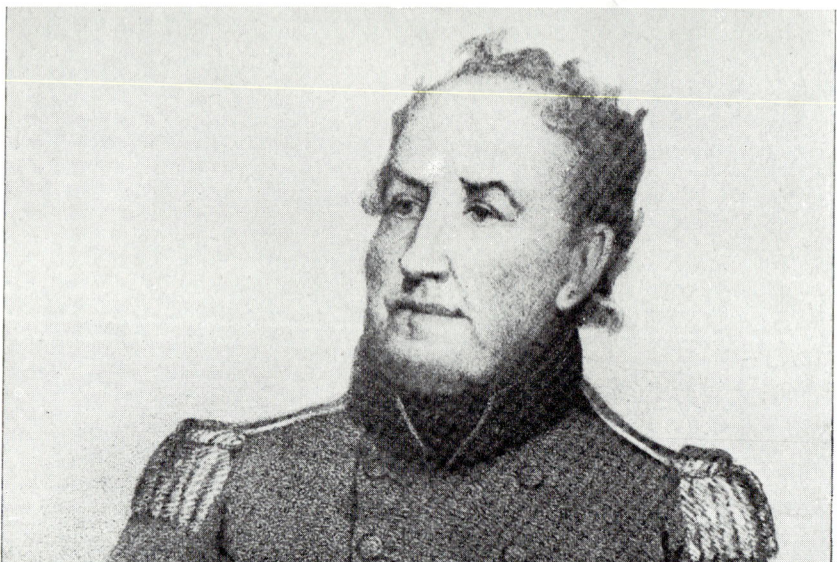

3 (*Top*) Surgeon General John Hunter

4 (*Bottom*) Inspector General of Hospitals Robert Jackson

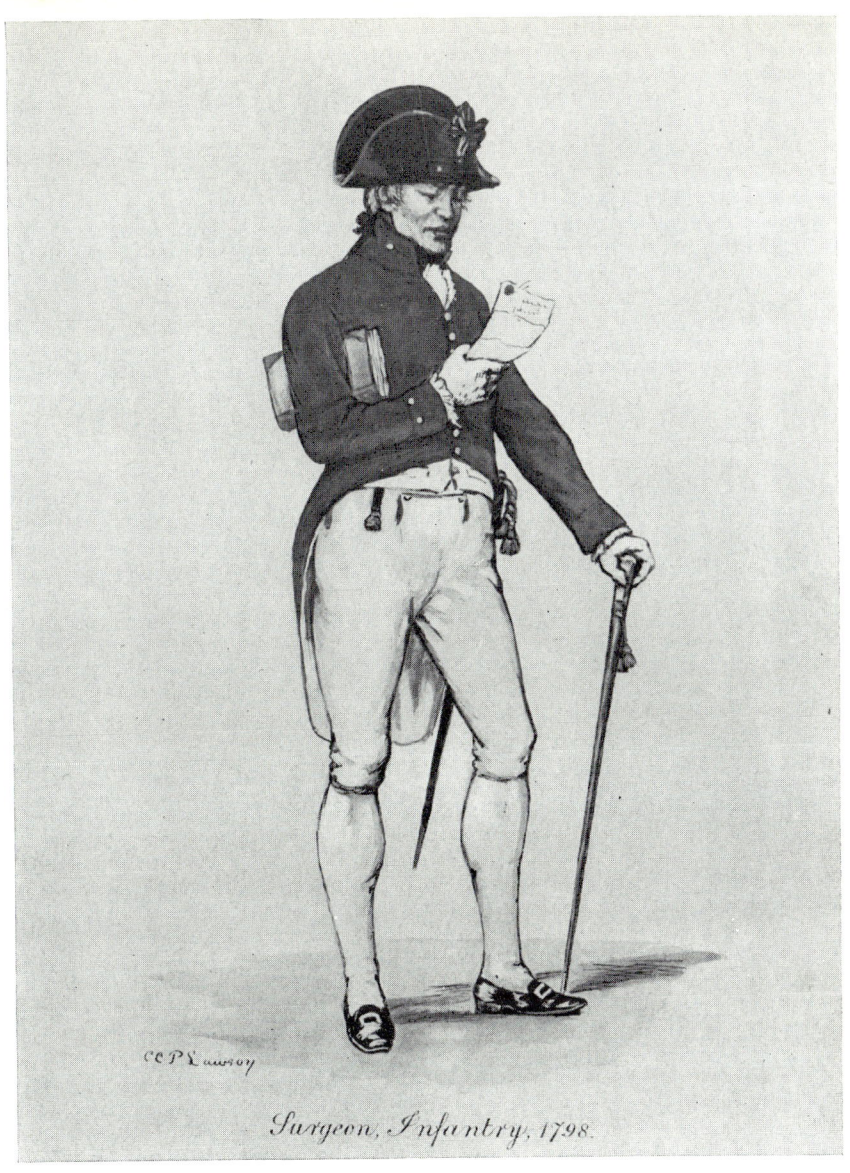

Surgeon, Infantry, 1798.

5 Surgeon of Infantry, 1798

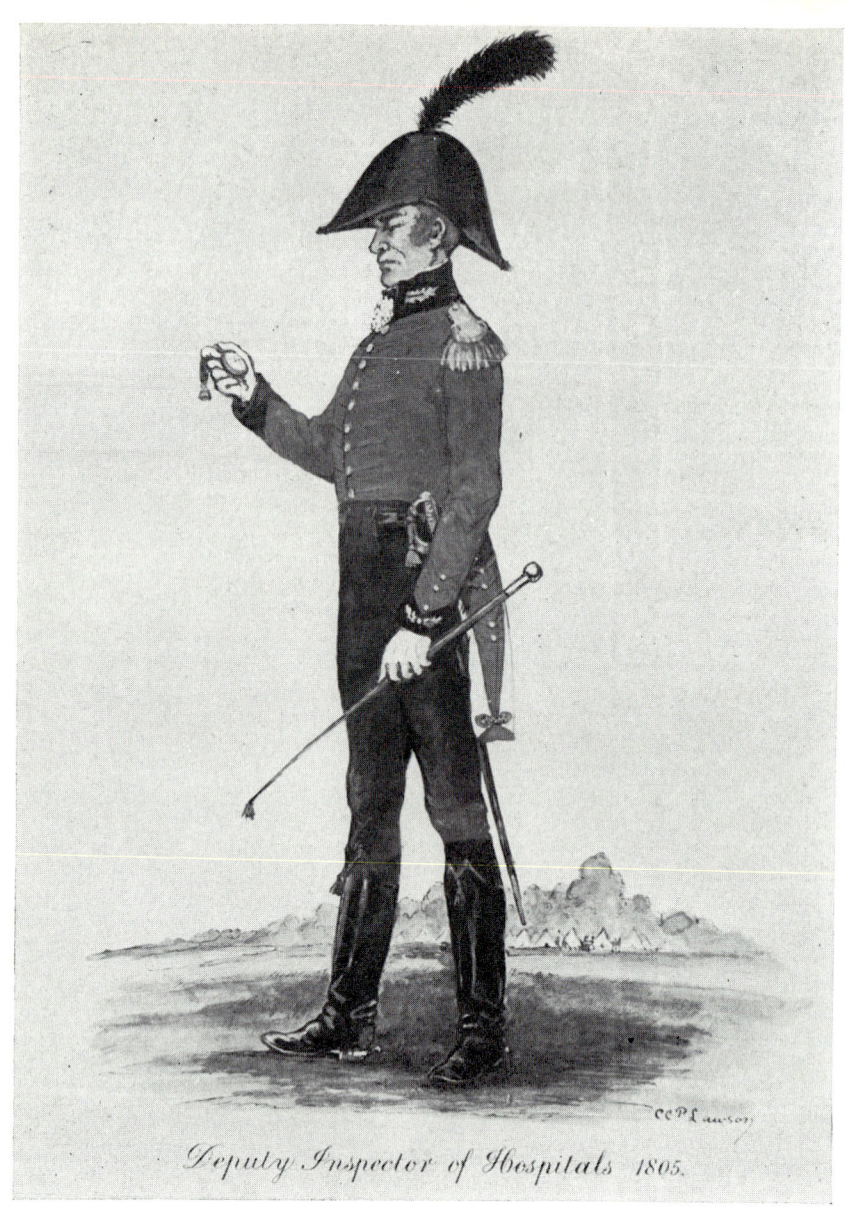

Deputy Inspector of Hospitals 1805.

6 Deputy Inspector of Hospitals, 1805

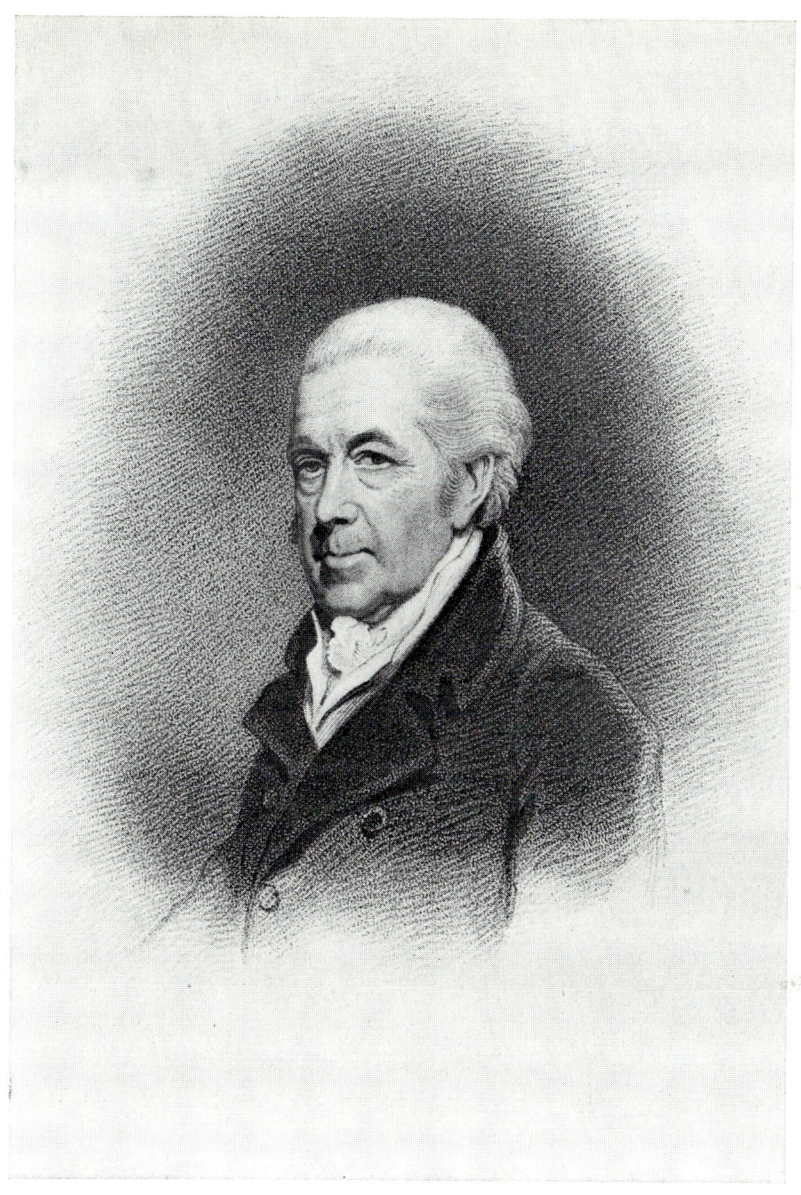

7 Physician General Sir Lucas Pepys
by kind permission of the Royal College of Physicians

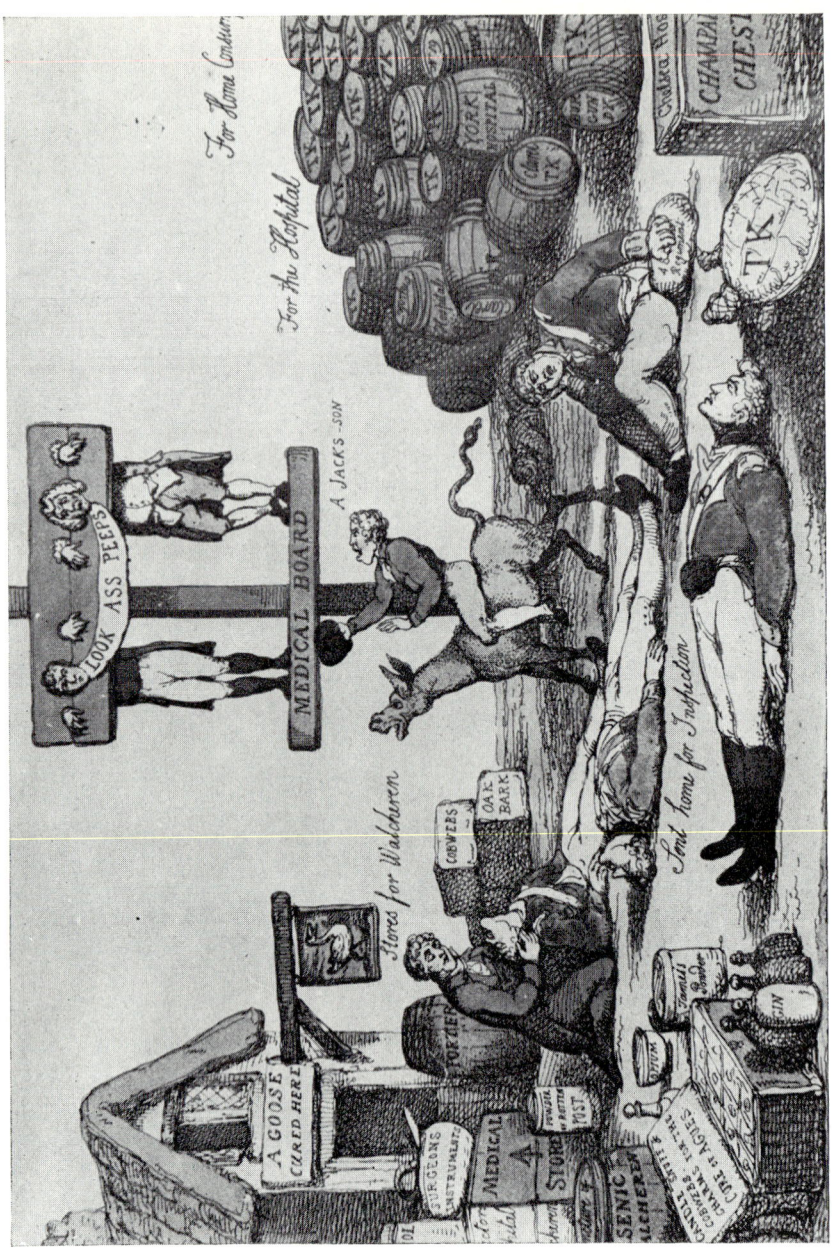

8 Walcheren Cartoon

'LOOK ASS PEEPS' stands for Lucas Pepys and shows the Medical Board being pillor-
ied for its inefficiency. The figure on the donkey represents Robert Jackson, a critic of
the Medical Board. The initials 'T. K.' stand for Thomas Keate, the Surgeon General. The
inn sign 'A GOOSE CURED HERE' probably means 'Agues cured here'.

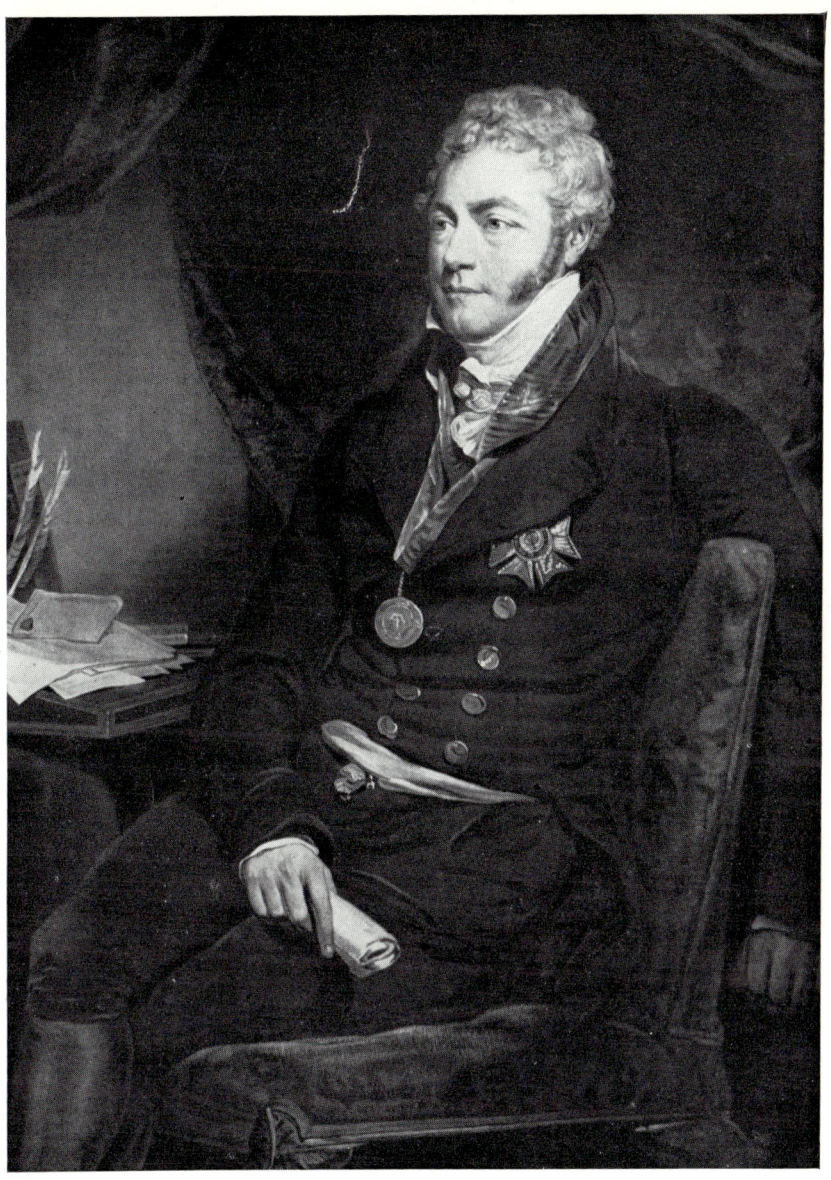

9 Director General Sir James McGrigor

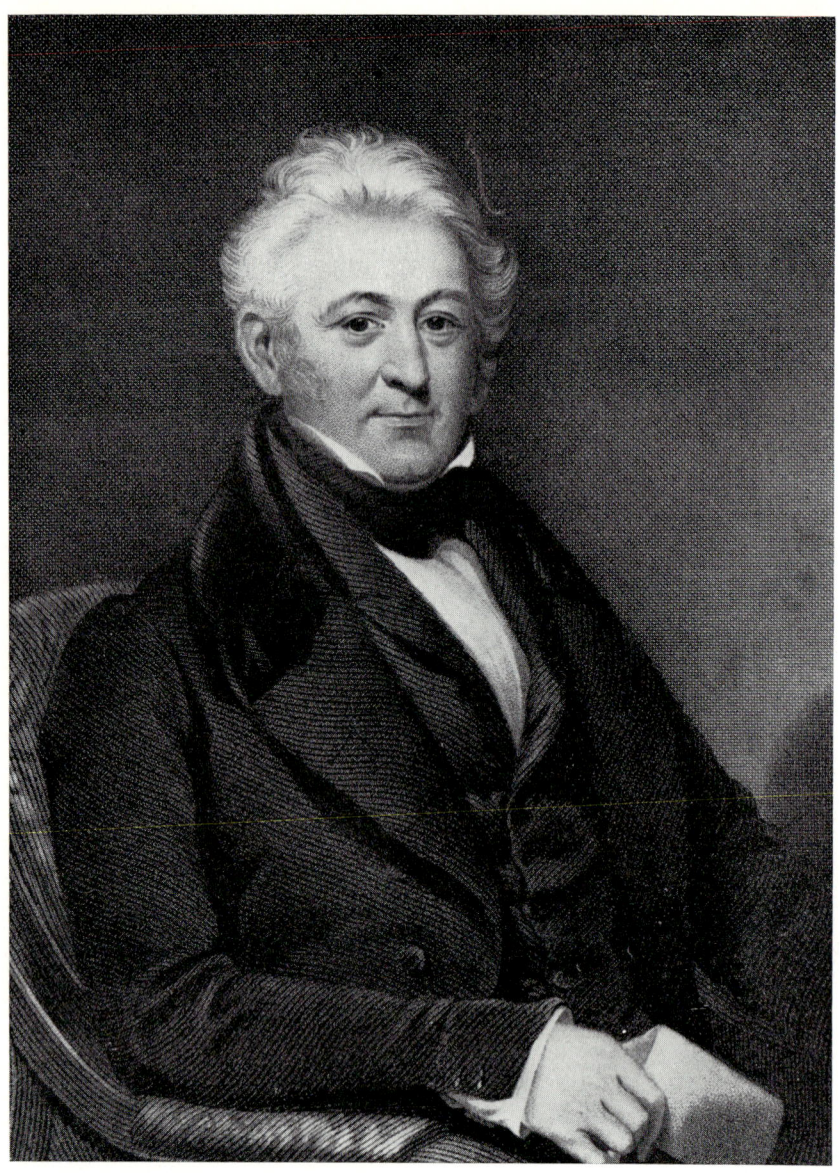

10 Deputy Inspector General of Hospitals James Guthrie

Among these 447 cases, 186 were classed as trachoma following Egyptian ophthalmia, and of these Adams claimed 96 were cured, 50 relieved, 2 not benefitted, and the rest still remaining under treatment. There is no doubt that Adams was a skilful and efficient operator and he invited members of the medical profession to attend his clinic at the York Hospital and compare his method of practice with that of others. Apart from trachoma he performed operations for artificial pupil after corneal ulceration, for the removal of cataract, and for inversion and eversion of the lids. But McGrigor continued to be hostile and unconvinced. He wrote to the War Office on the 3rd May 1819 and the utmost he would admit to was that Sir William Adams ... 'by means of certain operations long known and practised, but which never render one man fit for military service, some out-pensioners have had their vision improved.'[27] There was in fact no proof that any of the soldiers cured were able to resume military duty. It is true some were pronounced fit and actually rejoined their units but their condition soon relapsed from cold and exposure, and knowing now as we do how difficult it was to cure the condition until modern methods of treatment came into use, this is not surprising. When assessing Adams' claims McGrigor pointed out that he considered the results on cataract and for artificial pupils were no better than what could have been expected from military surgeons who had acquired experience, while for opacities of the cornea and trachoma he thought results in the main were unsuccessful. 'This opinion,' says McGrigor, 'is not meant to imply any disparagement of the Gentleman—it arises from the superior experience of the medical officers of the army in these diseases.'[28] And he follows this up by pointing out that Adams' chief assistant was Staff Surgeon Lindsay, one of his own more experienced officers. If Government policy was to render what he described as 'humane aid' to blind pensioners, there was no reason why this should not be carried out in the military hospital at Fort Pitt, or at the Detachment Hospital in the Isle of Wight, or at Edinburgh—the expense would be far less than treatment in a special hospital and at each of these stations there was a medical officer who was quite as competent as Adams. McGrigor's plea was however entirely ignored by the Adjutant General and Adams continued to treat patients gratuitously until 1821, although to suit his convenience they were moved to a building in Albany Street near London's Regent Park.

There were numerous instances where examinations were carried out by medical officers of the Department after treatment was completed, mostly between January 1818 and March 1819, and their reports show that although some had improved, in others blindness actually took place after operation. Dr. Gordon examined 13 men in 1818 after treatment; out of 9 operated upon—2 were successful, 1 not successful and 6 derived some benefit; out of 4 not operated upon—3 were improved, and 1 not improved.

Adams claimed that several soldiers pensioned solely for eye diseases in 1815, 1816, and subsequently, had been so far cured or relieved by treatment that had the same degree of relief been afforded prior to their being pensioned such persons would have been thereby either in part or wholly saved to the public.

In comparing the methods of treatment adopted by Vetch and Adams we have failed to discover any major difference. Vetch carried out extensive bleedings by both leeches and phlebotomy; irrigation with mild lotions; zinc sulphate and tincture of opium for local instillation; cold linen compresses to the eyes. He treated corneal ulcers with caustics, and for granular lids (trachoma) he used either escharotics such as silver nitrate, or excised the granuloma with scissors.

In the early stages of the disease Adams believed in promoting violent vomiting by giving tartar emetic for from eight to ten hours. His other methods of treatment appear to be much the same as those adopted by Vetch except the granuloma of the lids was excised with a knife instead of with scissors, and copper sulphate was applied to the inner surfaces.

Adams seems to have been unpopular with his civilian colleagues who it is interesting to note had already founded Moorfields Eye Hospital in 1805 to deal with the civilian population before he came upon the scene. Moreover his reputation appears to have suffered, a fact which he puts down to the hostility of the Services to whom he says he had imparted all his methods of treatment, and to the press. The enthusiasm of the War Office too appears to have evaporated after McGrigor's letter of criticism had been studied, although the Adjutant General wrote to Adams on the 28th June 1817 informing him that His Majesty appreciated his work.

Although he had given his services free over the years this did not prevent Adams from making an appeal to Parliament to make good his losses from private practice on the grounds that he had performed great public service and with Lord Palmerston's backing the House of Commons voted him the sum of £4,000. McGrigor undoubtedly would have belittled the extent of his 'great public service' and on this controversial issue it is unprofitable to judge. Suffice it to say that the acid test of cure as far as the soldier is concerned was whether he could resume duty in the ranks, and the final verdict appears to be that although many cases of trachoma were improved at least temporarily, this stage was never achieved.

As to the pathology of the disease, Duke Elder states that it was undoubtedly trachoma, proved by the presence of granulations and the chronicity and the cicatricial sequelae which followed. The initial conjunctivitis he puts down to a mixed infection which included the

Koch Weeks bacillus as well as some cases of gonococal origin.[29]

Leaving this controversial aspect of the rival claims to success let us look at some of the after results of ophthalmia generally. The figures quoted for Ireland showed some astonishing results. There were in that country no fewer than 1,859 soldiers drawing pensions for eye diseases and when in due course most were re-examined the following facts emerged.

Cases reported as incurable	315
Cases reported as susceptible to cure or relief	487
Cases reported to have recovered their sight.	1,043

Remarking on the last figure it seems that no further proof is needed that malingering was widespread and successful in spite of the lack of evidence from medical sources.

Ophthalmia continued to plague the army for many years and perhaps it is apt here to quote the Latin tag *Ex Africa semper aliquid novi*, for it amply corroborates the epidemic of Egyptian ophthalmia which left behind it so many distressing cases of blindness and threatened at one time to affect the morale of the whole army.

While the Egyptian campaign was in progress the first step in conquering another plague of mankind was being taken in the expeditionary force.

Vaccination

It was in August 1800 that the army adopted the recently introduced method of preventing smallpox by vaccination with cowpox. Jenner's discovery came about 1796, but this was not the first attempt to protect the population against the ravages of smallpox and as we have previously mentioned Lady Mary Wortley-Montague had introduced the Turkish procedure of inoculation with human smallpox. Although this method was in use it was a hazardous and sometimes a dangerous procedure, while the victims of this inoculation were of course themselves a source of infection to others. In the army it was only considered justifiable in time of war, and we have already seen in the American War of Independence how relatively less susceptible the British troops were owing to their protection. When new regiments were raised and encamped together inoculation was encouraged and practised although it was never compulsory. The regimental surgeon received a fee of a guinea for every inoculation provided he attended the soldier outside the bounds of the camp or garrison, a precaution which was necessary to limit the possible spread of infection from the inoculated victim.

For the first experiment in vaccination in 1800 two units were selected by the Medical Board, the Coldstream Guards in London and the 85th Foot in Colchester. The experiment at Colchester carried out by Jenner's nephew was unfortunately not as successful as had been hoped as many of the men were found to be suffering from itch which was evidently regarded as a bar to vaccination. Nevertheless the War Office under pressure from the Physician General paid Jenner the considerable sum of 100 guineas for his trouble.

Although precise details of the result of this initial experiment are not available the success of vaccination was by now firmly established, but as often occurs with new medical discoveries commanding officers were slow to take advantage of it and a General Order[30] was issued on the 15th November 1803 drawing attention to its benefits, and this had to be repeated by a further reminder the following year.

While this was the situation at home more active steps were taken abroad, and two civilian doctors, Walker and Marshall, were sent out to Egypt in 1801 to vaccinate all the troops in Abercromby's army. It was rightly thought that the risks of acquiring smallpox in Egypt were considerable. The doctors set sail in H.M.S. *Endymion*, employing their time on the voyage by vaccinating the sailors and marines on board as well as troops and civilian volunteers at the ports touched at *en route*, Gibraltar, Minorca and Malta. At Gibraltar the crew of an American vessel were vaccinated with matter taken from the arm of a sailor, while at Malta the volunteers for vaccination were encouraged by the enthusiasm of the local authorities—'these are some of the benefits you derive from the English'.[31]

When the exacting task of vaccinating the troops in Egypt was successfully accomplished the two doctors went on to Rosetta Hospital where they vaccinated those Turkish officials and soldiers who wished to avail themselves of this new discovery. Finally after receiving the thanks of the G.O.C. British troops, the two enterprising doctors, rather than sail home at once, elected to join the Principal Medical Officer's staff, and served in a military capacity until the end of the campaign.

By 1801 Britain had increased her forces immensely. The Navy had nearly 500 ships at sea with crews numbering 133,000 seamen; the Army had grown from 64,000 to 380,000 men, with in addition more than 100,000 volunteers. The country, however, was weary of war, weighed down with taxes and high prices, and the harvest was bad for the sixth year in succession. Addington who had succeeded Pitt as Prime Minister did not believe that the war could ever be won, and secret tentative peace proposals were put forward whereby France was to keep her continental conquests and Britain her colonial acquisitions. Napoleon too welcomed these proposals, and after the end of the Egyptian campaign a preliminary treaty was signed in October 1801 followed in April 1802 by the Peace of Amiens.

By the terms of the peace all the French and Dutch colonial possessions which had cost so many lives were handed back to France and Holland. For Napoleon the peace provided a much needed breathing space to rebuild his navy, but it was not long before he violated the terms of the Treaty and after a long period of tension, Britain on the 16th May 1803 once more declared war. This meant that the capture of the colonial possessions had to be undertaken all over again. The more immediate danger was the fear of invasion, and urgent measures had to be adopted for raising more men for the services because the army after the peace had been reduced to 150,000 men—a number barely sufficient to garrison Ireland and the Empire. The innumerable militia and volunteer units which were raised meant that fewer recruits were available for the regular army. Balloting was tried again without success and this was followed by the levy *en masse* which also failed.

The Addington ministry fell from power in 1804 and Pitt once again became Prime Minister. In 1805 the fear of invasion faded as the Third Coalition comprising Britain, Russia and Austria came into full play.

In 1806 Pitt died and was succeeded by a Ministry of all the Talents. The Whig Ministry which succeeded included William Windham who was in charge of the Department of War and the Colonies. In place of the old regulations for enlistment which had previously been for life he proposed that the period of service should be limited to seven years, a policy both bold and startling, but one which had been advocated by many officers for years. Now that the fear of invasion had been removed it meant that regular forces at home comprising 22,000 cavalry, 60,000 infantry and 10,000 artillery, with in addition some 200,000 militia, made it possible to spare a force of some 30,000 to 40,000 for offensive operations. Over the years 1803 to 1807 several expeditions were mounted to which we now refer, but from 1808 onwards almost all our military and naval strength had to be concentrated in providing the means to fight the Peninsular War.

West Indies

After the resumption of hostilities our forces in the West Indies retook the islands of St. Lucia and Tobago. This proved easy as the recall of the French fleet from the West Indies left these islands at Britain's mercy, and in 1804 the remnant of the French army in St. Domingo surrendered as the only alternative to massacre at the hands of the negroes. The Dutch colonies of Demerara, Berbice, Essiquibo, and Surinam which had also been returned to Holland by the Treaty were also re-occupied.

Scattered throughout the whole West Indies area there were 11,000 men of whom 2,000 were constantly in hospital even without any epidemics of yellow fever. As before, the principal hospital base was at Barbados with garrison hospitals throughout the islands, and further medical comment is unnecessary.

Ceylon

The Dutch colony of Ceylon had been originally seized in 1796 and its conquest is dogged by the familiar fight against disease. At first only the seaboard towns of Colombo and Trincomalee were occupied but after the Peace of Amiens an attempt was made to occupy the whole, and at the end of 1802, 1,400 British troops, with two battalions of natives, one Cingalese and one Malay, set out to accomplish the task.

After surmounting the almost impassable obstacles of the jungle tracks the columns, one from Colombo and one from Trincomalee, struggled into Kandy on the 21st February 1803. Then malaria struck men down so quickly that the strength was soon reduced to 1,800 bayonets, while the extended life line to Colombo along which supplies came was frequently cut by hostile attacks. Fever decimated all the occupants of the posts *en route* to such an extent that it was found impossible to maintain communications, and most of the troops were withdrawn to Colombo, leaving a garrison of 1,000 men including 300 Europeans of the Green Howards in Kandy.

By the third week in June the detachment was isolated and in parlous straits. The coolies still struggling to carry through supplies died off in large numbers. The few British in Kandy were perishing at the rate of six men every day, and their comrades of the Malay battalion were deserting as fast as they could. Elsewhere in Trincomalee itself the 51st Foot was reduced from 400 to 100 men within three months from malaria and smallpox. A relieving force of native infantry which attempted to evacuate the doomed garrison in Kandy failed. On the 24th June, when less than 200 of the British troops were left alive, and 120 of these were in hospital, the enemy attacked, and after a defence of ten hours the garrison capitulated on the terms that those who were able to stand were to be allowed to march unmolested to the coast. Accordingly 34 British and 350 Malays set out, leaving 150 sick behind. The party included the two surgeons, Holloway of the Artillery, and Hope of the 19th Foot. Soon they were waylaid; the Malays deserted; the rest were massacred, only a corporal escaping to tell the tale. The sick left in hospital in Kandy had been clubbed on the head as soon as the columns moved out, and one man alone was spared who was found alive when Kandy was reoccupied in 1815.

During the succeeding eighteen months the desultory fighting went on without achieving any military result, but at the cost of great hardship to the sick and wounded. The columns were often ambushed, the doolie bearers frequently deserted; the wounded were left untended and often perished. An officer wrote 'through the dreadful obstructions thrown in the way and the incessant attacks of the enemy it was found impossible to carry on the sick and wounded. These, along with the doolies, fell into the hands of the enemy. Many were taken, their hands and feet bound, their mouths stuffed with grass to prevent their cries, slung upon a bamboo pole, and thus borne off to be butchered like sheep. When the army had occasion to stop, however shortly, numbers secured in this means were rescued by their comrades, when missed in time, by a hasty charge with the bayonet.'[32]

Fevers, dysentery, and wounds almost decimated the regiments involved; the mortality rates of the 19th Foot were 400 per 1,000 in 1803, 200 per 1,000 in 1804, and 83 per 1,000 in 1805.

The final episode in the subjugation of Ceylon came in 1818 after guerilla warfare in swamp and jungle had taken a heavy toll of lives. In that year the 73rd Foot sustained 356 deaths, nearly all from disease, while in the island as a whole three British regiments lost 300 dead within a space of three months. Such was the cost of Empire.[33]

Gibraltar

At Gibraltar the year 1804 marked the centenary of its capture, while the late eighteenth century had been marked by an epic four year siege which lasted from 1779 to 1783. The garrison of some 5,000 troops under the command of the able but eccentric Governor, General Elliott,[34] steadfastly resisted the combined assault of the Spanish army and navy which culminated in the Grand Attack of the 14th September 1782. An army of 40,000 men, 44 enemy ships of the line, a bombardment by 10 naval floating batteries together with the land batteries of 100 pieces of cannon all failed utterly to capture the Rock.

During the siege there were 438 killed or died of wounds and 1,008 wounded,[35] while 1,034 perished from disease. As in the siege of 1727 scurvy was rife and 500 died, but the preventive effects of lemon juice was now realized and from time to time cargoes of limes and oranges from Tangier ran the blockade while the troops were encouraged to cultivate gardens of fresh vegetables. The naval hospital treated the bulk of the sick and wounded but there were 5 British and 3 Hanoverian regimental hospitals to augment the accommodation.

The centenary of its capture was marked by the outbreak of a severe epidemic of yellow fever which wiped out nearly a quarter of the garrison. Fifty four officers and 864 other ranks as well as 164 women and children succumbed; the civilian population also suffered nearly 5,000 deaths. The cause presented a medical problem of the first order and as in the West Indies much discussion ensued as to whether the disease was or was not infectious. Dr. Pym whom we have already met in the West Indies was we know convinced it was infectious and Dr. Fellowes[36] agreed with him, but Dr. Nooth Inspector of Hospitals thought it was not, and to prove his point he courageously attended the worst cases and survived. Tented camps were set up to thin out the military and civil population; discharges of artillery and bonfires were used to purify the atmosphere, 'but the great heat they occasioned and the terror they inspired turned out to be most detrimental'. So wrote Deputy Inspector John Hennen in a memorandum published two years after he himself had died of the disease in the further outbreak of 1828 which had been preceded by others in 1813 and 1814. In the 1828 epidemic there were 432 deaths in a garrison of 3,600, a mortality of 12 per cent, and Hennen's self sacrifice is commemorated in a monument erected by the Government and citizens of Gibraltar whose tribute is recorded in the following memorable words: 'Erected by his personal friends, not with a view of perpetuating his name, for that lives in the more imperishable memorials of his own genius, but as testimony of regard for a man whose zeal was indefatigable, and who, in the day of general calamity, sacrificed all consideration of his safety for the public weal.' In Arduis Fidelis.

Dr. Pym had a distinguished civil career after leaving the army. He received his knighthood in 1830, and during the cholera outbreak of 1832 in England he was chairman of the Central Board of Health.

Italy

We briefly mention Major General Sir John Stuart's audacious landing in southern Italy and the victorious battle of Maida in July 1806 chiefly for its military significance for it was the first time the redcoats, deployed in lines and superlatively trained in musketry, crushed a superior French force attacking in columns and drove them in flight from the field. The 282 wounded presented no special medical problem with the ships at hand and the base in Sicily close by where a general hospital was in being.

Cape of Good Hope

The recapture of the Dutch colony of the Cape of Good Hope was undertaken and successfully accomplished with surprising ease by Sir David Baird in January 1806 with a force of 6,000 men.

Buenos Aires

For some years there had existed plans for an expedition to support a revolution against Spain in the South American countries. With troops to spare after the capture of the Cape, Sir Home Popham the naval commodore on the station set this plan in motion, and persuading Baird to lend him a Scottish regiment—the 71st Highlanders—and borrowing another 400 men from the garrison of St. Helena, he sailed across the South Atlantic and landed at Buenos Aires which was quickly mastered at the cost of a dozen casualties. The only medical aid on this daring enterprise consisted of one regimental surgeon of the 71st Foot, and one assistant surgeon of the St. Helena regiment. Unfortunately the latter was reported missing after the affair. When the exhilarating news of this success was received in England a reinforcement of 4,000 men was dispatched under Major General Auchmuty followed later by a further expedition under Lieut General Whitelocke. But in the meantime Beresford's detachment at Buenos Aires had been overpowered and captured so that when additional reinforcements of over 2,000 men sent by Baird from the Cape in answer to Beresford's request arrived in October 1806 they found to their amazement that he and the whole of his men were prisoners. In England popular clamour had now made the Government enlarge their ambitious South American schemes and as Fortescue says, 'Windham evolved one of the most astonishing plans that ever emanated from the brain even of a British Minister of War.'[37] This was an expedition to conquer Chile, and to carry it out Colonel Craufurd was entrusted with the task with another small force of some 4,800 men.

Meanwhile Auchmuty had arrived, and finding that he was too weak to attack Buenos Aires decided instead to capture Monte Video on the opposite side of the Rio de la Plata. The P.M.O. of this force was Deputy Inspector Redmond and he had with him 2 staff surgeons and 4 hospital mates for staffing a small general hospital. Auchmuty with over 6,000 men now under his command was backed up by 1,400 sailors from the naval squadron, which from the medical standpoint provided valuable assistance in the way of naval surgeons and hospital accommodation on board. Monte Video was captured after a night of desperate slaughter under the breached walls; certainly a fine piece of work, but our losses were not small, totalling nearly 400 of whom 271 were wounded, the latter including two assistant surgeons—one from the 38th and one from the 87th Foot.

An unhappy complication was the number of cases of tetanus among wounds of the lower extremities all of which proved fatal and included two commanding officers.

For his zealous conduct in this relatively small affair Auchmuty recommended Redmond for promotion to Inspector of Hospitals a proposal which the Board regarded as unacceptable.

It was now the turn of General Whitelocke to arrive with his small contingent of 1,800 men and he was followed by Craufurd whose Chilean enterprise had now been cancelled. When he arrived on the 14th June 1807 some of his men had been on board ship for nine long months. Whitelocke's total force now amounted to some 12,000 men in all with an ample number of medical staff officers from these united expeditions. Inspector of Hospitals Theodore Gordon now took charge as P.M.O. and with him there were 2 deputy inspectors, 2 physicians, 6 staff surgeons, 2 apothecaries, 1 purveyor, 2 deputy purveyors, and 18 hospital mates with some 186 tons of hospital equipment and medical stores.

The task set Whitelocke to capture Buenos Aires was no easy one, and in the operations he showed himself both weak and incompetent. There was much marshy ground to traverse from the landing place thirty miles below the city, and no real effort was made to tackle the difficulties of supply and transport. Only sixty horses were provided to carry the 8 tons of reserve rations and most of these kicked off their loads in a scene of wild confusion so that only 1 ton was forwarded to the army the remainder being ruined in the swamps; this too was the fate of the rum ration, for the cart wheels stuck in the mud and the commissary was fain to broach the casks. After months on board ship the majority of the men were unfit to march, the route lay through swampy ground with streams to ford which took them up to their armpits in water, and they arrived at the end of the day hungry, exhausted, and dispirited having lost all confidence in their leader. Contact was made with the fleet at Reduction 20 miles from the start and thence the sick and lame were transferred.

The attack on the town was made on the 5th July 1807 and some 4,500 men divided into thirteen separate columns were planned to fight their way through the streets and unite in the centre of the city. Most of these detachments encountered strong opposition from the enemy sheltered behind houses and barricades while pouring a heavy fire on the invaders. A few reached their objectives and captured 1,000 prisoners, but when day dawned on the 6th July Whitelocke had lost touch with many of the columns and it was discovered that several had been overthrown and captured. The casualties turned out to be heavy. Over 400 had been killed, 649 wounded, and 1,924 were prisoners including 250 wounded, a total of nearly 3,000 or more than half the force engaged. On the 7th fighting ceased and an agreement was reached whereby all prisoners on both sides should be returned and that the British should evacuate the province within ten days.

We know nothing of the precise medical arrangements for the battle, and we can only surmise that the regimental hospitals of the ten different units engaged must have been established in the suburbs of the city which was the starting line for the attack. It is well known that 500 soldiers were told off to guard these hospitals as well as any prisoners captured. Of the medical officers who accompanied the assaulting columns Assistant Surgeon Fergusson of the 88th was killed, Assistant Surgeon Baxter of the 87th dangerously wounded, and four others captured. There is no information on the location of a general hospital, and it is probable that ships lying in the River Plate were used instead of opening one ashore. Gordon appears to confirm this when he says the best results were achieved in the hospital ships.

The figures available for the period of nine months from January to September 1807 show that the troops on the whole were healthy. There were 4,426 sick admissions to hospital in a strength of 10,508; this represents an average monthly admission rate of 492, which is 4·7 per cent, or 47 per 1,000 per month. Almost half these admissions were due to bowel diseases (2,136), followed by continued fever (599), and ophthalmia (458). This last figure is significant of the continued presence of this affliction, although considered medical opinion regarded a large proportion of the cases were self inflicted. The small number suffering from intermittent fever (76) shows that malaria was no problem. The wounded during the campaign totalled 1,095 of whom 198 died, a mortality rate of 18 per cent; tetanus and hospital gangrene were not infrequent, and ascribed at the time to the effects of climate.

The details of disease and wounds are given in the table below:

Disease	Admissions	Discharges	Died	Remaining
Continued fever	599	525	35	39
Intermittent fever	76	58	—	18
Dysentery	1,550	1,324	101	125
Diarrhoea	586	567	—	19
Pulmonary aff.	87	61	8	18
Hepatitis	16	15	1	—
Visceral obstr.	19	15	1	3
Rheumatism	148	144	—	4
V.D.	82	66	2	14
Ophthalmia	458	264	—	194
Wounds	1,095	699	198	155
Ulcers	218	148	2	68
*Casualties	249	228	5	16
Punished	338	312	—	26
Total	5,521	4,426	353	699

* The diagnosis of casualties is inferred to include accidents and injuries.

That the medical staff carried out their duties in a satisfactory manner may be gathered from General Whitelocke's tribute to Inspector Gordon when he thanked him for his 'assiduous work and utmost exertion of skill' as well as his 'professional talent and unremitting attention'.[38]

The end of this unhappy enterprise came when all the troops were embarked and sailed for England. Whitelocke had an untimely end to his career for he was court martialled and cashiered.

Egypt

There was an expedition to Egypt in 1807 to effect the capture of Alexandria, for the Government was obsessed with the idea that Napoleon meditated the occupation of Egypt in spite of his previous disastrous failure a few years previously. It was also essential to aid Russia in her struggle against the invading French armies, and the Tsar had chosen this moment to quarrel with the Turks, so that an expedition against their Egyptian possessions would help Russia. Some 6,000 men were in Sicily after the victory of Maida, and there were dispatched under Major General Fraser to Alexandria in March 1807. The town was captured with ease, but 1,600 men sent to capture Rosetta were repulsed with heavy loss in its narrow pestilential streets and a column hastening to its relief was forced to retire to the coast after losing a third of its strength. Finally this foolishly planned exhibition was recalled to Sicily having suffered nearly 1,000 casualties and having achieved nothing. The medical officers shared in these disasters. Two assistant surgeons, one of the 20th Dragoons and one of the 2/78th Foot were captured and of the medical staff officers under the superintendence of the P.M.O., Deputy Inspector Green, one was killed.

Denmark

The expedition against Denmark was primarily with the object of preventing the Danish Fleet coming under French domination. In July 1807, 20,000 men set sail under Lord Cathcart, but fighting the Danes was distasteful to our forces, and it was only after every effort had been made unsuccessfully to bring pressure on the Danes that Copenhagen was attacked by Sir Arthur Wellesley and occupied after casualties so trifling that fewer than 200 were killed and wounded. With the seizure of the Danish fleet and the completion of the objects of the enterprise the force returned to England. The medical arrangements are unimportant.

REFERENCES

[1] The unit had only been created on the 15th August 1799.

[2] Fortescue. *History of the British Army*, book XII, chapter XXIV, p. 701. Macmillan, London (1910).

[3] Kempthorne. *The Egyptian Campaign of 1801*. Journal, *R.A.M.C.*, vol. LV, p. 221

[4] *Diary of Sir John Moore*, II. 16. Maurice Edwin Arnold, London (1904).

[5] Sick present with the force 3,082; sick evacuated to hospital ships 1,182; total 4,264; fit for duty 11,156; total strength 15,420. Sick percentage 27·6.

[6] Kempthorne. *The Egyptian Campaign of 1801*. Journal, *R.A.M.C.*, vol. LV, p. 223.

[7] The troops neglected to adopt the Turkish custom of having a water carrier attached to each company.

[8] Gore. *Our First Campaign in Egypt*. Pamphlet, Muniment Room, R.A.M. College.

[9] The wine was probably Madeira which was universally drunk in India.

[10] Kempthorne states that nine men of the 86th Foot died on a 70 mile march from Suez to El Hanka. Journal *R.A.M.C.*, vol. LV, p. 225.

[11] 284 at Rosetta, and 838 at Exhove.

[12] One inspector, 3 assistant inspectors, 1 field inspector, 2 physicians, 11 staff surgeons, 1 apothecary, 1 purveyor and 20 hospital mates.

[13] This officer was given a special yearly allowance of 160 guineas for these services during his lifetime.

[14] P.R.O., W.O. 1/346.

[15] Edmonston, 1806.

[16] Edmonston, 1806.

[17] Fergusson. *Notes and Recollections of a Professional Life*, p. 110. Longman, Brown, Green & Longman. London (1846).

[18] Farrell. *Observations on Ophthalmia*, 1811, p. 13.

[19] P.R.O., W.O. 6/56. p. 142.

[20] Dr. Fergusson in an attempt to limit the infection had suggested separate washing tubs for every man, but the local G.O.C. demurred in such an expensive procedure until every other method of combating the disease had been tried.

[21] Later Sir William Adams.

[22] They were also to receive a gift of 36 guineas apiece.

[23] Facts and documents relating to the establishment of the Ophthalmic Hospital. R.A.M. College Muniment Room, pamphlet 51, p. 2.

[24] Facts and documents relating to the establishment of the Ophthalmic Hospital. R.A.M. College Muniment Room, pamphlet 51, p. 3.

[25] Pamphlet 51, p. 4.

[26] First Annual Medical Report of the Ophthalmic Institution. Appendix, p. ii. Pamphlet 51. Muniment Room, R.A.M. College.

[27] Report on Out Pensioners under treatment for diseases of the Eyes. Pamphlet 51, p. 5. Muniment Room, R.A.M. College.

[28] Pamphlet 51, p. 5.

[29] Duke Elder. *Diseases of the Outer Eye*, part 1, p. 260. Henry Kempton, London 1965.

[30] P.R.O., W.O. 3/152.

[31] P.R.O., W.O. 40/14.

[32] Kempthorne. Journal, *R.A.M.C.*, vol. LXI, p. 225.

[33] The best account of this forgotten war is given by Dr. Henry Marshall who was S.M.O. at Colombo from 1816 to 1821 in his 'Notes on Medical Topography of Interior of Ceylon 1821'.

[34] Afterwards Lord Heathfield.

[35] *Gibraltar besieged*. Russell 1965 (Heinemann), p. 278.

[36] Afterwards Sir James Fellowes.

[37] Fortescue. *History of the British Army*, book XIII, chapter XII, p. 377. Macmillan, London (1910).

[38] P.R.O., W.O. 40/27.

Chapter 10

PENINSULAR WAR I (1808–1811)

The Peninsular War originated from Napoleon's designs upon Portugal, and was calculated to force her into the continental system, with the closure of Lisbon and other ports to British shipping. In July 1807 she was ordered to declare war on England and a French force under General Junot was collected at Bayonne to enforce Napoleon's orders. On Portugal's refusal Napoleon declared war, and Junot occupied Lisbon. This was followed by a further declaration of war against Spain, where Napoleon had designed to replace the Spanish Bourbons by his brother Joseph as King. Additional French troops to the number of 70,000 crossed the Spanish frontier and to the dismay of the Spaniards seized the frontier towns and fortresses of Burgos, Pamplona, St. Sebastian and Figueras. Marshal Murat then occupied Madrid. Charles IV of Spain and his son Ferdinand were deported to France, and Joseph proclaimed King in June 1808. But now the whole nation rose in arms to drive the French out, and for the remainder of 1808 the Spanish armies fought with considerable success.

Meanwhile in England the Whig Ministry had fallen and in March 1807 Windham was replaced as Secretary for War by Lord Castlereagh. Castlereagh's plans for recruitment had raised the regular army to some 200,000 men. The type of recruit had improved. No longer were the majority the sweepings of the alehouse and the prison, and the men, although drawn from the poorest and less educated classes, were tough and enduring. Rifleman Harris wrote of them 'they are a strange set, and so determined and unconquerable that they will have their way if they can'.[1] Under the able guidance of the Commander-in-Chief the Duke of York much had been done to improve army administration and training and under General John Moore, the son of a Glasgow doctor, the elements of the first light infantry had been formed, a *corps d'élite*, some of them armed with the new Baker rifle, and disciplined by example instead of by flogging.

It was now decided to agree to a request to help the Spanish patriots and a British force of 10,000 men under Sir Arthur Wellesley sailed from Cork in July 1808 for Portugal. Accompanying them came 19 medical staff officers: Dr. J. Warren as Deputy Inspector of Hospitals,

2 physicians including Dr. Adam Neale, whom we will hear of again, 4 surgeons to the force, 1 apothecary, 1 deputy purveyor and 10 hospital mates, with the equipment and stores for general hospitals.

As the force crosses the Bay of Biscay on its voyage to Portugal to undergo the supreme test of the Peninsular War—a war which was to endure for six years and cause the death of 55,000 of our soldiers— let us take the opportunity of reviewing the organization of the Medical Department when taking the field in an operational role.

The Department embraced two principal groups of officers—the medical staff officers and the regimental medical officers. The principal medical officer of the Department in the field was the Inspector of Hospitals who was the advisor to the Commander of the Forces. He lived at Army Headquarters where he was in close touch with the military situation and issued his instructions from there through the Adjutant General's branch, or on strictly professional matters through medical channels. The medical staff officers were employed in administrative duties and in the general hospitals, and were under the direct command of the Inspector of Hospitals. The regimental medical officers held regimental commissions and were under the command of their colonel.

The medical staff officers were always referred to by Wellington as 'the medical gentlemen', which was in fact the correct term applied to the members of a Civil Department, for they held only relative military rank. These 'officers' included administrators, physicians, surgeons, apothecaries and hospital mates. The senior administrators were the deputy inspectors of hospitals, appointments which were created in the year 1808 by Mr. Knight, the Inspector of Army Hospitals and proved of great benefit to the service. These deputy inspectors held various appointments—they might be the principal medical officer of an independent force, of a division in the field, or the medical superintendent of a large general hospital. There were also administrative officers of the rank of staff surgeon who acted as senior medical officers of brigades, and co-ordinated the medical arrangements of the regimental hospitals and in battle organized a brigade dressing station. Here they combined administrative and professional duties, for they were called upon to operate upon the wounded and were in fact often selected because of their surgical skill. The S.M.O's issued recommendations on clothing, messing, cleanliness, and disease prevention, including weekly skin inspections, and reports were sent to G.O.C's brigades and divisions. They were also responsible for applying to the Commissary General for the transport needed to evacuate the sick and wounded to the rear, and the supply of equipment for units. Regimental surgeons were instructed in the duties of staff surgeon of brigades on a monthly rota, and assistant surgeons acted as regimental surgeons.

Passing now to the purely professional classes of medical staff officers we deal first with the physicians. As a class they could no longer claim the superior position they had previously occupied on account of their educational attainments when they were automatically selected as medical superintendents of general hospitals. The wars in Flanders showed their utter incapacity as administrators without previous military knowledge, and they were now employed in their true capacity of physicians to the forces in charge of the medical division of general hospitals. They were however eligible for promotion to the rank of deputy inspector equally with the surgeons. After the overthrow of the Medical Board in 1809 the appointment of physicians exclusively from civilian sources was changed, and although the majority still came into the army in this way, there were also promotions from the ranks of the staff surgeons and surgeons. They were still drawing a handsome salary of £1 a day.[2]

The surgeons employed in the general hospitals were often referred to as 'surgeons to the forces', and they added greatly to their reputation as skilful clinicians and operators as the war proceeded. We will see in due course that several profiting by the vast experience they were able to acquire became outstanding in their profession, and it is a historical fact that the advances in surgical treatment in the army during the period of any major conflict have usually outstripped that of the civilian profession.

The role of the apothecary is self-evident and need not detain us further except to remind the reader that they were commissioned medical officers selected from the regimental surgeons of the older type, and were eligible for promotion to the higher ranks.

Hospital mates were recruited from the regimental mates or direct from civil life and we have already noted that the demand for them was so pressing that the standard of acceptance had to be lowered. Their lack of knowledge of military custom and procedure on first joining as a raw Scottish or Irish student made them rather the laughing stock of the army, and a story is told of the master of a transport being asked at Lisbon what he had on board and replying 'horses and hospital mates for the army'.[3] The recruitment of hospital mates may be judged from the experience of Dr. Walter Henry, which is typical of many. After study at Trinity College in Dublin he had passed a year in London as a pupil of Sir Everard Home and Sir Benjamin Brodie, which in due course brought him a licence from Surgeon's Hall. 'There was,' he says in the year 1811, 'little difficulty . . . for a medical youth, duly qualified, to obtain a commission in the army; for Talavera, and other bloody fields . . . and camps and cantonments on the unhealthy banks of sluggish rivers . . . had caused a great demand for doctors. In times of yore, and not very remote either, young men of respectable families, good conduct, and fair classical education, when entering the army and navy as medical officers, were not looked upon as gentlemen, but considered as so many hospital drudges, scarcely ranking with the wardmasters or sergeants. They were despised' he says, 'by every new ensign, far their inferior in every estimable quality.'[4] After his appointment he disliked the designation of hospital mate, which 'grated on my ear at first and sounded odious and cacophonous to the last degree . . . It has sunk beneath the growing intelligence of the age, as the last relic of the times of the barber surgeons.'[5] This feeling against the designation of mate became so strong and widespread that it was eventually changed to hospital assistant.

Although the purveyors were exclusively employed in hospitals and were posted and transferred by the Inspector of Hospitals, the Department was financially responsible through the Purveyor in Chief direct to the Treasury. They were in charge of the hospital equipment and responsible for the arms, accoutrements, clothing and necessaries of the patients; they also provided the rations and medical comforts, and these and other stores were obtained through the Commissariat Department, or if unobtainable through that source of supply by local requisitioning. Formerly appointments were made to this branch from the regimental surgeons lists, but with the extreme shortage of medical officers this could no longer be entertained and they were now made from purveyors' clerks. The job was not an easy one and the temptation of making money considerable; it seems only too true that some feathered their own nests. These therefore were the different grades of officers of the medical staff. Their numbers in the year 1807 amounted to 303,[6] increasing six years later in 1813 to 362.

From the medical staff officers we turn now to consider the regimental surgeons. The keystone of the medical arrangements in the forward area was the regimental system where the establishment now included three medical officers, for a second assistant surgeon had been added in 1803 to all battalions with a strength of 500 men and over. After the fiasco in the West Indies to form a medical corps on a limited scale, no further attempt had been made, and in all hospitals the attendants of subordinate rank such as ward masters, stewards, cooks and ward orderlies were drawn from units in the field. These men were inevitably of poor quality and their nursing ability of the crudest kind; Sergeant Cooper of the 7th Fusiliers tells us the hospital orderlies 'were brutes'.[7]

For regimental medical equipment the principal items were the two panniers containing drugs, dressings, surgical instruments and medical comforts.[8] Hennen says he never omitted to carry a canteen of good wine or diluted spirits, for 'many men sink beyond recovery for want of a timely cordial before, during, and after operations; and many of the primary operations would be rendered much more favourable in their results, by the administration of a single glass of wine'.[9] The panniers were carried on a mule purchased by the surgeon from the sum of £20 allowed as bat and forage allowance, and not being Government property, its replacement was the responsibility of the surgeon.

Then there was the regimental hospital equipment consisting of 12 sets of bedding, 24 stretchers, cooking, feeding and ward utensils carried on a bullock cart provided under regimental arrangements. The hospital was equipped to treat 60 cases, the 12 sets of bedding being reserved for those severely ill, while the remainder were placed on improvised beds made by the unit of mats of straw, twigs or rushes. At each temporary halting place one regimental hospital for each brigade was always opened in a house or hut, but in cantonments or winter quarters bedsteads were obtained by local requisition, or beds of boards and trestles constructed locally.

Every M.O. had to provide his own pocket case of instruments, and it was usual to issue a certain number of field tourniquets to officers and some of the N.C.O's and drummers, with a warning that a medical officer must be called as soon as possible to avoid long continued pressure. No recognized body of stretcher bearers accompanied the regiment into action but drummers and other non-combatants were employed to bring in the wounded, although too often they were helped to the rear by their comrades.

At the commencement of the Napoleonic Wars the regimental surgeons were largely of indifferent quality and Hennen is emphatic that this was the fault of poor pay and conditions. 'He must,' he says, 'have been indeed possessed of a most glowing enthusiasm, and an utter contempt for self interest, who would have buried his talents and his industry in a situation where obscurity, poverty, and neglect spread all their miseries before him. These were, for years, the position of the army surgeons; their situation was looked upon as the lowest step of professional drudgery and degradation.'[10]

This is condemnation of a strong order, but the long and testing period of six years of active service brought confidence derived from constant experience. Their worth began to be recognized by their brother officers, and the camaraderie engendered by the hazards and dangers in the field and the essential role which they played in the heat of battle tended to improve their standing in the eyes of their comrades. To the increased morale which their own merits brought them was added in due course the able reputation which the Head of the Department came to acquire. We will see that Dr. James McGrigor became one of the Duke of Wellington's most trusted officers and such recognition of the merits of the Medical Department was undoubtedly reflected throughout the medical officers of the army.

The regimental mates or assistant surgeons had often a very poor reputation, and contemporary historians such as Napier and Colonel Hall severely criticized the employment of these young men in positions for which their experience rendered them unfitted. Sergeant Donaldson of the 94th Foot described them as 'apothecaries' boys, who, having studied a session or two, were thrust into the army as a huge dissecting room, where they might mangle with impunity'.[11] As so many operations were performed at the regimental level this criticism is likely to be a fair one.

The only medical units which accompanied the army were the general hospitals, for no mobile field unit existed in the forward area. The larger hospitals were located at fixed bases such as Lisbon and other large towns and the smaller hospitals sometimes known as intermediate general hospitals were opened in areas occupied by the army when static, or on the lines of communication; the latter generally had provision for 300 patients. Medical stores were supplied by the Inspector of Hospitals from depots held at the base, and transport for their move was provided by the Commissary General's department.

It must be acknowledged in passing that the French army were superior to the British in their field units, for their system included the 'ambulance volante' which set up a divisional dressing station, was staffed by a trained medical corps, and included its own ambulance waggons.

As medical officers had no executive power, hospitals were commanded by *military* officers of field rank with junior officers responsible for the discipline of the subordinate staff. The supervision of these military directors was vested in an officer of senior rank located at Lisbon. Also under military as distinct from medical control were the convalescent wings or depots where convalescents were sent on discharge from hospital. The staff consisted of a captain as commandant, a subaltern as adjutant, and an officer from both the Commissary and Provost Marshal's departments. Here the convalescents were inspected by a medical officer once a week. Wellesley complained there was much indiscipline at these institutions, and we shall see that many stringent orders were issued to control them.

When the army was on the move the disposal of the sick unable to march presented a difficult problem. In the absence of any mobile field medical unit they had to be left behind in the towns or villages through which the army passed; if they were few in number an N.C.O. was put in charge and they were handed over to the care of the local civil magistrate until either the general hospital arrived or they were evacuated to it by bullock waggon; when the sick were numerous a military officer was placed in charge with sometimes an assistant surgeon to supervise medical treatment. No duty was regarded by subalterns as so unpleasant as the charge of a convoy moving sick and wounded to the rear, and the reason is not far to seek as the following account shows: 'The eternal screeching of the ungreased wheels of the Portuguese bullock carts, which too often irritates the sick man into a fever, if he has not one already; the breaking-down of the carts, or the escape of the drivers with bullocks belonging to others, the upsetting

297

the "waggon train" waggons from the badness of the rocky roads, the assembly of the sick in the morning, the only novelty being some new misery, such as to become sexton and bury a man who died during the night, or on the road, are daily occurrences; and if, by chance, he has conducted the whole to the general hospital without having forfeited his commission, the only prospect before him is, that he will be ordered to conduct back from the hospital to the army the recovered men of twenty different battalions, who, having been free for some time from regimental military restraint, give trouble that no one can describe.'[12]

For the sick or wounded officers, regulations did not provide hospital accommodation. He was billeted out with his soldier servant to look after him, and as a result the nursing care and attention he received was often minimal. Wellington we will see became concerned at the lengthy periods officers were reported sick or wounded in billets and ordered medical boards to sit three times a month to make certain that their absence was justified.

We must refer for a moment to the complicated subject of the soldier's stoppages. In the field each man had 6d. a day stopped from his pay to provide his ration of meat and bread. This consisted of 1lb. of meat and 1lb. of bread or the equivalent in biscuit; if bread was not available the meat ration was increased to $1\frac{1}{2}$ or 2lbs.; when there was no fresh meat on the hoof salt meat was issued in lieu. Rice was supplied when available for making soup, and wine was issued at the discretion of the G.O.C. To these items potatoes, vegetables, and fruit were added, purchased out of the soldiers' pay and bought by the unit in the local market. In Portugal and Spain game abounded, and hares, partridges, bustards, and other game found their way into the soldiers' cooking pots, while in spite of constant orders to the contrary there was a good deal of pilfering of the local pigs and poultry. The soldiers fed together in small messes, and the iron canteen in which they cooked their rations was a constant source of trouble, it was heavy and cumbersome, and was carried in turn by each soldier in the mess; later, a mule was provided on a company basis and iron canteens gave place to tin.

When the soldier was admitted to hospital the stoppages were at first 10d. a day, which in 1809 was reduced to 9d. This paid for his ration and for the extras which he consumed in the shape of medical comforts.

The payment of these stoppages differed in general and regimental hospitals and it is necessary for the student of history to understand them. In a general hospital the diets were provided by the purveyor, and the stoppage account for each man was sent to the regimental paymaster monthly, and paid by him into the military chest to the credit of the Medical Department. When the soldier became convalescent, stoppages had still to be paid, and the ration then often included wine on the M.O's recommendation. In a regimental hospital on the other hand it became the surgeon's responsibility to feed the patients from the stoppages which the unit paid him in advance; he purchased this food in the open market or if he was not near a market he was allowed to obtain it from the Commissariat on repayment.

Finally let us briefly describe the soldiers living conditions in the field. Blankets were first issued at the end of 1809, withdrawn in the summer months, and issued again when winter arrived; when in use they were carried on blanket waggons. Greatcoats were worn during the winter months but returned to store each summer. Tents, although issued to officers in 1809, were not made available for the rank and file until 1813, but tents and marquees were in common use by hospitals. Whenever troops halted in wooded country they immediately set to work to build for themselves huts of boughs and leaves and in this they became remarkably expert, looking upon the task more in the light of a game than a duty; when wood was unprocurable they bivouacked in the open country or in bad weather were billeted in villages or towns.

In conclusion a domestic note. Ross Lewin tells us that shortly after arriving in Portugal the men's short hair queues were cropped, so abolishing for ever the tiresome business of each soldier spending half an hour every morning having his hair dressed.[13]

Wellesley's force having arrived off Portugal in the first week of August 1808, disembarked at Mondego Bay some 80 miles north of Lisbon. Here they were joined by 5,000 men under General Spencer, whose force had been lying in transports off Cadiz. With these 15,000 troops he advanced southwards towards Lisbon keeping his route close to the sea from which his supplies were drawn.

It was at Rolica on the 17th August that the first battle of the war was fought. The French held a line of rocky hills, which were successfully stormed. Our losses amounted to 487, of which 20 officers and 315 men were wounded.

On going into action the regimental medical officers divided their duties. The surgeon with one assistant surgeon went forward with the regiment and the surgeon positioned himself seven paces behind the regimental colours. Distinguished by the black feather in his cocked hat and furnished with a haversack of dressings he was here in the most central point to which casualties would be brought and where first aid and the control of haemorrhage could be applied.

The second assistant surgeon remained at the regimental dressing station, or if, as sometimes happened, this was combined with others to form a brigade dressing station, he worked with the brigade staff surgeons on the immediate amputations. After the battle of Rolica, as no brigade staff surgeons had as yet been appointed, Surgeon Guthrie of the 29th Foot was given the task of operating on the wounded, not only because he was the senior regimental surgeon in the field but also because he was the most experienced in surgery. His task took three days of unending toil. In the absence of a general hospital ashore, the wounded were evacuated to the hospital ship *Enterprise* which had already been utilised for the reception of the sick during the advance.

Three days after the fight at Rolica, Wellesley was further reinforced by two brigades landed on the coast near Vimeiro, and this brought his strength up to some 17,000 men, with 1,500 Portuguese Auxiliaries. The medical staff was also thus increased by an additional physician, 2 staff surgeons and 6 hospital mates.

Meanwhile Junot with 13,000 men, a force which he considered ample to drive the British into the sea, had marched from Lisbon and encountered Wellesley at Vimeiro. Wellesley's army occupied ridges on each side of the town. A series of attacks by Junot's force were all repulsed, and by midday it was in full retreat, with the loss of some 1,600 men, and 15 of their 23 guns captured. The British casualties numbered 720, of whom 37 officers and 497 men were wounded.

Dr. Adam Neale a physician of the hospital staff watched the French attack from a farm which became a brigade dressing station, but he felt he could not stand idly by in the heat of the battle, and offered his assistance to the wounded, although as he says, this was 'interference in a duty not strictly my own. I found I could be of assistance to a great many who might have remained for hours in excessive pain. To several, a simple inspection of their wounds with a few words of consolation or perhaps a little opium was all that could be done or recommended. Of those brave men the balls had pierced organs essentially connected with life, and, in such cases, prudence equally forbids the rash interposition of unavailing art, and the useless indulgence of delusive hope.[14] There were no medical comforts available but with the help of a soldier's wife he found some meal which was made into gruel. All the wounded were collected in the church at Vimeiro which was turned into an operating centre for both British and French alike. 'On entering the churchyard my attention was arrested by very unpleasant objects—one, a large wooden dish filled with hands that had just been amputated, another a heap of legs placed opposite.'[15] Next morning forty bullock carts were secured, and Neale was given the task of conveying the wounded to the hospital ships which now provided the means of evacuation to a general hospital opened at Oporto.

Wellesley's immediate plan was to take advantage of this victory by pressing on to Lisbon, but at this moment he had been superseded in command by the arrival of Lieut General Sir Harry Burrard. Slow and cautious by nature, Burrard vetoed any such movement until further reinforcements expected under Sir John Moore had arrived. On the following day Burrard was himself superseded by Lieut General Sir Hew Dalrymple, who took a similar view. Then on the 22nd August General Kellerman arrived under a flag of truce with Junot's proposal for a convention, whereby the French would evacuate Portugal. This was agreed by all three generals, for Wellesley now saw that the opportunity of quickly destroying the French army had gone. The signing of the Convention of Cintra allowed all French troops to be returned to France in British ships taking with them all their plunder and equipment. Wellesley, Burrard and Dalrymple now returned to England. The British troops in Portugal, some 30,000 strong, were now left under the command of Sir John Moore. He, with his force of 10,000 men, had recently returned from the abortive expedition to Sweden, and with him came a substantial number of medical staff officers; Dr. Franck was Inspector of Hospitals, and Dr. William Fergusson Deputy Inspector; there were also 2 physicians and 4 surgeons to the forces, 1 apothecary, 1 purveyor, 1 deputy purveyor, and 12 hospital mates.

With the movement of the army towards Lisbon, Oporto hospital was closed and another opened, first at Torres Vedras, and then at the picturesque palace of Mafra.[16] The beds were soon filled, for outbreaks of diarrhoea were rife, put down to the cold nights, the eating of excessive quantities of fruit, and the drinking of new wine. But bowel infection carried by flies was obviously the cause. Schaumann himself was cured by opium pills and rice water, but mercury in the form of repeated doses of calomel was the common remedy. Fergusson quotes Sir John Pringle in advocating ripe grapes as a cure; other doctors prescribed orange and lemon juice;[17] and these bland fluids, combined with avoiding the ingestion of indigestible food could be nothing but beneficial. The outbreak was so severe that local medical practitioners were called in to help when the army arrived in Lisbon, and where the principal general hospital was now established.

Throughout Spain the French continued to suffer serious reverses, and the Spanish armies were full of warlike enthusiasm. But there was no central commander-in-chief to co-ordinate strategy or tactics, and there was no central government; each province had its own army under its own generals, and their horizon was limited by the mountains which separated one province from another. British arms and money they received with enthusiasm, but Spanish national pride made them reluctant to allow British troops on their soil, for they considered that their own armies could fight and overcome the French. Thus when Sir David Baird arrived in October 1808 with a new reinforcement of some 14,000 British troops at Corunna in northern Spain to link up with the Spanish troops he was not received with any enthusiasm, and was forbidden to land until authority had reluctantly been given by

Madrid, a proceeding which involved weeks of delay. The medical staff included in his force brought Deputy Inspector Hogg, 2 physicians, 4 staff surgeons, 1 apothecary, 1 deputy purveyor and 12 hospital mates, with general hospital equipment and stores.

By the middle of 1808 the operations in the Peninsula, the Mediterranean, and Madeira had absorbed 2 inspectors of hospitals, 7 deputy inspectors, 6 physicians, and 20 staff surgeons. Considering the overall shortage of medical officers, the Medical Board were distinctly worried whether so many senior medical staff appointments were justified. One distinct handicap which the Board suffered was the reluctance of Whitehall to inform them of the destination of these various expeditions, either for security reasons or because they could not or would not appreciate why they wanted to know. They were simply told to provide medical officers and stores for 5,000 or 10,000 men, as the case might be. They were kept in the dark as to whether they were independent expeditions or sent as reinforcements to join other forces. Madeira was a case in point. In December 1807 Major General Beresford had taken over the island with a force of 4,000 men, and the Board had provided a deputy inspector, a physician, 2 surgeons to the forces, 1 apothecary, 1 deputy purveyor and 6 hospital mates. Subsequently, when the troops moved to Portugal, the Board, if it had been informed, could have re-employed the medical staff to better advantage.

The orders now sent to Sir John Moore were to unite with Baird's force landed at Corunna, and co-operate with the Spanish armies to drive the French out of Spain. His plan was to join Baird in the region of Valladolid in the Castilian plain, which meant an advance of some 300 miles over mountains 4,000 feet high, and along roads and tracks of which he knew nothing. Further, he was without adequate transport, for a lack of bullion prevented him hiring sufficient mules, horses, or oxen for baggage purposes. But in October he began his march to Salamanca, leaving 10,000 men in Lisbon. 'I am advancing,' Moore wrote, 'without the knowledge of a single magazine being made, or that we may not starve when we arrive.'[18] He was however forced to move before the winter rains began, and he had to trust to Spanish promises to furnish his 20,000 men with supplies. The advance was made on three roads and it was with high spirits that his troops set out on their march—'the men seemed invincible and nothing I thought could beat them'.[19] But the roughness of the mountain tracks compelled Moore to send his twenty-four guns, protected by four battalions and all his cavalry, by a wide sweep to the south and east.

While Baird's force at Corunna waited in their transports for permission to disembark, the sick were confined in the dark and ill ventilated sick bays between decks. Even after the troops had commenced landing on the 25th October a frigate converted for hospital use was the only accommodation provided, and this unsatisfactory arrangement had to be continued until the Spanish objection to handing over any building ashore for hospital use was overruled. Nothing could have been worse for the sick—the frigate was soon overcrowded, the accommodation devoid of comfort, the dieting of patients impossible and in bad weather all contact with the shore was cut off. When 'malignant' dysentery broke out and the sick had little else but salt rations and rum to live on the two physicians Dr. Faulkner and Dr. Knight complained bitterly. At length an additional ship was made available for convalescents, but this made but little difference, and only when a convent ashore was requisitioned were the doctors able to treat their patients with any degree of success.

But with the troops ashore Baird's difficulties had only just begun. The surly Spanish authorities made no arrangements for feeding, and here also the Treasury had omitted to provide bullion to hire forage and transport waggons and oxen. There was not even money to pay the troops. Consequently, Baird's advance over the 200 miles of mountain roads to Astorga was of necessity painfully slow.

Both commanders were faced with complete ignorance of the real situation in Spain, and as there was still no Spanish Commander-in-Chief to issue orders, they could only get news from the Supreme Junta in Madrid who appeared to be quite unpractical, and talked of encircling the French with Spanish armies which were in their excitable imagination much exaggerated in numbers, and were moreover entirely independent in their actions.

Since his reverses in Spain Napoleon had hurried troops into the country from all quarters, until by the 1st November he had a force of some 120,000 under his personal command. He struck at once. Burgos was captured, and on the 13th November he entered Valladolid, the city where the armies of Moore and Baird were to have met. The British commanders were entirely ignorant of this as they advanced into the heart of Spain.

On the 6th November the rain began to fall over the mountains on the road to Almeida which Moore was following, and as the men struggled over the rocky tracks he received disturbing news of the real state of the Spanish armies—weak, illtrained and unequipped—and moving away to the north and the east, far from his proposed point of junction with them. But his army, in excellent heart, reached Cuidad Rodrigo on the 13th November, having covered 250 miles in three weeks; but at Salamanca two days later he learned he had arrived too late, for Valladolid 60 miles to the north-east was already in French hands. Baird was still 100 miles away to the north-west, and Hope with the artillery another 100 miles away to the south-east.

Moore was now in a serious position. By the end of November the whole reason for his advance to co-operate with the Spanish armies had disappeared, for Napoleon had already destroyed one army, he was threatening Madrid, and was about to destroy another of their armies at Tudela. The British general was completely devoid of precise information either of the Spaniards or the French, for nobody troubled to send him information. He was in command of the only British army in existence, and to engage some 80,000 French forces before joining up with Baird would have risked a disastrous defeat. The situation was in fact no longer that which had prompted the Government to send its army to Spain, which was to combine with the Spaniards and not to cope unaided with the whole might of France. Until his guns and cavalry arrived Moore's position was indeed dangerous for not until then did he have a balanced force. His immediate inclination was to retire to Portugal, and he ordered Baird to fall back on Corunna, but he then delayed his move because fresh news arrived that the Spaniards in Madrid were in revolt, the Spanish peasants were in arms, and there was still a chance of saving Spain from destruction. This hope soon proved groundless, for Napoleon shortly after entered Madrid while the Spanish Junta was still clamouring for Moore to move to the aid of the capital.

By an unusual stroke of luck a captured French dispatch gave the momentous news that Napoleon had not 80,000 but 300,000 men in Spain, and the main French army was advancing towards Badajoz and Lisbon in which direction Napoleon thought Moore was retreating. Further important news was that Soult with a corps of 18,000 men was isolated from the main army and was operating to the north of his present position. His men were still in excellent fighting mood so Moore recalled Baird to Astorga, and on the 20th December, after the two forces were united, he moved north to attack and destroy Soult's Corps or at least strike a shrewd blow before retiring to the sea. Meanwhile Napoleon, having discovered his mistake, gathered his forces and hurried northwards to encircle and destroy the British.

Before we follow Moore's movements further, let us refer to the medical picture. On arrival at Salamanca Dr. Warren the Deputy Inspector of Hospitals with the force had been informed that a general hospital was not to be opened as the stay was unlikely to be prolonged. For the sick the result was lamentable. The regimental hospitals were herded together in an ecclesiastical college and each regimental surgeon attended his own sick and provided his own orderlies. Further, each surgeon had to feed his own patients from the stoppages of 10d. a day for each man. To simplify the purchase of food in the market it was decided that the regimental surgeon with the most cases in hospital should buy for all. But no sooner was this arranged than his regiment was ordered off and he went with it and took his orderlies as well. A second surgeon was appointed and the same thing happened, and a third and a fourth. Amidst this confusion the patients, according to Dr. Adam

Neale, the physician who accompanied the army, went without food except for some bread and water; what little nursing there was ceased, and the wards were in a filthy state. Dr. Warren appeared powerless to avoid this breakdown, and Dr. Shapter the Inspector of Hospitals was far away in Lisbon. It must be remembered however that with the system in force even with the necessary medical staff officers present it was impossible to administer a general hospital without a military superintendent, and it may well be that Sir John Moore under the difficult circumstances in which he stood was unwilling to lose the services of a field officer for the purpose. This was one of the disadvantages of not giving medical officers executive control.

When eventually Moore decided to sever his lines of communication with Lisbon this hospital with its patients was left in the air. They were told to pack up and take the road to Lisbon and with junior medical officers to take care of them on the way some 1,500 sick started their 300 mile journey in bullock carts exposed to the elements and crawling along at the rate of 2 miles an hour. There were still a further 2,500 sick to be dealt with, and these, mostly suffering from minor disorders, had to be carried forward with the army.

The attack on Soult was just about to begin when Moore received the unwelcome intelligence that Napoleon's advance troops were only 20 miles to the south. Only one thing now could save him from destruction and that was to withdraw to Astorga and take the mountain road to Corunna. So on the 24th December the retreat began. With the thought of a fight after months of marching the morale of the troops had been high but the unlooked for retreat was a shattering blow to discipline. The countryside afforded neither food nor fuel, and winter had set in with frost and snow. The columns struggled on day and night with the French cavalry in close pursuit cutting off the stragglers. Discipline soon lapsed, and scenes of drunkenness and pillage followed the trail of the army. The route over the mountains, deep in snow and slush, was marked by the bodies of men, women and children, dead from exhaustion or frozen to death. The carcasses of hundreds of horses and oxen which had to be destroyed encumbered the ground. The depots of food and clothing *en route* were largely pillaged and lost before they could be fairly distributed, and at every village the wine stores were broken open and consumed. In spite of every effort by the rearguard to force them along the route, many of the drunken stragglers were left behind and rounded up by the French Cavalry, but the rearguard itself never wavered or failed in their duty.

The state of the sick and wounded was terrible. Ever since Salamanca these had been carried along with the army in bullock carts as there was no route of evacuation now to Lisbon. As the bullocks died of famine and exhaustion the sick and wounded in the carts had to be abandoned to their fate. At Astorga when Romana's Spanish army joined the retreat, sixty or seventy of his men were admitted to hospital with typhus every day, and the contagion spread to the British troops. The medical staff officers who had come with Baird had opened hospitals at Ponferrada and Villa Franca where there was also a depot of medical stores, and here some 2,000 sick had been collected. But the retreat made it impossible to keep them open, and Neale tells us—'it was still attempted to carry forward our sick and wounded; the beasts which dragged them failed, and they were of necessity left in their waggons to perish amidst the snow'.[20] 'That no degree of horror might be wanting, this unfortunate army was accompanied by many women and children—of whom some were frozen to death on the baggage waggons which were broken down or left upon the road for want of cattle; some died of fatigue and cold while their infants were vainly sucking at their clay cold breasts.'[21]

At last after eighteen days and nights of unending toil and struggle the army arrived at Corunna on the 11th January 1809. In a retreat of nearly 300 miles carried out under appalling conditions in the face of a superior foe and without the slightest help of the Spaniards, they had not—for all their insubordination—lost a gun or a colour. Unfortunately the transports which would have carried them away to England without French interference were detained at Vigo by contrary winds, but there were hospital and store ships in the harbour and all the medical staff officers and the sick were embarked at once. By the 14th January when the transports arrived, the French were upon them and the British turned to fight. There were barely 15,000 effective troops, for thousands had been lost in the retreat, and on the morning of the battle there were 4,035 sick in Corunna. But at the prospect of action, discipline at once revived, and the French failed to overcome their resistance. But in the moment of victory Sir John Moore was mortally wounded. On the morning of the 17th January 1809 the army, unhindered by the French, embarked for England.

When the ragged, filthy and exhausted soldiers, riddled with typhus, landed in England the country was horrified. Of the 34,000 who had gone to liberate Spain some 28,000 returned. The losses in the campaign amounted to 5,998, of whom 3,809 perished on the road or in hospital and 2,189 were left as prisoners in French hands.

The acute problem which faced the Medical Board was how to deal with such a flood of cases. Their arrival was not altogether a surprise. Keate had received advance news from Spain that 1,570 sick and wounded had been embarked at Corunna and another 400–500 were ready to follow, while the final battle was likely to furnish a further 1,000 wounded. From Lisbon another 1,000 were expected, many of them serious cases. All this amounted to some 4,000, but in fact some 6,000 arrived. Owing to Knight's senseless policy of closing the general hospitals at Gosport, Plymouth and Deal on the grounds of economy there was not a single bed ready to receive them. It is true that the York Hospital in Chelsea and the Depot Hospital on the Isle of Wight were functioning, but the latter was filled with sick recruits, and the York Hospital was far away in London.

On receipt of the news Pepys and Keate had not been idle but had addressed an urgent letter to the Secretary at War on the 21st January demanding the immediate re-opening of the three general hospitals which they said had been built at great expense and would hold 500, 400 and 300 respectively, while the York Hospital which was reserved for wounded should be increased by a further 500 beds. To this request Knight refused to answer and as relations between the members of the Board were strained to breaking point the reason was not far to seek. Their personal quarrels were plainly leading to a break-down in effective administration, and even the Secretary at War had the sense to agree that hospitals should be re-established and equipped ready for such emergencies.[22] But the pressure of events was to overtake the steps proposed, although luckily the Portsmouth area had a very efficient Inspector in Dr. James McGrigor who tackled the problem with energy when the transports arrived. Immediate steps were taken to set up temporary hospitals in barracks, and in hulks, transports, and prison ships anchored in Spithead; the Royal Navy offered the use of Haslar Hospital, and some 1,400 cases were found accommodation here, while the regimental hospitals landed with the troops were expanded in hired buildings. Additional medical officers were provided by ordering the surgeons of the Guards down from London, and every civil practitioner around Portsmouth was employed.

All this however could not be done in a moment and in the meantime the typhus ridden victims were condemned to remain cooped up in the dozen transports which had brought them. Dr. Adam Neale, one of the physicians who was on board, estimated that the delay in treat-ment caused the unnecessary loss of a thousand lives. 'Without diet and stores, in filthy surroundings and parched with thirst,' he says, 'some had to remain in these conditions for weeks.'[23] Typhus raged through the ships and as batches of patients were sent off to different forts and barracks the contagion soon spread far and wide amongst both the military and civil population. Some transports were diverted to Plymouth and to Ramsgate and Dr. Knight the physician in charge at Ramsgate described the overcrowded conditions in converted bar-racks there as scandalous. Twenty patients or more all with typhus were crowded together in one room which, he says, should not have held more than five. It was no wonder that out of 38 orderlies only 5 escaped, and that 12 out of 15 doctors employed contracted typhus and one paid the penalty with his life. It had been known since Pringle's day that the only way of treating typhus successfully was by ample spacing and good ventilation. Neale, remembering Salamanca, condemned what he called the preposterous policy of the regimental system by which regimental surgeons had to act as purveyors and feed their patients from stoppage money as well as prescribing for them, keeping accounts, and rendering returns.

For all this Mr. Knight was to blame. Abolishing general hospitals on the grounds of economy he had earned the appreciation of the Treasury, and was quite unrepentant in rejecting Dr. Neale's criticism that they should be re-opened on the grounds of humanity. He was so furious that he demanded a court of inquiry which was in fact held at Portsmouth with five General Officers as members. Not only the conditions at Portsmouth but the criticisms of the physicians on the lack of proper hospital arrangements at Salamanca and in the transports at Corunna were investigated, although Knight, of course, was not concerned with Spain, which came under Surgeon General Keate.

The Board chose to set aside most of the complaints put forward by the four physicians who gave evidence, and Neale's report that the typhus patients were kept on board for three weeks was disbelieved.[24] In fact they whitewashed the whole affair. Salamanca they admitted might have been faulty but no one deserved censure. At Corunna the conditions were inevitable under the circumstances existing; six ships were finally put to hospital use and a purveyor was provided, so if the physicians did not get proper diet for their patients it must have been due to some misunderstanding.[25] Even at Ramsgate they said the accommodation was judicious and successful. 'Upon the whole we are of the opinion that the sick and wounded have met with every possible care, comfort and attention,'[26] and they were, they said, surprised so many were so well provided for. There was no undue mortality amongst the 6,000 sick, and in this connection the only figures that are available are those for Haslar, where 205 died out of 1,400 admissions, a mortality of 14·6 per cent. The important question of whether Knight was to blame for not having hospitals already established was shelved, and in fact he appeared to have come out of the investigation with a clean sheet, for the Board said the hospitals at Gosport, Deal, and Plymouth accommodating 1,200 between them had been re-opened with little or no delay. In fact it was Pepys and Keate who were blamed for believing the physicians reports before they had been fully investigated.[27]

Keate, for his part, was inclined to censure Shapter for the chaos at Salamanca, for with a physician and a purveyor present a general hospital could easily have been established. Shapter's refusal to do so was regarded as 'not quite satisfactory'[28] and in fact he had already been recalled from Portugal and Deputy Inspector William Fergusson was acting in his place. The Surgeon General was satisfied that there were no complaints of any deficiences of medical officers, of medicines, or hospital stores, although lack of transport created shortages during the retreat, and much had to be destroyed or abandoned.

On the 15th April of the same year, Sir Arthur Wellesley was on his way back to Portugal. Sir John Cradock with the 10,000 British troops left in Lisbon had expected a French advance, but the enemy were so actively engaged in supporting themselves in the bare Iberian hills that Soult did not move until March, and it was the city of Oporto in the north that was stormed and sacked. By that month reinforcements were on their way to Lisbon, and by the end of April Wellesley could muster an army of 20,000 British, 3,000 Hanoverians of the King's German Legion, and an uncertain element of 16,000 Portuguese. He was far from being overawed by the French superiority in numbers. Neither of the French armies in and near Portugal were concentrated for battle but spread out over the countryside supporting themselves by pillage, and Wellesley with masterly strategy seized the chance of attacking Soult at Oporto before he was aware of his danger. By the 4th May he had concentrated 16,000 British and 4,000 Portuguese at Coimbra 100 miles north of Lisbon, and on the 11th May he was opposite Oporto on the banks of the Douro. By a bold and brilliant operation his troops crossed the river by seizing Portuguese river craft in the face of the unsuspecting enemy, and occupied a large seminary in the town before the enemy were fully awake to their danger. Beating off the French counterattacks the British forces stormed into the town and Soult beaten at every turn was forced to retreat. The fight had been won at the cost of only 123 casualties including 98 wounded, and these were treated in a general hospital hastily formed in the town.

Here Guthrie again made himself conspicuous. He had been with his regiment in Cadiz during the Corunna campaign but rejoining the army at Oporto he had managed to be present at the front when the staff surgeons were still in the rear. Speaking fluent Portuguese he persuaded a boatman to ferry himself and his horse across the Douro, and was the first mounted officer to arrive in the town. While busily occupied in assisting at the general hospital he became separated from his regiment, but went forward later with a Portuguese battalion, which were mistaken for French when they came up with a British regiment. They were about to be shot at when Guthrie tore off his greatcoat and displayed his red tunic. This saved the day. Subsequently riding forward, our adventurous surgeon came on a French gun which the drivers were abandoning, and cutting the traces with his sword he captured it single-handed and handed it over to his astonished colonel.

The spring months of 1809 in Portugal were singularly healthy ones and at Coimbra on the 6th May the morning state shows there were 2,634 sick out of a strength of 27,231, a figure of 9·7 per cent. As the army set out on the march to Oporto we quote a General Order laying down the routine which was commonly adopted for the sick. 'The regimental surgeons of the brigades about to march will immediately report the number of sick they intend to leave behind to Staff Surgeon Morrell charged with the duty of superintending them. An assistant surgeon from each regiment will remain with the sick till they are properly given over; and one or more assistant surgeons per brigade according to the numbers will remain at Coimbra to take care of them.'[29] This last paragraph draws attention to the drain which so frequently reduced the number of regimental medical officers, a drain which the presence of a field medical unit in close support would have avoided.

At this date with over sixty medical staff officers in the country there was an ample number to man the general hospitals. Dr. Franck had taken over from Shapter as Inspector of Hospitals, and there were 2 deputy inspectors, 5 physicians, 15 staff surgeons, as well as apothecaries and purveyors and 30 hospital mates. Apart from a deputy inspector with Wellesley's headquarters and staff surgeons serving as senior medical officers to each of the brigades, the remainder were divided between the general hospitals where Franck was located, at Coimbra and now at Oporto. The subordinate hospital staff was provided in the usual manner by detailing men from regiments, and a General Order issued on the 24th May gives the proportion of officers and N.C.O's sent for hospital duty in respect of the sick of each brigade.[30] There is no reference here to the number of ward orderlies, which according to Hennen numbered 1 ward master and 6 orderlies to every 100 beds. An officer of field rank was detailed to act as the military superintendent, and there were precise instructions on his rendering weekly and monthly returns to the Medical Department. Hospital stoppages at the rate of 10d. a day for each man[31] were charged and accounts kept by the purveyor and settled monthly.

Whether soldiers' wives were employed in the general hospitals is doubtful and Hennen held no brief for women. 'The employment,' he wrote, 'of females is one of the greatest sources of irregularity . . . every species of excess, idleness, and plunder is carried on under their auspices.'[32] In regimental hospitals they were constantly employed performing the duties of cook and the washing of linen, and two wives per company were authorized to accompany their husbands overseas.

But now the accepted policy of treating sick and wounded in the regimental hospitals had to be abandoned when Wellesley ordered the bullock carts carrying the equipment to be withdrawn on the grounds that they interfered with the movement of the army, and all their bedding was ordered to be returned to Coimbra. This meant there was no bed in which to treat a sick man nearer than the general hospital and all cases had to be sent to the rear. Only a single cart was retained to carry the sick or the packs of men who fell out on the march, and beside it rode one of the assistant surgeons. These slow moving oxen plodding along at 2 miles an hour drawing their screeching carts with solid wheels gave anything but a comfortable ride for the sick and were torture for the wounded. Schaumann says, 'when a number of these carts are moving together, it (the noise) is enough to drive one mad'.[33]

Our narrative must return to the operations after Oporto when Soult's army was pursued beyond Braga 30 miles to the north. Here a further hospital was opened, but by the 24th May Wellesley decided to abandon the attempt to follow the French into the wild mountainous country through which they were retiring, and consequently the Braga hospital was closed and all cases were sent back to Oporto. Wellesley now turned south to engage the French under Victor, and the army was concentrated at Abrantes early in June, where a general hospital was established. Whenever the supply of hospital stores was inadequate to meet the demands, recourse was had to requisitioning, and a General Order of the 12th June lays down the procedure: 'When bedding is required for the sick, whether for regiments or general hospitals, and it cannot be supplied by the general stores, the surgeon in charge of the hospital must make a requisition in writing for what he requires on the commissary of the brigade or the Commissary General. The officer of the Commissariat will make a requisition upon the magistrate of the place for what will thus be required for the surgeon.'

It was always a complicated administrative problem to deal with the sick left behind in hospitals distant from the army area, and the following detailed orders are quoted in order to give an example of how this was tackled. The General Order published at Abrantes on the 13th June 1809 runs as follows:

(1) The senior officer in charge of the sick at Oporto and Coimbra will, once a week, send by the post to headquarters, a return of the sick, specifying the number of recovered men able to march. Whenever forty men at either hospital are sufficiently recovered to be able to march, an order and a route will be sent for their march by easy stages.

(2) They are to take with them, at setting out, three days' bread, in biscuit, which they are to keep by them as a reserve.

(3) The Commissary General will arrange that they shall be fed at the different halting places.

(4) An officer must be sent in command of every detachment of 40 men, and 2 officers if the number should amount to 80 and so on; 1 officer for every 40 in addition. One N.C.O. must be sent for every 20 sick.

(5) The senior officer of the hospital will report to the Quartermaster General the departure of the recovered men; and officers commanding

the parties of recovered men must report their progress to head-quarters at every opportunity.

When patients became convalescent they were under the military superintendent of the hospital for exercise and discipline. But misconduct became so widespread amongst these convalescents that a stern rebuke from Wellesley was contained in a General Order issued at Abrantes on the 17th June, dealing with such matters as quarters, dress, bounds and parades. Copies of these orders were sent to every hospital and a weekly report made that they had been carried out.

The provision of hospital attendants, the control of the convalescents, the return of the recovered sick to their units, all these tasks made an extensive call upon the manpower of regiments, and this denuded them of both officers and men which the establishment of a medical corps would have made unnecessary. Such however was the accepted policy, short sighted as it may now seem.

Before any further operations which involved an advance into Spain could be undertaken immense difficulties over the provision of transport had to be overcome. This was partly due to the negligence of the Treasury in not providing sufficient specie to buy animals, but in any case horses and mules were scarce and the allotment to units was minimal. One mule was allowed to every troop of cavalry, and every company of infantry, to carry the camp kettles; out of the five additional mules to each infantry battalion one was provided to carry the surgeon's two panniers. No unit transport was allowed for provisions, the standing order being that each infantryman would carry three days' bread, while meat was driven along or bought locally on the hoof. No supply column therefore existed, all rations being carried forward by bullock waggons to a supply park from which they were distributed through regimental or brigade stores.

With the arrival of further reinforcements it was now possible to re-group the army into four infantry and one cavalry division. On the medical side this meant the appointment of a deputy inspector or staff surgeon to each division to act as senior medical officer. The chain of command was therefore regimental surgeon, staff surgeon at brigade, staff surgeon or deputy inspector at division, inspector of hospitals at force headquarters.

On the 27th June 1809, Wellesley marched from Abrantes with 23,000 men and 30 guns, after the regimental hospitals had got rid of their sick into the general hospital. By the 15th July the army was at Plasencia, and the men were in high spirits after their march of over 120 miles. But although they were in good heart there were cases of contagious (typhus) fever due it was thought to lack of cleanliness, and a General Order was published based on a report by the Deputy Inspector of Hospitals, insisting on a better standard of hygiene. 'Many men have been lately sent to the hospital both here and elsewhere, in a state of the utmost filth, some with no shirts at all, and others with only one, which had not been washed for a very considerable length of time; greater attention to cleanliness and the state of the men's necessaries seems, therefore, called for in some brigades of the army; and bathing, whenever practicable, at an early hour of the morning, and at no other time, ought to be universally practised during the hot season. The present species of contagious fever is infallibly generated among the troops by the neglect of personal cleanliness. New-killed meat without salt is very prejudicial; and the mode of issuing and conducting the rations has been productive of much annoyance, exhaustion and disappointment, and consequently of disease to the soldiers.'[34] Personal cleanliness, however, was not such an easy matter with daily marches in the heat and dust of the Spanish roads, bivouacking in the open fields without tents, and the scarcity of water in a dry land. When marching in wooded country the men were expert in building huts of boughs and leaves to provide shelter, and on occasions houses and farms in the Spanish villages provided a night's rest, but the people were generally unfriendly, and as Schaumann says, 'hardly offered us a glass of water'.[35] A limited number of tents were in fact now available for officers, but a general issue of tents for the rank and file was not possible for another four years.

Wellesley now joined forces with a Spanish army under General Cuesta, and the allies arrived at Talavera on the Tagus some 60 miles from Madrid on the 22nd July. Six days later the battle of that name was fought. The defensive position taken up by the British and Spanish armies was some 3 miles in extent, with the Spaniards on the right amongst embanked gardens and olive groves; the British lines extended over open country devoid of cover until it reached a steep conical hill, the Cerro de Medellin. To hold this line against the 46,000 veteran French troops opposed to him Wellesley had only 17,000 British, very few of them seasoned troops, and 3,000 of the King's German Legion; the Spanish army of 32,000 strong which was confined to the defence of the town was incapable of manoeuvre and could be easily contained by the enemy. Even when drawn up two deep the British could barely cover the ground. On the road from Lisbon, Brigadier General Crauford's Light Brigade was hurrying forward by forced marches, but arrived too late for the battle. Moreover, the soldiers were hungry, for the provisions promised by the Spaniards had never materialized, and Wellesley was rapidly discovering that promises and performances were two very different things on the part of his unreliable allies. If the French decided to attack, the Commander-in-Chief felt that disaster could only be averted by relying on the courage and coolness of every man.

Before the battle is described let us review the tactics generally adopted by both combatants. The French army carried out attacks in massed formation and relied upon weight of numbers, while the British with their higher standard of discipline favoured formation in line and concentrated on fire power. Wellesley often avoided exposing his men to enemy artillery fire by positioning them behind the highest point of a defended ridge and brought them forward into view of the advancing enemy infantry only at a late stage in the attack. Then a crashing volley fire at close range was followed by a charge with the bayonet.

Marshal Victor was so certain of his prey that he spurned the idea of delaying his offensive, and as soon as it was dark attacked and gained the top of the Cerro de Medellin, but was quickly repulsed by a counter attack. At dawn on the 28th July the two armies faced each other across Portina brook, and throughout the day the French launched attack after attack against the British line all of which were repulsed after heavy fighting. As it grew dark the dried grass on the slopes of the Cerro de Medellin caught fire and hundreds of helpless wounded were engulfed in the flames. The French had now had enough and drew off at the end of the day leaving 7,000 dead and wounded and 17 guns on the field. So ended the battle of Talavera, one of the hardest ever fought by the British army. The casualties totalled 5,363, or a quarter of the force engaged, and of these, 3,915 including 196 officers were wounded.

The biggest task which had yet fallen to the lot of the medical service now became the responsibility of Guthrie, recently promoted to staff surgeon, who was called to act because Franck the Inspector of Hospitals was laid low by an attack of dysentery. All along the front the regimental hospitals had been opened up some 700 yards behind the firing line, out of the range of cannon and musket shot; several were concentrated behind the Cerro de Medellin area. Medical officers dealt with the lightly wounded who were able to make their own way back to the dressing stations, but the severe cases had to be left until the fighting was over. With such an immense number it took forty-eight hours before the collecting parties detailed from regiments were able to bring in both friend and foe alike; the Spaniards refused to help clear the battlefield, but their soldiers and civilians found better amusement in beating out the brains of the French wounded until the British opened fire on them. Franck had made all preparations beforehand for a general hospital to be opened in a great convent in Talavera, and here the purveyor's staff had prepared the building and provided beds and equipment both from army stores and local sources; but this building proved much too small, and the wounded overflowed into every church and convent in the town.

The colossal task of treating 4,000 British casualties as well as the French wounded was made easier by the inability of the army to pursue the French, which set free every medical officer to help. Certainly the army was in no fit state to move, for although the Spaniards had supplies of food, they refused to share them with the British, and the hungry troops were down to one-third of their full ration. This shortage, however, did not affect the sick and wounded, for a General Order of the 30th July ordered the Commissary General to attend in full to the requisitions of the Inspector of Hospitals for provisions and other articles. So although the wounded were tortured by the heat and the flies they were not allowed to go hungry, albeit this was at the expense of their comrades. To help in the hospital wards the standing practice was adopted of ordering brigades to detail officers, N.C.O's, and privates for duty in proportion to the numbers of each unit under treatment, but to save the fighting ranks being denuded of fit men the General Order laid down that they should be selected from those who were slightly wounded and likely to require detention in Talavera.[36] A field officer from the 1st Division was detailed to superintend the hospital, an essential step to preserve discipline and order amongst the subordinate staff drawn from at least a score of different regiments. It cannot be doubted that all these *ad hoc* preparations must have resulted in anything but the orderly and smooth running hospital system which trained personnel could have provided.

For forty-eight hours the wounded, friend and foe alike, were brought in on bullock carts, on horseback, and on muleback, and the surgeons, immersed in their task had hundreds of amputations to perform. Schaumann describes how in passing the convent he saw both dead and wounded dumped round the entrance, while from the front windows issued the cries of those whose limbs were being amputated, and from time to time arms and legs were flung out in the small square below.[37]

While Wellesley was awaiting supplies and transport to move forward on the road to Madrid he received alarming tidings that a threat to his communications was developing from Soult, who with 50,000 troops was coming down from the north. It was impossible to ignore this danger to his vital lines of supply from Lisbon, and Wellesley was compelled to turn back to Oropesa on the 3rd August, handing over the severely wounded to the care of his Spanish allies, but with some of his own medical officers left in charge. He did, however, delay his march for a few hours to cover the arrival of as many as were fit to be moved, and he sacrificed a quantity of baggage to procure carriage for some 2,000 of them, while 700 more were left to hobble along as best they could on their own feet, until many gave up the struggle. 'Wounded and sick men,' says Schaumann, 'who a moment previously one would have thought incapable of moving, suddenly recovered the power of their legs, and staggered, limped, and hobbled away so that they might escape falling into the enemy's hands. But rescued from Scylla they will only fall into the hands of Charybdis; for many of them, if they do not remain with the bulk of the wounded, will only be killed by the Spanish marauders and stragglers, or by Spanish peasants, who always scent money and heresy whenever they spy an Englishman.'[38]

At Oropesa Wellesley learnt that Soult was threatening to capture the crossings over the Tagus in his rear, and there was nothing he could now do but forestall the French by seizing the bridge at Arzobispo and move his army to the south bank of the Tagus. He did this without an hour's delay, and on the 4th August the units and corps, accompanied by artillery, muleteers, and carts piled high with wounded, poured over the bridge. Half starving and in insufferable heat the army marched westwards, and the Light Brigade reached Almaraz just in time to prevent Marshal Ney forcing the river. For the next fortnight the Brigade remained in the hills close by, living on wild honey and dough cakes made by pounding coarse corn between stones. The main body of the army, camped a day's march away in cork and oak forests fared little better; the countryside in the burning heat was destitute of every necessity, the men were famished and discouraged, and Wellesley wrote to his brother that the army would have to leave Spain if its present treatment continued. 'No troops,' he said, 'can serve to any good purpose unless they are regularly fed.'[39]

For the reception of the throng of wounded and sick a general hospital was opened at Truxillo and here some 2,000 drifted in, the remainder had either expired by the wayside or been captured by the French. Guthrie called this hospital 'the slaughter house of the wounded' and strongly criticised surgeons for performing too many amputations especially on the upper extremity. His outspoken remarks made him distinctly unpopular with his brother surgeons but although often inconsiderate in speech his growing reputation in surgery made his remarks worthy of attention. So opposed was he to allow the wounded of his division to be operated upon by anyone but himself that at Talavera he had refused to allow them to be admitted to the general hospital, and had established his own divisional hospital at Dallitosa on the road to Truxillo.

The Spanish army had already evacuated Talavera on the 6th August, and Cuesta the Spanish commander although bound in honour to do all that he could to save the British wounded falling into French hands had only provided Colonel MacKinnon the military superintendent of the hospital with seven bullock carts and a few mules, and if it had not been for some forty carts which came from British sources the numbers got away would have been small. As it was the carts were only enough to carry a tithe of the serious cases and nearly 1,500 had to be abandoned to the enemy. Two staff surgeons and four assistant surgeons were left with them, amongst whom the name of Staff Surgeon Summers Higgins is deserving of mention. The wounded British officers left under his care were so impressed with 'the unshakeable constancy with which he offered up Liberty and Expectations at the Shrine of Humanity and Public Duty' that these words were engraved upon a handsome silver cup which they presented to him; this is now a proud possession of the R.A.M.C. Headquarters Mess in London; and here also hangs a portrait of this handsome young surgeon by De Brie. Their chivalrous French captors treated the wounded prisoners with every consideration; the stores of food which the Spaniards had hidden they were now made to disgorge, and the wounded of both nations amply supplied. The French Marshal Mortier on visiting the wounded in hospital congratulated Higgins on their condition, and said he wished his own were as well attended.[40]

At this time the status of captured medical officers was not clearly defined, and Wellington later proposed that they should be immediately returned by either side without exchange. But the matter was never clearly settled, and Higgins and his brother officers were first sent back to Verdun and then released a year later.

By the middle of August the British army in the area south of the Tagus could endure starvation and exposure no longer. The drought and heat was so intense that the men's lips split and the skin peeled off their faces, while hunger, dysentery, and fever had reduced men and horses to the point of exhaustion. With the regimental surgeons treating so many of these cases their medical panniers were soon emptied, and authority was given to purchase locally those medicines absolutely required, the regimental paymasters advancing the money.

But Wellesley succeeded in averting the danger to his communications. Ney's corps had been recalled to the north to fight the Asturias and Galician patriots, and Soult's army was nearly as hungry as the British, so that he too was compelled to retire. With the Spanish armies now routed and dispersed there ceased to be any object in the British remaining. So the famished and discouraged soldiers were, to their great relief, led back to the fortress of Badajoz in the Guadiana valley, where supplies were available from depots at Elvas and Lisbon. But this area was highly malarious in the autumn months, and although Headquarters had been warned of its unhealthiness, no heed was paid. When the inevitable epidemic of malaria broke out the effect upon the soldiers weakened by their weeks of famine and exposure was disastrous, and on the 1st November there were 9,016 in hospital, an incidence of 28 per cent. The cause of the outbreak puzzled medical officers. Hitherto, malaria had always been thought to be associated with marsh miasma, a poison caused by the agency of the humid decay of vegetable matter or aqueous putrefaction; here the country was as dry as a bone, there were no weedy swamps but only dry river beds interspersed with pools of clear water; camping grounds had always been selected close to these rocky pools to provide drinking water, and now as Fergusson put it, these areas proved 'as pestiferous as the bed of a fen'.[41] The truth of course was that anopheles mosquitoes found the pools perfect areas for breeding. The fever which occurred was 'of such destructive malignity that the enemy and all Europe believed that the British host was extirpated'.[42] Aggravated cases were reported as resembling in severity the worst type of yellow fever met with in the West Indies, and no fewer than 500 men died. The general hospitals which had been opened at Elvas, Estremoz, and Villa Vicosa were overwhelmed with 5,843 patients, a number which included 1,500 of the Talavera wounded, while the regimental hospitals which had been reissued with their bedding and equipment were filled with over 3,000. For this immense task large local purchases of hospital bedding, clothing, and even medicines had to be made although Franck had already demanded from home large supplies of medicines and purveyors stores. For convenience of issue these were made up in blocks or divisions based on the quantities required for 500, 1,000, or 2,500 cases for one year. During the war there was in general no shortage experienced in the supply of these items and they were shipped out at regular intervals; it was only when the demand was excessive in such epidemics or when transport in Portugal failed to deliver supplies that local requisition had to be resorted to.

There was, however, another serious handicap to the effective treatment of the sick and this was an acute shortage of hospital mates, so that regiments had to be deprived of their already overworked assistant surgeons to help in the hospital wards. Every spare medical officer at Lisbon as well as new arrivals from England were hurried to the front. Wellesley, who after his victory at Talavera, had been elevated to the peerage as Viscount Wellington, had already asked at Franck's request for a reinforcement of 5 staff surgeons and 40 hospital mates.

In spite of his stern nature Wellington was acutely aware of the effect which an adequate and efficient medical service had on the morale of his troops. 'Indeed,' he writes, 'one of the reasons which induced me to cross the Tagus on the 4th August instead of attacking Soult was the want of surgeons with the army, all being employed with the hospitals, and there being scarcely one with each brigade, and if we had had an action we should not have been able to dress our wounded.'[43] 'Some effectual means should be taken to increase the medical staff. Not with gentlemen of rank but with hospital mates. The duty of the general hospitals in every active army ought to be done by the general medical staff and the regiments ought to have their surgeons and assistants entirely disengaged for any extraordinary event or sickness that may occur. We have not now one surgeon or assistant with each regiment instead of three, the others being employed at general hospitals instead of hospital mates, and we have always been equally deficient.'[44] Wellington asked in vain. Although the Medical Board had managed to send out twelve staff surgeons in August, the Walcheren crisis was now at its height and there was not a single medical officer to spare for Portugal.

By the middle of December there was a slight drop in the numbers of sick to 8,280 or 27 per cent, and there were many convalescents at Elvas where the accommodation was excellent and at Estremoz. Situated as they were on the main road to Lisbon, which was distant 100 miles from Elvas, it was possible to relieve the congestion by the use of the returning supply carts and mules. In Lisbon there were three main hospitals, the Estrella, the St. Francisca and the St. Jeronimo, with another in the suburb of Belem. These together had a total bed capacity of some thousands and in addition there were convalescent barracks both in Lisbon and Belem.

The numbers of sick led to considerable problems of discipline and several General Orders were issued from Badajoz on the subject. Hospital patients were forbidden to straggle about the towns and a roll call was ordered every hour, when all absent men were punished. Hospital stoppages which had been in abeyance in Spain were reintroduced, as medical comforts and extras were now freely available for the sick, and would have to be paid for.[45]

Wellington reiterated his request for thirty more hospital mates in December for 'The number of sick in the army,' he writes, 'is still very large, but the diseases of the soldiers have not lately been so violent as they have been or so fatal, and I hope the movement of the army will be beneficial to their health.'[46] This movement to the north took place the same month, and by Christmas Day the army was once again in the area of the Mondego river east of Coimbra. To foil any attempt by the French to invade Portugal by the southern route through Badajoz, the 2nd Division was left at Abrantes. As the army went into winter quarters the chief lesson of the campaign was brought out by Fortescue. 'The great military question in the Peninsula was that of feeding the troops, and final victory was practically assured to that army which should first vanquish the difficulties of transport and supply. Wellesley . . . perceived this truth after Talavera, and by recognizing it forthwith assured himself of ultimate success.'[47]

While Crauford and his Light Brigade kept watch along the Spanish frontier the remainder of the army spent the winter months in training and sporting activities. There was still a great deal of sickness and Wellington's hope that the move of the army to northern Portugal would shake off the ill health unfortunately proved vain.

Date	Strength	Sick in Regimental Hospitals	Sick in General Hospitals	Total	Percentage of sick
1810					
9th January	30,220	927	7,826	8,753	28·9
1st February	29,576	1,184	6,687	7,871	26·6
1st March	28,546	605	5,365	5,970	20·9
1st April	31,548	909	4,971	5,880	18·7

The regimental hospitals with their sixty beds apiece generally dealt with the minor sick but were also compelled to keep the worst cases who were unfit to stand a protracted journey, while the remainder were evacuated to one of the better equipped general hospitals which had now been established; at Coimbra in the north; at Santarem and Abrantes in the centre; and at Elvas, Estremoz and Villa Vicosa in the south; Oporto hospital too was in occasional use and Lisbon was of course the main base. Of these hospitals some like Santarem and Villa Vicosa were simply 'passing' or 'intermediate' hospitals whose chief function was to act as collecting centres for sick from the divisions. Under the static conditions which now prevailed orders were given to adopt the Standing Instructions for Hospitals which had been issued by the Medical Board on the 31st March 1800; these laid down the duties of the staff, the details of hospital routine and ward administration, and the payment of the subordinate staff.[48] At the same time the hospital stoppages were regulated by the Standing Orders of the 30th April 1800, so that advances hitherto sent with admissions were stopped and stoppages deducted in accounts kept by the purveyor and sent to the regimental paymaster monthly.

While the army spends its time preparing for the next campaign let us take the opportunity to turn to the part which the Medical Department played in the training of the Portuguese Medical Service. Early in 1809 a decision had been made to attach British officers to all the Portuguese units and General Beresford was placed in command with the rank of Field Marshal in the Portuguese Army. The Medical Board had also promised their assistance, and Deputy Inspector William Fergusson was appointed Inspector General of Hospitals, while on the 23rd May the Board had agreed to a dozen (later increased to twenty) medical officers being attached to Portuguese brigades as senior medical officers with the rank of staff surgeon.[49] Fergusson found the medical department hopelessly inefficient. The military hospitals were poorly administered, dirty and overcrowded, and Fergusson described them as the army's 'most destructive and dangerous nuisance'. Peculation was rampant in their provisioning and equipment, and every form of roguery, ignorance and prejudice existed. The sick suffered acutely from lack of bedding, poor food and want of medicines, and medical treatment was often antiquated; the use of calomel, antimony and strong purgatives was forbidden, and mercury had never been prescribed for syphilis. There were regimental surgeons it is true but they were forbidden to attend a medical case or compound a drug, and for the most part they lived remote from their regiments engaged in private practice to augment their miserable pay which was the same as that of army sergeants. Physicians, one of whom was on paper attached to each brigade, adopted a similar practice.

Fergusson's first task was to re-organize the existing hospitals and introduce regimental ones on the British pattern. From bitter experience of the failure of the general hospitals in Flanders he was a strong supporter of the regimental system, and he makes this abundantly clear in a letter to Beresford. 'The regimental hospital is the cardinal hinge on which the health of the army depends, the first resource of the sick soldier and best security for maintaining the health of the force. In actual war and during rapid movements of the troops, the sick must be left behind, and then general hospitals are necessary, but these ought not to be regarded as permanent, but only temporary expedients to meet the pressure of service, and in no respect essential under ordinary conditions to the proper care of the soldier. The plan of the general hospital should be precisely that of the regimental hospital on a more extensive scale. It is impossible that these can be well conducted unless by medical officers of good education who have acquired experience of medical practice and a knowledge of the soldier, his diseases, temper, and habits in regimental hospitals. Even under the circumstances mentioned, general hospitals will always prove a great though a necessary evil, destructive of the effective strength of armies. For diseases are with difficulty cured wherever a large body of such are aggregated together; new contagions are certainly generated, and discipline is imperfectly preserved because the dread of immediate punishment is removed. In all armies the sick should never under any circumstances be sent to the general hospital while their regiments are present on the spot.'[50]

This sweeping condemnation was based on the assumption that every general hospital was a hot bed of infection, but this was only true when overcrowding (which was at times inevitable) caused the spread of such contagious diseases as typhus and hospital gangrene. The answer to this question was not to condemn the general hospital system but by more generous planning in the provision of hospital beds to avoid the overcrowding. In fact as the war progressed and greater attention was paid to dispersion of sick and better ventilation, the general hospitals were transformed from necessary evils into acceptable institutions.

Fergusson's advice on hygiene was commonly ignored and in his experience this disregard of medical advice was not confined to the

Portuguese, for he criticizes equally the British army attitude when he cynically remarks, 'the convenience of the engineer, the whim of the Quartermaster General, or General Commanding, and the profit of the contractor, seemed ever to be consulted'.[51]

Over a period of three years the Inspector General diligently re-organized the department on British lines with the help of his A.M.D. staff surgeons. When war had broken out in 1809 there were not ten assistant surgeons in the army, and these had all deserted when they came to the Spanish frontier. Now, medical officers were adequately paid, and with their improved status their morale was enhanced. The whole department was re-equipped with stores, instruments and medicines sent from England and this was continued throughout the war. When Fergusson handed over his charge to rejoin the British forces, the Portuguese army could rely upon its medical department carrying out its task with an efficiency which did credit to its capable and energetic Inspector General.

It is time we took a look at the chief diseases which were characteristic of the Peninsula. Amongst the British forces the principal cause of sick wastage was fever, and this general term included four categories, simple continued fever, intermittent, remittent, and typhus. Both intermittent fever or malaria and typhus fever were distinct entities which were generally easy to diagnose, and well known from past experience. On the other hand simple continued fever and remittent fever embraced a multiplicity of diseases which were then indistinguishable; these included typhoid and para-typhoid fever, fever associated with dysentery, relapsing fever either tick or louse borne, and multiple malarial infections. The malaria season lasted from June to September and there were both benign tertian and malignant tertain types; from the former type relapses were frequent and recurred often for months. Typhus being louse borne occurred chiefly in the winter months when troops were crowded together for warmth. Dysentery and diarrhoea were other major causes of sick wastage which had a seasonal impact; it was in the late summer and early autumn months of August, September and October that these were at their height coinciding with the fly season, and due we now know to infection carried from excreta by flies to food and water. When dysentery attacked men already weakened from malaria or other types of fever the mortality rose alarmingly and treatment appeared to have little effect. During the winter months respiratory diseases appeared such as pneumonia and bronchitis, while rheumatism was common, due to exposure, wet, and lack of tentage, forcing troops to live in huts which were rarely weatherproof. Venereal disease which was largely syphilitic in origin was always prevalent with the ready facilities of civilian contact. Lastly, the skin affections and especially ulcers of the legs must be mentioned; these had been very common in past campaigns owing to rubbing by the gaiters, but even when these were discarded for trousers, ulcers continued to bring many men into hospital.

An insight into the work of the regimental hospitals is given in a return for May 1810, a comparatively healthy month. The total of 2,473 admissions gives a ratio of 82 per 1,000 per month and the prevailing diseases were intermittent fever or malaria, wounds and ulcers, simple continued fever and venereal disease in that order. Of typhus fever there were only seven cases. There were forty-two admissions as the result of 'punishment' and these were men with flayed backs after flogging.

Let us also take a look at the general hospitals. On the 1st April there were 4,257 patients occupying hospital beds: 1,563 at Lisbon, 615 at Coimbra, 1,881 at Elvas, Estremoz, and Villa Vicosa, 148 at Abrantes and 50 in other hospitals. It will be noticed that this figure is 714 less than the total of 4,971 given in the Appendix, and this is explained by the number of cases which were then in transit between the regimental and general hospitals, or as discharges from general hospitals on the way to rejoin their regiments.

From this short medical review we turn to Wellington's plans for the coming campaign. Reinforcements had been arriving from England during the winter, although the first contingent of 5,000 men sent to Portugal had to be diverted to Cadiz as we shall see in due course, and many of the new drafts had served in the Walcheren campaign and required a period of hardening before they were fit to take the field. However, when May 1810 came Wellington had a force of over 30,000 men, and although there were still more than 5,000 in hospital and the sick rate was just under 17 per cent this was not unduly high.

In reviewing future operations Wellington was in no doubt that he would be subjected to heavy and sustained attacks by Marshal Massena the new Commander whom Napoleon had nominated to conquer Portugal, and he had taken precautionary measures by constructing a very strong defensive position at Torres Vedras, 10 miles to the north of Lisbon.

The campaign of 1810 opened in the last week of May when Marshal Ney with an army of 30,000 men moved to attack the fortress of Cuidad Rodrigo. The fortress held out until the 10th July and his Spanish allies who had put up an effective resistance had gained for Wellington six valuable weeks; but this was followed by the unexpected and speedy fall of Almeida at the end of August. In the face of Ney's advance the British forces retired slowly, laying waste the land as they did so and removing the inhabitants, but at Busaco on the 27th September, Wellington and his 52,000 men made a stand on a steep ridge rising over 500 feet above the broken country around and some 9 miles in length. Massena launched his assault troops in massive columns, while Wellington, adopting his usual tactics, stationed his troops out of sight behind the crest of the ridge. The determined attacks of the French were hurled back each time they gained the crest by musketry volleys and cold steel, and by the end of the day Massena's force had suffered 4,600 casualties. The British and Portuguese casualties numbered 1,251, and here the 20,000 Portuguese troops in their first baptism of fire gained the confidence Wellington knew they so badly needed.

On the bare rocky ridge there was little shelter for the regimental hospitals strung out on a front of 9 miles, and only in the great convent at Busaco could reasonable accommodation be found. Here the chapel was soon filled with wounded undergoing treatment. But the road to it across the rocky ridge was so uneven that the jolting caused the wounded, who were being carried up in bullock carts, great suffering.[52] The general hospital at Coimbra was, however, only 8 miles away, and thither the wounded were transported for more extensive surgery.

Wellington's strategy, however, was not to be changed by the victory of Busaco, and the army continued to retire. Consequently Coimbra hospital had to be abandoned only three days after the battle, and many of the wounded were sent down the Mondego river by boat to Figueras where they were embarked in ships and carried to Lisbon. Others had to make the 100 mile journey to Lisbon in bullock carts and the sight of their pallid faces and piercing groans as the waggons bumped over the rough roads haunted Sergeant Donaldson for long after.[53] But now a more comfortable form of transport was making its appearance in the form of spring waggons of the Royal Waggon train. Three were supplied to each division and placed under the divisional staff surgeon for the transport of the worst cases. Temporary hospitals were opened in each divisional area as the army retired, and the Commissary General was made responsible that sufficient transport was provided to evacuate the cases daily to Lisbon.

In obedience to Wellington's orders the whole countryside was laid waste and civilians encouraged to accompany the army behind the defensive lines of Torres Vedras which were reached on the 10th October. When Massena saw what was before him he was astounded for he had no idea any serious obstacle lay in his path. Now he realized he had come upon an impregnable barrier. But although he could not go forward, he would not go back, and he kept his position in front of Torres Vedras for a month while his men starved and his draught animals died. 'I could lick those fellows any day,' remarked Wellington, 'but it would cost me 10,000 men and this is the last army England has got, we must take care of it.'[54] However, on the 15th November the

French began to withdraw, but only as far as Santarem, where to Wellington's amazement Massena managed to maintain his army for month after month.

The concentration of the army within the lines of Torres Vedras meant that the only hospitals were in the Lisbon area and the strain on the accommodation can be realized when in December there were 6,959 patients under treatment, with an additional 1,000 in the regimental hospitals. Between May and August the army had enjoyed the best of health and the sick rate on the 8th July was as low as 11·9 per cent with a total of 3,775 in hospital. This was in fact the lowest rate recorded throughout the whole war. In the succeeding months the incidence rose as it was apt to during the malaria and the fly breeding seasons, and varied between 15 and 19 per cent during the rest of the year.[55]

During the winter a great deal was done to tighten up control over the hospital administration. Without regular trained hospital attendants there was an understandable tendency on the part of medical officers to retain suitable convalescents in hospital to help in the wards, which meant exceeding the numbers of subordinate staff laid down. It was also tempting to employ such men as soldier servants. As long before as September 1809 a General Order had forbidden any medical officer to employ a N.C.O. or soldier on hospital duties except by permission of a board of officers presided over by Major General Peacocke, the Military Commandant at Lisbon and this was now rigorously enforced. The A.Q.M.G. was ordered to lay down the number of clerks, storekeepers, wardmasters and orderlies required in hospitals, while the employment of Portuguese as clerks and storekeepers was allowed. An order issued on the 23rd October 1810 commented on the fact that the number of men shown as sick in regimental returns was more than double those on the hospital books. At the large convalescent depot at Belem it was reported that many soldiers were walking round the town in perfect health although supposedly still on the sick list. Sick officers too were always a source of difficulty as they were never admitted to hospital but treated in billets where they were attended by their soldier servants and often lacked nursing care, and even regular medical control; consequently they were often kicking their heels on the so called sick list when they should have been back at duty. To stop this it had been laid down that all sick officers should appear before a medical board at regular intervals, and these boards were held three times a month at all hospitals.

Then the screw was put on medical officers, and the board instructed to 'advert to the necessity that the officers of the Medical Department should themselves attend the wards of the hospitals, and not have N.C.O's as wardmasters, at a period when the whole army are left at their posts day and night. The Commander of the Forces must insist upon the officers of the Medical Department being at all times in the wards of the hospitals.'[56] Even as a wartime measure this order if it was enforced must have been highly unpopular with the 'Medical Gentlemen', and was in fact unrealistic, for there was no medical mess or living accommodation in the hospital building as all officers had civilian billets. It was too exceeding the orders for hospitals which only stated that commissioned medical officers must visit the hospital twice daily, and only the orderly hospital mate had to remain on duty for a twenty-four hour period. The lash of discipline then fell on the hospital subordinate staff who were not on any account at any time to quit the square of the building in which the hospital stood. Convalescents at Belem were not there as the General Order states 'for their amusement, but that they may recover their health and return to duty. There appears therefore no occasion for them being in the streets and public houses at all hours of the day and night, but they ought to be made to lead a sober and regular life.'[57] Henceforth they were all to be confined to the depot yard and none to receive a ration of wine unless by a M.O's special authority.

The position of the medical staff officers especially the hospital mates was often unhappy and difficult. The majority of them seemed to be raw Scottish or Irish youths who from the time of their enlistment or appointment in England and while awaiting orders for service abroad had no headquarters which would afford them accommodation or any training in military procedure. They were left wandering about, acknowledged by none, unwanted by any, and without work or interest. When they arrived abroad they were ignorant of army customs, had neither a headquarters or experience of how to conduct themselves in a foreign country, were not allowed an army servant, and had to rely on civilians who might rob them at every turn. Fergusson quotes the case of a young mate who had all his clothes stolen by his Portuguese servant on the first night and was left naked in bed. Occasionally they cut ludicrous figures: a young dispenser of medicines or apothecary's mate appeared at Lisbon dressed in a brown ill-fitting surtout coat, blue trousers ending at the calf of the leg, pepper and salt coloured worsted stockings, and shoes, the whole surmounted by a cocked hat and straight black feather; in one hand he carried his sword, and in the other an umbrella.[58]

At last on the 3rd March 1811 Massena could maintain his famished troops no longer and orders for the retreat were given. When the British followed up, the dreadful consequences of their occupation became apparent; over the ravaged countryside dead soldiers, abandoned carriages, houses filled with sick and dying men, mutilated peasants, and violated women, were found everywhere. Wellington in his advance pressed Massena hard and there were many clashes between the opposing forces. In difficult country the pursuit went on for a month until the enemy had retired over the Spanish frontier to Salamanca, having lost 25,000 men from death, sickness and prisoners. Wellington too was at the end of his resources having advanced some 200 miles in twenty-eight days, and outmarched many of his supplies. Moreover the fortresses of Almeida and Cuidad Rodrigo, both in French hands, lay to the north and east, neither of which he could attack without a siege train which had not yet been disembarked.

Before the advance the Adjutant General had written to Dr. Franck, 'I am directed to inform you that in the advance of the army it will be necessary to provide for the establishment of general hospitals at different stations which will be fixed according to circumstances. They will be in the first instance on the Tagus. It is desirable therefore that you should immediately make arrangements for sending up the river bedding and other articles and medical attendants, in the first instance for a hospital of 300 men at Villa Nova, and nextly for 300 more at Santarem The men would be sent down from these establishments to Lisbon, and, in proportion as the army should advance, they would be broken up and others formed in more advanced situations. From what I have stated, you will see that your presence at Headquarters will now become essentially necessary.'[59] This shows the medical policy in a nutshell with the Inspector of Hospitals living as he always should at Army Headquarters.

In Wellington's rapid advance the absence of a mobile field medical unit was severely felt, for the general hospitals plodding along in bullock carts in the rear could not possibly keep pace with the troops, and collections of sick and wounded were dumped at Santarem, at Pombal and other towns until the hospitals arrived. But when Miranda de Corvo was reached on the 15th March the line of evacuation was switched to Coimbra where once again the familiar convents and colleges were taken over, and when the limit of the advance was reached another hospital was opened at Celorico, 60 miles to the north-east. Dr. Henry, who had arrived at Coimbra as a hospital mate, describes his experiences in this pleasant University town: 'the long corridors of the convent were occupied by a double row of beds containing the sick and wounded, classed into wards according to the nature of the case, with an M.O., ward master, and sufficient number of orderlies to each (1 for 8 or 10 patients), a common kitchen for the whole, a purveyor to provide supplies, and an apothecary to prepare medicines. Often I have stopped on entering to admire the picturesque perspective of the long corridors . . . now appropriated to the solace of pain, the preservation of life, and the best duties of humanity and benevolence.'[60]

Sick and wounded for admission to Coimbra were sent down in convoy from the army area at first once a week and later once a fortnight, and before long there were a thousand British and Portuguese patients in hospital and Henry who was keen on his profession expresses his satisfaction at having the opportunity to treat many bad surgical cases with not a few happy recoveries after terrible round shot injuries. Campaigning here, he thought, was a pleasant affair as he sat in his billet with a view of the city, the colleges, and the distant hills, drinking his ration wine over a dish of grapes and oranges, after a dinner cooked by his civilian servant of soup from the tough ration meat, fish from the river, and a roasted bullock's heart.[61]

In the south of Portugal General Beresford had been left with the 2nd and 4th Divisions guarding the area south of the Tagus. During March an unexpected disaster had occured. Soult captured the important frontier fortress of Badajoz, and Wellington now ordered Beresford to march to Portalegre and attack him. Accompanying the two divisions some 17,000 strong was the staff and equipment of two general hospitals, each calculated to hold 300 patients and one capable of expansion to 800. At the maximum this would only provide between 6 and 7 per cent of beds, but reliance was placed on the regimental hospitals treating all slight cases, and evacuating any overflow of patients to Lisbon via Abrantes. After an action at Campo Mayor the French retired, and Beresford invested Badajoz; but without a siege train the task was one of great difficulty and the siege was raised.

In the north, Massena had replaced his losses with amazing rapidity, and he felt his only chance of deflecting Napoleon's wrath against his previous failure was to attack and relieve the fortress of Almeida, which the British had invested, but which they could not attack without a siege train. The two armies faced each other on the 3rd May when the battle of Fuentes de Onoro was fought and where the French claimed the victory but did not capture Almeida.

The casualties amounted to 1,522 of whom 59 officers and 971 N.C.O's and men were wounded, and these were treated at a general hospital which had been opened at Villa Formosa 12 miles away. With over 1,000 wounded to dress and treat every house was requisitioned, but even then there was great overcrowding, and an outbreak of hospital gangrene was the inevitable result. Grattan has given a vivid description of the scene in the courtyard of a nobleman's house in the town: 'I looked through the grating and saw about two hundred wounded soldiers waiting to have their limbs amputated, while others were arriving every moment. It would be difficult to convey an idea of the frightful appearance of these men; they had been wounded on the 5th and this was the 7th; their limbs were swollen to an enormous size, and the smell from the gunshot wounds was dreadful. Some were sitting upright against a wall, under the shade of a number of chestnut trees and, as many of them were wounded in the head as well as in limbs, the ghastly countenances of these poor fellows presented a dismal sight. The streams of gore which had trickled down their checks was quite hardened with the sun, and gave their faces a glazed and copper-coloured hue; their eyes were sunk and fixed, they resembled more a group of bronze figures than anything human. There they sat, silent and statue-like, waiting for their turn to be carried to the amputating tables. A little further on, in an inner court, were the surgeons. They were stripped to their shirts and bloody; a number of doors, placed on barrels, served as temporary (operating) tables; to the right and left were arms and legs, flung here and there without distinction, and the ground was dyed with blood.

Dr. Bell (staff surgeon 3rd Division) was going to take off the thigh of a soldier of the 50th and he requested I would hold down the man for him. He was one of the best-hearted men I ever met with, but such is the force of habit, he seemed insensible to the scene that was passing around him, and with much composure was eating almonds out of his waistcoat pocket, which he offered to share with me. The operation was the most shocking sight I ever witnessed; it lasted half an hour, but the man's life was saved. Near the gate, an assistant surgeon was taking off the leg of an old German sergeant of the 60th. The doctor was evidently a young practitioner, and our staff surgeon took much trouble in instructing him. The narrator noticed that the first cut seemed to be far the most painful, after which the operation was borne with comparative indifference, or even boredom. When the arteries were being taken up, all the men said it felt like the application of a red-hot iron.'[62]

The delay which occurred before all the wounded were attended to after hard fought battles was inevitably the cause of much criticism. It was due to inherent faults in the medical organization. The absence of a recognized body of stretcher bearers, the want of a mobile field medical unit, the limited number of ambulance waggons, the slow evacuation over the bad roads, the lack of trained orderlies—all these factors combined to slow down the speed of attention to the wounded. And with 1,000 to be dressed and operated upon it was impossible to avoid delays before all were attended to. Sergeant Donaldson had a good deal to say on the matter. 'I have known wounded men often to be three days after an engagement before it came to their turn to be dressed, and it may safely be calculated that one half of these men were thus lost to the service. Those medical men we had were not ornaments of their profession. They were chiefly, I believe, composed of apothecaries' boys, who, having studied a session or two were thrust into the Army as a huge dissecting room, where they might mangle with impunity ... Without knowledge of anatomy they would cut down to extract a bullet and ten chances to one they severed an artery ... but this was no concern to these enterprising fellows, for clapping a piece of lint and bandage or a piece of adhesive plaster on the wound they would walk off very composedly to mangle some other poor wretch. The medical department of the French Army was much superior to ours at that time in every respect; this can only be accounted for by the superior opportunity they had of studying anatomy which in Britain is now almost prohibited—more the pity.'[63] This may be uninformed criticism, but the French 'ambulance volante', staffed by their own medical corps, was much superior to the British system; in their hospitals too they never had to rely on untrained orderlies from regiments, a policy which handicapped so disastrously the treatment in British units; Sergeant Cooper of the 7th Fusiliers says the hospital orderlies 'were brutes'.[64]

Meanwhile in the south Beresford in May 1811 had fought the bloody battle of Albuera. He could muster about 37,000 allied troops—only 10,000 of whom were British, while Soult had 23,000 men and was superior in cavalry and artillery. Abandoning Wellington's tactics Beresford had drawn up his men as if for a grand review in full view of the enemy.

Soult planned to sweep round the Allied right flank, cut their communications by capturing the bridge over the Guadiana and destroy them with his cavalry on the open plain. He was only defeated by the superb fighting qualities of the British soldier. In spite of suffering heavy losses from the French fire the battalions advanced steadily to within short range of the enemy and poured a murderous fire of musketry into the French infantry masses. The action is recorded in Napier's famous words—'Then was seen with what a strength and majesty the British soldier fights . . . their flashing eyes were bent on the dark columns in their front, their measured tread shook the ground, their dreadful volleys swept away the head of every formation.' At last the French could endure no longer 'and fifteen hundred unwounded men, the remnant of six thousand unconquerable British soldiers, stood triumphant on the fatal hill'.[65] The losses were terrible. Of the 6,500 British infantry engaged 4,159 or nearly two-thirds fell, and the total allied loss was 5,916 out of 35,284 engaged. Individual regiments suffered tremendous losses—the 57th Middlesex lost 428 officers and men, the 29th Foot 336, the three Fusilier regiments 1/7th, 2/7th, and the 23rd Royal Welch Fusiliers lost roughly 350 men apiece. The 1/5th Foot lost 4 officers and 212 men killed, 14 officers and 234 men wounded and 2 officers and 177 men made prisoner, a total of 648.

George Guthrie who had been promoted staff surgeon of the 4th Division was once again the medical hero of the occasion. Under fire all day, his assistant surgeon was killed at his side, and he gave shrewd advice to the regimental surgeons against opening their dressing stations too soon. Many of the wounded lay on the battlefield during the night amidst the piles of corpses with storms of rain sweeping over them, for there was hardly a man left to remove the wounded, and it seems the

Spanish troops would lend no assistance. The total transport available consisted of only four waggons, and after infinite pains 3,000 wounded were collected in the village of Valverde. Here Guthrie assisted by his regimental surgeons was kept operating eighteen hours a day for many days on end. This may have been due to his proverbial obstinacy in refusing to allow the wounded of his own division to be treated by anyone except himself, but this independent attitude inevitably led to delays in treatment which provoked the Adjutant General to accusing Guthrie of all people of neglecting the wounded. However, the officers he had treated protested so volubly that the A.G. had to withdraw his accusation.

Of the two general hospitals with Beresford's force one had been opened in excellent accommodation at Elvas 25 miles to the west and the other farther distant at Estremoz. Elvas was already busily occupied, for Wellington, who had arrived there while the wounded were coming in, wrote to Dr. Franck at Lisbon on the 20th May—'My dear Sir, you will have heard that Sir William Beresford fought a severe action on the 16th. The result is a great number of wounded in hospital, in addition to a considerable number already here. The gentleman here appears to be doing everything that is in his power, and has written to Lisbon for further assistance. I have written also to General Peacocke the Military Commandant and have desired that all possible assistance may be sent here, and 2,000 sets of bedding. It is impossible to calculate the number of wounded there will be, but I should think at least that number. You will know best whether from the state of the hospitals elsewhere it will be possible to send assistance from other quarters. P.S. I have desired Mr. Hogg to take care not to allow his hospital to become too crowded, and to evacuate upon Estremoz in time.'[66]

From this letter it appears certain that these preparations could have relieved the heavy burden which Guthrie and his surgeons had chosen to undertake at Valverde, but the work here rendered a service to surgical technique which proved of great benefit for it was after Albuera that he adopted the principle of ligaturing both ends of a divided artery. This was contrary to the teaching of John Hunter and of every practising surgeon, but it was nevertheless in course of time accepted as the correct procedure.[67] Guthrie said later that Hunter and Bell had such great reputations that their mistakes took him seven campaigns and thirty years of teaching to overcome.

During the summer of 1811 there were certain movements of the opposing forces but no major engagements except the sharp action of the Coa in September. Guthrie had collected some 300 wounded of all arms from the two days' fighting which he was uncertain how to deal with, as a further retreat was ordered; however, having cleared the last of the wounded by midnight, early the next day he came across a bewildered Dr. Franck, the Inspector of Hospitals, sitting on a pannier by the roadside and apparently keeping guard over some twenty or thirty more. Guthrie describes him as somewhat frightened and unhappy and asked him what he was doing in such unusual surroundings. 'I am,' he replied, 'here taking care of the medical stores of the army whilst the apothecary is watering the mules lest the muleteers should run away with them. I have seen a great many wounded passing. Are they yours?' Guthrie bowed and asked him if he had told them where to go. No, he had not interfered for he did not know where to go himself.[68] Having persuaded Franck to allow him to take what he wanted from the panniers Guthrie advised him to find his way to Sabugal with his stores.

Although this incident shows him in an unaccustomed role and under the circumstances rather ineffectual, Franck in Wellington's estimation was a capable Inspector, for when he was invalided to England on health grounds five weeks later the Commander of the Forces was concerned at his departure, 'and this concern is occasioned not less by my feelings for you personally than by my sense of the inconvenience and injury which the army and the public interests will suffer by the loss of your valuable services'.[69] When at a later date Franck had been criticized in certain newspaper reports and his ability questioned Wellington wrote on the 7th January 1812, 'You may be assured I shall be happy to avail myself of every opportunity of bearing testimony to the zeal, ability, and success with which the duties of the Medical Department of this army have been invariably carried on under your superintendence.'[70]

We have previously mentioned that 5,000 men of the reinforcements which Wellington had received early in 1810 had been diverted to Cadiz, a port some 60 miles west of Gibraltar. This was looked upon as a potential base for operations against the French in southern Spain. By June 1810 the British garrison under General Graham had been increased to 9,000 men, and together with Spanish troops was besieged by a French force under Marshal Victor. Wellington was not unduly concerned to leave the French to pursue their operations in this quarter for it relieved the pressure on his main forces further north. Graham, however, was an active and energetic commander who was determined not to remain cooped up in a fortress when he might assume a more military role. He therefore decided to attempt a sortie from Cadiz by constructing a bridge over the river Santa Petri, although the opposite bank of the river was in French hands. To assist this operation he planned to create a diversion in the rear of the French lines, and with the command of the sea in the hands of the British Navy a small force from the port of Tarifa was ordered to advance with this object in view. We give an account of this minor engagement because it involves the bravery in unusual circumstances of a medical officer.

The 28th Foot, 470 strong, moved out of Tarifa to threaten the towns of Vejer and Medina Sidonia and after a short campaign of less than a week achieved some success in drawing away some of the besiegers from Cadiz. But Graham's attempt to construct a bridge was never accomplished owing to bad weather, and with the main objective thus failing Graham had to order the 28th Foot to return to base to prevent annihilation. A frigate carrying this order arrived at Tarifa, and the naval officer in charge was strictly enjoined to give his dispatches to no other hands than Lieut Col Browne of the 28th, or in his absence to a commissioned officer who should be held responsible for their delivery to the Colonel. The only other officer of the Regiment left at Tarifa was sick, so Assistant Surgeon Johnson gallantly volunteered to act as the dispatch bearer. He immediately set forth. Owing to mistaken information, Johnson arrived at the gate of a convent only to find it held by the French and he was instantly fired on from within. Retiring on his horse at full gallop he took the wrong road and fell in with some Spanish guerrillas who from his blue coat mistook him for a French officer. One of them struck Johnson with a lance, broke his forearm, and unhorsed him. As he lay on the ground he was attacked and received several stab wounds, until pulling aside his great coat his attackers discovered to their surprise that his red tunic revealed him as a British officer. Luckily his life was spared, and his important message having been delivered, the 28th Foot retired in safety to Tarifa. For this gallant act he received from the Spanish King the decoration of Knight of the Order of Charles III, but as far as the British Government was concerned nothing was done to mark his self-sacrificing devotion to duty.[71]

On the 5th March 1811 the bloody and successful battle of Barrosa was fought. The operations were commanded by the Spanish General Lapena under whom Graham had generously agreed to serve. But Lapena proved timid and hesitating. The British troops comprised two brigades some 5,000 strong. The combined British and Spanish force set out from Tarifa as a base, captured Medina Sidonia, and encountered a superior force of two French divisions at the Hill of Barrosa. The British regiments showed a magnificent fighting spirit and in a confused battle the enemy by bayonet charges and hand-to-hand fighting were driven from the Hill, losing 2,000 men, 6 guns, and an Eagle. If Lapena had been resourceful or competent the enemy would have been completely destroyed, but he did nothing and was afterwards cashiered. The British loss was over 1,200 killed and wounded out of 5,200 engaged, and the casualties were treated under regimental arrangements and evacuated to a general hospital at Cadiz where Staff Surgeon Sir James Fellowes was in charge.

In November 1811 the French unsuccessfully attacked Tarifa, and by August 1812 the siege of Cadiz was raised and the French army withdrawn to face Wellington in the north. It is to his command that our narrative now returns.

In the early months of 1811 the admissions of sick had not been numerous and Wellington in February had pronounced the army very healthy except for the men in the Walcheren units who were still suffering from malaria relapses fifteen months after the original infection. In March the sick rate was only 13·2 per cent but from this month the rise in the incidence of disease followed almost the same pattern year by year. After the comparatively healthy spring months the period from June to October saw an increase in the incidence of malaria and with the heat and flies of summer, diarrhoea and dysentery predominated. With the late autumn and winter came the respiratory diseases such as pneumonia and catarrh, while rheumatism followed exposure to the cold and rain. This yearly sequence takes no account of the explosive outbreaks of typhus fever which usually but not always occurred in the winter, and followed spells of excessive hardship, exposure, hunger, lack of warm clothing, and contact with the dirt and squalor of civilian billets. From April 1811 onwards the sick rate steadily mounted; from 13 per cent to 20 per cent in May, and 24 to 26 per cent in June and September. Between[72] April and June the numbers in hospital doubled—from 6,160 in the former month to 12,392 in the latter. Much of this increase was due to the number of wounded of whom some 4,000 were then under treatment. The sick rates of the Portuguese Army were always lower by some 30 per cent, because the troops were partially immune to the endemic diseases especially malaria and the bowel infections which laid low the redcoats.

The month of October found the army in winter quarters dispersed over a wide area of central and northern Portugal. The main hospital centre in the north was at Celorico where all the surrounding villages were taken over to form a huge sick enclave; it was a wretched town without good accommodation and the buildings were crowded and insanitary. For the other divisional areas there were general hospitals at Abrantes, Castello Branco and Castanheira.

The sick rate for October was in fact unprecedently high at 32 per cent with over 17,000 men in hospital and Wellington became seriously alarmed. In a letter to the War Office he pointed out that the chief diseases were fever and bowel infections due he said to eating unripe fruit and excessive drinking. On the 16th October he wrote, 'I was twice last week at Celorico and I saw no bad cases, but the numbers are astonishing.'[73] Some figures will illustrate this point. At one time half the 4th Division was sick; in the 77th Foot there were only 287 men fit and 414 in hospital; the 40th Foot had 652 men sick out of 1,419, and the whole of the recruits recently arrived from England were in hospital. It was in fact the recent arrivals and especially the units from Walcheren who were struck down; the seasoned soldiers were 'salted' or in other words had acquired a degree of immunity. It is Colonel Hall who contradicts Wellington's statement that there were no bad cases, for he tells in his diary that before he arrived there were between 50 and 100 deaths daily, and at Celorico when he was there between 10 and 20 men died every day. He describes how the dead bodies were carried through the streets with scarcely the fragment of a tattered cloak or a few boughs to shroud their ghastly remains; 'death', he remarks 'was too common a guest to be treated ceremoniously'.[74]

Although the mortality rate is very suspicious of typhus there is no evidence to suggest that there was in fact an extensive outbreak of the disease at the time, and we account for it by the effects of active service conditions on the new arrivals from Walcheren who were already debilitated by chronic malaria and freshly attacked by the local form of dysentery. Be that as it may, Hall as an outside observer blames the death rate on the ignorance and inattentiveness of the hospital mates. He points out that the low pay and the unattractive prospects, added to the heavy demands of the service for doctors, had compelled the Medical Board to accept mates with a smattering of knowledge and education; moreover with pay always months in arrears they were tempted to augment the bare ration of tough beef, bread or biscuits and sour wine, by helping themselves to the medical comforts provided for the patients. Even the sick officers were deplorably situated, for the billets they occupied had been stripped of all furniture by their civilian owners and they were condemned to sleep on the bare floor.[75] October proved to be the peak of ill health for in November the number in the sick returns had fallen to just over 15,000, though Wellington said they were still so numerous that in his opinion the army was quite unable to take on any task of magnitude.

The Commander-in-Chief's secret intention was the capture of Cuidad Rodrigo, and to this end the siege train which had at length arrived at Oporto was brought up the river Douro and over the mountains to Almeida. Active preparations went on through the autumn and early winter; a new variety of bullock cart with iron axles was turned out in hundreds, and the mule train increased; equipment for the assault such as fascines and gabions were put in hand, and by the end of the year 1811 all was ready.

REFERENCES

[1] *Recollections of Rifleman Harris*, pp. 101–2. P. Davies Ltd., London (1929).

[2] Rates of pay in 1807 were: inspector of hospitals £2, deputy inspector £1 5s., physician £1, staff surgeon 15s., hospital mate 7s. 6d.

[3] *The Military Sketch Book by an Officer of the Line*, vol. II, p. 277.

[4] Henry. *Events of a Military Life*, p. 16. Pickering, London (1843).

[5] Henry. *Events of a Military Life*, p. 16. Pickering, London (1843).

[6] Eight inspectors of hospitals, 18 deputy inspectors of hospitals, 17 physicians, 60 staff surgeons, 26 surgeons of recruiting districts, 16 apothecaries, 8 purveyors, 14 deputy purveyors, 136 hospital assistants. The total pay roll of these officers came to £86,107 6s. od. a year.

[7] Cooper. *Seven Campaigns*. Smith Elder & Co. (1869).

[8] The chief items included in the panniers were lint, surgeon's tow, sponges, linen, both loose and in rollers, silk and wax for ligatures, pins, tape, thread, needles, adhesive plaster ready spread and in rolls, opium both solid and in tincture, submuriate of mercury, antimonials, sulphate of magnesia, volatile alkali, and oil of turpentine. There was in addition a capital case of surgical instruments including scalpels, saws, tourniquets, artery forceps, bullet forceps, tenaculum and catheters. Hennen advised great care of instruments by smearing with oil and keeping them in a waterproof bag. Medical comforts included tea, chocolate, portable soup, lemon juice and sometimes wine.

[9] Hennen. *Principles of Military Surgery*, p. 27. Constable, London (1820).

[10] Hennen. *Principles of Military Surgery*, pp. 1–2. Constable, London (1820).

[11] Donaldson. *Recollections of the Adventurous Life of a Soldier*. The author in later life became a surgeon. Edward West & Co., Edinburgh (1827).

[12] Gurwood. *The General Orders of the Duke of Wellington*, p. XII. John Murray, London (1851).

[13] Ross Lewin. *With the 32nd in the Peninsula*, p. 103. Simpkin Marshall, London (1904).

[14] Neale. *Letters from Portugal and Spain*, quoted by Kempthorne. Journal, *R.A.M.C.*, vol. LXI, pp. 230–231.

[15] Ross Lewin. *With the 32nd in the Peninsula*, p. 109. Simpkin Marshall, London (1904).

[16] Schaumann (1824). *On the road with Wellington*, p. 40. W. Heineman, London (1929).

[17] Fergusson. *Notes and Recollections of a Professional Life*, p. 104–105. Longman, Brown, Green & Longman, London (1846).

[18] Fortescue. *History of the British Army*, book XIII, chapter XXII, p. 296. Macmillan, London (1910).

[19] Harris. *Recollections of Rifleman Harris*, p. 71. P. Davies Ltd., London (1929).

[20] Neale. *The Campaign of 1808*, p. 190. Constable & Co., Edinburgh (1828).

[21] Neale. *The Campaign of 1808*, p. 190. Constable & Co., Edinburgh (1828).

[22] P.R.O., W.O. 1/641, p. 13.

[23] P.R.O., W.O. 1/641.

[24] P.R.O., W.O. 1/641, p. 199.

[25] P.R.O., W.O. 1/641, p. 185.

[26] P.R.O., W.O. 1/641, p. 199.

[27] P.R.O., W.O. 4/408—letter of 12th July 1809.

[28] P.R.O., W.O. 1/237.

[29] General Order, Coimbra 6th May 1809.

[30] If these totalled 100, a captain and a subaltern were detailed; if thirty, one subaltern; if under thirty, one sergeant, and for each thirty above that number, one sergeant and one corporal in addition to the officer.

[31] Reduced to 9d. a day by G.O. 7th June under War Office instructions.

[32] Hennen. *Principles of Military Surgery*, p. 61. Constable, London (1820).

[33] Schaumann. *On the Road with Wellington*, p. 9. W. Heineman, London (1929).

[34] General Order, Plasencia, 15th July 1809.

[35] Schaumann (1824). *On the Road with Wellington*, p. 165. W. Heineman, London (1929).

[36] General Order, 30th July 1809.

[37] Schaumann (1824). *On the Road with Wellington*, p. 193. W. Heineman, London (1929).

[38] Schaumann. *On the Road with Wellington*, p. 195. W. Heineman, London (1929).

[39] Bryant. *The years of Victory*, p. 338. Collins, London.

[40] Kempthorne. Journal, *R.A.M.C.*, vol. LIV, p. 138.

[41] Fergusson. *Notes and Recollections of a Professional Life*, p. 188. Longman, Brown, Green & Longman, London (1846).

[42] Fergusson. *Notes and Recollections of a Professional Life*, p. 188. Longman, Brown, Green & Longman, London (1846).

43 P.R.O., W.O. 1/242, p. 300
44 Kempthorne. Journal *R.A.M.C.*, vol. LIV, p. 139.
45 General Order 4th September 1809.
46 P.R.O., W.O. 4/409.
47 Fortescue. *History of the British Army*, book XIII, chapter XXI, p. 289. Macmillan, London (1910).
48 Soldiers acting as stewards were entitled to draw 1s. a day extra, wardmasters 6d. a day, and ward orderlies 3d. a day.
49 P.R.O., W.O. 1/641, p. 107.
50 Gore. *Our Services under the Crown*, p. 133. Balliere Tindall & Cox, London (1879).
51 Fergusson. *Notes and Recollections of a Professional Life*, p. 67. Longman, Brown, Green & Longman, London (1846).
52 Schaumann (1824). *On the Road with Wellington*, p. 250. W. Heineman, London (1929).
53 Donaldson. *Recollections of the Adventurous Life of a Soldier*. Quoted by Kempthorne. E. West & Co., Edinburgh (1827).
54 Fortescue. *History of the British Army*, vol. VII, chapter XXXIV, p. 547, Macmillan, London (1910).
55 Sick returns for 1810 are given in Appendix A.
56 General Order, Pero Negro, 23rd October 1810.
57 General Order, 23rd October 1810.
58 Fergusson. *The Military Sketch Book by an Officer of the Line*, vol. II, p. 277.
59 Kempthorne. Journal *R.A.M.C.*, vol. LIV, p. 142.
60 Henry. *Events of a Military Life*, p. 30. Pickering, London (1843).
61 Henry. *Events of a Military Life*, p. 30. Pickering, London (1843).
62 Gratton. *Adventures in the Connaught Rangers*, p. 143. Henry Colburn, London (1847).
63 Donaldson. *The Adventurous Life of a Soldier*, p. 258. E. West & Co., Edinburgh (1827).
64 Cooper. *Seven Campaigns*. Smith, Elder & Co., London (1869).
65 Napier. *The Story of the War in the Peninsula*, Book XII chapter VI, p. 170. Warne, London (1850).
66 Kempthorne. Journal *R.A.M.C.*, vol. LIV, p. 144.
67 Guthrie. *Surgery of the War*, p. 189–193. Renshaw, London (1855).
68 Kempthorne. Journal *R.A.M.C.*, vol. LIV, p. 145–146
69 Gurwood. *Wellington Dispatches*, p. 480.
70 Gurwood. *Wellington Dispatches*, p. 480.
71 An account is given by Blakeney in *A boy in the Peninsular War*, p. 161. John Murray, London (1899).
72 Sick returns for 1811 are given in Appendix B.
73 P.R.O., W.O. 1/251.
74 Colonel Hall. Journal of *R.U.S.I.*, no. 48.
75 P.R.O., W.O. 1/251.

Chapter 11

PENINSULAR WAR II (1812–1814)

Wellington moved early in January 1812, despite the fact that there were nearly 12,000 still in hospital and by the 7th of the month Cuidad Rodrigo was invested. The French were unprepared for an offensive in the depths of winter and their troops were widely dispersed. The fortress was stormed after a short siege, when despite heavy losses with the leading attackers blown to pieces and the breaches piled with corpses the assault columns pressed on and gained the ramparts at the cost of over 1,000 casualties. One of the gateways into Spain was conquered.

Details of the medical arrangements for the assault are scanty, but a General Order issued at Gallegos on the 8th January stated: 'Each Division will be attended by the medical staff belonging to it. A place will be fixed upon to which men who may be wounded are to be carried, and means will be provided for removing them from thence to cantonments.' In these assault operations the recognized position for the medical officer was at the foot of the breach, and many must have performed their first-aid duties at the risk of their lives exposed as they were to the holocaust of fire which swept the approaches. The majority of the wounded after receiving immediate operative treatment in the regimental or brigaded hospitals were sent away to the excellent accommodation which Coimbra could provide, although this was to expose them to a journey of over 100 miles, partly by road and partly by boat on the Mondego river; the remainder of the wounded were sent to Celorico and Castanheira. But Guthrie as usual got into hot water by defying the Adjutant General's order, and retained all his 4th Division casualties in his own regimental hospitals round Gallegos. Frostbite added to the sufferings of many of the wounded, for snow had fallen occasionally and the weather was bitterly cold.

On the 10th January 1812 Dr. James McGrigor landed at Lisbon to assume the duties of Inspector of Hospitals in relief of Deputy Inspector Bolton who had been acting since Dr. Franck's departure. Wellington had written to the Duke of York, now happily reinstated as Commander-in-Chief at the Horse Guards, requesting His Royal

338

Highness to send him an inspector in whose talents and judgement he could place entire confidence—or to quote his own words, 'should have the most active and intelligent person that can be found to fill his station'.[1] The Duke had no hesitation in sending him McGrigor. He was then 42 years of age and had been commissioned in the army by purchase as surgeon to the 88th Foot (Connaught Rangers) in 1793. He had served as a regimental surgeon for eleven years in Flanders and the West Indies, in India and Egypt. After a short time as surgeon to the Royal Horse Guards he came under the personal notice of the Duke of York, and was soon promoted over the head of several of his seniors to be Deputy Inspector of Hospitals, serving first in the Northern District at York and subsequently in the South Western District at Portsmouth. Here his outstanding administrative ability in dealing with the emergency occasioned by the sudden arrival of the 6,000 sick and wounded from Corunna had brought his name prominently to the notice of the Medical Board, and this was followed by an enhanced reputation when he unravelled the chaos of the hospitals in the Walcheren expedition. But his capabilities as an organiser did not detract from his reputation of being an experienced physician with a pronounced regard for the well being of his patients, and his inherent gift of sympathy was combined with a jealous attention to the welfare of his own officers.

He was now to undertake by far the most important post his career had so far offered, and it is not to decry the ability of Dr. Franck when we say that with McGrigor's appearance on the scene a new era began for the Medical Department in the Peninsula. With him came Staff Surgeon James Forbes as his personal assistant, a man whom he describes as one of the ablest officers he ever met.

During the three years the war had already lasted the Department at the Horse Guards now under Director General Weir had been gradually overcoming its troubles which were largely due to inexperience. Men like Guthrie and Fergusson were coming to the fore both as clinicians and administrators, and the staff surgeons of divisions were becoming increasingly efficient both in organizing the regimental arrangements and the transport of casualties, although their advice on matters of hygiene seldom obtained unqualified support. The hospital mates who were the weakest links in the medical chain were gradually learning their trade in a hard school, albeit this was at the expense of the sick or wounded soldier. What the Department now needed was the hand of an administrator who would be respected for his firmness and admired for his ability, and both were combined in the person of James McGrigor.

He lost no time in getting to grips with the problems, and his first task was to investigate the conditions at the base hospitals at Lisbon and at Coimbra, for at home he had already picked up rumours of irregularities and peculation in hospital stores. These complaints he found to be partially justified, for much of the accounting was in disorder, possibly due to slackness and lack of method than to wilful misconduct.

At Lisbon he thought many of the sick were only too ready to stay on in hospital with little incentive to return to their regiments once they were so far from the front. Franck's policy had been to allow all sick and wounded officers to be treated under the better conditions which Lisbon afforded, and McGrigor thought many were abusing this and enjoying the attractions of the capital and the company of their wives and ladies. The convalescents at the depot at Belem had come to be known as the Belem Rangers—a byword for shirkers who avoided being found fit for duty. The accumulation of so many sick immobilized a large number of medical officers who also much preferred the comforts of the capital to the hills of Cuidad Rodrigo. In July 1811 there were 70 medical staff officers on duty under a deputy inspector of hospitals; this included 7 physicians, 7 staff surgeons, and 43 hospital mates. By September the number had risen to 96, with 13 staff surgeons and 70 hospital mates, and this did not include a further 17 Portuguese and Spanish medical officers. When in November the demand for reinforcements came from the front many had been dispatched to the forward area, but when McGrigor arrived in January 1812 there were still 49 of a staff. As a result of his new proposals this was reduced in the following March to 41 British, with 10 foreign medical officers, and at about this number it remained.

At Coimbra the establishment was so extensive that McGrigor spent a week in inspecting both the British and Portuguese hospitals and administration and the care and comfort of the patients. But Celorico was highly unsatisfactory with a great deal of overcrowding in very poor accommodation.

After receiving a pressing order from Wellington, he reported to his headquarters at Frenada, and got a friendly welcome, renewing their acquaintanceship begun in Bombay in 1801. McGrigor's specific recommendations on the changes in medical policy which he now proposed were three in number. First, that only special cases of wounds and sickness should be sent to the rear, and such only as were approved by the Inspector himself. Second, that sick and wounded officers should be similarly treated. Third, that as in future no sick or wounded would be sent to Lisbon except those who would be ultimately invalided to England the great bulk of the medical officers should be ordered up to the front. Let us look at his first proposal more closely. The evacuations to general hospitals amounted to 90 per cent of admissions, and the compelling argument to eliminate or even reduce this as far as practicable was the hardship the sick and wounded had to endure in the long journey in bullock carts, a journey which often lasted from one to three weeks. Forced to live on unsuitable food and deprived of medical treatment many patients suffering from dysentery and fever either died or arrived in such a serious condition that recovery was out of the question. The corollary was that soldiers were absent from their units and corps for weeks and months before they rejoined. Moreover, most soldiers hated the general hospitals where they believed no one cared whether they lived or died, and much preferred to be treated in their own regiments amongst their comrades. The exceptions were the malingerers who eagerly grasped the chance because they could simulate illness with a greater measure of success amongst medical officers who did not know them. To reduce evacuations, the remedy lay in treating more cases in the forward area, and to do this the capacity of the regimental hospitals had to be utilized to their full complement of sixty beds, and supplemented wherever this was possible by a brigade hospital. To this end McGrigor devoted all his energies.

Some writers have hailed his proposals as something quite new but this is far from the truth as the regimental hospitals throughout the years 1810 and 1811 were always treating an average of 1,000 patients, and in November 1811 when the pressure upon all accommodation was so intense the figures had gone up to nearly 3,000.

Excellent though these proposals were in theory the original plan had soon to be modified. While the army was in winter quarters no sick or wounded were evacuated to the general hospitals without permission of the divisional or brigade senior medical officers, and this applied to sick officers also. But while Wellington heartily approved of this plan, for it effectively limited the drain on manpower, as soon as McGrigor proposed that transport should be provided to carry all the hospital equipment when the regiment moved it was immediately rejected on the grounds that this extra transport would impede the movement of the troops. This was a disappointing blow to McGrigor's hopes, but there for the moment he was compelled to leave the matter.

Wellington was in the habit of seeing the heads of his administrative services daily but when McGrigor arrived on the first morning he was stopped by the Adjutant General who told him he would receive his report himself and it was unnecessary to trouble his lordship. McGrigor replied bluntly that he was instructed to see his Commander personally and at that moment Wellington summoned him within. From his daily contacts with his Commander there soon grew a warm personal relationship, and McGrigor became the confident of Wellington's future operations. This information gave him the inestimable benefit of planning effective medical arrangements in advance, and so avoiding the hindrances and delays that the withholding of intelligence so frequently imposed upon the medical branch. When it is remembered that some 20 per cent of the strength was generally absent through sickness and wounds the drain on manpower was a constant cause for anxiety, and Wellington fully appreciated how much the success of his operations depended upon the administrative services. Would that all commanders were so medically conscious. How difficult it has often proved for the head of the medical department to break through the closed ring of the General Staff.

With Cuidad Rodrigo in his hands, Wellington, without waste of time turned south and by March 1812 had invested Badajoz. The capture of this fortress proved a sterner task, for it was defended by 5,000 veteran French troops and Wellington was hindered in his operations by a lack of engineer units due to a parsimonious Treasury refusing to provide the necessary funds. Badajoz suffered the same fate as Cuidad Rodrigo being taken by storm after a brief siege at heavy cost to both sides. Five thousand British fell, over 3,500 of them in the actual assault. Six generals were wounded. Some regiments suffered terribly; the 43rd and 52nd Foot of the Light Division lost 347 and 323 men respectively, while the 4th Foot lost nearly half its strength.

In expectation of casualties, McGrigor before the operation had arranged for a third general hospital to be opened at Alter de Chao in addition to those at Elvas and Estremos. At Elvas too depots of medical and purveyors stores were established. Other preparations included setting up a small field hospital to provide immediate aid for the headquarter staff at Badajoz, and allotting two spring waggons to each unit to speed up the evacuation of cases to Elvas. Although heavy and cumbersome and only capable of carrying four lying cases they were a great improvement on the primitive bullock carts.

During the assault McGrigor had been in close attendance on Wellington, 'Being with his Lordship the whole time the business went on I saw everything and heard everything . . . when the account came that our people had been repulsed from the two breaches, it was an awful moment . . . During the time the thing lasted, about five hours, Lord Wellington was extremely anxious to know the number of men that came wounded to the different posts, and I went from one to the other and occasionally informed him. When the thing was over and I told him what I believed the actual number he really cried. . . .'[2]

For the attack of the 4th and Light Divisions a dressing station was established in a quarry which proved to be well within musket range, and the medical officers' efforts were not rendered easier by the fact that the wounded understandably showed a marked reluctance to remain under fire while their wounds were being dressed. The severely wounded could not be reached until the assault was over, when they were collected at the convent of San Andre in the town, but the fatigue parties detailed to bring their unlucky comrades to shelter and treatment had no scruples in disappearing to search for loot after making but a single journey.

Both when under fire during the assault and afterwards in the care and attention which they gave to the 4,000 wounded, the surgeons performed sterling work and McGrigor was determined in his own mind that their efforts should not pass unnoticed. 'Nothing,' he said to Wellington, 'could more gratify these officers, nothing could be a greater incentive to their exertions on future occasions, than his noticing them in his public despatches.' 'Is that usual?' the Commander asked. McGrigor replied, 'It would be of the most essential service; really their extraordinary exertions gave them in justice a claim to this.' Wellington rejoined, 'I have finished my despatch, but very well, I will add something about the doctors.'[3]

Camp at Badajoz. April 8th 1812.[4]
'My Lord

It gives me great pleasure to inform your lordship that our numerous wounded officers and soldiers are doing well. I have great reason to be satisfied with the attention paid to these by Mr. McGrigor the Inspector General of Hospitals and the Medical Gentlemen under his direction, and I trust that the loss to the Service upon this occasion will not eventually be great.

> I have the honour to be
> My Lord
> Your lordship's obedient servant
> Wellington.

The Earl of Liverpool'

Although in accordance with Wellington's nature this despatch was not particularly effusive in its terms, it is of historical interest as it was the first occasion the Medical Department had ever been mentioned in despatches. Needless to say it gave great satisfaction and encouragement to the medical officers throughout the army and this was reflected in public opinion at home.

With so much surgical work on hand it is an appropriate time to consider the rough and ready surgery which conditions in the field allowed. The requirements were simple—a house or barn, sometimes a tent, straw for bedding, water, an improvised operating table made from a door or wooden planks; these together with instruments, splints, lint, bandages, opium and brandy constituted the essentials for the immediate and life saving operations undertaken at the regimental hospitals. It is no part of this history to describe the details of treatment of the different types of wounds and these can be studied in the works on the surgery of the Peninsular War by Guthrie and Hennen, but certain general principles must be mentioned. Although most soldiers believed that surgeons lopped off limbs in cart loads to save themselves trouble, this accusation was unjustified except perhaps in the early period when undoubtedly there was a tendency to sacrifice limbs too freely. The basic choice of performing either primary or secondary amputation had long been settled in favour of the former, and this was impressed upon all surgeons by Mr. Gunning, who was the senior surgeon of the medical staff; it was also the accepted practice of the most famous of all contemporary French military surgeons Baron Larrey. Amputation in suitable cases was therefore performed with as little delay as possible, the only exception being to postpone operation for a few hours in cases of severe primary shock; but as experience was gained, definite rules were formulated to amputate only when certain criteria existed: (a) where there were extensive injuries to joints; (b) in compound fractures close to joints; (c) in extensive loss of soft tissue with loss of circulation to the part; and (d) when there were fractured or dislocated bones with great injury to ligaments and vessels. Experienced surgeons such as Guthrie and Hennen were noted for their dexterity and speed, for both were paramount to reduce pain and shock, and Guthrie could amputate a limb in a matter of minutes. But the toughness displayed by some soldiers was astonishing as Corporal Wheeler records:

'This man had been severely wounded in one of the Batterys by a shell. It was necessary to amputate an arm and both legs. Dr. Webster commenced the operation with a leg, this done the arm followed. It was thought proper that the man should rest awhile before the other limb should be cut off, but the man insisted that the doctor should proceed, observing, "It's no use to make two bites at a cherry, what use in making so much fuss about a leg that will be of no service to me or anyone else again."[5] It was soon off and he dropped into a deep sleep. Early the next morning the doctor visited him and found him leaning on the only elbow he had left, smoking a short black pipe, and was apparently as comfortable as if the amputations had taken place a month before.'

The sacrification or dilatation of wounds which originated in the idea that they were poisoned had been abandoned for some time although among foreign surgeons and particularly the French it was still practised. British surgeons following Hunter's teaching used the knife chiefly for extracting balls or splinters of bone and other foreign bodies, or for ligaturing blood vessels.

Turning to the treatment adopted for other injuries we find that in penetrating wounds of the chest and abdomen both entry and exit wounds were dressed and 16 to 24 ounces of blood taken from the arm; if the intestines were cut and protruding they were stitched to the edge of the wound; if the gut was sound it was replaced, and the wound closed with ligatures and strapping. Dressings were of the simplest, lint soaked in cold water was used and adhesive plaster applied; clean open wounds were strapped up or stitched and bandaged. As nearly all wounds suppurated, healing was a long process, while hospital gangrene and tetantus were complications about which we will have something to say later. For fractures, whalebone splints were in common use, and fractures of the legs were often treated with the patient lying on the side to relax as far as possible the pull of the muscles. When Guthrie later became the chief surgeon at Lisbon he claims he was the first to employ a long straight splint for fractured femurs with the patient lying on his back. For below knee fractures there were alternative methods with the knee either bent or straight and the patient lying either on his side or back. Hennen writes, 'though I recommend the splints, I have seen numerous cases where they have been omitted and the patient has done perfectly well, the parts being merely covered with compresses moistened with cold water'.[6] With such masterly inactivity it would be hard to expect nature to do more.

After a major engagement such as Badajoz the greater burden of surgery was borne of course by the general hospitals. John Hennen who was both chief surgeon and principal medical officer at Elvas had 2,500 wounded under his care and could proudly boast that not a single case of hospital gangrene or typhus occurred due to the care taken to preserve cleanliness and ventilation. The number of deaths and severely wounded in the general hospitals are given below.

	Badajoz	Elvas	Estremoz	Alter de Chao	Santarem	Total
Deaths	72	126	40	2	—	240
Dangerous Wounds	34	30	98	12	20	194

If the figure of 4,000[7] is taken as the total number of wounded the death rate comes to 6 per cent and the dangerously wounded to 5 per cent. This however is not the complete figure, as the deaths in regimental hospitals are not included.

Before we leave the account of the military operations at Badajoz let us quote again some of the experiences of Dr. Henry. Posted as assistant surgeon to the 66th Regiment, he covered the 500 miles from Coimbra to Badajoz on horseback, joining his unit in April. No sooner had he arrived than he was dispatched with a convoy of 140 sick to the general hospital at Alter de Chao, amidst the roar of artillery from the siege. Scores of his patients were so ill with fever that they had to be tied on the mules' backs, with a guard to prevent them falling off; but strangely enough by the second day they felt so much better they were able to ride by themselves. 'I am convinced,' Henry asserts, 'that the lives of several were saved by this march, and the recovery of all was materially accelerated.'[8] Here is a sniff of something we have heard of before—Robert Jackson's 'gestation in fresh air.'

Such heroic treatment was either kill or cure, but heroic treatment was the order of the day, as witness Henry's own experience when he got malaria. When the headache became severe he had his hair shaved off and three to four dozen leeches attached to his scalp; a few hours later he was carried into the yard, made to stand erect, and twenty-five buckets of cold water were poured over him from a third storey window to drive away all the blood left in his head; wondering whether his head was still on his shoulders he had a violent reaction in the night and became delirious in the morning. Henry does not tell us if he took bark to supplement his cold water cure, but when in the following spring he had the usual relapses he tried gestation again and took to horseback every second day just when the paroxysm was about to begin. After three days it went, never to return.[9] Highly unorthodox we must admit but clearly effective.

Leeches are not commonly associated so much with Spain as with more tropical climes, but Henry gives an account of an unusual incident which happened to the men of his regiment when after a long march on a hot and dusty day the thirsty soldiers had drunk avidly from a fountain, and as he puts it 'quaffed away like fishes'.[10] Down went some 3–400 leeches which attached themselves to the mouth, throats, gullets, and even the stomachs of the eager drinkers. 'We certainly had a bloody day at the hospital although no lives were lost except the leeches, and they were attacked in all manner of ways, both by stratagem and open force. Some were noosed by the tail with a silk ligature and torn off leaving the head sticking; several were dislodged by a strong solution of salt, and tobacco was used to others. Powerful emetics were necessary to oust the knowing ones that had reached the citadel of the stomach . . . At last the enemy were finally beaten from all their positions with great slaughter, and the doctors of the brigade washed their hands and went home to dinner.'[11]

Before we resume the account of Wellington's operations after Badajoz let us summarise the medical situation. While the southern group of hospitals were principally concerned with the wounded, by the month of May 1812 there were over 14,000 sick or nearly 30 per cent of the strength absent from their units. The spring relapses of malaria, the 'continued' fevers, the pneumonias, catarrhs and cynanche[12] comprised the majority of cases. There were eleven general hospitals now established for British troops, the largest at Lisbon and Coimbra, with the latter in communication with Lisbon through Figueras, the port at the mouth of the Mondego river where sick were embarked. In the north there were general hospitals at Celorico and at Vizeu, in the central area at Abrantes, which was a hub of communications, and at Castello Branco, with a 'passing' hospital at Santarem; and in the south at Badajoz, Elvas, Estremoz and Alter de Chao. McGrigor's passionate desire to increase the scope of the regimental hospitals was meanwhile frustrated because of the Commander's refusal to provide the necessary transport to carry the equipment, but some commanding officers did at times accept the risk of incurring official censure by appropriating waggons for the purpose.

Wellington's original idea after the fall of Badajoz had been to advance into Andalusia and drive out Soult, but he had to abandon this plan because of a new advance by Marmont in the north. The general hospital at Castello Branco had to be closed and Celorico itself was threatened. Wellington countered this threat by moving his divisions to the north of the Tagus, and pushing northwards he compelled Marmont to retreat.

Now that he had regained the initiative the Commander-in-Chief was free to choose his line of advance and in June moved up to Salamanca with 43,000 men. For several weeks the two armies manoeuvred, often in full view of each other, until Marmont was convinced that Wellington had lost his power of offensive. Throwing discretion to the winds, on the 22nd July he attempted to move his army across the Allied front with the object of turning their right flank and cutting off their communications. In a moment Wellington seized his opportunity and with his forces concentrated launched them against the French divisions strung out across his front. In the ensuing battle of Salamanaca the French suffered a severe defeat losing over 14,000 men including 7,000 prisoners. But the day was only won at the cost of 5,200 Allied casualties of whom 252 officers and 4,078 were wounded

McGrigor's arduous task was concentrated on providing accommodation for such a large number of wounded in the colleges and convents in the city of Salamanca some 10 miles distant. Thither the wounded both British and French were by degrees conveyed and treated, the most severe cases being sent down in due course to Cuidad Rodrigo. Wellington wrote from Flores de Avila on the 25th July assuring McGrigor that he was very sensible of the diligence and attention of the Medical Department, 'of which I have reported my sense to the Secretary of State'.[13]

Guthrie was the senior surgeon at Salamanca and is given the credit of carrying out the first operative treatment on a case of phlegmonous erysipelas which was cured by making multiple incisions in the swelling. Besides the many Allied wounded under his care he discovered some 300 sick and wounded French prisoners in the Convent of San Carlos who were being horribly neglected by the Spanish until by browbeating and threats he forced them to a more humane line of conduct. The good relations which always existed between the British and

French in the compassionate handling of their wounded prisoners is illustrated in the following incident. Under Guthrie's care was a severely wounded French officer who in due course recovered sufficiently to be exchanged as a prisoner-of-war, but this occurred when Guthrie was away and he had soon forgotten the case. In the following year Guthrie on one occasion was suddenly surrounded and taken prisoner by a body of French cavalry in command of whom he recognized in the nick of time his former patient. Needless to say he was immediately freed and received the French officer's grateful acknowledgement for his previous care and attention.

On the 30th July 1812 Valladolid was taken and 800 sick in hospital captured; this was followed by the triumphal entry into Madrid on the 12th August amid scenes of wild enthusiasm, and the capture of much booty.

After having satisfied himself that all was going well in Salamanca, McGrigor took the road to Madrid and found his attention immediately drawn to the considerable numbers of sick and stragglers who had been left behind in the army's wake, many incapacitated by dissipation and drunkenness. In addition there were groups of both officers and men wounded at Salamanca who had insisted on accompanying their units on the march and had given up when their strength had failed. Without medicine or medical treatment and destitute of provisions, their situation was deplorable, and many were 'fast sinking in the last stage of disease and not a few officers as well as men had died without having been seen by a medical man. I everywhere went round and visited them, but was powerless to help them.'[14] Determined to prevent further unnecessary suffering and 'obeying the dictates of humanity' he immediately ordered medical and purveying officers to be sent from Salamanca, and wrote to the Commissary asking for provisions to be dispatched under commissariat control. This, on the face of it was a very reasonable and natural act but it brought him nothing but a severe censure. When he reported what he had done to Wellington he was greeted by a violent outburst of rage. At the time his lordship was sitting for his portrait by a Spanish painter,[15] and the temper he displayed made the artist look aghast. 'I shall be glad to know,' exclaimed Wellington angrily, 'who is to command the army, I or you? I establish one route, one line of communication for the army; you establish another, and order the commissariat and the supplies by that line. As long as you live, sir, never do so again; never do anything without my orders.'[16]

While the British army occupied Madrid, Clausel the new French commander had re-entered Valladolid, but when Wellington advanced from the capital in September 1812 the French fell back to Burgos. There, after a triumphant march of 160 miles through a cheering and excited countryside but in a blistering heat of 90° the Allied forces invested the town on the 19th of the month. Along the route of advance hospitals were established in succession at Medina, Valladolid and Segovia, while from Madrid, where a force under General Hill had been left to watch the army of Soult, the long line of evacuation to Portugal went by way of Toledo, Talavera and Truxillo, where passing or intermediate hospitals were opened, the last named in the magnificent palace of the Count of Medina Sidonia.

The siege of Burgos did not go well, for Wellington was still short of engineers, and failed to order up enough heavy artillery. After a month's effort and the loss of 2,000 men in five minor assaults, the siege was abandoned. As the hospital accommodation in the vicinity of Burgos was woefully inadequate McGrigor had sent the sick and wounded back by every returning commissariat waggon and mule the 80 miles to Valladolid where the general hospital which had been opened was only established in spite of determined opposition from the Spanish bishop.

Throughout the late summer months the sick rate had as usual been gradually rising. From a percentage of 29·9 in May it had fallen to 25 per cent in June and 24 per cent in July, but with the inevitable outbreaks of dysentery, diarrhoea, and malaria in the heat and the rain, it had increased sharply to 34·7 in August and to 35 per cent in September with 18,000 shown on the sick returns, and over 16,000 of this number in general hospitals. It is a noteworthy fact that for the three months period between the 25th June and the 24th September there were no fewer than 55,346 admissions to hospital, a total greater than the whole strength of the British force. Strange as it may seem the army was marching and fighting a great deal of this time. Obviously the great majority of the sick were slight cases who were quickly cured and returned to duty. Of all the hospitals Salamanca was the busiest, for during the same three months there were over 13,500 admissions, which of course includes the Salamanca casualties and accounts for the deaths reaching a total of 1,024 or 7.5 per cent.

The failure to take Burgos was now to prove disastrous, for the enemy was soon threatening Wellington from two sides; reinforcements had swelled the troops facing him to a number half again as strong as his own, and Soult and King Joseph with 60,000 men were approaching Madrid from the south. To escape the danger of being crushed between these two powerful forces an Allied retreat was imperative, so Wellington once again turned his back on the enemy and the troops, disgruntled and bewildered, for they had suffered no defeat, took the road which they had advanced along with such high hopes a month before. Within five days the army was back at Valladolid, notwithstanding some anxious moments due to the skill and daring of the French advance in capturing some river bridges before they were blown.

Strong justification for McGrigor's energetic policy of evacuation was endorsed when Wellington told him confidentially that the army was about to retreat from Burgos and that he was deeply concerned at abandoning the sick and wounded. His Inspector was able to reassure him that all casualties fit to be moved had already been sent away and only a small number of wounded would be left behind with two medical officers and a purveyor to attend them. Relieved by this assurance Wellington could not refrain from praising his forethought and initiative.

From Valladolid to Salamanca the retreat went on and the 2,000 sick and wounded which had filled the hospitals at Valladolid had to be brought back by every available waggon and mule, or sent back on their own feet to Salamanca. When the Commander was told that not more than 100 under the care of three medical officers would have to be left behind Wellington replied, 'And you have made Salmanca choke full. I cannot stop there.'[17] Salamanca it is true had 4,000 cases in hospital but when reassured that orders had already been issued to the medical superintendent there and at Cuidad Rodrigo to clear their cases back to Celorico, Coimbra and Oporto, Wellington exclaimed, 'This is excellent, now I care not how soon we are off.'[18] Still nettled by his previous rebuff at Madrid, McGrigor could not resist reminding Wellington how much he had been blamed before for taking steps to help the sick on his own responsibility, but Wellington's only rejoinder was, 'It is all right, as it has turned out, but I recommend you still to have my orders for what you do.'[19]

Events in the south had also gone ill, for Hill's force at Madrid was unable to bar the Tagus to Soult's superior strength and the British had fallen back northwards through the Guadarrama pass to join forces with Wellington on the 8th November near Salamanca. Guthrie who had now been promoted acting deputy inspector of hospitals[20] was in charge at Madrid with 287[21] sick and wounded on his hands under Spanish doctors and orderlies. When the order for evacuation came he had already dispatched the chronic cases to Salamanca. With only fifty mule carts earmarked at twelve hours notice for medical use and hardly a single spring waggon, he tackled the crisis with his usual energy and determination and managed to get all his cases away. Furthermore, by coercing his medical officers and adopting every possible means of conveyance he carried along with him a further 2,000[22] sick accumulated on the line of march. On arrival at Salamanca half of these were returned fit to their regiments, and the remainder sent on to Cuidad Rodrigo in convoy instead of being allowed to wander about and plunder the countryside. Out of the 4,000 at Salamanca only 60 cases unfit to be moved were left in French hands, with 3 medical officers and a purveyor's clerk provided with money to look after them, and with a letter to the French Commander recommending them to his care.

On the 15th November at Salamanca the order to resume the retreat was given and the day it began the equinoctial gales set in and the rain fell in torrents turning the primitive Castilian roads into muddy rivers. Still perplexed at retiring in the face of the enemy without a fight, the soldiers became angered and embittered. Bivouacking in the open, soaked through by the rain for no greatcoat could keep it out, foot sore, and weighed down with 60 pounds of kit, the men trudged on, while dysentery and malaria thinned their ranks. The climax came when for four days the rations went astray and the men fed on acorns and the carrion from dead bullocks. From sheer exhaustion 3,000 men fell out on the march and were gathered up by the French.

Wellington was furious with the Commissariat Department for their inept handling of the ration problem and contrasted them with the Medical Department, which he said, 'is the only one which will obey orders; on them I can rely for doing their duty'.[23] And it was not only by words that he showed the regard he felt for his principal medical officer, for when McGrigor had received a kick on the knee from a horse which caused such pain that he was unable to ride, Wellington, hearing of the accident, sent his own carriage to convey him, the only one in the army.

Marshal Soult fortunately hesitated to press his advance so that Wellington was able to continue his withdrawal westwards. It was not until he reached the fortress and base at Cuidad Rodrigo that he called a halt, and when the infantry struggled into the town they had been over thirty days on the march, and had lost in killed, wounded and prisoners some 9,000 men. Very quickly it became apparent that the perils of the retreat had had a disastrous effect upon the men's health for by the 29th November 1812 there were 19,540 men shown on the sick returns or 36 per cent of the strength.[24] The incessant moves to prevent the sick and wounded falling into enemy hands had made it impossible to provide them with proper food and treatment while on the road, and this had proved disastrous to those who were already seriously ill. Many of the cases of dysentery reached hospital in an advanced stage of the disease only to die. Fever cases too took on what is described as the 'typhoid state' which often terminated fatally from an attack of enteritis. The strain on the hospital accommodation became overwhelming and every spare medical officer from general hospitals in the rear was hurried to the front; Spanish medical officers were engaged, and captured French doctors who were offered and accepted pay at British rates were employed at the base hospitals in relief of those who were sent up country. There were in fact on the establishment 343 medical staff officers, but leaving out those who were sick, on leave in England, and accompanying the transports carrying invalids home, it appears the effective number for duty was only about half that number, and this was barely sufficient to staff the twelve general hospitals now in being.[25] In the last two years some 80 medical staff reinforcements had been sent from England, 70 of them mates: the latter were always preferred, for the more senior posts on the medical staff could always be filled by local promotion of the more capable and experienced regimental surgeons.

With so much pressure upon the general hospital beds the policy of increasing the scope of the regimental hospitals to the maximum became of vital importance, and by a General Order of the 29th November McGrigor was given a free hand to effect this and to control the transfer of cases to general hospitals. As the officers of the Medical Department had no executive power, such control had previously been in the hands of the Adjutant General, but McGrigor's ability and clear thinking had so impressed Wellington that he was now allowed a degree of freedom to direct his own Department which so far had never been permitted. And this continued throughout the war.

Under McGrigor's drive and exertions the regimental hospitals were soon adequately housed and more generously equipped so that within a few months the patients increased from 2,000 to 5,000, and the evacuations to general hospitals became a mere trickle. But the dread that typhus fever might attack men who were famished, exhausted, and crowded together in billets for warmth was soon realized. It was the 1st Guards Brigade who suffered most. Their regimental hospitals managed upon their own system had always been considered superior to those of the rest of the army but here it was a question of numbers, and a general hospital had to be opened for them at Vizeu. The 1st Guards who marched into the town 2,000 strong suffered terribly from typhus of the most malignant type with all the classical symptoms of fever, petechiae of the skin, depression, delirium and gangrene. But there was another type of case which though equally deadly had jaundice as its prominent feature, and when this was associated with many recurrences of temperature the combination of symptoms were highly suspicious of relapsing fever. For both types remedies were tried without avail; Peruvian bark was often combined with camphor, or with aromatics or opium, leeches, blisters, sinapisms, and cathartics were all administered. But the mortality was not stayed, and finally in an attempt to shake off the contagion the whole Brigade of Guards were moved in March 1813 to Oporto. 'Roughly speaking 700 marched out of Vizeu, 700 remained in hospital, and 700 were in their graves.' So said Fortescue.[26] Typhus, however, was not the only cause of this heavy loss of life for dysentery had acquired a lethal power amongst these worn and exhausted soldiers, and taking the year 1812 as a whole dysentery caused two and a half times as many deaths as typhus, the figures being

2,340 for dysentery, and 999 for typhus. The Guards Brigade did not leave Oporto until June 1813 when it rejoined the army after the battle of Vitoria.

The rest of the army suffered less severely, but even so the deaths from the middle of December until the end of January are reported to have totalled 400 to 500 a week,[27] due mainly to the two diseases we have already mentioned although 'continued' fever which was mainly typhoid in origin also claimed many victims, and 2,020 men died from it during the year 1812. The soldiers who had served in the Walcheren expedition and were riddled with chronic malaria displayed less resistance than the rest, while typhus ran its deadly course through all the medical staff—medical officers, ward masters, orderlies, and nurses alike—and 11 medical officers died, while amongst the local inhabitants 1,200 perished. The 3rd, 4th and 5th Divisions in the Mondego Valley were better off for billets, which meant less overcrowding, and the 4th did not have a single case of typhus, while the 6th and 7th Divisions occupying the high ground of the Sierra de Estrella amidst frost and snow and icy winds suffered more from respiratory troubles than from fever. Hill's 2nd Division in Estramadura with headquarters at Coria also appeared to escape the worst with only 1,400 in hospital and 7,000 fit for duty and the Light Division, perhaps due to the superiority of its discipline, also suffered fewer losses. In the period of three months ending the 24th December 1812 the figures for admissions to the three hospitals which dealt with most of the cases showed that Cuidad Rodrigo had 4,006 admissions and 289 deaths, Coimbra had 3,408 admissions and 301 deaths, and Celorico with 2,847 admissions and no fewer than 611 deaths had the appalling mortality rate of 21·4 per cent. In all there were 38,888 admissions to both general and regimental hospitals and 2,231 deaths.

Of the innovations which McGrigor introduced none was more important than a new system of comprehensive returns of the sick and wounded. However unpopular such measures were on active service, regimental surgeons were made to render weekly, monthly and quarterly returns through medical channels to the Inspector, and as a result from the date of his arrival we get the first accurate picture of the state of health of the army. Further, there were monthly reports on medical equipment and transport. The annual return from the 24th December 1811 to the 20th December 1812 shows that during the year the total number of admissions to both regimental and general hospitals was 176,180 made up of 95,075 admissions to general and 81,105 admissions to regimental hospitals. Of this number there were discharged fit 119,798 or 68 per cent, and there were 7,193 deaths, a rate of 4 per cent.

The causes of admission and the number of deaths are given in detail in the Appendix[28] but the principal causes are listed below.

Unfortunately the return is incomplete for we are unable to quote the number of direct admissions to general hospitals as only the figures for regimental hospitals are available. The deaths for both regimental and general hospitals are however included.

Disease	Admissions to regimental hospitals	Deaths in Regimental and general hospitals
Continued fever	16,923	2,020
Intermittent fever	13,759	148
Dysentery	3,241*	2,340
Remittent fever	1,826	67
Typhus fever	331*	99

* A large number of dysentery and typhus fever cases were admitted direct to general hospitals.

There were also 905 deaths from wounds, 35 from hospital gangrene and 4 from tetanus.

With the sick more numerous than at any other time during the whole of the Peninsular War it is an appropriate moment to indicate the lines of treatment in two of the commoner diseases, dysentery and malaria. Dysentery was still regarded as being caused by chills and the suppression of perspiration, but amongst other theories put forward was one that it arose from water in its early stage before it attained the qualities of miasmata, which was then looked upon as the cause of ague. It was treated by immediate venesection followed by pulv. ipecac. co. grs.xii every hour, and repeated on three separate occasions; every second night 3 grs. calomel and 1 gr. opium was given, and in the intervening days 2 ozs. of magnesium sulphate dissolved in a quart of light broth. Venesection was repeated until the stools were free or nearly free of blood; warm baths were given if there was much tenesmus, and tonics and light diet used to complete the cure. Relapses were not infrequent and if chronic dysentery developed a cure was very difficult to achieve. Amongst the drugs then used were ipecacuanha and calomel, salts, castor oil, jalap and pulv.creta cum opio, astringents and demulcents. When the patient was convalescent, bitters were given to restore the tone of the gut, warm clothing was advocated, and flannel round the abdomen to guard against chills.

Intermittent fever or malaria was not difficult to cure in the first instance provided bark was given in sufficient quantity; there were two varieties of bark, cinchona cordifolia, and cinchona lancifolia, and they appear to have been equally efficacious. But the great number of relapses points to the benign tertian type of fever being predominant and it appears to have been the custom to give $\frac{1}{2}$ to 1 oz. of bark six hours before the rigor was due. Ensign Bell describes how he suffered a relapse every second day for months after his first attack, but he still remained with his regiment throughout and fought in all its engagements. He described the bark treatment as useless, but probably never took enough. Arsenic was the most favoured remedy second to bark, venesection was carried out in plethoric cases, and mercury was administered in chronic malaria if it was associated with hepatitis.

After the troops had settled into winter quarters, Wellington issued strict orders on discipline and man management, fresh clothing and blankets were issued and provisions made abundant. The soldiers were set to work to repair and rebuild the damaged villages in which they passed the winter. McGrigor for his part was so concerned at the spread of infection whenever there was the least suspicion of over-crowding that strict orders were issued on ventilation and dispersion. At one stage he went so far as to stop all evacuation to the general hospitals, and even chronic cases were sent back to the regimental hospitals. Each of these was equipped with 12 sets of bedding for the worst cases and 6 palliasses, the rest sleeping on locally made straw mattresses, 4 inches thick, 7 feet long, and 3 feet wide. Sheets were occasionally in use and ward equipment was of local construction. Every division was reinforced with hospital mates, an apothecary at divisional headquarters to dispense medicines and supply medical stores, and a purveyor to provide hospital comforts and extras which were difficult to obtain under the normal regimental system. For the basic supplies of bread and meat 6d. was paid in hospital stoppages daily, but rice and wine were issued free, supplied from purveyors stores in the nearest general hospital.

Now a more ambitious scheme was hatched in McGrigor's mind. After his experience at Burgos he was worried about the lack of good hospital buildings in a future campaign, and recollecting his service in the West Indies he suggested to his Commander that sectional wooden hutted hospitals which were movable might be constructed. Without saying a word of approval or objection Wellington appeared to take little interest in the scheme but some weeks later he told McGrigor that the huts, which he did not omit to emphasise were extremely costly, were on their way out from England. After being landed at Oporto and conveyed up the river Douro by boat the huts, capable of holding 4,000 patients, were erected at Escalhao hard by Castello Rodrigo.

By the month of February 1813 the worst was over and the typhus epidemic on the wane; the sick rate dropped to below 30 per cent for the first time in six months, by April it had fallen to 20, and by May to 16 per cent with a total of 2,000 in the regimental and over 7,000 in the general hospitals.

William Fergusson had now finished his three years of training the Portuguese, and had become Principal Medical Officer of the 2nd

Division, but he still retained his former title of Inspector General of Hospitals. Endowed with immense experience he threw himself enthusiastically into the task of improving hygiene and increasing the efficiency of the regimental surgeons, and the comparatively good health of the 2nd Division may be attributed to his efforts. When the spring came all was in high order, and Fergusson addressed his surgeons in a stirring appeal. 'During the approaching campaign,' he wrote in a memorandum, 'the upholding of the effective strength of the army in the field must in a great degree depend upon their exertions to meet and overcome the difficulties which warfare in this or any other country inevitably presents. Every possible assistance will be given them from the public stores, but they well knew how limited that assistance must be, and the Inspector feels bound to say that whoever will not or cannot find measures for succouring and preserving the sick beyond those put into his hands from the public stores is unfit for the service of the Army in this or any other country and will be so reported to the Inspector of Hospitals.'[29] The emphasis in this trenchant appeal was on the important role which the regimental surgeons could play in the prevention of sick wastage and the necessity to maintain the units' strength in the field.

Before the army takes the field let us look for a moment at the distribution in March 1813 of the medical staff officers whom McGrigor had at his disposal both as principal medical officers of field formations and to staff the general hospitals. There were 9 deputy inspectors of hospitals, 2 of whom were serving as principal medical officers of field formations, 1 with the Cavalry Division and 1 with the Guards. The remainder were superintending general hospitals, Mr. Gunning the Chief Surgeon to the Force at Coimbra, and the others at Lisbon, Celorico and Vizeu. At Coimbra too was stationed Dr. Lucas, the Physician-in-Chief, and all the 14 physicians under him were distributed among the general hospitals except for the physician appointed to Army Headquarters. Staff surgeons numbered 44; 10 of these were principal medical officers with divisions and field formations and the remainder except for one at Army Headquarters were surgeons at the general hospitals. There were 10 apothecaries, 59 hospital mates with commissions and 44 with warrants, 22 dispensers, and 20 purveyors and deputy purveyors. This makes a total of 293 medical staff officers actually in post out of the establishment of 343. In addition there were 4 medical officers with the different companies of the Royal Waggon Train and about a score of Spanish and Portuguese doctors and mates employed with British hospitals.

The Ordnance Medical Department under its own Deputy Inspector General exercising an independent command had 23 surgeons attached to Royal Artillery batteries.

With the disasters of the winter months now behind them all were prepared to play their part in the events which lay ahead.

When the campaign of 1813 opened the Spanish guerillas' war was at its peak of ferocity, and the French troops were widely dispersed fighting them. The enemy opposite Wellington were thereby reduced to 50,000 men, while on the Allied side the British by April had 52,000 and the Portuguese 29,000 troops in the field—a striking force of over 80,000, not counting some 20,000 Spaniards. Some of the credit for this must go to McGrigor, for his plan to augment the regimental hospitals was paying a handsome dividend. In the first four months of the year nearly 20,000 patients were treated in the forward area thereby saving hundreds of lives by sparing the sick the exposure and exhaustion of a journey to the general hospitals. Regimental surgeons and their commanders co-operated in devising comforts for their patients. Moreover the irregularities and outrages which had long disgraced the return journeys of the discharges from hospital came to an end. From the purely medical angle too there was a gain, for by limiting movement the spread of infection was reduced. As a result of all this there were more men with the colours than ever before, and Napier's opinion was that McGrigor's efforts added the equivalent of a division of fighting troops to the army at the battle of Vitoria. By such results the conservation of man power showed the true role of the Medical Department.

McGrigor did not believe in sparing his officers and although their work was arduous, and not a few sacrificed their lives in carrying out their tasks, they continued to give of their best and to serve him with skill and devotion to the end of the war. Nor did he spare himself or his personal staff, for in 1813 appeared a volume of Hospital Regulations and Standing Orders running to 150 pages and this included a formulary of over 200 prescriptions. In general hospitals it was laid down that separate ward accommodation was to be provided for cases of continued fever, for dysentery, and for surgical patients, although the last could be used for cases of intermittent fever. All patients were to have bedsteads. Separate hospitals were also now to be provided for sick and wounded officers although this was on a voluntary basis, and they could still be treated in quarters if this was preferred. Convalescents were to be housed in a special building apart. In the regimental hospitals, when the unit was stationary, the same orders for separation of the different categories of sick were also to apply, although the authorized beds were limited to sixty. But the P.M.O. of the Division was now given authority to nominate the number of hospital servants to be employed, a step which usurped the hitherto overall control exercised by the commanding officer. Moreover, in spite of the hospitals being non dieted, medical comforts such as tea, sugar, sago and port wine were to be issued on a limited scale. Weekly skin inspections were to be held and regimental surgeons were ordered to extend their authority to advise on the clothing, messing facilities and meals.

Every one of these changes was beneficial in the highest degree and being within Wellington's powers of command were readily accomplished. It was quite another matter when the advancement of deserving medical officers was in question. In vain McGrigor strove to bring promotion to those who, by their ability showed their capacity to be advanced in rank. Director General Weir at the War Office was understandably opposed to give accelerated substantive promotion to officers who were serving in the Peninsula when the seniority of those in other parts of the far flung British forces had to be considered. But this policy annoyed Wellington, and he not only wrote officially to the Commander-in-Chief in his usual trenchant manner, but in a private letter did not conceal the fact that he entertained the poorest opinion of the Medical Director General. 'The Duke of York,' answered Torrens, 'entirely agrees with you. The Medical Board is the torment of his life and the Director General—a good man in his time—is an old driveller, but so long as they continue as a Board, the Duke must suffer them.'[30]

During the winter reinforcements had been flowing in from England, for Castlereagh staked everything on success in Spain and the Government only retained 25,000 regular troops to resist invasion. Even a trained corps of sappers and a properly organized siege train arrived. There were, too, improvements in equipment. Tin kettles which had to be carried by the men themselves were substituted for the iron ones, and the mules which had been used for carrying the iron kettles were now utilised to carry tents, for the army was now to encamp to remove it from the temptations of towns and villages and to safeguard its health. Another benefit which the rank and file experienced was the order at McGrigor's suggestion that they should be relieved of the burden of carrying great coats, as the relief in weight would more than compensate for any mischief from cold. With regard to discipline, the Commander hoped that the floggings and the hangings of deserters which the insubordinations of the retreat had forced him to adopt would act as a deterrent to future disobedience.

With the initiative firmly in his hands and with the command of the sea in the possession of the Royal Navy, Wellington adopted a new strategy. His plan was to strike in a north-easterly direction towards the northern coast of Spain and establish supply bases at the Biscay ports. This would not only shorten his line of communication by hundreds of miles, but by driving north he would outflank the French positions on the Douro. With these possibilities in mind and in the utmost secrecy, supply ships, guns, and ammunition were accumulated at Corunna as a preliminary to forming a base at Santander which lay 250 miles to the east. As a diversion to this main plan of operations Lieut General Sir John Murray who was commanding a force of 18,000 men of various nationalities on the east coast of Spain was ordered to attack Tarragona.

Accordingly on the 22nd May Wellington divided his forces, and with 30,000 men advanced on Salamanca, while the main Anglo-Portuguese army threaded it way northwards through the mountainous defiles and precipices of the province of Tras-os-Montes. For this difficult operation the regimental hospitals were streamlined; bedding was reduced to four sets and the surplus returned to the general hospitals; three mules only were allotted to carry equipment, and the bullock carts and spring waggons withdrawn to a rear echelon. Medical officers had a haversack with medicines for use on the march, and a first-aid kit which included 2 field tourniquets, needles and 12 ligatures. In the lid of one of the panniers Peruvian bark and only the medicines and dressings which were easily portable were carried.[31]

As Wellington had foreseen, the French were powerless against this unexpected march and finding their Douro defences outflanked by superior forces were compelled in June to abandon in succession Valladolid, Palencia and Burgos. After many brushes with the enemy but without any major engagements a further sweep to the north was made, and having covered 300 miles the sweating dusty columns arrived at the river Ebro spoiling for a fight. Never had the army been in better health; the rations were abundant in quantity and excellent in quality; fever had almost disappeared, and in one division with a strength of 5,700 there were only 58 sick in a space of seven days.

It was originally planned to send back all sick and wounded to Castello Rodrigo but the pace became too rapid for this to be found practicable and hospitals were opened in succession for the northern column at Miranda do Douro, Zamora, Toro and Palencia, and for the southern column at Salamanca and Valladolid. At Salamanca the hospital was as before opened in one of the numerous colleges of this ecclesiastical town with a staff surgeon supplied by the cavalry division to treat the wounded, and a deputy purveyor and 3 hospital mates to look after the sick of the divisions and the French prisoners.

It was in the valley of Vitoria that the French armies at last stood at bay and on the 21st June 1813 battle was joined. The French army numbered some 50,000 men with 150 guns, while against them the Allies had a strength of some 72,000 sabres and bayonets, including 11,000 Spaniards.

The Allies made a three-sided attack from the north, west and south, the northern attack planned to operate against the enemy's right rear and cut the main road to Bayonne. The French resistance was stubborn

359

and the fighting fierce and prolonged; but they were finally driven back on all fronts and King Joseph's army accomplished its retreat by the road to Pamplona after abandoning all their guns and baggage. Darkness and exhaustion put an end to the Allied pursuit. The subsequent follow up of the enemy was ineffective for the victorious troops were delayed by the spoils of war and by gorging themselves after days of privation on the hoards of provisions. The total French losses were over 7,000 and although only 2,000 prisoners were taken, Vitoria was one of the decisive battles of the war for it finally liberated Spanish soil.

The Allied casualties amounted to something over 5,000 of which 230 officers and 3,940 other ranks were wounded. The severest losses were sustained by the British, whose wounded numbered nearly 3,000 officers and men, and some regiments suffered very heavily. The 71st Highlanders in the 2nd Division lost 316 officers and men and several other regiments had more than 200 casualties.

A glimpse of the medical work which must be typical of what went on all along the battle front is afforded us by Assistant Surgeon Henry who was now acting as assistant to Staff Surgeon Wasdell who was in medical charge of the 2nd Division. This division was engaged on the southern flank in the neighbourhood of Puebla, and after watching the progress of the battle from an advantageous hill Henry was soon called to sterner work. 'Almost immediately afterwards General O'Callaghan's brigade consisting of the 28th, 34th and 39th Regiments marched to attack the village of Subijana D'Avala, half a mile to our front, and having there suffered a heavy loss, I was ordered to the assistance of the surgeons, and soon after this, being the most pressing point, Mr. Wasdell joined us himself. We collected the wounded in a little hollow out of the direct line of fire, but within half musket shot of the village, unpacked our panniers and proceeded to work. The brigade had four or five hundred men killed and wounded in the course of an hour or two, so we were fully employed. A stray cannon shot from a battery firing on the village would occasionally drop among us by way of an incentive to expeditious surgery, and after one of these unpleasant visitors had made its harmless appearance, a young chirurgeon of my acquaintance became so nervous that although half through his amputation of a poor fellow's thigh, he dropped the knife, and another hand was obliged to complete the operation. But this was only a temporary weakness. At my suggestion he lay down on the grass took a little brandy and soon recovered, and did good service the whole day. Spring waggons were in attendance in which we placed the worst patients and sent them to Puebla village where Dr. McGrigor had, early in the day, made the most judicious arrangements for their accommodation.'[32]

No sooner had these casualties been seen to when a message arrived from the 1st Brigade that medical assistance was required and Henry is sent on horseback to help. 'I reached the top in time to witness the last moments of Colonel Cadogan of the 71st. Such was the loss sustained in this part of the field, not more than 2 acres square, I counted 150 men killed or badly wounded. The wood being now abandoned by the French light troops and the artillery withdrawn from the hill behind, Mr. Wasdell, two other surgeons and myself, set to work afresh, after swallowing some wine and bread, and we remained collecting, dressing, amputating, packing the wounded into spring waggons and sending them to the temporary hospital till seven o'clock. When our work was done and we had packed off every wounded man in the neighbourhood of the village we pushed on to join the Division now far in front.'[33]

In Vitoria a general hospital spread over many buildings was opened. The stretcher bearers told off to collect the wounded after the battle had behaved disgracefully by joining in the search for booty but at length the 4,000 casualties were collected and for many days every available surgeon was at work under the direction of John Hennen.

The liberation of Spanish soil meant that the old line of evacuation to Portugal which now stretched for over 300 miles could be abandoned and general hospitals brought forward to suitable ports on the coast of the Bay of Biscay. Of the general hospitals in existence all were still back in Portugal except for two on Spanish soil at Salamanca and Toro, the last the nearest to Vitoria but still over 150 miles away. A shorter line of evacuation was essential and on the 15th July 1813 orders were issued for a major redistribution of general hospitals.

Santander was now to be the site of the principal hospital with a total of 4,000 beds; the accommodation here had been increased by the arrival of portable wooden huts capable of holding 750 patients which had been brought in by sea. Vitoria hospital which was over-crowded with 4,800 British, Portuguese, and French sick and wounded was to be reduced in numbers by evacuation to Bilbao, which was to be equipped for 2,500 beds. Here the new hospital centre had obtained the use of a fine convent for medical cases while the surgical cases were accommodated in a cordelaria or rope factory. Bilbao was ordered to evacuate cases as necessary to Santander so that it could be closed at short notice. A hospital at Corunna was to be prepared to receive invalids and any surplus cases from Santander.

The hospitals at Santarem, Viseu, and Celorico had already been closed and the hospitals at Salamanca, Toro, Palencia, Reinosa, Villadiego and Elizondo were now to follow suit, except that the first four were to be allotted a role as Passing Stations, together with the hospital sites at Gallegos and Villarcayo. The general hospital at Escalhao (500 beds) was to remain open until its cases had been evacuated to Oporto. Lastly the hospital at Figueras (500 beds) was to evacuate its invalids to Lisbon and dispatch the remainder by sea to

Santander. The great base hospital at Lisbon was now after five years no longer required except as a holding unit for invalids, and closed its doors on the 24th August 1813. Guthrie, who had been the senior surgeon there since the retreat from Salamanca in November 1812, was to his joy transferred to more active duty at Santander. The medical store depot at Castello Branco was to remain open for the time being, but the depots at Elvas, Badajoz, Estremoz, and Alter de Chao were to close after dispatching their stores to Lisbon via Abrantes.

A week after the battle the Allies were on the French frontier, occupying a front of some 50 miles stretching from the pass of Roncesvalles on the right through the valley of Bastan in the centre to the Bidassoa river on the left, with the army split into separate columns facing the frontier passes. On the left stood the fortress of San Sebastian while behind the front lay the city of Pamplona which was now under blockade by a Spanish force. Wellington's strategy for the moment was a defensive one except for the capture of San Sebastian which he ordered to be attacked without delay. The construction of batteries to bombard the southern defences of the fortress was commenced on the 14th July and the convent of St. Bartholomew stormed and captured on the 17th with no great difficulty. But the assault on the main fortress failed, and it was not until a second attack was mounted six weeks later that the Allies were victorious. The date was the 31st August 1813 and a costly price in lives was paid, the casualties for the two attacks numbering 3,000

Before this date, however, Marshal Soult who had replaced Marshal Jourdan after the defeat of Vitoria was putting into operation an attempt to relieve the fortress. This was to attack the Allies right at Roncesvalles with an overwhelming force of 35,000 men and cut Wellington's communications by advancing westwards towards the coast. Simultaneously another column was to storm the Maya pass further to the west, and dominating the roads through the Bastan, intervene between Wellington and his threatened right in front of Pamplona, where the capture of the besieger's stores was an essential part of the operations as the French were devoid of transport after Vitoria. It was a daring plan and initially it succeeded. Wellington had expected an attack against the left and was away at San Sebastian when it erupted on the 25th July 1813. On the Roncesvalles front where 6,000 British, Portuguese and Spaniards were confronted by 35,000 of the enemy the pass was captured after fierce fighting; but at the Maya pass farther to the west 2 British brigades successfully resisted 3 French divisions.

Wellington, who had immediately returned to the east at the sound of the guns found the situation at Maya under control and pressed on all day at a hand gallop to Roncesvalles where the situation was now perilous. Soult had penetrated to Sorauren only 6 miles from Pamplona but providentially hesitated to press his attack, and on the next day 4 British divisions arrived and a counter attack drove the French from Sorauren. Under continued pressure Soult was now forced to withdraw to the north, and the Allies won their way to the highest ridges of the Pyrenees. The French counter-offensive ended in utter failure with the loss of over 13,000 men, while the Allied casualties amounted to 7,000, exclusive of the Spaniards. Fortescue says, 'the British soldier has seldom shown himself to greater advantage than during this eventful fortnight'.[34]

Although the number of wounded approached the 5,000 mark the medical problem was eased by the fact that the casualties were spread over a period of some ten days' fighting. The main hospital centre was established at the church at Berrioplano some 3 miles from Pamplona on the route to Vitoria, where the general hospital eventually received and treated all the casualties. Assistant Surgeon Henry was working at Sorauren where for five days and nights the wounded poured in so that he had scarcely an hour's rest, 'razorless and clean shirtless . . . snatching half an hour's sleep on a heap of wheat in a barn which was literally my bed and board, I worked away amidst as much surgical practice as would have set up a hundred young sons of Aesculapius if shared amongst them'.[35] Getting casualties away from Sorauren itself presented a difficult problem which called for all McGrigor's ingenuity, and eventually it fell to the horses of D'Urban's Portuguese cavalry brigade to carry them to Berrioplano. Thence in spring waggons and carts they were sent off to the general hospital in Vitoria over 50 miles away. John Hennen so well organized the care and attention paid to the wounded that Wellington was duly complimentary and on the 1st August he wrote, 'Although our wounded men are numerous, I am happy to say the cases are in general, slight, and I have great pleasure in reporting that the utmost attention has been paid to them by Inspector of Hospitals, Dr. McGrigor, and the Department under his direction.'[36]

The same month of August 1813 found Bilbao hospital in the grip of a deadly epidemic of hospital gangrene. This had first made its appearance among the wounded amidst the crowded conditions in Vitoria and it was carried far and wide by the patients evacuated to Bilbao, Santander and the other hospitals, all of them crowded not only with British but with Portuguese, Spanish and French casualties.

Although hospitals had often been badly overcrowded on many previous occasions the number of cases of hospital gangrene had never been enough to present a worrying problem. There were a few cases after Albuera and more at Salamanca in 1812, and there were thirty-five deaths during that year. Now this dreaded contagion struck with fatal effect, and nearly 500 men succumbed.

Hennen, who was in charge of the surgical work in the Cordelaria at Bilbao has given an accurate account of the outbreak. In the last week of August 1813 he went there from Vitoria to find it packed with 1,000 wounded crowded together on straw and with but scanty supplies of bedding. The rapid advance of the army had left the general hospital stores far behind, and the hope of obtaining any assistance from the Spaniards was negligible; even the drugs and dressings, although purchased principally from local chemists, were of the very worst description. Most of the wounded cases had arrived in successive waggon convoys, in carts, or had even accomplished the whole journey of some 40 odd miles on foot, but some had come by sea from the storming of San Sebastian and these proved the worst cases. Benefiting from his long experience Hennen realised the danger of infection and took every measure to enforce cleanliness, provided ventilation, and divided the hospital into separate wards. He had enforced similar precautions at the general hospital at Elvas in 1812 when with 2,500 wounded under his care his proud boast was that not a single case of gangrene or typhus fever had occurred. But by the time he arrived at Bilbao it was too late to prevent the infection taking hold. The premonitory symptoms were severe headache, want of sleep, loss of appetite, fever and a quick pulse; then the wound which had previously been healthy and granulating became tumid, dry and painful, losing its florid colour and taking on a dry and glossy appearance. Within twenty-four hours the affected area became circular with hard prominent edges and a black slough, and the limb became oedematous. The patient's general condition now quickly deteriorated, venous and later arterial bleeding occurred from the wound, and incessant vomiting, hiccough, involuntary stools and coma closed the scene. Hennen describes the remarkable case of a soldier just landed from England who was under treatment with mercury for a venereal complaint, and died within forty-eight hours after admission, gangrene having attacked an open bubo in his groin, eroded the great vessels in the neighbourhood and destroyed the abdominal parietes.

Fergusson writes of its prevalence and cause—'Few of our general hospital stations have escaped a visitation at one time or another of this terrible distemper. Confined to crowded hospitals from accumulated exhalation from human bodies causing an impure and vitiated atmosphere.'[37] His observations led him to believe it was contagious through other ulcerated surfaces, and capable of being propagated into any fresh wounds, 'by breathing vitiated air the poison comes out through the wound, which otherwise in the absence of a wound would have caused constitutional disease'.[38] We now know hospital gangrene is a bacterial infection caused by an anaerobic bacillus carried from one case to another by the contaminated hands of dressers, by instruments, and by dressing materials such as sponges. It attacks those with open wounds such as amputation stumps.

The details of treatment can be studied in Hennen's *Military Surgery*[39] so we confine our remarks to mentioning the general remedies employed. External applications included poultices moistened with opium, or camphor in oil, or dilute nitric or citric acid. The ulcerating wounds were exposed to the fumes of nitrous acid gas which was also constantly diffused throughout the wards; all dressings were repeatedly washed and cleaned. French surgeons used the actual cautery, or sprinkled the wound with nitrate of silver.

Internally the patients were given emetics of antimony, and purgatives of mercury; Peruvian bark, opium and wine, what in short was described as the 'antiphlogistic' or anti-inflammatory treatment. In the long run, however, the measures which were found most effective were the break-up of any hospital with many cases in its wards, the wide dispersion of cases in tents or huts, and the provision of adequate ventilation. It can readily be understood that these measures proved beneficial when the cause was the spread of infection directly from case to case.

We will anticipate the chronology of our story and round off this account of hospital gangrene by giving the figures up to the end of the year 1813.

Hospital	Number	Discharged	Died	Remaining
Santander	160	72	35	53
Bilbao	972	557	387	28
Vitoria	441	298	65	4
Passages	41	2	2	—
	1,614	929	489	85

The mortality here is 30·3 per cent.

Tetanus was another complication which now occurred more frequently than before, and there were twenty-three deaths throughout the year 1813 as compared with four in 1812. Treatment here was opium often combined with camphor, but the mortality was 100 per cent unless we can believe an account of Assistant Surgeon Brown of the 57th Regiment who claimed treating two officers successfully by bleeding, antiphlogistic remedies and emollients to the wounds.

Apart from these two distressing complications all surgeons were unanimous that in the main field of surgery the improvements in technique and methods of treatment after five years of experience had greatly improved the standards of recovery and led to a decrease in mortality.

In the early months of 1813 the army had rarely been healthier.[40]

In the months of May and June during which the army marched for twenty-six consecutive days the rate had fallen to 16 per cent of the strength, the lowest figure for over two years. With the arrival in the mountainous region of the Pyrenees, the months of July, August, and September brought an outbreak of diarrhoea and dysentery which were blamed on the mountain air and the cold nights, and such bowel diseases accounted for half the 13,000 cases who were under treatment each month. As we would expect at these high altitudes there were few fresh cases of malaria but continued and remittent fevers which were happily mild in nature were the next principal causes of admission. In the quarterly return June to September, 16,000 cases were admitted to the regimental hospitals more than half of whom were discharged to duty, and 5,000 were evacuated to Vitoria which was the only general hospital in the forward area to receive cases, except for those from the 5th Division near San Sebastian which went direct by sea to Bilbao. It was on Vitoria, Santander and Bilbao that the bulk of the work fell and in these three months they dealt with nearly 10,000 admissions, half of whom were discharged to duty and nearly 1,000 died, a death rate of 10 per cent.

By September the regimental hospitals were installed in good buildings and treating over 2,000 patients who were provided with diet tables and enjoying extras and medical comforts. The sick from the high slopes of the Pyrenees were brought down by Spanish peasants in blankets slung between poles. Throughout most of the war there is no mention of the use of stretchers, and it appears that these were only authorised as an article of supply towards the end. Guthrie mentions that they were quickly found useless as they were too heavy. But improvised stretchers were continually in use, and these were made by the pikes which all sergeants carried acting as side poles with a blanket forming the bed of the stretcher.

At this point it is necessary to leave the Peninsular War and bring the reader up to date in the European situation, for this was affecting Wellington's strategy. A temporary truce had been agreed between Napoleon on the one hand and the alliance of Austria, Russia and Prussia on the other, and while it lasted Wellington had hesitated to risk following up any of his successes because Napoleon's overwhelming strength might have been turned against him with fatal results. But on the 3rd September 1813 came the news he had been waiting to hear. This told him that the armistice was over. Napoleon had refused to consider the offer of the Rhine as the frontier of France, and hostilities had recommenced. Without further delay Wellington decided to invade France. His plan of campaign was to attack Soult's line of defence at its western extremity where the river Bidassoa runs into the sea, and to this end during the early days of October he unobstrusively moved unit after unit to his left flank, until more than 25,000 men had been concentrated. For his part Soult had only 10,000 men on this front for he expected the attack would be made at Roncesvalles.

It was on the 7th October that the crossing of the Bidassoa was achieved. The troops surprised the French by fording the river up to their armpits in water and the enemy fought with little spirit. The casualties amounted to 1,500, half of them Spanish, and the wounded included two of the divisional staff surgeons who were hit during the passage of the river.

Then when Pamplona had capitulated to the Spanish army Wellington felt free to strike a further blow. Soult had constructed a strong defensive position south of the Nivelle and Wellington's main attack was launched against the heavily fortified French centre at Sare. The Allies' attack proved irresistible and succeeded all along the line although the casualties on both sides were about equal, the Allies losing 145 officers and 1,903 rank and file wounded, but the trophies captured included 69 guns.

Now at last Wellington had gained access to the Plain of Gascony for his winter quarters, and the situation was sensibly improved. The army too was at the peak of its power—well disciplined, in excellent health and more effective than any British continental army had ever been before. Thanks to a proclamation forbidding all plunder and ordering all requisitions to be faithfully paid for, it was not long before the French civilians returned to their homes. This was most welcome but it presented a difficult problem in the further employment of the Spanish army, for, short of pay and rations as they were, and with many injuries to avenge, it was not likely they would spare plundering the French peasants. Wellington who did not deny their good fighting qualities decided that the only way to preserve this good relationship was to send the majority back to Spain. By adopting the policy of civil fraternisation it became possible to leave the lines of communication free from garrison troops, a measure which added at least two divisions to the effective strength; moreover the sick and wounded could be safely treated in the French hospitals in every town without guards being required.

For a whole month the bad weather stopped further movement but on the 9th December Wellington struck again to force the passage of the river Nive. The Nive joined the river Adour at Bayonne where there existed an entrenched and heavily fortified camp occupied by some 12,000 enemy troops.

The passage of the river led to a stubborn fight lasting for two days with Soult counter attacking fiercely, a counter stroke which took Wellington by surprise. This action was as well contested and bloody as any of the Peninsular War. Three brigade commanders were wounded and almost every officer of two brigade staffs were struck down; the total Allied loss in the fighting was 5,061, of whom 233 officers and 3,674 rank and file wounded, nearly half of them Portuguese.

General hospitals were opened at Cambo for 1,300 of the wounded, and at Espelette. Although the facilities at Cambo were decidedly inadequate, it was well situated on the lines of communication and did in fact remain open until the end of the war.

As the British advance liberated the coastal area the sea ports which had been freed were in succession utilised to bring in supplies and act as hospital bases. So we find general hospitals springing up at St. Andero; then at Passages, where a medical store depot was also installed; and finally at Fuenterrabia. These materially shortened the line of evacuation, and it was to Fuenterrabia that the cases were evacuated from Cambo and Espelette.

The numbers absent sick each month from September to December remained fairly constant at between 13,000 and 14,000, or between 23 and 25 per cent of the strength. With the rain and the cold, and with frost and snow at times, the respiratory diseases, catarrhs, colds and rheumatism predominated. A few cases of typhus had occurred, caught from civilians on the banks of the Ebro, and even cholera was at one time reported. There were 30,196 admissions this quarter, the general hospitals chiefly concerned being at Santander (2,471), at Bilbao (3,770), at Passages (3,363) and at Fuenterrabia (1,363); there were over 17,500 discharges to duty and nearly 1,500 deaths. The initial shortages of hospital beds and bedding which Hennen had reported at Bilbao had now been made good with the arrival of 5,000 sets of bedding from England and medical supplies also poured into Passages so that the army was now amply provided for.

If we look at the year 1813 as a whole we find the number of patients treated in both regimental and general hospitals amounted to 123,019 which was some 50,000 less than in the disastrous year of 1812, and is a measure of the healthier state of the army and the improvements in sanitary discipline and prevention of disease which the year had brought forth. Such measures as abundant food, better and warmer clothing, (with cloth pantaloons for winter wear, linen trousers for summer, and waistcoats) all tended to this end. It was a maxim that the best clothed regiments were always the healthiest regiments. It was requested that the arrival of recruits from England should be limited to the winter months to allow them to become acclimatised before the unhealthy autumn period when malaria and dysentery were so rife. As regards regimental discipline and man management McGrigor said a lesson could be learned from the German Hussars who on the retreat from Burgos in 1812 never sent a man to a general hospital. There were several judicious measures in medical administration which had tended to improve the lot of the sick and wounded. In hospital the separation of the different diseases had limited infection and increased the recovery rate. There was now a spring waggon permanently attached to each unit, and in addition a tilt cart for carying the kits of sick men.

During the year, 64 per cent of admissions were discharged to duty and there were 6,866 deaths, a rate of 5·6 per cent. Dysentery with 1,629 deaths again proved to be the cause of the greatest mortality, closely followed by continued fever with 1,598, the great majority of whom were undoubtedly suffering from diseases of the typhoid group. There were 971 deaths from typhus, the great majority due to the continuance of the disastrous epidemic begun in the late months of 1812, and there were 1,095 from wounds; hospital gangrene accounted for 489, and there were 23 from tetanus; a further point of interest is that the malaria deaths numbered 139 although we are not able to give the total number of admissions. The detailed figures will be found in the Appendix.[41]

To return now to the operational side: for nearly two months activity was suspended by the winter weather and it was not until February that Wellington was able to make his next move. This period was a welcome rest for the troops who were snugly ensconced in the villages and farms and were suffering few hardships except that there was a lamentable shortage of pay and of replacements for worn out clothing. But on the 14th February 1814 the advance began. Soult's army held a line to the north of the river Nive with the formidable entrenched camp at Bayonne still forming his right wing, and in the course of the next ten days the army with insignificant loss had forced the passage of the river Gave D'Oloron and compelled Soult to retire to Orthez, where after breaking down all the bridges on the river Gave de Pau he took up a new position. While these movements were in course of execution there were intricate operations afoot to achieve a crossing of the Adour at Bayonne. After a daring feat when the Guards were got across the estuary under the unsuspecting noses of the French, a bridge formed of coasting vessels was established with the co-operation of the Royal Navy, and by the 27th February Bayonne was encircled.

At Orthez Soult held a strong position with 37,000 troops against Wellington's 33,000 and regarded the Gave de Pau as an impassable barrier, but again the British after severe fighting drove the enemy into retreat with the British cavalry in pursuit. The Allies' losses were just short of 2,000 including 133 officers and 1,594 other ranks wounded.

On the 2nd March the town of Aire was entered after a feeble resistance, for the French were now disintegrating when attacked. 'It was all in vain,' wrote Bell of the 34th. 'The blood of the old bricks was up and we drove them into and right through the town.' Soult with his army reduced to 25,000 infantry and 1,000 cavalry, marched away towards Toulouse until all contact between the contending armies was lost.

It is at Aire that once again we find Guthrie. He had been sent forward from Santander, which although still open in order to dispose of its cases was now replaced by the general hospitals nearer at hand which included St. Jean de Luz and Orthez. The pressure was now on the hospitals at Passages, Fuenterrabia, and Orthez, each of which had over 2,000 admissions in the period between December 1813 and March 1814 while St. Jean de Luz had over 1,600. In all there were 23,744 admissions, 16,792 discharges and 1,871 deaths. At Aire, Guthrie, besides the care of the British and Portuguese wounded had a large number of French to look after, men whose wounds either from faulty surgery or neglect were sloughing; most of their stumps had to be re-amputated.

Suddenly the campaign had become a picnic, with fowls to roast at camp fires, wine at fifteen sous a bottle, and riflemen slicing slabs of bacon on their bread.[42] Beresford was sent off to Bordeaux, and seized the city with two regiments of hussars, the mayor tearing off his tricolour and declaring for the Bourbons. This meant that the estuary of the Gironde was now open to British shipping.

We have already mentioned that Wellington had ordered subsidiary operations to be undertaken on the east coast of Spain as a diversion to the main thrust and we must briefly refer to these.

The troops employed came from Sicily where British forces were in occupation and the army included not only some British infantry regiments but Italians, Germans, Spanish and Portuguese elements under British commanders. The operational area ranged from Barcelona in the north to Valencia in the south and there were various actions, notably at Castalla, Tarragona and Ordal, the former a French defeat and the siege of Tarragona an allied reverse. The latter was chiefly due to the faults of Lieut General Sir John Murray who proved himself an ineffective commander and was later court-martialled. It is not the intention to enter into a detailed account of these operations and it is only necessary to state that Staff Surgeon Boyle was the P.M.O. of the force, and that general hospitals were established at different times at Alicante, Castalla, Valencia and Barcelona.

Napoleon's armies in the north had disintegrated under the combined attacks of the Russian, Prussian and Austrian armies, but Wellington knew nothing of the Emperor's defeat when his troops at last stood before the fortress of Toulouse on the 26th March 1814. The city was impregnable on three sides with the river Garonne sweeping round it, and on the east where it was approachable Soult had strongly fortified the defences of a ridge dominating the surrounding plain.

Wellington had a force of 49,000 men available against Soult's

42,000 but he never hesitated to attack, for according to Bryant his moral ascendancy over the enemy was complete and his soldiers engrafted with a seasoned confidence that made them invincible.[43]

An initial attack made by the Spanish army ended disastrously, but the British redeemed this failure when they repelled Soult's counter-attack, and fought their way to a foothold on the ridge which succeeding attacks enlarged until the British guns now on the ridge paved the way for the Allies to gain their last victory of the Peninsular War.

The casualties amounted to 4,200 of which 1,850 were British, 530 Portuguese and 1,800 Spanish. The 6th Division upon whom the bulk of the fighting fell sustained severe losses. The 42nd lost 26 officers and 386 rank and file; the 79th 18 officers and 215 men, and in the 61st only the adjutant and 2 ensigns remained unwounded.

When the wounded British, Portuguese, Spanish and French prisoners were all collected in Toulouse they numbered 6,000, and occupied all the suitable accommodation the city could provide; civil hospitals, convents, nunneries, churches, and large houses were all put to use as well as a camp outside the town. This vast hospital area was separated into two divisions under the two ablest surgeons, Guthrie and Murray, and their duties were arduous indeed, for McGrigor tells us that after no previous battle were so many operations done and never was more skilful surgery performed. To quote Guthrie's own words: 'Nearly all the wounded had every possible assistance and comfort. The hospitals were well supplied with bedsteads, the medicines and materials were in profusion. The sick and wounded, 1,359 in number including 117 officers,[44] were in charge of 2 deputy inspectors, 10 staff surgeons, 6 apothecaries, and 51 assistant staff surgeons, and the whole worked from morning to evening with the greatest assiduity. The surgery of the army was at its highest pitch of perfection it attained during the war, every broken thigh was in a straight splint and the success greater than ever before.

Wellington entered Toulouse the day after the battle and the troops with drums beating and colours flying received the acclamation of the inhabitants. Then on the 12th April came the news that Napoleon had abdicated. Although the principal campaign thus came to an end, the city of Bayonne did not surrender until the 26th April, and not until then was the Peninsular War finally over.

It was not until June 1814 that the general hospitals were finally able to close and the casualties disposed of by evacuation to Bordeaux; while the surplus hospital stores and the huts were loaded on transports to be dispatched to America where the war which had broken out in 1812 was still being fought. From January 1814 onwards the health of the army had been good in spite of much fighting, long harassing marches, and bad weather early in the year. Between January and June the principal diseases were continued fever with 5,007 admissions, malaria with 952, dysentery with 865, remittent fever with 436, and 155 cases of typhus. The diagnosis of 'cynoche' is also used, described as an 'un-remitting' fever.

The general hospitals which were now closed included Santander, Bilbao, Vitoria, Passages, Fuenterrabia, St. Jean de Luz, Cambo, Orthez, and Toulouse, while away in Portugal there were still details of invalids to be disposed of from Lisbon and Oporto.

Finally, to complete the account of the Peninsular War let us analyse certain points in the statistics which will be found in the Appendix. Unfortunately these figures do not cover the whole span of the war but only a period of two and a half years from December 1811 to June 1814. For the three and a half years from August 1808 no comprehensive system of returns had been instituted. We know however that the average sick rate over the whole period of the war was 21 per cent, while the period from December 1811 onwards for which detailed statistics are available was 25.9 per cent. Further, the figures under the various Appendix tables do not always agree, and only general rather than particular observations can be made; they do however give as accurate a picture as is possible of the health of the army.

Under Table 1 the total number treated was 346,108, divided almost equally between the regimental and general hospitals, a fact which reveals how extensively the regimental hospitals were able to limit sick wastage by treatment in the forward areas. If the number transferred in column 5, i.e. 95,042 is subtracted from the total discharges of 324,672 in column 4, the number discharged to duty is 229,630 or 66 per cent.

The total deaths amounted to 18,513 or 5·3 per cent, and this death rate was some four times greater in the general as compared with the regimental hospitals; this is understandable if it is assumed that the more severe cases were evacuated to the general hospitals and therefore constituted poorer risks. There was however the contention that deaths were more numerous in the general hospitals because of overcrowding with the consequent spread of contagion.

In the Divisional Sick States the numbers shown as absent from their regiments in general hospitals were always much greater than the figures those hospitals showed as being under treatment, and the difference was due to the cases in transit to and from hospitals. The distances to be covered between many of the regimental hospitals and the general hospitals amounted at times to hundreds of miles and the rate of progress of the sick convoys was only some 15 to 20 miles a day. With admissions and discharges averaging between 600 and 1,000 a week from Lisbon alone the numbers actually occupying hospital beds might be some thousands less than the numbers reported as absent in the Divisional Sick States.

Table 2 deals with regimental hospitals only and shows the prevailing diseases which are: (a) continued fever with over 40,000 admissions, (b) intermittent fever with nearly 23,000 admissions, (c) diarrhoea 15,677, (d) leg ulcers 12,167, and (e) dysentery 7,526. If dysentery and diarrhoea are added the total bowel diseases amount to 23,203, which would take second place in the list. Unfortunately the Table does not include direct admissions to general hospitals, and in static periods and while the army was in winter quarters these may have been considerable.

Table 4 shows that 1812 was the most unhealthy year with over 176,000 admissions compared with 123,000 in 1813. This is confirmed by the average monthly percentage sick rate for each year based on strength which reads:

> 1811 24·3 per cent
> 1812 29·4 per cent
> 1813 24·0 per cent

This Table also shows the chief causes of death from disease which are (a) dysentery 4,717, (b) continued fever 4,005, (c) typhus 2,277, and (d) hospital gangrene 603. There is however a statement which shows that the total deaths between 1808 and 1814 numbered 24,930 from disease, and 8,889 from battle casualties or 33,819 in all.

Another report gives the mean strength in the Peninsula from January 1811 to May 1814 a period of forty-one months as 66,772. In the same period the deaths amounted to 35,525, of whom 9,948 fell in battle or died of wounds. There were therefore 25,577 deaths from disease and therefore nearly three times as many men died from disease as died from wounds.

On looking at Table 5 we see that 1812 was much the worst year for malaria, and 1813 the worst for continued fever and typhus fever, the latter due to the epidemic after the retreat from Burgos, when over 30 per cent of the army was continually sick. By adding the figures for the admissions to general hospitals quoted in the Appendices for the particular years 1810 and 1811 we get the nearest possible number of admissions for the period from 1810 onwards. These are as follows:

Admissions in 1810	75,268
Admissions in 1811	164,964
Admissions between 1811 and 1814	339,870
Total	580,102

This however still omits the years 1808 and 1809 for which returns are not available.

There is no record of the total number of equipped beds in the general hospitals, for no fixed establishment existed, and beds were added as circumstances demanded; but if we take the total strengths and compare the total admissions to general hospitals shown in the Divisional Sick States the figures are as follows:[45]

1810   16·1 per cent bed cover
1811   23·6 per cent bed cover
1812   27·2 per cent bed cover
1813   19·6 per cent bed cover

On the surgical side Guthrie's *Gunshot Wounds* and Hennen's *Military Surgery* give accounts of the work of the surgeons in the Peninsula and here we can only briefly refer to a few points. Guthrie had amputated the first of his wounded cases at Rolica in 1808 and the last at Toulouse in 1814. Starting medicine at the age of 13, at 15 he was a hospital assistant at the York Hospital, and when Surgeon General Keate gave instructions that all hospital assistants who had not been examined and approved by the College of Surgeons should be removed, Guthrie immediately passed the examination at the age of 16.[46] By birth a Scot, in appearance he was robust and active with keen energetic features and piercing dark eyes. In manner he was shrewd, quick, and outspoken, and often inconsiderate in speech, although behind his brusqueness was much real kindheartedness. Surgically known as the English Larrey,[47] at the end of the war he was still only 29 years of age, but from his vast experience had introduced many new surgical techniques. He was the first to use the straight splint for fractures of the femur. He distinguished himself by extracting a musket ball from the bladder and later was the first to use the lithotrite to crush stones. He averred that the great danger of secondary haemorrhage from gun shot wounds was groundless. Guthrie's experience taught him that in the field amputations were performed too commonly and he became more conservative as the war went on. He rarely amputated the upper extremity but performed excisions of the head of the humerus and the elbow joint; he gave up using the tourniquet in amputation cases and relied on digital compression.

The early criticism that surgeons lopped off arms and legs wholesale had some real substance, but when we come to the statistics published after the battle of Toulouse (Table 6) we see that by then amputations were uncommon. Out of 1,242 capital (major) operations only 48 times were amputations performed, or 4 per cent of the total; and out of 304 wounds of the upper extremity there were 7 amputations or between 2 and 3 per cent. The mortality in these 1,242 operations, performed we must remember without any anaesthetic, amounted to 146 or 11·7 per cent; in the upper extremity the mortality was 1 per cent; in the lower extremity 4 per cent; but in secondary amputations for compound fractures it was 33 per cent. With the excellent care and attention which all the casualties received at Toulouse there was not a single case of hospital gangrene.

A different picture is presented by statistics for the period between the 21st June and the 24th December 1813, when the hard fought engagements of Vitoria and the Pyrenees were causing many casualties. In the general hospitals of Vitoria, Santander, Bilbao, Passages and Vera there were 584 capital operations performed of whom 287 died, a mortality of 49 per cent. Over the same period 317 capital operations were performed in the divisional areas with only 27 deaths, a mortality of 8·5 per cent; such a disparity seems to point again to the discredit of the general hospitals, but is probably due to them treating the severer cases with a lesser chance of recovery.

John Hennen, an Irishman, second only to Guthrie in his fame as a surgeon is chiefly remembered for his comprehensive work on *Military Surgery* published in 1818. The treatment which he adopted for the slighter types of wounds is remarkable for its simplicity. These were dressed with lint moistened with cold water or mixed with spirits, wine, or vinegar, and left in place for three days. Subsequent treatment might follow the same lines, or moderately warm emollient poultices might be applied, made either of bread, bran, pumpkin, or carrot, and removed twice daily until the sloughs loosened and pus appeared showing that suppuration had commenced. Poulticing was then stopped and cloths applied moistened in acidulated water or simply cold water. 'With cold water,' Hennen says, 'one is never at a loss for a remedy.'[48]

We can close this surgical aspect of the war by quoting McGrigor's cautious praise. 'Great experience and reflection had at this time created among us a body of operators such as never were excelled, if ever before equalled in the British army.'[49] The results of this were twofold—one, that military surgery made great strides in advance of previous knowledge, and the other that after the war this advance was reflected upon civil surgery with the greatest advantage.

We come now to the administrative lessons the Medical Department could learn from six years of continual warfare. Undoubtedly the greatest was the need for a field medical unit which could clear the cases from the regimental hospitals and evacuate them to the general hospitals. It seems strange that the lessons of former wars had been forgotten and the flying hospital which had acted as the link was never introduced. With this complete gap in the field organisation regiments were continually being denuded of their medical officers for other duties, and as Wellington said after Talavera when scarcely one medical officer was left with each brigade, this had a decidedly adverse influence on his tactical operations. It was certainly bad administration to remove doctors from the battle area where their presence was essential for units in action, and to employ them in looking after sick left behind in towns and villages, or conducting convoys to the general hospitals. And further, the heaviest demand came after a battle, when they were sent back to assist in the general hospitals owing to the shortage of hospital mates. A field medical unit or a flying hospital would have resolved these difficulties and McGrigor says, 'I once proposed an adoption of it in Spain to Lord Wellington, but he would have none of it.'[50] Wellington's firm rejection was due to his determination not to allow slow moving transport in the divisional area which might hinder his tactical freedom of action.

It was the lack of transport provided for the sick and wounded which caused the greatest hardship and Fergusson wrote, 'Our means of transporting sick and wounded have ever been deficient and cruel, as all can testify who attended the bullock carts of the Peninsula.'[51] As the war progressed the Royal Waggon Train with its spring waggons was reorganised to release the maximum number of vehicles for the conveyance of the sick and wounded; these carried 8 sitting or 2 lying cases and were drawn by 4 horses with 2 drivers. But they were heavy and cumbersome and often blocked the roads, which was precisely one of the reasons that Wellington would not employ them on a scale sufficient to satisfy the medical authorities. 'We have indeed a few spring waggons but not a tithe of what an army enaged on actual service would require,' wrote Fergusson. But later when operations were developing successfully the Commander-in-Chief relaxed his orders and one spring waggon was regularly issued to regiments.

The French medical establishment was well organized to render effective first aid to troops in action compared with which the British system was crude and defective, and credit must go to the French nation for being the first to provide a trained medical corps. Their *ambulance volante* moved with the divisions and rapidly transported the wounded to the rear hospitals. It had an establishment of 113 officers, N.C.O.'s and men, including 14 surgeons, all mounted and under the command of a surgeon major of the 1st Class. All personnel who were trained in their duties wore distinctive uniforms and carried instruments or dressings in pouches on their person or on horseback. Naturally, with conscription, the man power problem in France was never acute as with the British who were constantly short of recruits for fighting units and unable to spare men for full time duty as trained medical attendants. But in due course the French organization was followed by every civilized nation, although the British were tardy in adopting it, and fifty years later in the Crimean War the British army was still completely unprepared and were often forced to call on the French to come to their aid. Soldiers' lives in the British Army were too often sacrificed to political expediency or financial stringency.

As the war progressed there were several improvements in the British

field organization. The first was the establishment of passing or intermediate hospitals established on the lines of communication as a link
between the regimental and general hospitals. These took care of the
casualties which occurred amongst the sick convoys passing along to
the general hospitals, or from the discharged men going up to the front.
A staff surgeon with some hospital mates served the needs of a medical
staff. Another sensible innovation was the setting up of a receiving
hospital at the general hospital centres to which all wounded were at
first admitted, where nourishment was given, particulars taken, soiled
clothing removed, and patients classified according to their injuries.

Hospital wards were divided into medical, surgical, and convalescent;
dysenteries and infectious cases were given separate accommodation
usually in tents.[52] Bedsteads were sometimes in use but generally boards
and trestles were used to raise patients off the floor, and close attention
was paid to the preparation and ventilation of wards. The ward staff
varied in different hospitals but was generally 1 wardmaster and 6
orderlies for every 100 beds.

Although Fortescue condemns the general hospitals as 'hotbeds of
waste and dishonest dealing'[53] when McGrigor inspected those at
Lisbon and Coimbra in 1812 he was agreeably surprised at their order
and regularity. No major administrative scandals were ever brought to
light and the Commander-in-Chief on his visits never had adverse
comments to make.

Supplies of medicines, purveyors stores, and hospital equipment
arrived regularly throughout the campaign, and although at times
there were temporary shortages these were due more to difficulties of
transportation in keeping up with the advance of the army than by any
lack of medical planning. In Portugal too it was easy to make good any
shortages by requisitioning from local sources, but in Spain the authorities always proved difficult.

As we have said the authorised stretchers were never really
satisfactory. There were no traverse bars so that the patient rested on
the ground when the stretcher was lowered. At times looped blankets
were used, the pike which sergeants then carried being used as side
poles.

With regard to personnel, the shortage of hospital mates was one
of the constant difficulties throughout the war, and a corollary was the
criticisms of inefficiency on those who were sent out, due to the Medical
Board being quite unable to obtain candidates of a suitable standard.
Undoubtedly the sick and wounded suffered at times from their
ignorance and neglect, while owing to their low rate of pay some could
not resist the temptation of appropriating medical comforts for their
own use. But as Guthrie remarked, 'Young men sent out to the Peninsula incapable of performing any operation in military surgery,
became able operators in a short time, from the practical lessons

377

inculcated in the dissection room, hospitals and fields of battle.'[54]

Let us now give the views of some of the senior medical officers. Inspector of Hospitals William Fergusson who from his seniority held equal rank with McGrigor was an able administrator and a keen sanitarian. He deplored the want of a proper headquarters for the medical staff officers or as he puts it, 'there being no ambulance with the British army at which the young medical officer might find a home, nor an hospital corps to furnish him with means of conveyance and service'.[55] This was especially evident in such stations as Lisbon or Coimbra where medical staff officers who had to live in civilian billets, looked after by a civilian servant, and feeding individually, felt the want of an officer's mess where the juniors would come under the influence and guidance of their more senior colleagues and build up the feeling of a corporate unit.

Guthrie's views on organization also deserve attention. 'Nothing,' he writes, 'could be more inefficient than the Medical Department of the Army during the first two-thirds of the war. It was only when it reached the summit of the Pyrenees that its Medical Department approached perfection . . . And why was it so? Simply because the necessary means of every kind were at hand, and the medical men were numerous, young and efficient. The confidence the Duke of Wellington reposed in Sir James McGrigor . . . in giving him the uncontrolled management of the Department, enabled him to enforce military discipline amongst us on the one hand, whilst he encouraged ability, excited emulation, and rewarded merit on the other. Every officer of the Department endeavoured, by keeping the army effective in the field, to prove to their brethren at home that although they were less profitably, they were not less honourably employed in the service of their country.'[56]

With the end of the war few honours came the way of the Medical Department for medical officers did not possess executive rank and were not entitled to receive the Order of the Bath, the sole military decoration which was given to commemorate outstanding service. Medals and clasps for the different actions were awarded to those holding the equivalent of field rank and above. It would however have been ungracious not to have acknowledged McGrigor's outstanding services and he was honoured by a Knighthood (Kt.) although in his auto-biography he acknowledges he had hoped for a Baronetcy.[57] Added to the accolade he was created a Knight of Hanover (K.H.)[58] His popularity with the officers of his Department whom he had commanded with such universal success was made evident by their presentation of a handsome service of plate at the cost of a sum approaching 1,000 guineas.

After dealing with the aftermath of war problems, McGrigor was placed on the half pay list with a special allowance of £3 a day, and he now contemplated setting up in practice as a physician in London. To this end he determined to renew his study of anatomy and chemistry, and attended the Hunterian school in Windmill Street. But these plans were soon eclipsed when Director General Weir was taken ill, and McGrigor was informed by the Military Secretary that the Duke of York had appointed him as his successor.

POSTSCRIPT

Before we take leave of the Peninsular War let us give a short account of the future of some of the principal figures who have engaged our attention. Inspector of Hospitals William Fergusson was dispatched on duty to the West Indies, and went on half pay in 1817. He took up private practice first in Edinburgh and later at Windsor, where several members of the Royal Family were among his patients. Much of his spare time was devoted to writing, and we are indebted to him for valuable comments on his army experiences which have come down to us in his *Notes and Recollections of a Professional Life*.

George Guthrie profiting by his wide experience embarked on a flourishing surgical practice in London and a distinguished civilian career—surgeon to the Royal Hospital at Chelsea, founder of the Westminster Ophthalmic Hospital in 1816, F.R.S. in 1826, and in 1827 surgeon to the Westminster Hospital. He was elected a member of the Council of the College of Surgeons in 1824, and was President of the College in 1828 and on three subsequent occasions. It is said a knighthood was offered him by the Duke of York but was declined for want of means. He continued his army connection by retaining the charge of wards at York Hospital for the purpose of demonstrating surgical cases to newly joined medical officers, while his lectures on surgery were open to all service officers without fee. Guthrie had always been impetuous and had a reputation for outspokenness which at times got him into trouble When ordered to rejoin the colours during the Waterloo campaign he refused, but he could not resist visiting and treating the wounded in the hospitals in Brussels as a civilian. Later at York Hospital he performed one of the few successfully recorded cases of amputation at the hip joint, and this was done without previous ligature of the artery. It was the type of operation which, in the absence of anaesthesia, required speed and dexterity of the highest order, attributes which Guthrie possessed in full measure. His memory is kept alive by the institution of a Guthrie medal at the Royal Army Medical College which is awarded biannually to the most outstanding of the civilian consultants to the army. As a writer he is best known for his book *On gun shot wounds of the extremities* which went through several editions.

John Hennen was recalled to the colours from half pay in 1815 and served as surgeon at the Jesuit's Hospital in Brussels. He was promoted Deputy Inspector of Hospitals and while serving at Gibraltar lost his life in 1828 fighting an epidemic of yellow fever.

REFERENCES

[1] Gurwood (1852). *Despatches of Duke of Wellington*, vol. VIII, p. 365.

[2] McGrigor to Grant. Muniment Room, R.A.M. College, 8th April 1812.

[3] McGrigor (1861). *Autobiography*, p. 278. Longman, Green, Longman & Roberts, London (1861).

[4] P.R.O., W.O. 1/254.

[5] Wheeler. *Peninsular Diary*. Michael Joseph, London (1851).

[6] Hennen (1820). *Military Surgery*, p. 144 footnote. Longman, Hurst, Rees, Orme & Brown, Edinburgh (1818).

[7] This includes Portuguese wounded.

[8] Henry. *Extracts from Events of a Military Life*, p. 61. Pickering, London (1843).

[9] Henry. *Extracts from Events of a Military Life*, p. 139. Pickering, London (1843).

[10] Henry. *Extracts from Events of a Military Life*, p. 78. Pickering, London (1843).

[11] Henry. *Extracts from Events of a Military Life*, p. 78–79. Pickering, London (1843).

[12] A term used for affections of the throat.

[13] Gurwood (1852). *Despatches of Duke of Wellington*, vol. V, p. 760.

[14] McGrigor (1861). *Autobiography*, p. 301. Longman, Green, Longman & Roberts, London (1861).

[15] Probably the Goya portrait.

[16] McGrigor (1861). *Autobiography*, p. 302. Longman, Green, Longman & Roberts, London (1861).

[17] McGrigor (1861). *Autobiography*, p. 311. Longman, Green, Longman & Roberts, London (1861).

[18] McGrigor (1861). *Autobiography*, p. 311. Longman, Green, Longman & Roberts, London (1861).

[19] McGrigor (1861). *Autobiography*, p. 311. Longman, Green, Longman & Roberts, London (1861).

[20] The Medical Board refused to confirm his appointment because of his youth. Guthrie was only 27 years of age.

[21] Another report gives the number as 800.

[22] *The Healing Art*, vol. II, p. 291. Ward and Downey, London (1887).

[23] Kempthorne. Journal *R.A.M.C.*, vol. LIV, p. 215.

[24] The sick returns for 1812 are given in Appendix A.

[25] Lisbon, Coimbra, Cuidad Rodrigo, Celorico, Vizeu, Santarem, Abrantes, Castello Branco, Niza, Estremoz, Alter de Chao, Elvas.

[26] Fortescue. *History of the British Army*, book XV, chapter III, p. 102. Macmillan, London (1910).

[27] Fortescue. *History of the British Army*, book XV, chapter III, p. 102. Macmillan, London (1910).

[28] Appendix D, table IV.

[29] Fergusson Papers. Muniment Room R.A.M. College, (18th April 1813).

[30] Wellington MSS. *Torrens to Wellington*, 17th February 1813.

[31] Powders: ipecacuanha, jalap, jalap and calomel, jalap and chrystal tartrate, antimony, rhubarb.
Pills: opium, mercury, calomel and colocynth, calomel and antimony.
Ointments, plaster, linen, sponges, calico bandages, pins, caustic, alum, and white vitriol.

[32] Henry. *Events of a Military Life*, p. 152–153. Pickering, London (1843).

[33] Henry. *Events of a Military Life*, p. 155–156. Pickering, London (1843).

[34] Fortescue. *History of the British Army*, book XV, chapter IX, p. 304. Macmillan, London (1910).

[35] Henry. *Events of a Military Life*, p. 174. Pickering, London (1843).

[36] Kempthorne. Journal, *R.A.M.C.*, vol. LIV, p. 218.

[37] Fergusson Papers. Muniment Room, R.A.M. College.

[38] Fergusson Papers. Muniment Room, R.A.M. College.

[39] Hennen. *Military Surgery*, chapter XIII, p. 210. Longman, Hurst, Rees, Orme & Brown, Edinburgh (1818).

[40] Hennen. *Military Surgery*, chapter XIII, p. 210.

[41] The sick returns for 1813 are given Appendix B.

[42] Bryant. *The Age of Elegance*, p. 90. Collins, London (1950).

[43] Bryant. *The Age of Elegance*, p. 95. Collins, London (1950).

[44] Bryant. *The Age of Elegance*, p. 95.

[45] This must refer only to the British wounded.

[46] It is said that in the French army the hospital beds were first based on 3 per cent, raised later to 6 per cent, and finally to 12 per cent.

[47] There was no restriction as to age at this time.

[48] Hennen (1820). *Military Surgery*, p. 66. Longman, Hurst, Rees, Orme & Brown, Edinburgh (1818).

[49] McGrigor (1861). *Autobiography*, p. 340. Longman, Green, Longman & Roberts, London (1861).

[50] McGrigor (1861). *Autobiography*, p. 353. Longman, Green, Longman & Roberts, London (1861).

[51] Fergusson. *Notes and Recollections of a Professional Life*, p. 62. Longman, Brown, Green & Longman, London (1846).

[52] Regulations for military hospitals in 1813 is given in Appendic C.

[53] Fortescue. *History of the British Army*, book XV, p. 194. Macmillan, London (1910).

[54] Guthrie (1815). *On gun shot wounds of the extremities*, preface p. v. Burgess & Hill, London (1820).

[55] Fergusson. *Notes and Recollections of a Professional Life*, p. 65. Longman, Brown, Green & Longman, London (1846).

[56] Guthrie (1815). *On gun shot wounds of the extremities*, preface p. xi and xii. Burgess & Hill, London (1820).

[57] McGrigor (1861). *Autobiography*, p. 357. Longman, Green, Longman & Roberts, London (1861).

[58] Knight of Royal Hanoverian Guelphic Order.

Chapter 12

WATERLOO

While Wellington was successfully driving the French before him in southern France the armies of the Allies operating on its eastern boundaries had advanced 250 miles in a month and were sweeping towards Paris. Intent on reviving the policy of supporting their Allies in the Low Countries the Government decided to send a force of some 5,000 troops under Lieut General Sir Thomas Graham to Holland early in 1814. The main objective was the capture of Antwerp, but the only important battle was the attack on Bergen op Zoom in March. Although the assault was initially successful and the ramparts of the city were captured, the tactics employed were faulty and the French after heavy fighting in the narrow streets drove out the British troops with heavy loss. Out of 4,600 men engaged nearly 3,000 were lost, 1,600 of them prisoners, and many perished from drowning when the ice was broken up by the French cannonade.

Deputy Inspector of Hospitals Robert Grant was chosen as P.M.O. and with him came the staff of a general hospital[1] which was opened in buildings at Willemstadt, supplemented by specially fitted transports in the harbour. Hospital attendants on this occasion were provided by a Veterans battalion sent from England, but they seemed generally as inefficient and undisciplined as ever, for we read from the account of Dr. Walsh a physician that on the death of a French prisoner, 'while in articulo mortis, the savages of the same ward took from his person the sum of £15.'[2]

Due to the severe wintry conditions respiratory diseases and bowel infections soon filled the hospital with 500 patients, while an epidemic of typhus necessitated many evacuations to England. When after the attack on Bergen op Zoom some 200 wounded were added to the number a third of the town was taken over for hospital use, and additional accommodation was opened in outlying stations.

Although Paris was entered by the Allies on the 30th March 1814, hostilities in Holland continued until the end of April. On the 5th May Antwerp and Bergen op Zoom were occupied and the campaign ended with headquarters being established at Brussels. The hospital was not able to close until the 10th July. This according to Dr. Walsh was partly due to the Treasury insisting that the invalids had to be detained in Holland until the regimental accounts for hospital stoppages had been settled. This meant a six weeks delay which inflicted untold suffering on the sick and wounded and led to the death of seventy of these victims of government red tape.

This was the fourth time within a period of twenty years that a campaign in Holland had ended in a reverse for British arms. Moreover the Government had engaged in this useless expedition forgetting that if Napoleon was defeated in the field, Antwerp and Holland itself would fall anyway.

Meanwhile in France the armies of Prussia and Austria had entered Paris on the 30th March 1814. Napoleon at Fontainebleau abdicated and was banished to Elba.

By February 1815 the great powers known as the Concert of Europe had agreed on a European settlement. Britain retained St. Lucia, Tobago, Trinidad, Demerara, Essequibo, and Guiana on the western shores of the Atlantic, Mauritius and Ceylon in the Indian Ocean, Malta and the Ionian Islands in the Mediterranean, and the Cape of Good Hope. Joined to her existing possessions these gave Britain's fleets untrammelled control of the world's seaways. On the 7th March a great victory ball was to be held in Vienna but that night news was received that Napoleon had escaped from Elba; by the 10th March he was in Lyons, and by the 20th in Fontainebleau near Paris. Such a direct threat to revive Napoleon's hegemony and plunge Europe once more into the throes of war led to immediate mobilisation of the continental armies, and the onus of the defence of the Low Countries devolved on the British and Prussians.

The Duke of Wellington was appointed to command the forces which gathered in Belgium and occupied the country between Brussels and Ostend, while Field Marshal Blucher with a Prussian army 110,000 strong had his headquarters at Namur watching the line of the Meuse and the Sambre beyond Charleroi. By June 1815 Napoleon had concentrated in northern France an army 70,000 strong, most of them veterans.

Owing to the disbandment of units and the requirements of the war against America, the entire strength of the troops which Ministers had been able to place at Wellington's disposal did not at first exceed six regiments of cavalry and twenty-five battalions of infantry, many of them second battalions which were both weak and inefficient. But until troops from America and Canada could be recalled nothing more could be done to concentrate a striking force in time. Only a few regiments were veterans of the Peninsula and the army as a whole was far less efficient as an instrument of war. To the 6,000 cavalry and 20,000 infantry which made up the British contingent was added a polyglot array comprising German Legion, Belgian, Hanoverian, Brunswick and Nassau troops, 'an infamous army' Wellington called it, numbering in all some 15,000 cavalry and 70,000 infantry with 192 guns. But of this total a third were Belgian troops most of whom were regarded as unreliable. The Duke divided his army into two corps comprising ten divisions, in each of which foreign troops were intermingled with the red coats.

Some changes had taken place in the soldiers' dress; the coatee had taken the place of the long skirted coat, trousers and ankle boots were worn, and the shako had been adopted as a headdress. Each soldier carried a blanket which he was prepared to use as a bivouac tent; great coats were held in store at the base. Tents on the scale of thirty per battalion were brought but only issued as required. The ration scale was bread 2 lbs., meat $\frac{1}{2}$ lb., barley or rice $\frac{1}{4}$ lb., and brandy $\frac{1}{8}$ quart.

As Principal Medical Officer, McGrigor selected Inspector of Hospitals James Grant, who was already on the spot in Brussels after the short lived campaign in Holland. He was initially allotted a total of 52 medical staff officers[3] for the administrative heads of the field formations and for the general hospitals, but this number had to be successively increased. The Ordnance Medical Department with its own battery hospitals was under the independent control of Deputy Inspector Wittman, while the Hanoverians although they had their own regimental organisation were treated in the British general hospitals.

Regiments had the usual establishment of medical officers and each now had a spring waggon to carry the sick and wounded. Each brigade had a staff surgeon as S.M.O. and each division a deputy inspector or staff surgeon as P.M.O. Several of these officers were old hands of the Peninsula.

The British troops were landed at Ostend where a general hospital was opened, and by June four more had been established at Brussels, Bruges, Antwerp and Ghent. To act as hospital attendants a complete garrison company of four officers and 107 N.C.O's and men of a Veteran's battalion were sent over with the army.

Napoleon's aim was to capture Brussels, and his plan was to strike at the junction of the Allied and Prussian armies and destroy each of them in turn. His offensive began on the 15th June with an attack on Charleroi and on the 16th June he also engaged the Prussians at Ligny. The British at Quatre Bras held their ground after a hard fight costing some 3,000 Allied casualties of which 2,380 were wounded. The lying cases were collected during a night of heavy rain and evacuated to the general hospitals in Brussels where the best of accommodation was available.

Napoleon gained a victory over the Prussians, and was convinced he had accomplished his design of driving a wedge between the two armies. But in fact Blucher had fallen back to Wavre where he was only

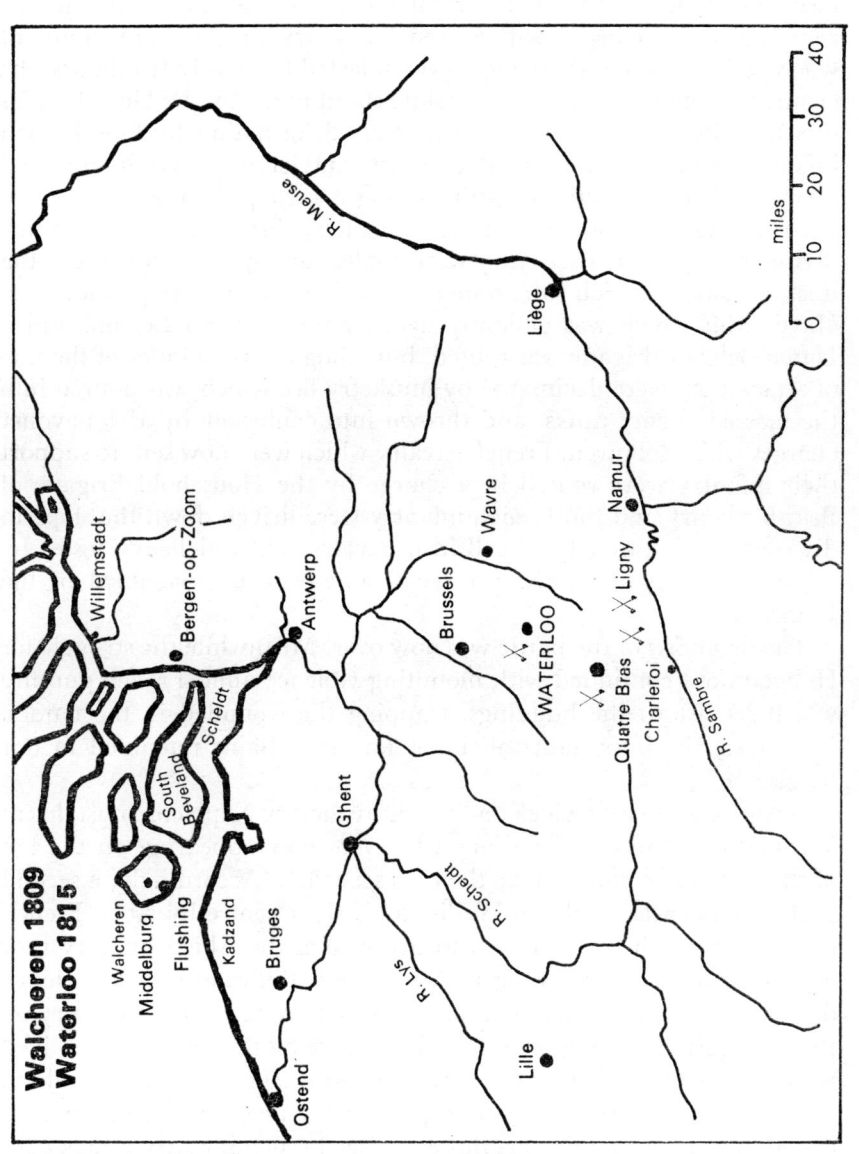

Walcheren 1809
Waterloo 1815

miles
0 10 20 30 40

R. Meuse

Liège
Namur
Ligny
Wavre
Quatre Bras
WATERLOO
Brussels
Charleroi
R. Sambre

Willemstadt
Bergen-op-Zoom
Antwerp
South Beveland
Scheldt
Walcheren
Middelburg
Flushing
Kadzand
Bruges
Ghent
Ostend
R. Scheldt
R. Lys
Lille

some 15 miles from Waterloo, the position which Wellington had chosen to stand on the defensive and receive Napoleon's attack.

On June 18th the Allied army was drawn up for battle on a ridge south of the village of Mont St.Jean with forward elements holding the farms of Hougoumont on the right flank and La Haye Saint in the centre. The battle began with a French infantry attack on Hougoumont where, after a desperate struggle which lasted for nearly two hours, the enemy were hurled back by a resolute stand made by the Guards. This was then followed by an attack in massed formation by four French infantry divisions on the Allied left centre and left wing. Wellington had adopted his usual tactics of withdrawing his troops behind the crest of the ridge to minimise the effects of artillery fire, and as the French divisions topped the ridge they were confronted by every musket in the lines of infantry which rose to meet them. The enemy swept round La Haye Saint which was gallantly held by the German Legion, and a Dutch Belgian Brigade was routed, but along the remainder of the line of attack they were decimated by musketry fire which was poured into the massed enemy ranks, and thrown into confusion by the bayonet charges which followed. French cavalry which were now sent to support their infantry were routed in a charge by the Household Brigade of British cavalry and the French infantry were driven down the slope in disorder. Unfortunately, the British cavalry suffered heavy losses by refusing to obey the order for recall and were overwhelmed in the French lines.

The first crisis of the battle was now over. Meanwhile the struggle for Hougoumont continued with mounting violence amid French gun fire which set fire to the buildings, trapping the wounded in the flames. Moreover, the important salient of La Haye Saint remained in our hands.

It was now after 3 o'clock and to ensure victory Napoleon must defeat Wellington before the Prussians who were now appearing on the left of the Allied line could make their presence felt. Accordingly, a second grand assault was made on Wellington's right centre by 5,000 French curassières which tried in vain to overwhelm the Allied infantry now formed into squares bristling with bayonets. Refusing to acknowledge defeat, this was repeated by a further attack by some 9,000 cavalry on the area between Hougoumont and La Haye Saint which was received with volleys of musketry and salvoes of grapeshot from the artillery. This employment of cavalry unsupported by artillery fire or infantry ended once more in disaster. But a further French infantry attack captured La Haye Saint, and with this key position in their hands the French launched further assaults on the weakening Allied centre. The situation became dangerous. Wellington called in fresh troops from his left and right wings and was able to hold on while the Prussian attack on his left was developing more strongly every minute. Finally the remaining French on the ridge were thrown back.

Napoleon's last throw was now at hand. The finest soldiers at his command, the battalions of the Old Guard, were thrown against Wellington's right centre and their attack was preceded by a bombardment which reached a new peak of intensity. 'Hard pounding this, gentlemen,' Wellington observed, 'but we will see who can pound the longest.' In the 27th Foot 450 of the 700 men were lying where they had been struck down; in the 40th both ensigns and fourteen sergeants had been killed or wounded round the shot torn colours; everywhere the casualties were on a similar scale; almost every member of Wellington's staff had been killed or wounded. His grip on the battle however never for a moment relaxed.

As the regiments of the Imperial Guard strode majestically forward to the attack through the fields of trampled rye the British Guards sprang to their feet, and pouring in a volley which shattered the front ranks, the Guards continued to rain on the enemy an unceasing torrent of lead. Even the veterans of the Imperial Guard became unsteady and at the order to charge the British hurled their enemies in confusion before them. The rout was completed by the 52nd Foot which took the Imperial Guard in flank and rapidly pressing on was joined by the 71st and the 95th, which shattered the enemy ranks in succession. As Wellington with hat raised on high gave the signal for the whole line to advance the Allied counter attack strode forward into the valley and under it the French army wavered and dissolved into rout. Within a month Napoleon had abdicated for the second time and was exiled to St. Helena where he died in 1821.

It was a formidable task which the medical service was called upon to undertake in a battle of such magnitude. Within an area of some two square miles lay over 40,000 dead, dying or wounded men. The number of British[4] wounded was 7,016, but to this number must be added the losses at Quatre Bras and the sick. The figures are as follows:

Wounded	At Quatre Bras	2,380
	On the retreat from Quatre Bras to Waterloo	132
	At Waterloo	7,016
		9,528
Sick	In general hospitals on the 18th June	3,046
		12,574

In addition there were 2,500 sick and wounded French prisoners, so that the formidable total of 15,000 hospital beds had to be provided. A significant footnote in Wellington's despatch says there were 1,875 men reported missing, but the greater number of these had gone to the rear with wounded officers and soldiers. Although this practice was rigidly forbidden, an appreciable number were able to slip away in the turmoil of battle. It illustrates the loss of fighting man power due to the absence of recognized stretcher bearers.

Behind the battle front the regimental hospitals were generally brigaded together for mutual assistance and nearly every suitable building out of the range of cannon fire was made use of. The village of Mont St.Jean on the main road to Brussels provided shelter for a host of dressing stations of all nations. Into action with each unit went an assistant surgeon armed with dressings and tourniquets to render first-aid and control haemorrhage, and the numbers of wounded they had to attend to in the shattered battalion squares must indeed have been overwhelming. Streams of walking wounded made their way back to the dressing stations during the fighting and the worst cases were as we have seen often helped by their comrades, 'the attendants' as the Rev. Gleig remarks, 'more numerous than the wounded'.[5]

Deputy Inspector Gunning who was P.M.O. of the 1st Corps was located at the farm on Mont St. Jean where he ran a small field hospital of his own which served the casualties from Wellington's headquarters. The Hon. Fitzroy Somerset[6] who was Military Secretary arrived with a shattered elbow and Gunning decided on immediate amputation. The Prince of Orange described the scene. 'Not a word announced the entrance of the patient, nor was he conscious of his presence until he heard him call out in his usual tone, "Hullo, don't carry that arm away till I have taken off the ring." Not a groan, not a sigh, not a remark had been extorted either by the wound or the operation.'[7] Lord Uxbridge whose leg was amputated showed equal fortitude. General Picton after his death was found to have been hit by a spent bullet at Quatre Bras which broke two ribs and caused a huge haematoma which he had concealed. Deputy Inspector Hume who was attached to Wellington's headquarters roused the Duke on the morning of the 19th to read out to him the list of casualties, a list so long and grievous that the Duke was in an agony of grief. 'What victory,' he said, 'is not too dearly purchased at such a cost.'[8]

Considering the fierceness of the fighting the medical officers appear to have come off remarkably lightly, for only one, George Denecke, P.M.O. of the 3rd Division was wounded, and of regimental medical officers only the assistant surgeon to the 92nd Foot was hit. Whymper of the Coldstream and Good of the 3rd Guards were in the thick of the fight at Hougoumont and came off unscathed.

The experiences recorded by medical officers shows how much they shared the dangers of the battle field. Assistant Surgeon Gibney attached to the 15th Hussars tells us he was compelled to shift his aid post while dressing his wounded and seek shelter in Mont St.Jean. 'Shot, shell and bullets flying about in all directions.'[9] As he made his way along a sunken road to the village 'the huge cannon balls hissing and whistling over our heads, lodging with a terrible thud into the opposite bank or striking the surface and rebounding, committed havoc and destruction in most unexpected quarters.'[10] 'Nothing could exceed the misery exhibited on this road which being the highpavé . . . leading to Brussels was crowded to excess with our wounded and French prisoners, shot and shell meanwhile pouring into them. The hardest heart must have recoiled from the scene of horror, wounded men being rewounded, many of whom previously had received the most frightful injuries. Here a man with an arm suspended by only a single muscle, another with his head mangled by a sabre cut, or one with half his face shot away, received fresh damage.'[11]

The colonel of Gibney's regiment having had his leg shattered by a round shot was desperately wounded and in need of immediate amputation. 'After obviating all danger of haemorrhage I endeavoured to get him to a more suitable place for operation; so removing a door from an outhouse, we placed him upon it, and as we were leaving the dreadful room I came across Mr. Carson who suggested his being taken to Waterloo . . . The misery to be seen in that room was more than dreadful . . . It was crowded to excess with wounded officers, many of whom were dying, and melancholy it was to hear the cries for relief, and to know that in only too many instances nothing could be done. There was not even a drop of water to be had so as to assuage their burning thirst, nor apparently any of the usual provision made for wounded men.'[12]

An assistant surgeon of the 7th Hussars, after collecting as many of his own wounded as possible from the field had them carried into Mont St. Jean with the forcible help of peasants who had to be taken from their more gruesome task of pillaging the dead. He found himself in a gathering of a dozen other assistant surgeons with 500 wounded on their hands. His regimental surgeon had been called to the front to attend to his colonel and was no more seen that day or for several days after, for he went with him to Brussels.[13]

For the first twenty-four hours nothing effectual could be done, for assistant surgeons only carried a small pocket case of instruments and they were without their amputating knives. But while awaiting their arrival the doctors were not idle for with their lancets, 'we bled our fellows all round'.[14] 'No respite next day' writes Gleig, 'nor for many a day afterwards to these ministers of health and ease. Indeed the demand upon their skill was so multitudinous and so incessant that the marvel is how they succeeded to any extent in paying heed to it.'[15] Three days went by while the wounded were treated without regard to friend or foe, but their attitude to surgical interference differed, the British clamouring for amputation while the French resolutely declined the knife. One morning says Gleig all pain and suffering was forgotten in a drunken orgy, after a hidden store of wine in a cellar had been rifled during the night. As wine was never prescribed for wounds because it was thought to increase inflammation the news of this self administered carousal was badly received by the doctors.

Many of the French wounded had to endure hunger and thirst for several days, and some kept themselves alive by eating the flesh of the dead horses which lay around in thousands, their carcases polluting the atmosphere until Prussian soldiers compelled the local villagers at bayonet point to dig huge pits and bury not only the horses but the decomposing bodies of the dead. A visitor to Quatre Bras noted in his journal, 'Coming from Waterloo passed forty waggons of wounded crying out. The men had been in cottages and not able to be removed before. Many died instantaneously, others were in a putrid state—a kind of living death.'

Every wounded man who could somehow make the long journey of twelve miles to Brussels did so on his own feet, on horseback, or in any kind of vehicle, but for most of the lying cases it was not until the following morning that any aid was possible. Spring waggons, carriages, and carts of all kinds were used to convey the cases to Brussels but it took four days to clear the wounded from Mont St. Jean. A field hospital had by then been set up in the village but until it opened, Gleig tells us 'the wounded just continued to die'.[16]

Every house in Brussels sheltered the injured men and a week after the battle they were still uncounted. Additional orderlies were supplied on the scale of one N.C.O. and three men for every hundred patients, but there was no lack of voluntary assistance for 'Delicate women waited upon them and dressed their hurts—every door was open to receive the wounded.'[17] Patients were showered with gifts of food and wine. Five large hospitals[18] in the capital were quickly filled and many more wounded were sent off by canal barges to civil hospitals and hotels in Antwerp where Deputy Inspector Summers Higgins of Talavera fame was the P.M.O.; while 1,000 French wounded were accommodated in the Corderie factory under the care of Belgian surgeons. Unfortunately the spare hospital beds at Bruges, Ghent, and Ostend could not be made use of through lack of transport. James Simpson an advocate who landed at Antwerp noted 'a general air of comfort and comparative ease in the accommodation, clothing and appearance of the men'.

Additional staff medical officers poured out from England but the Director General was glad, too, to receive assistance from many civilian surgeons. James Guthrie was horrified to find how the special surgical technique of dealing with battle casualties had been forgotten. 'I found the assistant surgeons doing everything they should not have done . . . Amateur surgeons flocked over from London . . . Nothing could recall . . . the irretrievable mischief insufficient care had occasioned in the first few days.'[19] From the great number of wounded it was impossible he said to give them anything like proper attention. John Hennen was busy at the Gendarmerie Hospital operating on the French wounded, many of whom were not brought in until between the eighth and thirteenth day; amongst those desperately ill there were 140 compound fractures. Charles Bell of Edinburgh operating for twelve hours a day found that 'All the decencies of performing surgical operations were soon neglected; while I amputated one man's thigh there lay at one time thirteen all beseeching to be taken next. It was strange to feel my clothes stiff with blood and my arms powerless with the exertion of using my knife.'[20] Such experience could well apply to surgeons throughout all wars.

Mr. Thomson who hurried over with Bell from Edinburgh (his only passport being a case of operating instruments) has recorded his experiences in his '*Report on observations on the military hospitals of Belgium after the battle of Waterloo*'. In spite of the good accommodation which the hospitals provided where both cleanliness and ventilation were strictly observed, hospital gangrene and a small outbreak of typhus occured. Treatment of the former followed the lines of the Peninsula, caustics such as strong mineral acids, solutions of potass, corrosive sublimate, and arsenic,—while the actual cautery was popular with the French. Bell gives the figures as 146 primary amputations with 40 deaths (27·4 per cent) and 225 secondary amputations with 106 deaths, a mortality of 47·1 per cent. Thomson tells us that many surgeons afterwards regretted that more primary operations had not been done.[21] Compound fractures of the femur presented the greatest problem and Guthrie estimated that two-thirds of all these cases died and only one sixth survived with a useful limb; if the fracture was above the middle of the femur all died from septicæmia or shock. As Guthrie had taught in the Peninsula the prolonged application of tourniquets was coming into general disfavour because of the mortification of the limb which followed, surgeons were now substituting pads, sponges, bandages and digital pressure. Of the total of 9,528 wounded 856 or 9 per cent died of wounds.

At the end of June there were still nearly 5,000 wounded remaining in Brussels and Antwerp and several months elapsed before all were removed to England. Hospitals in many places had to be utilised and at Haslar the naval authorities, as always, extended their full co-operation and provided the best of accommodation and treatment. It was a year later before the final disposal of the cases was completed. In April 1816 the figures showed:

Total cases	6,831
Rejoined	5,068 or 74 per cent
Discharged the army	506

Posted to Veteran battalions 167
*Amputations 236
Remaining in hospital 854

* These figures evidently refer to the cases which had survived amputation on the date in question.

Since the battle of Blenheim our narrative has never mentioned the grant of prize money for medical officers after a victory. That it was given after Waterloo was due to the successful plea made by Knight when he pointed out that this was a serious grievance which must be remedied, and a comparative table with officers of combatant rank had been worked out.[22] Only those officers who served in the actions of the 15th, 16th, 17th and 18th of June were eligible and these were found to number 72 out of the 206 medical officers who served in the campaign. These too as a mark of Government approbation were permitted to count two years additional service.[23] As a personal award Gunning the senior surgeon received the Order of the Belgian Lion.

Paris was triumphantly entered by the Allies on the 7th July and the occupation forces remained in France for the next three years. The British contingent was stationed in the Cambrai Valenciennes area, and general hospitals were opened in both these towns as well as at St. Denis in Paris.

The only reasons we have for referring in our narrative to the death of the Emperor Napoleon at St. Helena is because his medical attendants during his last illness were for the most part doctors from the Navy and the Army. There are circumstances surrounding his death which are still the subject of controversy and into which we do not intend to enter.

The position of the Emperor's medical attendant was no easy one for such bitter hostility existed between Napoleon and his entourage and Sir Hudson Lowe the Governor of St. Helena that there was no personal contact between them. The unfortunate doctor was inevitably drawn into this quarrel. Deputy Inspector of Hospitals Baxter whom Napoleon refused to see was the P.M.O., and at his own request Dr. O'Meara a young naval medical officer who had been surgeon in H.M.S. Bellerophon (the vessel which conveyed Napoleon to St. Helena) was assigned as personal physician and attended him for three years before he became involved in quarrels with the Governor and was ordered home. O'Meara found the Emperor suffering from abdominal trouble which he diagnosed as inflammation of the liver. Surgeon Verling of the Artillery was ordered to succeed O'Meara, but Napoleon would have none of the Governor's choice, and Stokoe, another naval surgeon, took his place. He was a well meaning but weak man and quickly found himself in such an impossible position that he obtained leave to go home where on arrival he was court martialled for breach of discipline and disobedience to his Admiral's orders and dismissed the Navy. As he was within a few months of his retirement this harsh order was modified later to the extent that in view of his long service he was allowed to receive his pension.

Napoleon on O'Meara's departure had asked if he could be attended by one of his own countrymen and in September 1820 Dr. Antommarchi arrived. The choice made appears to have been an unhappy one. Although for a time he gave satisfaction, he was young, inexperienced, and frivolous, and Napoleon had little confidence in him; and after he had on one occasion administered an emetic which caused agonies of pain the Emperor called him an assassin and would have nothing more to do with him. Surgeon Arnott of the 20th Regiment was now called in by Marshall Bertrand of Napoleon's entourage and attended the patient from April 1821. The doctors had continued to diagnose inflammation of the liver but Arnott could find no evidence of this, and by this time Napoleon's illness was soon to prove mortal for he died some six weeks later. The autopsy was performed by Antommarchi under the supervision of Dr. Shortt who was now P.M.O. The greater part of the stomach was found to be infiltrated by a cancerous growth and at the pyloric end there was a large ulcer; the liver was reported to be unaffected. Five doctors signed the report and two other assistant surgeons were amongst the dozen officers from the Emperor's suite and the military authorities in the island who attended.

Arnott who wrote an account of the last illness[24] appears to have received Bonaparte's appreciation, for he was given a snuff box on which the Emperor scratched with his own hand the letter N.

REFERENCES

[1] Two physicians, 5 staff surgeons, 1 apothecary, 11 hospital assistants, 3 hospital mates, 3 dispensers, 1 purveyor, 1 deputy purveyor, 3 purveyors clerks.

[2] Dr. Walsh's Diary.

[3] Three deputy inspectors, 3 physicians, 13 staff surgeons, 22 hospital assistants, 1 purveyor and 3 deputy purveyors, 3 apothecaries and 4 dispensers.

[4] Including the King's German Legion.

[5] Gleig. *Battle of Waterloo*, p. 250. John Murray, London (1849).

[6] Afterwards Lord Raglan.

[7] Dorsey Gardner quoted by Kempthorne. Journal *R.A.M.C.* Vol. LX, p. 55.

[8] Gleig. *Battle of Waterloo*, p. 278. John Murray, London (1849).

[9] Gibney. *Eighty Years Ago*, p. 191. Bellairs & Co., London (1896).

[10] Gibney. *Eighty Years Ago*, p. 191. Bellairs & Co., London (1896).

[11] Gibney. *Eighty Years Ago*, p. 196. Bellairs & Co., London (1896).

[12] Gibney. *Eighty Years Ago*, p. 200. Bellairs & Co., London (1896).

[13] This is a problem which at all times has confronted medical officers. Any self respecting medical officer naturally feels he cannot refuse to go forward to the front line when the demand comes, and would be branded as a coward if he did not comply; the regiment expects it of him. But the only proper place for the regimental officer in battle is at the regimental aid post where every wounded man may expect to receive first aid. When he is called away to attend to an individual case, be he the colonel or any other soldier, none of the

wounded who come to the dressing station in his absence can receive treatment. In order to attend to one, many others will suffer and some perhaps die. This is a dilemma which a regimental medical officer should never be called upon to face but it is one which will often occur in the future as it has in the past. To illustrate the point the experience of the author in World War I, may be quoted. After the colonel of his regiment had been hit in the front line the R.M.O. was sent for and was promptly killed; the colonel survived and was taken prisoner. The only result was the loss of an indispensable medical officer.

[14] *An English Army in France*, p. 164.

[15] Gleig. *Battle of Waterloo*. Bellairs & Co., London (1896).

[16] Gleig. *Battle of Waterloo*, p. 255. Bellairs & Co., London (1896).

[17] Gleig. *Battle of Waterloo*, p. 257. Bellairs & Co., London (1896).

[18] Jesuits, Elizabeth, Annonciata, Orpheline, Notre Dame.

[19] Kempthorne 'The Waterloo Campaign,' Journal *R.A.M.C.* Vol. LX, p. 56.

[20] Pichot. *Life of Sir Charles Bell*. Bentley, London 1860.

[21] Gordon Taylor and Walls. *Sir Charles Bell*. Livingstone, Edinburgh (1958).

[22]
Inspector General		share as a colonel.
Deputy Inspector		if the head of Department share as lieut. colonel, if not share as major.
Assistant inspector, physician, purveyor, surgeon, apothecary }	..	if the head of Department share as major, if not share as captain.
Deputy purveyor, assistant staff surgeon }	..	share as lieutenant
Hospital assistant and mate..	..	share as ensign.
Dispenser, and purveyor's clerk	..	share as sergeant.

[23] P.R.O., W.O. 4/313.

[24] Arnott (1822). *An Account of the Last Illness, Disease and Post Mortem appearances of Napoleon Bonaparte.*

Chapter 13

BOTH EAST AND WEST

It is now necessary to look back to the campaigns which were taking place in other parts of the world while the main conflict in the Peninsula was being waged. We refer in this chapter to the Walcheren expedition to Holland, to Java, to North America, and to the first account of the numerous campaigns which were fought during the creation of our Indian Empire.

Walcheren 1809

A classical example of a military operation foundering under the impact of disease is furnished by the expedition to the Scheldt in July 1809, known as the Walcheren expedition. Within a period of just over four months 4,000 soldiers died of disease while the total of those killed in action amounted to the insignificant total of 106. The magnitude of such a disaster brings to mind memories of yellow fever at Carthagena and in the West Indies. But this was no tropical expedition, and only served to show that the mosquito in Holland could under certain conditions prove as destructive as its fellow in the tropics.

The operations were primarily undertaken to help the Austrians who were fighting Napoleon on the Danube, the object being to attract French reserves who might be sent to that area by forcing them to resist this threat to their domination of Holland. Moreover the British nation had always proved sensitive to the occupation by a hostile fleet of the harbours in the Low Countries, and a third reason was the desire to help the insurrectionists in the Netherlands expel the French from their country, for it was hoped that the local garrisons and the nation at large would rise and support our invasion. The same wishful thinking by the British Government and the same unfulfilled hopes had been raised at the expedition to the Helder in 1799.

The immediate objectives of the expedition were to capture Flushing and the town and arsenal of Antwerp, destroy the French fleet, render the Scheldt unnavigable to shipping, and then withdraw to England after leaving a garrison at Walcheren. Success depended upon the promptness, secrecy, and vigour with which the operations were carried out, but none of these conditions were fulfilled. However, in the early

395

summer of 1809 we find an army assembled in the Downs, 40,000 strong, incomparably the greatest armament which had ever left these shores. After the inevitable delays in providing 100,000 tons of shipping, the expedition sailed in July escorted by a fleet of men of war, which carried half the troops on their decks. As this was a combined operation everything depended on the closest co-operation between Lord Chatham who commanded the army and Admiral Strachan of the Royal Navy, but before the end these gentlemen were not on speaking terms, an unfortunate state of affairs with which we have not been unfamiliar in the past. The army comprised six infantry divisions organised into two wings, and as this has a medical impact we notice there was a small waggon train of 132 vehicles and 238 carts,—a number quite inadequate, but intended to be supplemented by local requisition after landing.

Surgeon General Keate who was responsible for the arrangements had gathered a considerable medical staff under the superintendence of Inspector of Hospitals John Webb, which included 3 deputy inspectors of hospitals, 7 physicians, 22 staff surgeons, 2 apothecaries, 4 dispensers, 4 purveyors, and more than 30 hospital assistants, a total of nearly 80 in all. Medical stores were provided sufficient for 41,000 men for six months, made up of seven divisions for 2,500 men, three divisions for 1,000 men and extra medical and surgical chests.[1] Hospital stores included marquees and tents, nearly 4,000 palliasses, over 9,000 sheets more than 5,000 blankets, together with bolsters, coverlets, and hospital clothing, etc.[2] sufficient to provide 4,000 hospital beds or ten per cent of the force, a figure which was considered reasonable but in the event proved entirely inadequate.

Keate had shown commendable activity in his preparations, and asked for hospital ships which the authorities were so slow to provide that he protested to the Agent of Transports in letter after letter; eventually only one ship, the *Asia*, 480 tons, was forthcoming, but two transports for convalescents were also made available. He was equally concerned at the delay in embarking the medical staff officers at Deal. For hospital accommodation in England the Secretary at War had authorised medical officers and stores to staff general hospitals to be set up in barracks or buildings at Yarmouth and at Plymouth, each for 500, and at Harwich, Deal, and Portsmouth for 1,500 apiece; these, together with 800 beds available at Haslar Naval Hospital made a total of 6,300 beds or nearly 16 per cent of the expeditionary force.

Before going further we must here remind the reader that at this time, following the recent unhappy Corunna affair, the quarrel between Pepys and Keate on the one hand and Knight on the other was at its bitterest. Knight in fact refused to have anything to do with the hospital arrangements within the United Kingdom and it was only after a positive order from the Secretary at War that he would provide the apothecaries and purveyors for whom he was responsible. Matters came to such a pitch that the Secretary at War issued a warning obviously directed at Knight: 'It is necessary to caution the members of the Army Medical Board from permitting any difference of opinion among themselves interfering in the slightest degree with the performance of their duty for the execution of which they are responsible to the Service and to His Majesty.'[3]

The expedition arrived off the mouth of the Scheldt on the 30th July and after landing in open boats on the island of Walcheren, Middleburg was captured with only slight opposition. The enemy was pursued to the gates of Flushing which was shortly afterwards surrounded on the landward side, while awaiting the arrival of the fleet to complete its investment by sea. On the 1st August another division landed on South Beveland and advanced without any serious opposition, both operations having been achieved at the cost of 300 casualties, 200 of whom were wounded. But now difficulties arose. A force detailed to capture the island of Kadzand lying south of Walcheren was unable to obtain enough boats from the fleet to make a surprise landing in force, and the garrison having been rapidly increased by the enemy the whole of this important phase had to be abandoned. This placed the whole operation in jeopardy, as until the southern channel of the West Scheldt was opened the fleet would have to wait until the fall of Flushing had cleared the north channel, and this meant that the enemy would have ample time to reinforce Antwerp. The French too were free to keep reinforcing Flushing with the British helpless to prevent them, and before long between 7,000 and 8,000 of the enemy were in the town. This meant that the investing force had to be strengthened, and two more divisions were landed after such delay that when they were in position the French forces in the whole area had risen to 40,000 men. Then came a further hazard when on the 10th August the French opened the sea dykes and the water began to rise in the innumerable channels and ditches which intersected the countryside; added to the rain which was heavy and prolonged, the troops up to their knees in water became soaked through, so that they began to suffer from the effects of exposure and from bowel complaints. More significant still twelve days after landing the first cases of intermittent fever or malaria appeared.

Helped by a change of wind the fleet now successfully risked the passage of the West Scheldt despite the guns of Kadzand, and Flushing was so effectively bombarded from both land and sea, that on the 16th August it surrendered with 5,800 prisoners. The battle casualties between the 30th July and the 17th August totalled 738 killed, wounded and missing. This success opened the way to the next stage which was the attack on Antwerp, but apart from malaria which now took command, there were on the operational side other good reasons for abandoning the whole enterprise. Chatham had been sent to take Antwerp because the city was insecurely fortified and weakly held. Now it was neither. The French fleet had sailed up above the city which could only now be taken by a regular siege for which the guns of the fleet would be essential. After Walcheren had been garrisoned there were only 13,000 troops free to besiege it and there were some 23,000 French in the city. The means of transporting supplies and ammunition had failed, as specie for hiring carts from the farmers was short, and Chatham resolutely refused to collect animals and vehicles by force, as Walcheren had surrendered on the understanding that all private property would be respected.

These compelling reasons were soon eclipsed by the epidemic of malaria; in South Beveland on the 20th August the victims numbered 1,600; on the 27th there were 3,400; the next day 600 more, and thereafter malaria struck down hundreds every day. The dead were buried at night by the light of torches and candles lest the survivors should see them and despair. Great anxiety prevailed at the War Office on the way operations were being hazarded by sickness and a report from Webb forwarded by Lord Chatham laid the blame on the putrid vegetable and animal matter which filled the ditches and canals of this flat and swampy country. The P.M.O. also pointed out that nearly one third of the local population was attacked with fever every sickly season which lasted from August until October, in spite of the greatest attention to cleanliness both in buildings and in person. At first he said the disease appeared as a low fever and spread with unexampled rapidity, but subsequently took a form similar to jail fever. No remedy could be devised to check the ravages.

It speedily became clear that further successful operations were impossible and Chatham decided on re-embarkation, except that the original plan to garrison Walcheren Island was adhered to, and the seven brigades totalling 19,000 men chosen for this duty took all their sick with them in waggons. Embarkation of the South Beveland troops began on the 1st September and on the 7th they sailed for England, by which date there were 8,000 sick, and from the hospital ships *Asia* and *Bulliver*[4] the invalids had overflowed on to forty transports. Two brigades which arrived at Deal on the 9th September had 3,658 effectives and 1,078 sick, and the sufferers were accommodated in the local barracks, and extra M.O's despatched to help the depleted regimental staff.

With half the force now returned to England, Chatham handed over the command to Lieut General Sir Eyre Coote at Walcheren where the fever was raging with equal virulence. In the 6th Foot the sick numbered 500, while the 23rd Foot could not furnish a man fit for duty. Nothing could stem the plague. By the 17th September over 8,600 men were in hospital, by the 1st October over 9,600, without counting the deaths within four weeks totalling over 1,000. With medical officers disabled by fever in every unit and in the hospitals at Flushing and Middelburg, there came a crisis in medical attendance, in hospital accommodation, in essential medicines such as bark, in bedding and equipment. The regimental medical officers were housing their cases in every house and farm, while the general hospitals at Flushing and Middelburg became vastly overcrowded and in the former there were thirty to forty deaths a day. Flushing had been so damaged by the bombardment that there was scarcely a room left to keep out the rain, and owing to the inundation the ground floors were uninhabitable. But the Royal Artillery who provided their own hospital were lucky enough to find good accommodation where the patients received excellent care and treatment. Middelburg had much better accommodation to offer in the former French hospital and the large and roomy warehouses of the Dutch East India Company. At Veere too there was a good hospital in a large and lofty church which would hold at least 400 patients, and there were additional hospitals at Arnemuidem, Zoutelande and Rammekens. In fact the whole island became a vast hospital.

For weeks past requests had been pouring in to the Medical Board for more doctors and more medicines. Both were met to the best of its ability, and on the 4th September a score of physicians and other medical officers, some of them temporarily employed, had arrived as reinforcements. Webb too was trying to enlist the help of local Dutch doctors but the language difficulty and their poor attainments made their help of little avail. What the Board was unable to do was to supply the full number of hospital mates demanded, for at this time it will be remembered Wellington in the Peninsula was continually asking for more, and the other world wide commitments of the British Army had to be met. One basic reason for the shortage was the better financial terms offered by other civil organizations and this therefore was not the Board's fault. Port wine, medical comforts, oatmeal, barley and porter, bark and medicines were sent over in quantity, and the depots of hospital stores at London and Portchester were increased to cater for 15,000 men apiece.

When by the end of September there were 9,000 in hospital at Walcheren and Webb himself had become a victim of fever, General Coote wrote to Chatham—'Something must be done or the British nation will lose the British army,—far more valuable than the island of Walcheren.'[5] At this, the Commander-in-Chief at the Horse Guards pressed Sir Lucas Pepys in his capacity as Physician General to go over and see things for himself. Pepys at once refused, excusing himself on the flimsy grounds that he was not acquainted with active service conditions. Keate was then approached and although he did not positively refuse he said his duties as Master of the Royal College of

Surgeons would be materially affected if he went. This was most discreditable and on the 28th September the Secretary at War wrote to Pepys—'Sir, I am directed to acquaint you that under the circumstances stated by you in your letter of yesterday's date the Commander-in-Chief and Secretary at War are of the opinion that your services at Walcheren may be dispensed with, a communication to this effect will be made to the principal officers of the Army Medical Board.'[6] Thus did the members fail their country in its hour of need. Not so Knight, the reviled member of the Board, who offered to go, but by then it was felt the task would be best carried out by those qualified as physicians, and three commissioners were dispatched. Foremost was Sir Gilbert Blane now a civilian but with former service in the Royal Navy; the others were two army medical officers, Dr. Borland and Dr. Lempriere. As Inspector of Hospitals, the man selected to deal with the crisis in the place of Webb was McGrigor. Keate was much perturbed at these choices as both Borland and McGrigor were opponents of the Surgeon General on many points of administration and he complained that his reputation would be damaged and his authority undermined as all army medical officers knew of their disagreements. But by this time no-one took any notice of what the Board felt or said, for Pepys' behaviour had been nothing short of disgraceful, and Keate registered his protest by going through the motions of resigning but not actually doing so, clinging to office on the grounds that at his advanced age he could not hope to regain the professional emoluments which he had sacrificed on taking up his army appointment. So in this way as we shall see the Medical Board settled its own doom.

To give him his due Keate as we have seen had striven to provide hospitals for the care of the invalids expected from Holland, and to augment this he now made a proposal that the hospital at Gosport should be re-opened and added to the 6,300 beds already established. Having sent every staff surgeon he could spare overseas he was concerned lest there should be a shortage in the hospitals opened at the coastal ports and he asked that the leading surgeons of the London Hospitals and their dressers might be asked to serve in these hospitals, granting them the pay of staff surgeons on foreign service. The Commander-in-Chief rejected this proposal, pointing out that there were twenty-one medical officers lying idle in the general hospitals opened in East Anglia. There was some reason in his refusal, for it was not surgeons and dressers who were required, the number of surgical cases being negligible.

McGrigor arrived on the 3rd October to relieve Webb who went home seriously ill, happily to recover, and we will meet him again as a future Director of the Ordnance Medical Department. McGrigor was lucky to arrive at all as the man of war in which he sailed went aground, and he was helping at the pumps all night to keep the ship afloat. Luckily their distress signals were seen by other ships and they were all taken off safely, his party including seven other medical officers. Although he found the medical situation critical owing to the totally unexpected extent of the calamity and the consequent deficiencies of personnel and equipment, the general hospitals although overcrowded were never disorganised as in the case of the Helder expedition ten years before. There were no conceivable steps he could take to control the epidemic but he set to work to do his best with the facilities available. There were only forty seven medical staff officers available for duty out of the original eighty, for several had accompanied the sick to England and the remainder were victims of malaria. At the outset of the expedition fifty men of the 7th Royal Veterans Battalion had been detailed as hospital orderlies and with the increase in sickness Coote had asked for 300 more; this was refused, and the General was instructed to hire Dutch civilians on the scale of ten per regiment; these were termed regimental pioneers and paid at the rate of a florin a day. The purveyors' accounts being in confusion owing to the number of clerks off duty with malaria a senior purveyor from England was sent out to put them in order. Amongst the most urgent problems was a shortage of bark, so vital to treatment, for although 1,460 pounds had been purchased by the Chief Purveyor only four days' supply now remained. While sending to England for a further quantity the gap was bridged by purchase from an American ship bringing wines for sutlers' stores, which, by the enterprise of some astute businessman had included bark in its cargo.

On the 12th October the sick were 9,614 and to look after this vast number the total of medical officers fit for duty on the 16th October had fallen to twenty-three and it was impossible to provide adequate care and attention. Happily there was excellent co-operation between the services, and naval surgeons were sent ashore to help. The only sensible course was to remove cases from the infected area by wholesale transfer to England and McGrigor advised assisting evacuation by using men of war after their guns had been removed and hammocks fitted in place. In fact 4,000 cases were sent off on the 21st, and a further 6,000 on the 27th October, but on the 30th there were still 1,300 fresh infections in hospital, and out of a total strength of over 9,000 left on the island on the 12th November, there were 4,900 sick, and the average number per regiment was 400. The 23rd Foot was quite unfit to march to Flushing for embarkation and they were conveyed in waggons from Middelburg.

The Commissioners headed by Sir Gilbert Blane in their report confirmed that the epidemic was entirely out of human control and gave the following figures:—

Date	Strength Rank and File	Sick	Died
25th August	37,737	2,702	114
10th September*	17,870	7,491	221
17th September	17,410	8,660	277
24th September	16,400	9,196	287
1st October	16,156	9,680	354
8th October	14,927	8,942	217
21st October	14,927	9,800	20 to 30 a day

*From this date the figures only refer to the garrison at Walcheren.

They affirmed there was no doubt the epidemic was due to attacks of intermittent and remittent fever with frequent relapses, and the symptoms of shivering and headache were entirely typical of malaria. Both dysentery and typhus were at the time of their inspection of little account although they were plainly on the increase. The hospital administration in conditions of extreme overcrowding and unexampled difficulties was better than the Commissioners had expected and all medical officers were striving to do their utmost. This favourable report was not however borne out by Dr. Wright who it appears had accepted temporary duty as a physician. 'Some', he said, 'even refused to do the duty and if they could effect their retreat to Flushing did not scruple to take leave to retire. This accounts for the difficulties and want of support felt but too severely by the temporary physicians in a duty which few would undertake.'[7]

This want of support which Wright complained of was largely due to the physicians' exclusiveness and inexperience of army hospitals. Although professionally competent, for Pepys only chose physicians from highly qualified men, their superior attitude is brought out by Dr. Fergusson. 'These physicians,' he said, 'could read Hippocrates in the original Greek but were ignorant of the grain scales and weights. To have touched a bleeding wound (with cannon booming in their ears) would have led to a loss of caste,—so superior were they. They quickly made themselves look ridiculous, for they had to learn from regular officers with years of service but who were much junior to the inflated ranks to which they had been appointed by the Physician General.'[8]

The only recommendations the Commissioners could make were that stoves should be installed in hospitals and barracks to dry and warm the buildings, that the rations should be augmented by providing hot breakfasts and a double ration of spirits, that vinegar should be added to the water, and warmer clothing provided.

But all this was soon irrelevant as it became plain that it was high time to evacuate Walcheren altogether as the French were planning to recapture it. In November preparations were made for destroying the works and docks of Flushing and on the 9th December the last man left the island. McGrigor was amongst the last to embark on the hospital ship *Asia* with several other medical staff officers and two companies of the Veterans' hospital corps under an officer. Landing at Deal on Christmas Day he promptly went down himself with an attack of fever.

The 6,300 beds which Keate had provided now proved anything but sufficient, for by the 1st February 1810 there were over 11,000 sick under treatment. At Deal where 5,625 were landed barracks had to be taken into use at Faversham, Margate, Ramsgate, Dover and Hythe. Hospitals were utilised at Dover, Shorncliffe, Hythe and Ashford, and at Harwich where 1,100 were put ashore, a new hutted barracks, well drained and well ventilated, provided accommodation for 400 patients from the Royal Artillery. Here Dr. Wright was appalled at their appearance. 'The pallid looks of the breathing spectres was so ghastly, they exhibited a type of resurrection, and their unhappy attendants, too few to administer relief to half the number through fatigue, were marked with melancholy little calculated to communicate hope or confidence in the sick.'[9] In the first convoy received twenty bodies were sent ashore for burial, and eighteen patients died on their stretchers.

A summary of the final figures of the epidemic is contained in the Adjutant General's report.

	Officers	Rank and file	Officers	N.C.O's and men
Embarked for service			1,738	37,481
Killed	7	99		
Died on Service	40	2,041		
Died since sent home	20	1,859	67	4,108
Deserted		84		
Discharged		25		
Total officers and men who returned and now borne on strength of corps—of which number are reported sick			1,671 217	33,373 11,296

Harry Calvert
A.G.

We may well ask if this was an epidemic of malaria why was the mortality so heavy? There were 3,960 deaths from disease amongst officers and men out of a strength of 39,219 which give a mortality of nearly 10·1 per cent. These deaths included of course those from diseases such as dysentery and typhus described by Webb as jail fever but these from all accounts were not numerous. Although the description of the patients arriving at Harwich would appear to be typical of typhus it must be remembered that many of the troops sent out were the survivors from Corunna, and a great number had already been victims of this disease; it is likely their constitution and powers of resistance were much below par, and they suffered more severely from malaria than men in prime health. Further, after a stay of some months in Holland with a water supply which must have been under suspicion there were probably cases of typhoid and paratyphoid fever and perhaps the combination of typhoid and malaria proved fatal to many. Wright describes the epidemic as a remittent fever but says there was also a continued type as well as quotidian, tertian and quartan fevers, the last two types characterised by many relapses with enlargements of the spleen or 'ague cake'. In a disease with such protean manifestations it is difficult to be precise but undoubtedly it was largely malaria which constituted the main cause of death and we can only assume that it was the malignant tertian variety with its cerebral complications which the harrassed medical officers had to deal with. Compared with malaria in Portugal and Spain the difference was remarkable, for there were only 291 deaths in a period of two and a half years in that campaign and the only explanation is that in the Peninsula the prevalent form was benign tertian.

In spite of Wright's opinion it appears that the regimental surgeons and the regular officers of the Medical Department as a whole showed great devotion to duty and emerged with credit, but the temporary physicians were inexperienced and the temporary mates who were employed were of very indifferent ability and many could barely write, spell or read a prescription. The Medical Board came out of it very badly and the ridiculous policy of employing civilians to manage the affairs of the army was shown up in all its fatuity.

When a Commission of Inquiry was held at the House of Commons Pepys was asked 'What acquaintance had you with army medical practice previous to your appointment to be Physician General in January 1794?' He replied, 'None.' 'What acquaintance have you had since your appointment with army hospital practice?' 'None personally.' 'Have you ever visited the York Hospital at Chelsea?' 'Never.' One can almost read into these replies the contempt with which the Presiden of the College of Physicians answered his accusers. But the Commission of Inquiry also blamed him for neglecting to check the quality of the medicines, which was one of his few responsibilities.

When Surgeon General Keate was giving evidence he made a spirited reply to the accusations of shortage of medicines. The force, he said, had six months supply of Peruvian bark for fever at the recognized rate of consumption, but Dr. Webb, the chief medical officer, asked for a further 1,000 lbs. on the 18th September, and on that day he gave orders for its supply, but as the request was not marked urgent there was a delay in shipping it abroad. As it had not been sent by October, he orderd 1,800 lbs. to be despatched by coach and packet to Flushing, and followed this up by 1,500 lbs. by the same means. Keate denied that any shortage of bark could have existed, because one supply which arrived was not opened until three months later. The total amount of bark dispatched was 6,954 lbs. and up to the 19th November only 3,132

bs. had been used. Moreover this was exclusive of 1,460 lbs. purchased
ocally.

However from the regimental surgeon's accounts there was at one
time a definite shortage, and this must have been caused by the shipping
delays and possible administrative muddles in Holland.

As regards bedding, Keate says no shortage was ever reported to him,
but he sent 1,000 additional sets on the 6th September and a smaller
amount on the 6th October. This quantity of course was nothing like
sufficient for thousands of sick. Again when asked why there were not
enough physicians and hospital mates, Keate wriggles out of this by
saying the physicians were appointed by the Physician General, and the
mates by the Inspector of Regimental Hospitals. The foolish division of
responsibilities in the Board made it very easy to apportion the blame
to another member. In any case the shortage of hospital mates was
world wide.

Finally, the epidemic itself was inevitably ascribed to those local
causes which, before science had unravelled nature's secrets, were the
only ones known,—poor billets, bad water, salt meat and biscuit
rations, unsuitable clothing, absence of blankets, too much fruit and
drinking too much spirits. The verdict was that no-one was to blame.

So ended one of the greatest medical disasters to befall an expedition
which in fact accomplished little or nothing of miltary importance.
It was unfortunate that the operations took place at the worst possible
time of the year for it was well known that Holland was notoriously
unhealthy in the autumn months, which was in fact the height of the
breeding season for the anopheles mosquitoes which carry malaria.
But no-one from Castlereagh downwards had ever bothered to consult
the Medical Board.

Java

We now turn to a country further afield than any the British army
had so far operated in. Java was the great seat of the Dutch eastern
empire, and Napoleon with designs upon the British territories of the
East Indies had sent out General Daendels, a capable and energetic
officer, to build up a strong base from which he could harass our
possessions. In the year 1811 the British and Indian Governments
agreed that this threat must be eliminated and in June a force of over
12,000 men including British and Indian units under Major General
Sir Samuel Auchmuty arrived at Malacca. The superintendent surgeon
was Dr. Hunter of the Bengal Establishment of H.E.I.C. and it was
usual with Indian Army forces to take one staff or field surgeon for duty
in the general hospital. The regimental medical establishments had
their normal organisation and there was a doolie corps of 100 bearers
to remove casualties. During the voyage 'the salutory regulations laid
down . . . by order of the Commander-in-Chief for the treatment of

both men and horses, and the provident care of Sir Samuel Auchmuty, who like an affectionate parent, was attentive to every suggestion that could contribute to the preservation of the health of the troops, were productive of the most beneficial effects.'[10] Be that as it may 1,200 sick including cases of sunstroke and exhaustion from the voyage, were left behind at Malacca.

Although the navigation was difficult and hazardous, a landing was safely made to the east of the town of Batavia and the city which had been evacuated by enemy troops was at once occupied. The French commander's plan was to tempt the invaders into Batavia which was regarded as so pestilential that the army would melt away from sickness, but Auchmuty foiled this scheme by proceeding to capture the enemy's cantonment at Weltevruden which had excellent barracks with large quantities of stores, guns and ammunition.

The enemy had now retired to the strongly fortified lines of Cornelis, garrisoned with a force 10,000 strong. After a week's preliminary bombardment by siege artillery the enemy guns were silenced, not however without many casualties from enfilading fire, and in addition to wounded the regimental hospitals were full of fever and dysentery cases. The task of assaulting the position was a formidable one, and the principal attack was made on the eastern side while other attempts were made on the west to cut off the enemy retreat. In a heroic action the defences were successfully stormed after severe fighting in which both armies lost heavily.

The British casualties numbered 633 of which 550 were Europeans, including 44 officers and 442 wounded and missing; the 59th lost 137 killed and wounded out of 400, and the 14th Foot over 100, an indication that the European regiments bore the brunt of the fighting. But 6,000 prisoners including 2 generals were captured, and their killed and wounded amounted to over 2,000. Shortly afterwards General Janssens the Dutch commander surrendered and the Dutch East Indian Empire ceased to exist.

In each regiment one of the regimental assistant surgeons went forward with the attack, furnished with dressings and tourniquets to give first-aid to the urgent cases of hæmorrhage. The surgeon with the second assistant surgeon took post at the regimental hospital to which the doolie bearers brought the worst cases while the walking wounded were left to find their own way back. In the town Dr. Hunter had organized a general hospital with the field surgeon in charge reinforced by naval surgeons from the fleet.

From a private soldier in one of the British regiments we are able to learn of his experiences after being wounded. It reveals the hardships which the wounded had to endure when no stretcher bearers or trained medical corps existed and it gives a sidelight on the tough and enduring qualities of the British soldier. Wounded by grapeshot in the face and body during the attack, our victim found no assistant surgeon or aid post where his wounds could be dressed, but removing the sash off a sergeant who lay dead beside him he bound up the wound in his arm, and together with some of his wounded comrades set off to find a surgeon. But his companions refusing to move until the battle was over he made his own way back until he fainted from loss of blood. Seeing his plight, an officer laid him in a shallow pit and bound up his wounds, but recovering consciousness he again set off, this time with an officer who was walking back with his arm almost shot off at the shoulder and hanging useless at his side. After passing the colonel of his regiment lying mortally wounded with his legs mangled by cannon shot and his horse expiring beside him the doolie bearers picked him up and carried him to a house used as a hospital for the severely wounded where he found 'two or three surgeons cutting and slashing and lopping off limbs'.[11] A surgeon came to dress him but to his annoyance immediately left him to attend to some wounded French officers, for which our writer roundly abused him. The only reply he got however was to be told to make his own way to the general hospital to have his arm amputated. So once more he set off on foot only again to fall unconscious through loss of blood. This time a carriage was found, which was shared with wounded French officers, and after reaching the hospital he was attended by a naval surgeon who removed pieces of cloth and a piece of Dutch copper money from his wounds. Lying in his bed in the ward on two occasions he was forced to get up to attend his fellow sufferers who were bleeding, for no mention is made of any hospital orderlies, and next day he went out for a walk with evidently no one to say him nay. His ward mates died off, some from wounds and some from dysentery, the latter brought on he says by their own intemperance and dissipation.

The hospital rations were so scanty that several patients clubbed together to have food and drink brought in from outside, and this continued until all their money was spent, but after a visit to the hospital by Lord Minto the Governor General of India who had accompanied the expedition, he was able to register his complaint to such purpose that a double ration of food was produced for all and what was still more acceptable a half pint of wine a day. His arm wound becoming septic a rice poultice was applied and amputation was threatened but averted after the wound had been slashed open and a piece of 'putrid' flesh removed; it was then treated with red precipitate of mercury which caused intense pain but relieved his symptoms and he ultimately recovered to record his experiences.

American War 1812-1814

While Britain was concentrating all her energies in ejecting the French from Spain, the United States on the 17th July 1812 declared war over the question of the impressment of British seamen serving on board American ships. The regular troops in Canada at this time consisted of four battalions some 4,000 strong, and there were a few regiments of Veterans and of Fencibles making in all a force of 6,000 to 7,000 men. But the enormous length of the frontier made such numbers seem ridiculous and the regiments were mostly divided up into small detachments dispersed over hundreds of miles in both Upper and Lower Canada. The great Canadian Lakes formed a barrier between the two countries in Upper Canada and the warfare here depended on operations both at sea and on land.

In the campaign of 1812 there were British successes on land at Amherstburg, Queenstown, and Frenchtown but the victory at Queenstown was saddened by the death of Colonel Brock, a commander of outstanding ability. There were however reverses on the Great Lakes where the American naval officers gained considerable credit from their success, while the American army commanders showed the poorest generalship, and according to Fortescue it was chiefly owing to their incompetence that Canada was not conquered.

The P.M.O. appointed in 1812 was Deputy Inspector Redmond whom we last heard of in the Buenos Aires expedition, and when he took over he found the medical resources in Upper Canada on a meagre scale. This was not surprising as there had been no replenishment since the War of Independence thirty years before. At the various outposts there were often neither hospitals nor medicines and where hospitals did exist they were poor and ill equipped. At York, the modern Toronto, which was then the capital city, the hospital was 'a miserable one . . . it was an old condemned house and could not hold more than twelve patients. Mr. Lee (the surgeon) had few medicines or purveyor's stores, particularly articles for wounded men.'[12] At Fort George near Niagara it was the same story, and he found the militia went off to their own homes whenever they were sick.

In the following year the Americans succeeded in driving the British from Lake Erie after a successful naval action where the heavier armament of the American vessels and on the British side the want of trained seamen turned the scale. But the several land actions which were fought mainly favoured our forces, and the most striking British success was gained in the fighting round Fort George on the Niagara river where the town of Buffalo and the surrounding country fell into our hands, and Fort Niagara on American territory remained in our possession throughout the war. At the same time a great stroke planned by the Americans on Montreal failed miserably but they did succeed in occupying York and burning the Government buildings. In all these engagements the forces on each side were never larger than a few thousand men, and the casualties rarely amounted to more than a few hundred on each side.

The end of the Peninsular War allowed reinforcements to be sent both from England and from France, and by August 1814 Sir George Prevost had 16,000 troops concentrated in Lower Canada. But in Upper Canada, General Drummond with only 4,000 men under his command was defeated at the fight at Chippewa and lost 512 officers and men, 321 of whom were wounded. This reverse was avenged by a successful action after stout fighting at Lundy's Lane, but at the heavy cost of 878 casualties, the wounded numbering 559. But disaster befell our naval and military forces on Lake Champlain, and the American despatch stated that the army retreated precipitately leaving the sick and wounded on their hands. When the campaign ended it was on the whole really discreditable to the American land forces that with all their resources they had not done better.

Additional medical staff officers and equipment must have been sent to Montreal with the reinforcements but details of any hospital arrangements have not been traced. There was little sickness in the healthy Canadian climate apart from a good deal of malaria round Fort Erie in the autumn months, while the long winters caused little trouble as the troops were well fed and amply supplied with protective clothing.

With the termination of the blockade of the French coast Britain had ample ships to send across the Atlantic to undertake amphibious operations, and a force of 4,000 men under General Sherbrooke entered Chesapeake Bay, sailed up the Patoxent river, defeated the Americans at the fight at Bladensburg and burnt President Madison's official residence and the Parliament House at Washington in retaliation for the Americans wholesale destruction of York the previous year. The force was then re-embarked bringing off some 200 wounded under the care of Staff Surgeon Baxter. Those unable to travel were left to the care of the inhabitants to whose credit it must be stated that they were well cared for. Half the army is reported to have been affected with bowel complaints. A similar attempt to capture Baltimore was called off in the face of some 15,000 American militia, and the field of operations was then transferred to New Orleans. This foolish undertaking was made at the instigation of the Naval Commander who it is said was desirous of prize money, and after picking up two more battalions at Jamaica a force of 6,000 men arrived off the mouth of the Mississippi river, with Deputy Inspector Robb as P.M.O. in place of Redmond who had been invalided.

Tactically the operation was a most difficult one and with the force available should never have been attempted; the troops had to be transported in small boats through many miles of shoal waterways, and when finally ashore they had to advance across swampy ground and confront an enemy strongly entrenched behind stockades. An American night attack was repulsed at a cost of 12 officers and 155 rank and file wounded, an occasion on which Deputy Inspector Thomson won praise 'for the care and attention shown to the wounded the whole of whom were collected, dressed and comfortably lodged before two in the morning'.[13]

The main battle took place on the 8th January 1815 when the American position was gallantly assaulted in a direct frontal attack. But the accurate enemy fire swept the men away in hundreds until some 2,000 dead and wounded covered the plain, and General Pakenham the Commander was killed leading his troops. For nine days longer the British held their ground while Robb the P.M.O. was overcoming tremendous transport difficulties in conveying casualties to the shores of a lake nine miles away, and Sir Harry Smith praised the creditable way he performed his task. 'The number of wounded was three times what he was told to calculate for, but never did an officer meet the difficulties of his position with greater energy or display greater resource. I firmly assert not a wounded soldier was neglected.'[14] The historian James also reports that Robb 'Met the embarrassments of crowded hospitals and their immediate remove with such excellent arrangements that the wounded were all brought off with every favourable circumstance.'[15] A few cases too ill to be moved had to be left behind under the care of an assistant surgeon.

This resounding defeat left the situation quite untenable, and the remains of the force, sick, weary, and dispirited, were re-embarked. The losses were so heavy that eleven transports had to be used each accommodating over 100 patients, and in addition every man of war received a proportion of the sick and wounded. Soon the news arrived that the expedition had been fruitless, as peace between the two countries had already been signed.

Although here again the hospital arrangements cannot be given in detail, from what has been said it appears certain that the officers of the Medical Department carried out their task efficiently under the most adverse conditions, and what is worthy of note is that both Deputy Inspector Thomson and Staff Surgeon Baxter were mentioned in despatches.

India

'Primus in Indis' is the proud motto of the 39th Foot (1st Dorsets) for this regiment arrived in India in 1755 for service with the Honourable East India Company. It was present at the decisive field of Plassey in 1757, when Clive brought 3,000 men into action of whom 900 only were Europeans, against a force of 40,000 infantry and 15,000 cavalry and with a loss of less than 100 men routed his opponents. Over the succeeding years there was a gradual increase in the number of British troops so that by the year 1800 three cavalry and seventeen infantry regiments were serving in India, a total of some 16,000 men with over 50 regimental medical officers.

It will be quite beyond the scope of our narrative to depict all the events which the turbulent history of India furnished during the 18th and 19th centuries and our task will be to concentrate only on the numerous campaigns in which British medical officers played their part. The hardships and dangers which British as well as Indian troops had to encounter and the diseases from which they suffered will lead us as far afield as Burma and China as the history unfolds and it will be necessary to describe briefly the military background of each campaign. Our narrative will range from the Mahratta Wars, the Afghan Wars, the Sikh Wars, the China and Burma Wars, to the Indian Mutiny and some of the Indian Frontier Wars. These will be described in due course in the order of their occurrence. But before they are recounted it is necessary to look at the medical organization of the Honourable East India Company since its foundation in the year 1600. Medical men were recruited into the Company from civil life and many came from the doctors in the ships which traded between the two countries. They were employed to look after the Europeans and others in the various settlements established in the country and many were men of some eminence who took part in advancing the Company's affairs. Some could wield the sword as well as the lancet and took part in various engagements; Dr. Fullerton took command in the defence of Patna in 1760 and others served both as medical officers and as lieutenants in the Company's military forces; Dr. Holwell who escaped alive from the Black Hole of Calcutta was made colonel of Militia by Clive. Their pay from the Company amounted originally to only £36 a year, but they had the right of private practice and this generally earned them a considerable sum.

By the middle of the 18th century the Indian provinces controlled by the Company were divided into the three Presidencies of Bengal, Madras, and Bombay, and the medical services for the military forces were similarly constituted by an order dated the 20th October 1763. In 1764 it became a regular medical service with surgeons appointed by warrant up to the year 1788 and by commission after that date. By this time there were 95 medical officers, with pay of 300 to 500 rupees a month for a surgeon, and 125 to 300 rupees for an assistant surgeon.

The Bengal Presidency which was the largest was divided in 1766 into military and civil branches under a Surgeon General and surgeons were liable to be transferred from one branch to the other. This was followed in 1786 by the creation of a Medical Board with a Physician General, who was also Director of Hospitals.

With the arrival of British regiments medical officers were interchangeable between European and Indian units although the establishment differed; British units had their surgeon and two assistant surgeons, while native units had one European assistant surgeon and one native doctor. There were hospitals for native troops and separate garrison hospitals for British troops staffed by surgeons and assistant surgeons of the H.E.I.C.

Throughout the 18th Century wars were continually being waged against the French possessions in India or against those native princes who supported the French. That great administrator Clive, by his victories at Arcot and Plassey, had established British power in the valley of the Ganges, and his successes were followed by General Eyre Coote, who was hardly surpassed as a soldier by Clive himself, and at the battle of Wandewash he destroyed the vestiges of French power. By 1761 after the fall of Pondicherry there was nothing left of their Indian Empire, but at the Peace of Paris in 1763 Pondicherry was returned to the French and before long was once more the seat of attacks and intrigues against Britain. Pondicherry was however recaptured in 1775 when hostilities broke out again, and for the next eight years (1775-1783) small actions were fought all over Southern India against the French and those Mahratta chiefs, Saraj-ed-Dowla, Hyder Ali, and Tippoo Sahib who were associated with them.

Peace with France was again proclaimed in 1783, but the wars against the native states continued until the storming and capture of Seringapatam in 1792 brought peace with Tippoo and the conclusion of the First Mahratta War. In this heroic action half the 500 casualties were sustained by the British regiments, and we should note that among the officers was Lt. Col. Arthur Wellesley of the 33rd Foot who distinguished himself in the fighting.

Now let us look at the medical organization which accompanied the troops in the field. In the earlier engagements this was solely on a regimental basis but in the Second Mahratta War which broke out in 1802 a field hospital makes its appearance for the first time. Administrative control lay entirely in the hands of a senior surgeon of the Honourable East India Company, and he acted both as administrator and as consultant. Under his command he had a field surgeon, a medical storekeeper, and sometimes but not always, a number of assistant surgeons. The field surgeon who was chosen for his operating ability controlled the field hospital; included on his staff were the assistant surgeons, but in their absence he had to rely for help on withdrawing medical officers from the regimental establishment. This often proved unsatisfactory, for at times as we shall see it led to inefficiency and delay in the treatment of the wounded. The field hospital was usually equipped for 200 beds and the equipment and furniture provided was, as in all Indian operations, on the most extensive scale, involving the presence of vast numbers of servants, followers, and baggage animals, which made any campaign a slow moving affair. We must not forget the medical storekeeper, really an apothecary, who safeguarded the medical and surgical stores, a task which was essential in a country where peculation and theft were common occurrences.

The regimental medical establishment of the British regiments in India at this time was very complete and self contained. Apart from three medical officers the staff also included a steward, a native apothecary, and a full menial staff, making up a total of forty-eight personnel. The surgeons acted as their own purveyors except for European medicines which were issued in kind, and we have Wellesley's testimony to the excellent order of their hospitals. The surgeons of Indian units were accustomed to make their own contracts for the hospital dieting and the supply of country medicines, and it was a common belief that they made considerable profits from these transactions. The carriage of sick and wounded on active service depended upon the use of doolies[16] and for British troops these were provided on the scale of 12 per cent.

We now pass to the year 1802 when owing to Napoleon's intrigues the Second Mahratta War became inevitable, and the British and H.E.I.C. forces with their Indian allies the chief of whom was the Nizam of Hyderabad fought the powerful Mahratta chiefs Scindia and Holkar. This long campaign which lasted for two years was contested over an immense area of country from Poona in the south to Delhi in the north, and was divided into a southern area where Colonel Wellesley was in command and a northern area where the British forces were under Major General Lake. Only a few thousand British troops took part, the bulk of the army being composed of Indian regular forces under British officers.

In planning his campaign Wellesley's chief problem was concerned with the transport of supplies and his organisation in this matter was detailed and highly efficient. Following the troops came thousands of slow moving bullock carts carrying food, forage, and baggage, and although both public followers and personal attendants were greatly reduced,[17] these were still counted by thousands.

The medical arrangements were under the control of Dr. Anderson the Superintending Surgeon of Mysore State and regarded by Wellesley as the ablest man of his profession in the country. As an innovation in Indian warfare a fully staffed and equipped field hospital accompanied the force, a contrast to previous campaigns when the staff of the hospital had been completed by drawing from the regimental establishments. Medical supplies for three months were carried in the bullock train and a similar quantity in reserve; particular attention was paid to provide sufficient bark, mercurial ointment, and calomel, while nitrous acid was regarded as an essential item for the fumigation of wards. The doolies instead of being detailed to units were here concentrated under the orders of the Superintending Surgeon to allow of more flexibility in their use.

In order not to hinder mobility the usual procedure of carrying

413

forward all sick on the line of march was forbidden and replaced by forming depots in which the sick and wounded were left under guard. This was disliked by commanding officers and surgeons alike but Wellesley's instructions on this point were emphatic. In an order issued to one of his column commanders he said at an early stage in the operations: 'You must immediately establish a hospital. Look for some secure place for this, and leave all the sick of the Scots Brigade that require carriage, otherwise the first action will be ruinous to you.'[18] Such meticulous planning was characteristic of all Wellesley's actions.

Hurryhur in Mysore was the concentration area for the campaign and here a British and an Indian hospital were set up. The first aggressive move was the occupation of Poona which was accomplished after a rapid cavalry advance, and this was followed by months of protracted negotiations with Scindia until Wellesley's patience was exhausted and open war was declared. Under his immediate command he could put into the field some 20,000 men and 5,000 native cavalry; while there were further forces on the east coast to invade the province of Cuttack, and on the west coast at Bombay. In all including garrison troops there were nearly 50,000 men of whom some 6,000 were British.

The first engagement was the storming of the fortified town of Ahmednagar in August 1803 where in a direct assault against a strong garrison the courage and élan displayed overcame the most formidable obstacles. The effect of this success was great. 'These English are a strange people and their General a wonderful man' wrote a Mahratta chief from Wellesley's camp after the action. 'They came here in the morning, looked at the pettah, (fortified town wall), walked over it, killed all the garrison, and returned to breakfast.'[19] The next day the fort itself was stormed and captured and the 141 wounded were left in a hospital opened in the town. Then followed the decisive battle of Assaye fought on the 23rd September when Wellesley with 7,000 men defeated 50,000 Mahrattas in a hard fought struggle. 'Assaye' Fortescue says, 'presents a roll of valiant deeds which is unsurpassed in our military history.' Wellesley himself had two horses killed under him. The 74th Foot lost 17 officers and 400 men, and the total casualties amounted to 650 Europeans including 53 British officers and 800 sepoys. A field hospital was set up at Ajanta twelve miles from the battlefield and the wounded conveyed by doolies or by carriage on elephants, horses, and bullocks.

With over a thousand wounded on their hands six additional assistant surgeons had to be ordered up and they were continuously at work for nearly a week before all were attended to; extra dressers were supplied by the regimental hospitals, and pioneers from units were provided. Wellesley attended personally to the patients' comfort, and each of the wounded officers of the 78th (Seaforth Highlanders) were said to have received a dozen bottles of Madeira from his private stock. The battles of Argaum and Gawilghur completed the downfall of the Mahrattas, and after the former the 304 wounded were treated in the field hospital which had been moved up to Ellichpoor.

Dr. Gilmour who was Superintending Surgeon of the Madras contingent served his commander well, but as only combatant officers at this time were entitled to a mention in despatches this honour escaped him. Wellesley however showed his appreciation by recommending him for promotion, asserting that 'those who do their duty to the army ought to enjoy its benefits and advantages,'[20] while the consideration which the Commander devoted to all his personnel is exemplified by his granting a special bonus to the kahars or doolie bearers.

We must now turn our attention to the operations in the northern area of the Mahratta territories which were conducted by Major General Lake, a Guardsman who had distinguished himself in Flanders in 1793. Lake set out in August 1803 from Cawnpore with a force of some 15,000 fighting men, the British element of which included only three cavalry regiments and the 76th Foot (2nd Bn. Duke of Wellingtons). With ten times the number of followers the army advanced across country in the form of a huge square covering many miles and at Aligarh came up with Scindia's army. By a bold and impetuous attack which was characteristic of the Commander, the fort was stormed and over 2,000 of the enemy perished by the bayonet or by drowning at a cost of some 260 killed and wounded.

Lake now took the road to Delhi, and on the 12th September he confronted and defeated 19,000 Mahrattas. On the British side there were 478 casualties of which 137 were sustained by the 76th. The capture of Agra followed, and then on the 1st November the last of the Mahratta hosts were crushed at the bloody battle of Laswaree. 'As fierce a fight', says Fortescue, 'as ever was fought by mortal men.'[21] The losses were over 800, including 29 officers and 623 rank and file wounded who were conveyed to the field hospital opened at Agra. The 76th again suffered so heavily that the total casualties of this gallant regiment amounted to 18 officers and 428 men between the 4th and 11th September.

The proud Scindia, beaten on all fronts, now sued for peace, but Holkar was still undefeated. His turn came at the battle of Deig where his army of 14,000 was heavily overthrown. But by then it was the month of May, and in their long marches to overtake the enemy, when the regulation tents were uninhabitable and the hot wind and driving sand blistered their hands and faces the British suffered disastrous losses from the heat. Within one period of four days fifteen men died.

After these successes Lake had to acknowledge defeat at the great stronghold of Bhurtpore. Four assaults were made over a period of some two months but all were thrown back at the cost of some 3,000 casualties. Holkar however finally capitulated, and the peace signed on the 24th December 1805 brought the long contest to a close.

Lake's Superintending Surgeon in this campaign was Dr. Cochrane of the Bengal Medical Department and although there are few details available of the medical arrangements a compliment was paid to the Army Medical Department when Surgeon Lyss and Assistant Surgeon Newman, (who also held a Cornet's commission), of the 29th Light Dragoons were called in front of their regiments after the battle of Laswaree to receive the thanks of their Brigadier for 'their humane and successful exertions in bringing off the wounded of the brigade at great personal risk'.[22] Kempthorne says the rate of sickness was high, amounting at times to nearly 25 per cent of the effective strength. Amongst the casualties suffered by medical officers, three of the H.E.I.C. surgeons were killed, and at Deig, Assistant Surgeon Bean of the 76th was wounded.

Leaving aside the Ghurkha Wars of 1814-1815, we come to the Pindari War, and the pacification of Central India between 1814 and 1819 which followed the risings of the Mahratta chiefs. The only battle of importance was Maheidpore fought on the 21st December 1817 in which three British regiments were engaged. Here the largest military force ever assembled in India numbering 120,000 troops and 40,000 followers had been decimated by the first serious visitation of cholera. For a fortnight the camp became a vast hospital and Lord Moira the Governor General gave orders that in the event of his death which happily did not occur, his body should be secretly buried lest the news give encouragement to the enemy.

The battle itself cost 800 casualties of which 621 were wounded and it is chiefly to recount the criticism which was heaped on the Company's medical service that we refer to it. The official historian quoting a contemporary writer says: 'In the field hospital there was scarcely a bit of sticking plaster for the wounded officers, and none for the men; nor was there a single set of amputating instruments besides those belonging to the individual surgeons, some of these without them; and we have the best authority for saying that, of those amputated, from the bluntness of the knives and the want of dressing plaster alone, two out of every three died in hospital.'[25] Doolies were few and villagers had to be impressed to carry the sick and wounded. These deserted whenever they could, leaving the wounded to shift for themselves; on one occasion they were all thrown into a river and drowned. Wastage from sickness was heavy and one regiment lost 340 men out of 800 between May 1817 and December 1818. The disgraceful lack of preparation showed the mistake of relying on the regimental surgeons to provide not only their own instruments, but medicines and hospital equipment as well. At a period when dishonesty was a prevailing sin it is perhaps understandable but none the less blameworthy that they put money in their own pockets instead of providing for future active operations. Unlike Wellesley's previous carefully laid plans in the Second Mahratta War the medical arrangements in this campaign appear to have been based entirely on the regimental system, and their failure brought home the fact that the previous lesson had already been neglected or forgotten. It is one that will be repeated in the future.

REFERENCES

[1] Thirteen regimental chests, 36 voyage chests, 32 field chests, 12 surgical chests, 24 light depot chests.

[2] Palliasses 3,710, sheets 9,340, blankets 5,420, bolsters 3,710, coverlets 2,710, hospital dresses 2,100, flannel sheets 669, linen sheets 2,140, sets of bedding 500.

[3] P.R.O., W.O. 4/408, p. 112, 113.

[4] This ship had recently been made available.

[5] Chatham MSS.

[6] P.R.O., W.O. 4/408, p. 289.

[7] Wright. *History of the Walcheren Remittent*. Bone, London (1811).

[8] Fergusson. *Notes and Recollections of a Professional Life*, p. 57. Longman, Brown, Green & Longman (1846).

[9] Wright. *History of the Walcheren Remittent*. Bone, London (1811).

[10] Thorne. *Memoirs of the Conquest of Java*.

[11] Author. *A soldier's life in barracks and camp*, p. 52. Starke, Montreal (1841).

[12] Diary of Inspector Redmond, quoted by Kempthorne, Journal *R.A.M.C.*, Vol. XVII, p. 544.

[13] James. *The Military occurrences of the late war between Great Britain and the United States of America*.

[14] Kempthorne. 'The American War 1812-14,' Journal *R.A.M.C.*, Vol. LXII, p. 140.

[15] James. *The military occurrences of the late war between Great Britain and the United States of America*.

[16] The doolie made of bamboo is a form of hammock or bed supended from a bamboo pole which is carried by four doolie bearers often called kahars.

[17] The allowance of personal attendants was ten for a subaltern and forty for a major.

[18] Kempthorne. Journal *R.A.M.C.*, Vol. LXI, p. 148. Quoting from Wellesley's Despatches.

[19] Fortescue, book XIII, chapter 1, p. 17. MacMillan, London (1910).

[20] Kempthorne. 'The Army Medical Services at Home and Abroad 1803-08', Journal *R.A.M.C.* Vol. LXI, p. 150.

[21] Fortescue, book XIII, chapter II, p. 65. MacMillan, London (1910).

[22] Kempthorne. 'The Army Medical Services at Home and Abroad 1803-08,' Journal *R.A.M.C.*, Vol. LXI, p. 151.

[23] Kempthorne. 'The Army Medical Services 1816-1825', Journal *R.A.M.C.*Vol. LX, p. 304.

Chapter 14

DIRECTOR GENERAL JAMES McGRIGOR

We have now to revert to the problems presented by the administrative control of the service following the collapse of the Army Medical Board. This is marked by the appointment of the first Director General and the beginning of the Army Medical Department. The chapter covers the years from 1810 to 1851.

From the Horse Guards on the 2nd March 1810[1] the following order was issued: His Majesty has been pleased to approve of the following officers being appointed and formed into a Board for the superintending and conducting the whole medical business of the Army, viz:

> John Weir to be Director General.
> Theodore Gordon ⎫ to be Principal Inspectors
> Charles Ker ⎭

The actual appointments were dated 24th February 1810 and all three officers were recalled to the colours from half pay as Inspectors of Hospitals. Weir had been on half pay for as long as twelve years, and why he was selected as the first Director General it is hard to say. A graduate of Aberdeen University, he had received his commission as a regimental surgeon in 1775, and passing through the grades of staff surgeon and purveyor he had been made Inspector General of Hospitals in 1795. Nearly ten years of his service had been spent in Jamaica, and now after twelve years absence from active duty his experience of the medical requirements of Continental warfare into which he was at once plunged must have been minimal. He was however a regular officer with a good military background and knowledge of the service, and therefore the antithesis of the part time members of the recently discredited Board. He was too the senior Inspector of Hospitals of fifteen years standing, and as the previous Board had paid so little attention to seniority with such devastating effects on morale it was understandable that the return to established custom was desirable.

The new policy which was to govern the action of the Board is laid down in the following statement.

'The chairman should be well acquainted with the details of military service both at home and abroad, and the two junior members should be medical officers who have served in the capacity of regimental and staff surgeons in different climates and on active service.' Every act of the Board was to be sanctioned by two members at least, which included the concurrence of the chairman, except when the Secretary at War might overrule him and adopt the opinion of the two junior members. Financial matters were to be the chairman's chief concern together with the general conduct of officers; the first junior member was to control the supply of medicines and overseas expeditions, and the second was to supervise hospital stores and accounts. The Board was to audit its own accounts, and bills would be inspected by the Comptroller of Army Accounts, while all expenditure was to be shown under one heading which should be part of the Army Estimates and approved by the Secretary at War.

From this it appears that Weir was not necessarily expected to be versed in the medical problems of active service, and personal evidence of his failure in these respects is contained in the remark made by the Duke of York in 1813 which described him as 'a good man in his time but is now an old driveller'.[2] The old driveller was however only 55 years of age! Fortunately to back him up he had two Principal Inspectors with much active service experience; the senior, Charles Ker had gone through the various grades for promotion from regimental surgeon to inspector of hospitals and had obtained the M.D. of Edinburgh in 1787, while Theodore Gordon, another Aberdeen graduate and a M.D., whom we last met at Buenos Aires, had a distinguished career during which he had been wounded on three occasions, the last time from a dangerous gun shot wound in the neck when called forward to the front line to attend to his commanding officer. He also suffered much from eye trouble and having lost the sight of one eye he was eventually compelled to retire and awarded a special pension of £600 a year in virtue of his meritorious service. To succeed him, William Franklin, again from Aberdeen was appointed; he had been surgeon, apothecary, assistant inspector and inspector of hospitals; a man of conspicuous ability he continued in office under Weir and his successor for the next twenty years.

During the five years which Weir's directorship lasted the biggest problems the Board had to face were connected with the Peninsular War, where the scale of the conflict imposed an unparalleled strain upon the Department's resources. And although the war on the Continent was the first priority there were world wide commitments from Canada in the west to Java in the east which absorbed both medical officers and equipment.

So in spite of the Duke of York's caustic remarks it would be quite wrong to assume that the Board itself was inefficient. It was Charles Ker who as the senior Principal Inspector was chiefly responsible for the overseas arrangements and the facts show that these duties were performed with ability and dispatch. Perhaps the personal capability of the Director General as compared with his Principal Inspectors is most clearly manifested by the fact that while both his assistants ultimately received knighthoods, this honour never came his way.

In accordance with the policy laid down, Weir himself was chiefly concerned with financial matters and expense, and after the scathing criticism of the extravagance of his predecessors it was perhaps natural that he paid undue attention to this aspect. This led to a degree of unpopularity with senior medical officers overseas and some chafed under the restraint. So we find friction arising with Dr. Francks the Principal Medical Officer in Portugal on certain payments to officers and extravagance in expenditure on medicines and dressings, although the requisitions were signed by Wellington himself.[3] A demand for 20,000 bandages, 500 sets of splints, 1,500 lbs. of lint, and 2,000 lbs. of tow which Francks sent home in 1811 was almost certain to be queried even although it referred to the aftermath of the bloody storming of Badajoz; while Sir James Fellowes the Senior Medical Officer at Cadiz came in for criticism both for excessive demands of medicines and extravagance in prescribing articles of diet.[4]

It may be remembered that Knight had closed the general hospitals at Deal, Gosport, and Plymouth between 1806 and 1809 thus throwing the burden of treating invalids from overseas on the regimental hospitals which were ill adapted for such long term cases. This shortsighted policy, even although it had the approval of the Commissioners of Inquiry solely because it saved money, was found to be totally unrealistic and was now abandoned. The need to re-open these hospitals was all the more urgent when Weir inherited from the old Board the aftermath of the Walcheren disaster with over 11,000 men in hospital, all of whom had to be found accommodation in temporary hospitals installed in barracks and buildings from Harwich in the north to Dover in the south.

When the general hospitals were reopened, Gosport, Plymouth, and the Army Depot Hospital at Newport in the Isle of Wight, which with the Army Recruiting Depot had been moved there from Chatham, were all well situated to receive the invalids pouring home from the Peninsula and other stations abroad. Deal however where the landing facilities were bad was closed in 1812 and the patients were transferred to York Hospital, Chelsea. Under Keate this hospital had been utilized for surgical cases only but a physician was now added to the staff to take charge of the medical cases. York Hospital was the centre where all newly joined mates spent their first few months in the army, and with its variety of both medical and surgical cases it afforded ample facilities for giving clinical instruction. This blossomed into a suggestion to start a properly constituted school of military medicine, thus reviving an old proposal which alas was destined to suffer the same fate of rejection. Assistant Surgeon Gibney who joined the Department in 1813 has described his brother officers at York Hospital as 'a comical set of fellows'.[5] He was impressed by the standard of instruction given by the hospital staff and not least by being initiated into the tricks of malingering attempted by patients; 'sores and slight wounds which under ordinary circumstances would have healed quickly became inflamed and daily worse. Tongues rubbed against the whitewashed walls certainly puzzled us doctors. Fits were common and constantly enacted in the barrack yard, lameness was a general complaint, and not a few declared themselves to be hopelessly paralysed.'[6] The officers' quarters and the food he found disgusting, the bedding was damp and dirty, with sheets so coarse as to act like 'nutmeg graters'. The messing consisted of 1 lb. of beef as tough as shoe leather, potatoes bad and badly boiled, 1 lb. of bread of the brickbat nature, and a pint of porter sufficiently sour to 'necessitate our practising on ourselves the cure for diarrhoea'.[7]

The Board were soon concerned at the number of deaths occurring amongst invalids sent from abroad and an instruction was issued in September 1810 criticizing the propriety of patients who were severely ill undertaking long sea voyages in bad and uncomfortable transport vessels, and suggesting it would be preferable for them to be kept in a warmer climate abroad.

A summary of the general hospitals from 1812 onwards includes an Ophthalmic Depot at Selsey and the number of beds are given in the following list:

York Hospital, Chelsea	385 beds
Plymouth	450 beds
Gosport	number not specified
Depot Hospital, Newport, Isle of Wight	283 beds
Bognor (Selsey)	about 500 beds (for ophthalmic cases)

All these institutions were now supplied with hospital orderlies from the Veterans Battalions.

Another problem which the Director General tackled was the running down of the immense quantities of reserve stores in Portchester Castle which McGrigor had criticized so adversely and these were now transferred to a transport vessel in Portsmouth Harbour. But the smaller depots both in London and in Falmouth were retained, the last a convenient port for shipping supplies overseas.

The immense strain of finding medical officers to fill all their world wide commitments compelled the Board in October 1812 to relax the regulations for commissions; surgeons now could be appointed direct to regiments of the Line without passing through the grade of hospital mate, and in April 1813 would-be entrants to the Department were accepted if they possessed an Edinburgh diploma on the same terms as the London Colleges, while instead of twelve months hospital attendance only six months was now insisted upon. But on the other hand civilian physicians on first joining were now compelled to learn ward duties and army procedure in the junior rank of hospital mate. They were however given a promise of early promotion to physician's rank without restrictions as to seniority. Moreover at the same time the tight rein with which Pepys had controlled the appointment of physician was relaxed when Weir in 1811 allowed any surgeon or staff surgeon who held the degree of M.D. to attain this appointment.

The further step taken to attract candidates as medical cadets by paying for their education was soon successful but others there were whose training was skimped and quality poor, and as we saw, many adverse comments came from Wellington in the Peninsula where the wounded complained, what was undoubtedly true, that they had to suffer being 'mangled' in order to provide these ignorant mates with experience. Happily at the same time some candidates came forward of good education and better qualifications which did a certain amount to redress the balance.

By 1814 when the Peninsular War was at its height the strain imposed upon the Board to obtain a sufficient number of medical officers to make good the wastage and provide a world wide service can be gauged by the fact that there were nearly 1,300 medical officers on the full pay list.

*Medical Staff Officers	354
Regimental Surgeons	313
Regimental Assistant Surgeons	573
Garrison Surgeons and Assistant Surgeons	23
Miscellaneous appointments	11
	1,274

* Includes 47 purveyors and deputy purveyors, of whom only a proportion were medical officers.

At the same time the independent Ordnance Medical Department under Director General Webb numbered a further 99 officers, while the Irish Establishment which is also in addition to the above figures was composed of:—

Physician Generals	Dr. Guinn, Dr. Harvey
Surgeon General	Mr. Crampton
Director of Hospitals	Dr. Renny

There were four medical districts with headquarters in Dublin, Athlone, Belfast and Cork respectively, each under a deputy inspector of hospitals with 34 medical staff officers serving in garrisons throughout the country.

One officer who was glad to see the downfall of the old Board was Robert Jackson who had resigned on half pay after the criticism over his administration of the Depot Hospital at Newport. Weir who had known him in Jamaica was well acquainted with his ability, and he was recalled to full pay as Inspector of Hospitals and despatched to take up the chief appointment in the West Indies where he remained for five years before his final retirement in 1815. We shall have more to say about this remarkable man in a later chapter.

Director General Weir retired from ill health in 1815 after forty years service, and from the fact that he was not honoured by the accolade his period in office must be regarded as undistinguished. But to his credit we must remember that he controlled the Department during the most onerous period which it had so far ever encountered, and during his directorship there were no Committees of Inquiry set up to investigate the misdeeds which had befallen his predecessors in office.

James McGrigor was forty-four years of age when he assumed the appointment of Director General on the 13th June 1815. In the prime of life, of proved ability, unrivalled experience, trusted and respected, there is no doubt that the choice was eminently suitable and universally popular. It was inevitable that there was disappointment and jealousy on the part of the Principal Inspectors above whose heads he had been promoted, and Dr. Ker resigned shortly afterwards, but Franklin who had already replaced Gordon, continued in office with the new Director General in a happy association which lasted for nearly twenty years. Somerville, who replaced Ker, held his appointment for only a year as in 1819 Government for economy reasons decided that only one Principal Inspector was necessary.

No sooner had McGrigor taken up his appointment than he was plunged into the preparations for the Waterloo campaign, but as Napoleon's freedom only lasted for the famous 'One Hundred Days', he was soon free to devote time to the reforms on which he had set his heart.

The period of his Directorship was a contrast to the turbulent years which had preceded it, and there were no major wars of importance to disturb the peaceful post-Waterloo period. There were it is true numerous campaigns in India and in the Far East, but here the Honourable East India Company held sway and assumed medical responsibility. For the rest there were wars in South Africa, in West Africa, and in Spain, and there were troubles in New Zealand, but these were all on a small scale and the largest of them did not involve more than a dozen battalions. McGrigor's term of office was therefore a comparatively tranquil one and the problems he had to deal with in a Department which numbered over 500 officers scattered throughout the Empire were nearly all concerned with internal administration. His personal friendship with the Duke of Wellington who was appointed Commander in Chief in 1827 served him well, for he continued to direct the affairs of the Department for the next thirty-six years, and was referred to by the Duke in glowing terms as one of the most devoted public servants he had ever encountered.

After Waterloo the Government began to reduce the size of the army. The Militia eventually disappeared, while the regular forces for the next forty years varied according to political pressure and numbered between 100,000 and 130,000, distributed as follows: in Britain between 20,000 and 30,000; in Ireland 20,000; in India 30,000; and in the Colonies between 40,000 and 50,000.

After 1815, barracks were built for most of the troops at home but their hygiene and the amenities provided were markedly deficient; un-flushed privies were associated with shallow wells for drinking water; there were no ablution rooms, and the wooden tubs used in barrack rooms as night urinals were actually at times the receptacles the men washed in under the pump.[8] Sleeping accommodation was usually over-crowded and beds were composed of wooden cribs in which men were huddled together four at a time, while the married women on the strength[9] brought up their families in the corners of the barrack room with curtains maintaining a most indifferent privacy. These wives undertook the soldiers' washing. The inveterate habit amongst troops for sealing up every aperture for ventilation generated foul air which increased the tendency to chest diseases such as pulmonary tuber-culosis, while the defective water supply often led to the dissemination of typhoid fever which was then frequent and widespread.[10]

The soldier's ration fixed in 1813[11] was 1 lb. of bread and ¾ lb. of meat daily, for which 6d. a day was stopped from his pay. The meat was invariably boiled, as only coppers were provided in barracks, two to each company, one for meat and one for potatoes. The men of each company took it in turns to cook. The soldier was therefore expected to subsist for his whole army life upon an unalterable diet of beef broth and boiled beef with boiled potatoes. And there were only two meals a day; breakfast at 9.30 a.m. and dinner at 12.30 p.m., so that for nine-teen hours he had no food at all. Not until the year 1840 was an evening meal made compulsory.

His uniform consisted of the scarlet coatee and dark serge trousers; in summer, duck trousers were issued, in itself the chilliest of materials and often made worse by the habit of pipe claying them and wearing them while still damp. The leather stock was universal.

Drinking was the commonest dissipation not only of the soldier but of all classes, but it affected the soldier the more because under its in-fluence most military crimes originated. The habit was encouraged by the regimental canteen system which was first instituted to prevent men smuggling drink into barracks. The letting of canteens to contractors brought to the State annually the useful sum of some £53,000; but the evil of it was that contractors made as large profits as possible by pro-viding veritable poison in the way of liquor. Drink led to crime, crime led to punishment and punishment often meant flogging, the maximum number of lashes permitted was now 200.

Most of the soldier's life was spent abroad, Government having fixed the proportion of ten years abroad to every five years home service. The periods abroad however were frequently exceeded. The army's stations varied greatly in climate and in health, from good stations like Canada, Australia and the Cape of Good Hope, to bad ones such as India and the West Indies, with the worst of all in West Africa. This is shown by the differences in army mortality which between the years 1816 and 1836 varied from around 13 per 1,000 annually at the Cape to 59 in India, 71 in the West Indies, 121 in Jamaica, while the West Coast of Africa was a death trap where the *annual* mortality ranged from 75 to 80 in every 100.[12]

In India the soldiers' life was one of monotony and boredom. After an hour's drill before breakfast there was little to do except when detailed for guards and pickets. To escape the effects of the sun the men were shut up in barracks from after breakfast until tea time, although the officers were never entombed to this extent and suffered no harm in indulging in sport of all kinds. But recreation for the rank and file hardly existed and drinking was perforce the chief relaxation. In the regimental canteen the soldier was allowed 2 drams of spirits which amounted to 8 ounces, but he could also buy arrack cheaply in the native bazaars. Old soldiers made a habit of priming themselves with a morning dram and many of them became so accustomed to their drinking habits that they would exchange into the relieving battalion rather than leave India.

On the other side of the world in the West Indies the problems of drink were similar. The men's only solace lay in rum, a quart of which could be bought for 6d. and when the visitations of yellow fever made life so uncertain—when the mortality in epidemic years rose as high as 275 in every 1,000 men—it is little to be wondered at. Moreover the salt meat which was issued five days a week was unpalatable, indigestible, and thirst promoting. The Commissariat was in the hands of a department which was concerned not with men but with money, and its method was to take the average price of provisions in all the colonies and to charge the soldier accordingly for his subsistence. In Australia for example victuals were cheap, but the men had to pay for them above cost price in order that the garrisons in the West Indies might cost the nation a trifle less.

All this makes the life of the soldier sound unendurable, but it was relieved by the regimental officers many of whom took a great interest in their men's welfare. Besides the Brigade of Guards who were generally in advance of most other units in this respect, many Line regiments adopted the system of giving regimental badges for faithful service and good conduct, and the hope of reward was gradually substituted for the threat of punishment.

Between the years 1830 and 1840 a new era of reform was introduced by Lord Howick, Secretary at War, by the grant of good conduct badges with additional pay. As Dr. Jackson many years previously had preached in vain 'In place of fear and punishment,—instead, honour, discipline, confidence and skill.' Reading rooms and saving schemes were set up and outdoor recreation encouraged. A new diet scale introduced in 1840 provided for the first time a supper of bread and tea; while the issue of salt meat was reduced or eliminated.

There were many changes in the ranks and titles of medical officers during the first half of the 19th Century and to make this clear we must take our reader back a few years.[13]

(1) *Hospital Mates*

By the Royal Warrant of the 22nd May 1804 hospital mates for duty in general hospitals were divided into two classes, a commissioned class and a warrant class. The former were commissioned as hospital mates for General Service, while the warrant class who were intended for Temporary Service only were designated either warrant hospital mates, hospital mates for Temporary Service or hospital mates for Local Service. Although the above Royal Warrant took effect from the 25th December 1803 the first commission did not appear in the London Gazette until the 25th July 1809, when twenty-three 'gentlemen' were gazetted hospital mates for General Service. The last batch received their commissions on the 20th April 1813, for on the 8th June of that year the designation of commissioned hospital mate was changed to hospital assistant. Those appointed by warrant however still retained the title of hospital mates.[14] The next change came about in 1830 when by the Royal Warrant of the 29th July the designation of hospital assistant was changed to staff assistant surgeon.

(2) *Apothecaries*

Apothecaries for general hospitals had been commissioned medical officers since the time of William III, and these appointments were given as a reward to senior regimental surgeons who thereby obtained improved pay and status. But by the Royal Warrant of the 12th March 1798 the status and pay of apothecaries was lowered, and appointments to this class were then made only from the junior classes of assistant surgeons and hospital mates. After the peace of 1815 when nearly all the general hospitals disappeared the need for apothecaries was eventually so small that further commissions were abolished by the Royal Warrant of the 29th July 1830.

(3) *Purveyors*

This rank also first appeared in the reign of William III and appointments to it were given to medical officers as a step in promotion. As they were well paid they were much sought after. It was laid down by a Royal Warrant in 1798 that they should be 'taken from amongst the senior staff or regimental officers whose pay was only 10 or 12 shillings a day'. During the Napoleonic wars when the shortage of medical officers became acute, purveyors after 1807 were selected from persons versed in accounts and were not necessarily medical officers. Deputy purveyors and purveyors clerks were added, all of whom were commissioned officers, the last class ranking as ensigns. As by then they were no longer medical officers the Commissioners of Military Inquiry in their Fifth Report of 1808 considered them to be overpaid. By the Royal Warrant of 29th July 1830 the purveyors branch was regarded as unnecessary, and in fact at that date there were only 5 deputy purveyors in the service, 1 stationed at Fort Pitt, 2 in Ireland and 2 abroad. Consequently no further appointments were made.

(4) *Staff Surgeons*

First established as a rank by Surgeon General Hunter in 1793, these officers primarily chosen for their operative skill either acted as medical staff officers of a formation in the field, or served in general hospitals or garrisons. In the field they were senior medical officers of brigades, and occasionally of divisions. In the former case they combined this administrative task with their duties as surgeon at the brigade hospital formed by the amalgamation of one or more regimental hospitals. In general hospitals their task was purely surgical, but garrison staff surgeons' duty included an administrative element. Staff surgeons were at first selected from a wide range of officers which included apothecaries, purveyors, hospital mates, regimental surgeons, or direct from the civil profession, but from 1830 onwards no officer could become a staff surgeon unless he had first served as a regimental surgeon. At first the rank was a wartime one only and when peace came staff surgeons disappeared from the active list, (apart from those with permanent garrisons) and went on half pay. From the nature of their employment they were usually on foreign service, thus in 1807, out of 60 staff surgeons all were abroad except seven.[15] But after 1815 the rank was adopted as a regular step in promotion on length of service, so that in later years when promotion became slow some staff surgeons were still employed on regimental duties. An important change in the Royal Warrant of the 14th October 1840 divided staff surgeons into first class and second class, the latter with pay corresponding to the regimental surgeons. The staff surgeons first class drew pay at a higher rate, and must have served three years at home and two years abroad before becoming eligible for promotion to deputy inspector. Staff surgeons second class and regimental surgeons could not be promoted until they had completed ten years service on full pay. A Horse Guards memorandum of the 17th September 1841 gave the staff surgeon first class the relative rank of major, and the second class that of captain.

To complete this review of surgeons employed as staff officers we must refer our reader back to the 18th century when we occasionally come across the designation of surgeon-major. This title indicated no positive rank but only the senior surgeon in a hospital, garrison, or command. This custom also obtained in India, where the senior surgeon of a force in the field was designated surgeon-major and later superintending surgeon, just as the senior surgeon of an army was sometimes called surgeon-general. These ranks were only temporary and local, but they did in fact carry a higher rate of pay. John Crane M.D., an apothecary, speaks of acting as surgeon-major in Minorca between 1769 and 1787[16], and in Gibraltar the senior surgeon held the title of surgeon-major throughout the 18th century. Finally, in this class we must mention the district surgeons who from 1802 were allotted to the recruiting districts into which the country was divided; from the year 1810 they were re-designated staff surgeons.

(5) Physician to the Forces

We have already seen that the appointment of physician which from 1793 was exclusive to graduates of Oxford and Cambridge had been extended in 1804 to include graduates of other universities such as Edinburgh and Dublin. Throughout the wars of the second half of the 18th century they had from their superior status acted as medical superintendents of general hospitals even although as civilians they were completely ignorant of medical administration. The chaos which resulted from the Physician General's absurd insistence on this prerogative resulted in would-be physicians being afterwards made to serve for a period as hospital mates before assuming the responsibilities and rank of physicians. A further widening of the field of recruitment came in 1811 when on the 29th July a Horse Guards letter announced that the appointment of physician would be extended to regimental and staff surgeons who possessed the degree of M.D. of a university in Great Britain. Finally, by the Royal Warrant of the 29th July 1830 came the order—'The title of Physicians to the Forces is to be discontinued and instead thereof that of Assistant Inspector of Hospitals is to be established.' And so after 170 years the designation of physicians came to an end.

(6) Assistant Inspectors of Hospitals

This rank had many vicissitudes after Robert Jackson received the first appointment on the 16th September 1795. Under the Royal Warrant of the 22nd May 1804 it was discontinued and those officers then serving on full pay as assistant inspectors received the new title of deputy inspector.[17] Then in 1830 the rank was re-introduced concurrently with the abolition of the title of physician, only to disappear finally on the 14th October 1840.

(7) *Field Inspector*

The Royal Warrant of the 22nd May 1804 abolished the title of field inspector, a designation which was applied to a few officers who were employed with armies in the field both in the American War of Independence and in Egypt in 1801. Their task had been to co-ordinate the work of the regimental hospitals and control the rearward evacuation of sick and wounded to the general hospitals.

(8) *Superintendent General, Inspector General, Deputy Inspector General*

These three ranks were done away with by the Royal Warrant of 1804 the last two classes by a change of name becoming inspector of hospitals and deputy inspector of hospitals respectively. The addition of the term 'general' to their titles was restored in 1830 when they again became inspector general and deputy inspector general of hospitals.

In illustration of the careless manner in which medical military titles were used it may be mentioned that when Inspector of Hospitals James Robert Grant had the honour of knighthood conferred on him by the Prince Regent at Carlton House on the 18th March 1819 he was described incorrectly as Inspector General of Hospitals.[18] Perhaps this mistake is hardly to be wondered at with the frequent and bewildering changes which went on. However, by 1840 the list of medical ranks had been standardised as:—Inspector general, deputy inspector general, staff surgeon first class, staff surgeon second class, regimental surgeon, staff assistant surgeon, regimental assistant surgeon.

The reduction in army strength after 1815 led to a corresponding fall in the number of medical officers, and the Director General who had always regarded the professional ability of his officers as supremely important now seized the opportunity to retain in the service only the best of them.

'The soldier' said McGrigor, 'should not be consigned to the ignorant and uneducated of the profession; he is clearly entitled to the same quality of advice as when he was a citizen.'[19]

From his previous experience McGrigor knew that under both Knight and Weir emphasis had principally been placed on finance and economy. Much of the Board's time and energy had been spent on what he regarded as relatively unimportant subjects such as expenditure on salt or oatmeal in the diet or the cost of poultices, and this was practised to such an extent that it became the chief subject of Departmental correspondence and the cause of much ridicule amongst all military officers. Primary attention was now to be devoted to the care of the soldier in sickness and in health.

Accordingly, a memorandum was issued on the 30th September 1816 which reads 'The Army Medical Board, solicitous for the improvement of the Department in its various branches, and considering the present a favourable opportunity for the selection and encouragement of well-educated persons, have thought it advisable to promulgate the course of instruction and the qualifications required from gentlemen entering the Medical Department of the Army, and during the progress of advancement in the service.'[20] Candidates for first commissions were to produce certificates of regular study at an established school in surgery, anatomy, practical anatomy, practice of medicine and chemistry during a full period of twelve months; materia medica and botany for six months; and the practice of medicine and surgery in a hospital or infirmary during at least one year, with a regular apprenticeship, or three years without an apprenticeship, in which case a certificate of having studied practical pharmacy was required. Courses on midwifery, eye diseases, and mental diseases were also recommended. 'A liberal education' the memorandum goes on to say, 'is indispensably requisite, and the greater the attainment of the candidate in the various branches of science, in addition to competent professional knowledge, the more eligible he will be for promotion; as selection to fill vacancies will be guided more by reference to such requirements than to seniority. By the established regulation, every gentleman must have served five years at least in the junior appointments before he can be promoted to the rank of regimental surgeon, and he who gives the best proofs of diligent exertion in the performance of his public duty, and of attention to the requirements of practical knowledge will be noted as the most eligible candidate for advancement.

Gentlemen already in the service are earnestly recommended to avail themselves of every opportunity of adding to their knowledge by attending universities or schools, for which purpose every facility will be afforded by the Director General, and every gentleman must be prepared for examination if called upon, before he obtain further promotion.

Medical officers are encouraged and recommended to look forward to the appointment of Surgeon to the Forces and of Physician to the Forces, and to endeavour especially to qualify themselves for either, ascending to the rank of their inclination, and to their previous study.'[21]

This then was the commencement of a new era in professional standards. No longer were certificates of attendance at lectures and at hospitals sufficient to enable a doctor to enter the service. No candidate for assistant surgeon or hospital assistant was accepted unless he had passed his examinations at the College of Surgeons in London, Edinburgh or Dublin, and in 1826 it was affirmed that a Diploma of one of the Royal Colleges must be produced.

McGrigor makes it clear that promotion in future was to be judged on knowledge and ability rather than seniority or patronage, and the first steps to create specialists in certain subjects is evident in his memorandum. The indifferent attitude which in the past many of the regimental surgeons had displayed to professional attainments had to be replaced by awakening their interest in the prospect of promotion by merit. Study leave for six to twelve months was readily granted and a new spirit of emulation appeared which was applauded by their brethren in civil life.

The Department called for a higher standard of entry than either the Royal Navy or the Honourable East India Company, for these services were willing to accept medical men who possessed only certificates of attendance. Moreover the Navy in 1838 was still suffering from assistant surgeons being appointed only by warrant, and in 1840 Burnett the Director General confessed that not a single candidate had appeared for entry to the service.[22] On the other hand the Ordnance Medical Department which always attracted a high standard of medical officer was the only branch which insisted on candidates presenting certificates of good moral conduct and character.

The vindication of his policy came later when McGrigor with no little pride was able to observe, 'in the ranks of the medical officers of the army men are to be found upon a level at least with those in the Colleges of Physicans and Surgeons of London, Edinburgh and Dublin,'[23] and 'Taking the profession in civil life generally, there are comprised in the body of the medical officers of the army, not fewer men of literary attainments and university education than in the ranks of civil life.'[24]

The actual reduction in the strength of the Department on selected dates after peace was proclaimed is given in the following table:[25]

Category	1814	1821	1831	1841
Medical staff officers	354	238	141	162
Regimental surgeons, regimental assistant surgeons, garrison surgeons and miscellaneous appointments	920	327	385	380
	1274	565	516	542

These figures include purveyors although after 1807 they were not always medical officers. Of the 238 medical staff officers in 1821, 182 were serving abroad, and their distribution in 1831 is given in the footnote, showing the responsibilities which the claims of Empire were making.[26] After 1840, Hong Kong, Australia, and New Zealand were added to the list of stations, while in India in 1845 a senior staff officer was making his appearance for the first time. The reason for sending an officer to India will be related in the chapter dealing with the First

Sikh War but reference must be made to it here. It was a matter which called for diplomacy on McGrigor's part for the Honourable East India Company was entirely responsible for the medical arrangements in India. Criticism had however been directed to the neglect of the British wounded after the battle of Ferozeshah, and a senior medical staff officer was sent out from home to hold a watching brief over the Queen's Troops. McGrigor carefully pointed out that this position called for much circumspection, moderation, and tact, to ensure that the amicable relations with the Medical Department of the Honourable East India Company should not in any way be jeopardized, and his task was to be confined entirely to the professional aspects of treatment and was not concerned with administration or finance; happily, no evidence of friction between the Services arose.

We must now deal with the questions of promotion and pay. The successive steps of promotion in 1831 were laid down as follows:— Assistant surgeon for 5 years before promotion to regimental surgeon; 7 years as regimental surgeon before promotion to staff surgeon; staff surgeon for 10 years before promotion to assistant inspector of hospitals; 2 years in this rank before becoming deputy inspector general, and a further 5 years before inspector general, making in all 29 years total service. As one would expect, there was constant pressure by the Department to improve the rates of pay over the years, a process which involved the customary long wrangle with the Treasury to justify the necessity for such increases. Following the Royal Warrant for 1830 the rates established are given below.

Rank	Daily rate of full pay	Daily rate of half pay
Regimental Assistant Surgeon	7s. 6d.	4s.
Staff Assistant Surgeon	7s. 6d.	4s.
Apothecary	9s. 6d.	5s to 7s. 6d.
Regimental Surgeon	from 11s. 4d. upwards, according to service, and 18s. 10d. if over 20 years service.	7s. and 10s. after 20 years service from ill health contracted on service. 15s. after 30 years service with unqualified right to retire.
Staff Surgeon	14s. 3d. to 18s. 10d. according to service.	As for regimental surgeon.
Physician	19s.	10s.
Deputy Inspector General	{ 23s. 8d. to 28s. 6d. according to service	12s. to 15s. according to service.
Inspector General	36s. to 40s.	20s. to 30s. according to service.

The titles of apothecary and physician were now abolished by this Royal Warrant, and physicians took the rank of assistant inspectors of hospitals.

The total cost of the establishment of medical staff officers amounted to between £40,000 and £45,000 a year, of which sum the Director General's Headquarters accounted for £5,614. 12s., including the Director General at £2,000 a year, one principal inspector at £1,200, one professional assistant at £410. 10s, one secretary and clerks at £600. The title of professional assistant had been added to the establishment when the second principal inspector had been abolished in 1819. At the same time there were many hundreds of officers on half pay, and there were even some venerable regimental surgeons who were still only drawing the old rates of 2s. a day; in 1826 there were 679 medical officers in the half pay category, but by 1847 the total had fallen to 357.

Ten years later the rates of pay were reviewed in the Royal Warrant for 1840 and to the lower ranks especially increases were granted after a fight with the Treasury which lasted for two years. These increases and the equivalent ranks accorded to medical officers are as follows:

	Daily rates of pay			
	Under 20 years service	*20 to 25 years service*	*Over 25 years service*	*Equivalent rank*
Regimental assistant surgeon, Staff assistant surgeon	7s. 6d. and 10s. after 2 years			Lieut.
Regimental surgeon 2nd Class staff surgeon	13s. and 15s. after 10 years	19s.	22s.	Captain
1st Class staff surgeon	19s.	22s.	24s.	Major
Deputy inspector general	24s.	28s.	30s.	Lt. Colonel
Inspector general	36s.	38s.	40s.	Brigadier

In addition to these rates additional pay was granted for field service; in a force of 10,000 men and upwards the Head of the Department received 20s. a day; in a force of 5,000 men and upwards, 14s. and if less than 5,000 men, 10s; while if serving in a Colony where the forces numbered 1,500 and upwards, 5s. a day.

The status of medical officers vis-à-vis their comrades of combatant rank was a matter of continual concern and argument. It was felt strongly that the rank of senior officers should be the same as that of combatant officers of corresponding rank, and it was stressed that although medical officers were the proper advisers on measures necessary to keep medical practice abreast of scientific progress and the problems of sick wastage, the rank and status officially accorded to them did not bear this out. Because of this their power to make their representation effective was weakened. Sir George Napier voiced this feeling when he wrote, 'It is a very general but unjust idea to think slightly of the medical men, for few officers receive so good an education or are so generally acquainted with science and literature. I am bound to state that if one takes the conduct of the whole Medical Department of the Army into consideration one will find few such large bodies of men who are more distinguished for their kindness, skill and indefatigable exertions for the health and comfort of the sick and wounded; and, as to danger, the medical officers of the British Army have, without exception, invariably shown an utter contempt for it either in the field of battle or, which requires a higher courage, in the hospitals of plague or yellow fever.'[27]

It came about in 1850 that one of these contentious questions of status was resolved. There was a long standing complaint that A.M.D. officers who shared the dangers of the battlefield were not eligible for those honours or awards which were open to combatant officers. There was a trenchant article in the *Lancet* in 1849[28] by an author who remained anonymous which strongly pressed the claim for medical officers to be eligible for the award of the Order of the Bath. Lieut General Sir Howard Douglas and General Sir de Lacy Evans were amongst the military advocates who supported the claim although the majority of senior officers were it is said not enthusiastic. But de Lacy Evans raised the issue with success in the House of Commons, and the measure was passed, but argument continued as to whether the Civil or the Military Order should be awarded. The Department was of course a Civil Department of Government but there was profound opposition from the military medical officers against the Civil award, and their civilian confreres also protested because they saw that the number of their own awards would be materially reduced. The *Lancet* supported the army doctors in emphatic terms and said they did not ask for the civil dignity and did not want it because they shared the same conditions of active service as the combatant officers in regiments, and in combat conditions and in the trenches were equally exposed to danger and death. Under this volume of protest Government finally relented and the award of the Military Order was confirmed. The *Lancet* expressed its satisfaction. 'We believe this signal triumph—for triumph it is—to be the greatest step ever made by our profession towards obtaining its just recognition by the State ... It is the removal of a profound stigma which has hitherto attached itself to those departments of the profession in the more immediate service of the Government. Surgeons are no longer to be treated as aliens to our fleets and armies.'[29]

General Evans' efforts to improve the image of the Medical Department took a further form. In the year 1807 a chair of military surgery had been instituted at the University of Edinburgh during the Napoleonic Wars. This chair owed its origin to a spirited memoir addressed to Government by Dr. John Bell who was shocked at the poor treatment of the wounded sailors after the battle of Camperdown. The original appointment was held by Mr. John Thomson, an able and experienced surgeon, but a man totally unacquainted with military medicine except for his experience in the military hospitals in Brussels after Waterloo. In 1822 he was succeeded by Dr. George Ballingall, a retired regular surgeon who widened the scope of instruction to include steps to improve the health of the soldier, the organisation of medical units in the field, and the transportation of casualties. After an uncompromising start when prejudice and misconception met him on every side his course became so popular that, when voluntarily taken, it became one of the subjects included in the graduation course.

Evans was now successful in having a bill passed through the House of Commons authorising similar chairs at Dublin and London and within a fortnight the College of Surgeons in Ireland had agreed to co-operate. This was not altogether fortuitous, for Mr. Tuffnell, an Irish surgeon, had previously in 1846 on his own initiative begun to teach military surgery as a separate branch with such success that the medical departments of the Navy and Army had already recognized it as equivalent to six months surgery in the professional qualifications required for entry. In 1852 the East India Board had also followed suit. It was now only London which lagged behind, but the establishment of a chair here was overtaken by the outbreak of the Crimean War. In due course we shall see that the creation of the Army Medical School after the war made the chairs of military surgery in the other capitals superfluous, and these were closed down, the funds being utilized for paying the professors of the new school.

The prospects of promotion were disappointingly slow as the best of the half pay officers were necessarily re-employed as vacancies became available. This delay in promotion, said Ballingall, prevailed to a most injurious extent and constituted an evil of no common magnitude; at one time there were assistant surgeons of 20 years standing, and one was quoted as dying at the age of 43 after 23 years service, while as late as 1851 there were seven regimental surgeons still serving who wore the Peninsular medal and had over 40 years service. To help the block in promotion earlier retirement was suggested with the promise of a better pension, for this was so wretched that officers were almost forced to remain in the service, and the Department carried many who were useless and worn out.

Officers were permitted to remain on half pay as long as they wished provided they conceded the right to be recalled when their services were needed, but numbers in private practice considered this a hardship, and it was extraordinary how, after drawing half pay for twenty years, many claimed that they were suffering from ill health contracted on service and should be allowed to retire on a pension of 10s. a day. Those who went on half pay naturally engaged in civilian practice and one of the advantages of army service was the knowledge that they could set up private practice, often in partnership with the local druggist, without having to undergo further examination beyond that which they had passed at the College of Surgeons on first joining. But in 1815 this much prized privilege was swept aside by the Apothecaries Act which permitted apothecaries to charge fees, but only if they became Licentiates of the Society after examination and a five year apprenticeship with evidence of instruction at a hospital. For the first time penalties were imposed on those who were unlicensed, and in this way the qualified practitioner came into being, an important step in medical ethics. This Act however created consternation amongst the half pay medical officers who saw their future livelihood dependant upon passing a further examination by the Society of Apothecaries and one retired surgeon expressed himself in the *Lancet* in the following terms:

'In 1816 the reduction of our military and naval forces was immense and hundreds of medical officers were thrown upon half pay, and among the rest the writer of this article. What did the Hags? ("The Hags of Rhubarb Hall" was a term invented by the editor, Wakley, to attack the Society of Apothecaries). Why, they promulgated a notice intimating that no persons, and of course neither army nor navy surgeons, could practise as apothecaries until examined by them!!! Had it been ordained by law that such examinations were to be conducted by Fellows of the College of Physicians, all would have submitted with cheerfulness, and many with pride; but I will not attempt to describe my feelings upon that occasion. I was one of a number who had been interested, many years, with the medical charge of 600 to 800 men, who had seen much disease in various parts of the world; had been painfully conversant with gunshot wounds; and had performed of the capital and minor operations of surgery, not a few;—I submit to examination by the drug-pounders of Blackfriars!!! My disgust and indignation was not singular; the sensation was universal in both services; and memorials were instantly forwarded to the heads of the respective departments, of which these shop-keepers were no sooner aware than they met, concocted and advertised a by-law exempting from the operations of their Act all medical officers who had served his Majesty!!![30]' It was not however until 1825 that in Mr. Brougham's Declaratory Act a clause was inserted which allowed army and navy surgeons to practise as apothecaries without having to undergo further examination or to receive any certificate from the Worshipful Company.[31]

In common with the pressure on all army departments to reduce expense an investigation was made into the headquarter establishment of the Army Medical Department.[32] Previous to 1810 the members of the Medical Board received pay of about £2 a day, which was partly staff pay and partly civil pay. After Weir became Director General staff pay was abolished and officers were paid entirely from civil sources; this meant that they were purely departmental officers and as civilians were entitled to a superannuation allowance. Under the new proposals contemplated the Director General was to be abolished and replaced by an Inspector of Hospitals, with one assistant graded as an Assistant Inspector; these would draw only staff pay and their salaries with allowances would amount to £1,788. 4s. thus constituting a saving of over £1,800 a year. But on further investigation it was found that under the terms of the superannuation allowance the amount of retired pay to which they were entitled would mean very little saving. At the same time the Horse Guards was impressed with the degree of responsibility which the Director General was now bearing, especially as we shall see with the emphasis on the methods leading to the prevention of sick wastage which would result in great financial economics. The Duke of Wellington therefore rejected the proposals.

In the case of the Irish Board however revision was agreed to, and in 1832 the Physician General and Surgeon General each drawing a salary of £320 a year, were abolished, and the responsibility transferred to the Director General in London. But Dr. Renny the Director of Hospitals was regarded as a special case on account of his long and meritorious service and he was allowed to continue in office until he retired; moreover the saving in his salary as compared with his rate of pension was negligible. After his retirement in 1847 administration of the Irish Establishment was controlled by one deputy inspector in Dublin and one in Cork. The Ordnance Medical Department also came under scrutiny but for similar retired pay reasons the proposal was shelved. These investigations extended beyond the medical branch to all departments and their rejection meant that the army organisation for many years remained as it had been in 1815. When the Crimean War broke out all had to be ruthlessly altered under the pressure of events. In fact the organisation of the army as an army did not really exist in time of peace. There were only a number of regiments which might be combined into an armed force. The regiment was everything, and units were usually scattered in small detachments over a wide area in the interests of internal security for there was no police force existing in the country until 1829. Not until 1853 was combined training ever attempted, and in that year the first camp of exercise was formed and three brigades of infantry with ancillary troops did a month's training together. A few years before this, in 1849, enlistment for unlimited service was once again abolished, and in this connection it is interesting to note that according to Marshall who was intimately concerned with statistics, by the time the soldiers had reached the age of forty, 95 per cent had either died, deserted, or been invalided for infirmities or by purchase. Now a short service period of ten years in the infantry and fourteen years in the cavalry was substituted; the object of this change being the compelling necessity to build up a regular army reserve.

The number of assistant surgeons in regiments now differed according to where the unit was stationed; in India and in the West Indies there were three in addition to the regimental surgeon; on the Colonial stations there were two, and at Home stations only one. In 1824 hospital sergeants were appointed to battalions of infantry at home and abroad except in India, and later the same year acting hospital assistants were abolished and their duties performed by hospital sergeants.

Coming now to hospital administration the most important change was the closing down of York Hospital at Chelsea and the establishment of the principal military hospital at Fort Pitt at Chatham. The reason for this change was solely a question of convenience of site. York Hospital which had originally been established by Surgeon General Keate because he wished to operate on the wounded from Flanders had now outlived its usefulness, for its location in the centre of London was inconvenient for the transportation of cases and a site directly accessible to shipping was needed where invalids from overseas could be easily landed. The port of Chatham at the mouth of the Thames provided these facilities and the barracks at Fort Pitt were regarded as suitable for conversion. The fort had been constructed during the Napoleonic wars and commanded a fine view of Chatham harbour. There were nine wards accommodating some 200 patients intended mainly for invalids from abroad. At Fort Clarence nearby the first lunatic asylum was opened in 1819; and many years later in 1845 wives and families were admitted to Fort Pitt. Although the conversion of barracks can never be ideal for hospital use a French visitor spoke highly of its organisation and the skill of its surgeons.

Here also the new depot was established where medical officers joined on first commissioning, and where they spent a period of probation receiving instruction in officers' duties, in medical administration, and in military medicine and surgery in the hospital wards. That a course of tuition in officers' behaviour was necessary we learn from Dr. Fyffe in his *Reminiscences*.[33] He describes most of his fellow officers as pretty rough specimens of the Scottish and Irish schools who badly required a course of mess instruction on how to use a silver fork or a finger bowl at dinner, and he says the time spent on meals was not the least part of their education. This instruction in the niceties of mess behaviour was in the hands of Inspector General James Forbes who founded the first medical staff officers' mess. One of Fyffe's complaints was its high cost when he was trying to live on a meagre salary of £126 a year. He praises the excellent arrangements for professional study as well as the classes of operative surgery on dead subjects, and the facilities of the library and museum.

McGrigor's museum was established in the underground chambers of Fort Pitt and was divided into a natural history section and an anatomical and pathological section. Here too was an anthropological collection of skulls some 458 in number known later as the Williamson Collection from the surgeon major of that name who became its curator. This collection of skulls was later handed over to the Natural History Department of the British Museum between 1841 and 1849. The museum itself acquired a reputation of importance and a medical journal of the period mentions visits by distinguished surgeons and naturalists.

One of the Director General's most cherished ambitions was to establish an army medical school where officers on first joining would undergo systematic instruction in all forms of army procedure and medical and sanitary administration as well as the diagnosis and treatment of the common diseases which afflicted the soldier. Such a school had been strongly advocated many years previously by such ardent reformers as Brocklesby and Jackson. But at the termination of a war which had involved vast expense any scheme which required financial expenditure was certain to be rejected, and Government refused to entertain it. Nearly fifty years were to elapse before it became a reality. McGrigor had to be content with what he regarded as the very inadequate instruction which the period of probation of a few weeks at Fort Pitt provided, where no systematic lectures by qualified instructors was possible. But in other ways he was able to promote the professional interest which was so dear to his heart, and a library was formed to which he contributed some 1,500 volumes of his own.

From his extensive experience in the Peninsular War McGrigor regarded accurate returns as of the highest importance and he was now in a position to initiate this on the largest scale. The reports were to embrace very aspect of the living conditions of the soldier; the rations and diets; the sites of barracks and cantonments; climate and conservancy, and the prevalence of disease in the various stations. From 1817 onwards these returns provided a record of valuable information on the state of health in all parts of the Empire, and the collection of 303 volumes of McGrigor's reports is housed in the Muniment Room of the Royal Army Medical College, providing unlimited scope for research on the life of the soldier in barracks and in the field. Sir James had once remarked 'The efficiency of an army must ever depend on the state of the health of the corps which comprise it, and no regiment will ever be found healthy when the internal economy is bad. It is a trite but true saying that a good C.O. will generally have a healthy and effective regiment. Whenever there was much attention paid to the discipline and exercise of the men, where they were well fed, personal cleanliness as well as of the quarters kept up, the men's clothing repaired, and the men regularly messed, that regiment was always invariably found healthy.'

In the early years of the 19th century the mortality rate amongst the troops at home was between 15 and 17 per 1,000 compared with a rate in the civil population of 10 per 1,000. Barrack hygiene and ventilation were defective and with the soldiers packed into overcrowded barracks contagious diseases such as typhus and infectious diseases such as lung tuberculosis were common. The Brigade of Guards who were often notoriously overcrowded had the highest rate in the Kingdom with 21·6 deaths per 1,000 in the period 1830-36, mainly caused by chest complaints. The admission rate was around 1,000 per 1,000 troops per annum, and amongst the causes of ill health venereal diseases mostly syphilitic in origin was the largest single factor with 20 to 25 per cent of admissions. Out of 5,861 patients in regimental hospitals in 1808 there were 1,308 venereal cases.

Outbreaks of cholera was one of the hazards of these years. The disease which was Asiatic in origin spread overland through the Middle East and Russia and appeared first in Europe in 1817-23, but it did not affect Britain until 1826 when it reached Sunderland and London by ships from the Baltic. During the next thirty years a succession of epidemics occurred; one in 1832 when there were 14,796 cases of which 5,432 proved fatal, and again in 1849-50, when there were 54,000 deaths 15,500 of them in London alone. The disease was regarded as being spread by 'atmosphere' until Snow in his famous Broad Street experiment electrified the profession by proving that it was water borne, although previously in India it was beginning to be associated loosely with drinking impure water. It was this discovery which led to early efforts in preventive medicine, although Pasteur's experiments which led to the foundation of bacteriology were still to come. During the 1832 outbreak the Director General had emphasized the need for the strictest sanitary discipline and this was so strictly obeyed that out of some 20,000 troops in the Kingdom only 108 contracted cholera, and 42 lost their lives. 'We are disposed,' said the Medical Board, 'to attribute the comparative exemption . . . to the strict and exemplary manner in which . . . the regulations were enforced by commanding officers . . . and the promptitude and judgment with which all incipient symptoms were detected and arrested by the medical officers in charge.' In 1846 a considerable stir was created in the corridors of the Medical Department following a disastrous outbreak of cholera in the 86th Regiment in Karachi. The Director General, struck by the vivid account given by Surgeon Thom, ordered his account to be circulated to all medical officers through the Adjutant General's branch and published in Parliamentary Papers.[34]

It was not until 1835 that the statistical information contained in McGrigor's returns was put to practical use when Dr. Marshall whom we last came across as S.M.O. Ceylon, became aware of their value. Marshall, now an Inspector General of Hospitals has truly been called 'The Father of Medical Statistics' and the importance of his work is difficult to exaggerate if only for the powerful effect it had in rousing public opinion. He was besides an intelligent and discerning writer on many military subjects such as recruiting and punishments, while his *Military Miscellany* which was published in 1846, although critical in many respects of prevailing methods was accepted by Lord Panmure when Secretary at War as 'my bible in all that relates to the soldiers' welfare'.[35]

Initially, Marshall was asked by the War Office to make enquiries regarding expenses incurred in the Colonies on replacing soldiers who died or were invalided, and while seeking this information he realized the opportunities provided by McGrigor's returns to extend this enquiry into a more general investigation. His chief object he tells us was 'to excite attention to the means which may ameliorate the condition of the soldier, and exalt his moral and intellectual character.'[36] Associated with him was Captain Tulloch of the 45th Foot who, before joining the army, had been trained as a lawyer, and as a subaltern had exposed various scandals with regimental pay and food and pension frauds tolerated by H.E.I.C. in Burma. He was now employed in the Recruiting Service and was led from an interest in pensions to an enquiry into mortality rates, in the course of which he first met Marshall. By the instigation of Earl Grey who was Secretary at War they collaborated in drawing up a report on the state of health of troops in the West Indies which was presented to Parliament in 1838.

Their researches which covered the years 1817 to 1836 brought to light certain facts affecting the health of the soldier which led to important conclusions. They showed that in the Windward and Leeward Islands the mortality was 78·5 per 1,000 and the admissions to hospital 1,903 per 1,000 for European troops each year. In Jamaica the figures were 1,812 admissions to hospital per 1,000 and mortality 121·3 per 1,000 per annum. Between the years 1817 and 1836 there were 86,541 admissions to hospital and 5,966 deaths, while in the four unhealthy years of 1819, 1822, 1825, and 1827, when there were epidemics of yellow fever the greatest mortality amounted to 259 per 1,000 per annum.

Amongst the causes of death, yellow fever proved to be the most deadly, with one man dying in two and a third cases; next to yellow fever came typhus with one death in every four and a third cases, and among the less deadly illnesses:

Remittent fever	—	1 in 9 cases
Common continued fever	—	1 in 23 cases
Intermittent fever	—	1 in 165 cases

Although all these facts had been known for many years, it was Marshall and Tulloch who turned on them the discerning eye of the statistician which led them to certain conclusions. The heavy wastage from sickness in the tropics had previously always been put down to exposure to a high degree of temperature; as Marshall put it 'atmosphere was everything'. But they were able to explode this theory at once because in the different West Indian islands with the same temperature, there were large differences in the rates of sickness, and the mortality in one year might be as much as twenty times greater than another year. Another theory that sickness depended on an excess of moisture was also proved to be false but the most important practical point was the discovery of the fallacy of what was known as 'seasoning', the theory that troops became accustomed to the climate as time went on and therefore suffered less from sickness. This was the reason that regiments were kept for as long as nine or ten years in the same station. Marshall showed this theory to be false and was able to prove that young soldiers lived longer in a bad climate and mortality increased with age, as the following statistics show.

1)	Age	Annual ratio of deaths per 1,000
	18—25	50
	25—33	74
	33—40	97
	40—50	123

2) Annual ratio of deaths per 1,000 according to length of residence	
Resident one year	77
Resident two years	87
Resident over two years	93

After the report had been digested by Parliament the existing policy of regimental reliefs was scrapped, and instead of remaining in one station for many years, units were now moved to successive foreign stations in turn. The benefit to health which this policy achieved can be appreciated from the fact that the mortality in the West Indies fell from around 80 per 1,000 to 62 per 1,000, and in Jamaica from 120 per 1,000 to 60 per 1,000.

Marshall had to retire in 1836, and after his place had been taken by Assistant Surgeon Graham Balfour of the Medical Department Tulloch and Balfour continued to initiate a series of reports which covered all the stations throughout the Empire, a summary of which is given in the table:

Station	Year	Annual admissions per 1,000	Annual mortality per 1,000	Ratio per 1,000 of mean strength constantly sick
Windward and Leeward Islands	1817—1836	1903	78·5	87
Jamaica	1817—1836	1812	121·3	63
United Kingdom	1830—1836	929	14	37·3
Gibraltar	1818—1836	966	21·4	41
Malta	1817—1836	1142	16·3	45
Canada	1817—1836	1097	16·1	44
Sierra Leone	1819—1836	2978	483	
Gold Coast	1823—1826	—	668	
Cape of Good Hope	1818—1836	991	13·7	
Ceylon	1817—1836	1678	69·8	143
Burma	1827—1836	1587	44·7	

Apart from the West Indies these statistics revealed the appalling wastage of soldier's lives in such stations as West Africa, Ceylon and Burma, and later we will give further details of the conditions in West Africa which exacted a toll of between 50 and 70 per cent of the garrison each year.

The authors then prepared a new sanitary proforma to be submitted annually by the P.M.O. of each station to the Secretary at War, stating how far sickness and mortality had been affected by:—

a) the duty and employment of the troops

b) the barrack and hospital accommodation

c) dieting

d) crime and punishment

e) intemperance.

A second series of reports commenced in 1848, but after the first one had been completed the outbreak of the Crimean War stopped further publication. In the year 1860 Annual Reports on Army Health were instituted.

From these reports the arousing of public interest and the emergence of proposals to improve the troops' living conditions can be dated and it is to Government's credit that in spite of the financial stringency from which all departments suffered, the logic that money spent in bettering the soldiers' health would save expense in soldiers' lives was a powerful lever to induce the Treasury to provide the funds.

A further step in the saving of public funds came about the same year that Marshall was carrying out his researches. This concerned greater care in the selection of men for foreign service, and was brought into force by a General Order published on the 25th March 1836. It arose from the fact that the hospitals abroad were being crowded with men who should never have been sent overseas because of disabilities such as tuberculosis, chronic bowel diseases, chronic ulcers, rheumatism (especially in old soldiers), and chronic eye disease, and the expense of invaliding them home again was considerable. The retention of so many soldiers who were unfit was largely due to the terms of enlistment for life which at this time prevailed, and in fact the commonest author-ised category for invaliding was 'worn out', although this was only applicable to soldiers with more than fifteen years' service; within a period of four years when the total invalids numbered 5,963, there were 2,195 or 36 per cent in this class; other common causes were fractures, dislocations, wounds, and hernia, which together amounted to 1,420; followed by chest diseases, 1,216; dysentery and hepatitis, 846; and rheumatism, 822; invalids due to venereal disease (which meant syphilis) were only 13 in number, so that the great majority of these sufferers continued to serve on.

When the only means of avoiding service was by invaliding it was inevitable that malingering was common, and warnings to medical officers to be on their guard against feigned diseases were frequent. Epilepsy and palsy, the instruction states, are often simulated, and under chest diseases we are told 'The stethoscope is highly useful in detecting the simulation of consumption, a class of imposters found in almost all hospitals'. In fractures the degree of disqualifying effect is sometimes entirely feigned. Rheumatism too was a fertile source of deception but the instruction astutely adds—'military exercise seldom aggravates this complaint and sometimes contributes to remove it.' Eye troubles were still far too frequent and medical officers are warned against 'not becoming the tools of unprincipled soldiers who voluntarily mutilate themselves'.

The regimental hospitals were the keystone of the medical organization and with only 20,000 to 30,000 troops scattered in individual locations throughout the country, they were quite adequate in dealing with the number of sick. General hospitals only existed at Fort Pitt at Chatham, the Depot Hospital at the Army Recruiting Centre at Newport, Isle of Wight, and for a short period one at Devonport. In Ireland there were general hospitals at Dublin and Cork. On the financial side the hospital stoppages of 9d. or 10d. a day were normally enough to cover the hospital expenses, but when patients were few in number and the stoppages would not cover the cost of hospital diets it was supplemented by a Government grant. Thus in 1818 the regimental hospital expenses at home amounted to £8,554 which was covered by £3,954 stoppages at the rate of 10d. a day from the sick, and a Government grant of £4,600. The cost of supporting each patient (including the pay of medical officers) was then £33 per annum. It was however only in peace when patients were few in number that Government grants were needed, for during an earlier war period of twelve years from 1804 to 1816 the hospital stoppages derived from patients exceeded the cost of running them by the following amounts:

General Hospitals	£21,034	14s.	3½d.
Regimental Hospitals	£34,409	2s.	3d.
Irish Militia Hospitals	£20,841	2s.	5¼d.
British Militia Hospitals	£5,054	13s.	9½d.
	£81,339	12s.	9¼d.

If we look ahead to the year 1847-8 we find that the cost of the general and regimental hospitals both at home and in all stations abroad amounted to over £50,000 a year, and when to this is added the cost of medicines and surgical instruments the total came to £68,000. But when we find that the total of hospital stoppages paid by the soldier came to over £61,000, and that the charge to the public purse only amounted to some £7,000,[37] we appreciate once more the truth of the old Government maxim that the army must pay for itself.

Let us see what kind of diet the soldier in hospital was getting for his money. The diets were five in number, full[38], half, low, spoon, and milk. As the cooking equipment only provided facilities for boiling, there was an unchanging diet of boiled meat, but there were a variety of puddings made of sago, rice, bread, sugar and milk, egg, and ginger or cinnamon.

Amongst the regulations for regimental and general hospitals which were issued on four occasions between 1820 and 1838 we refer only to a few of the more important. Soldiers' wives were still employed up to 1838 for nursing duties in regimental hospitals but after that date they were forbidden for male patients except by previous sanction of the Secretary at War. Female nurses were however sanctioned for attendance on sick families which were now allotted a dozen beds in every regimental hospital.

Regimental medical officers had to submit monthly sanitary reports to their commanding officers, but as it was always easy for the latter to ignore their recommendations it was decided to strengthen the authority of the R.M.O. by sending a copy of the report to the Inspector General. By this action commanding officers who neglected their duty in these matters would do so at the risk of War Office censure.

In a pre-anæsthetic age major operations were rare and regarded as incurring so much risk to life that it was stipulated none would be performed without the agreement of the hospital P.M.O., the Deputy Inspector of Hospitals, or the Director General himself. An event of such importance was then communicated to medical officers in the neighbourhood including those of the Ordnance Department and surgeons of the Royal Navy so that all would have an opportunity of benefitting.

A further concern of regimental surgeons was with the effects of punishment and they had to be present at all floggings to ensure that the soldier's constitution was strong enough to stand up to the lashes without risk to his health. Their position was often a delicate one, for the commanding officer of the unit was always anxious to see the full punishment carried out, and would often blame the medical officer for excessive caution if he gave orders to stop; on the other hand if the victim died from sepsis following the laceration of the tissues, a tragedy which though rare had been known to occur, the medical officer was held entirely responsible, and there was a case when a regimental surgeon had been chased by an angry mob of civilians. Queen's Regulations laid down that:—'Sentences of Corporal Punishment are to be inflicted in the presence of the Surgeon, or of the Assistant Surgeon in case of any other indispensable duty preventing the attendance of the Surgeon. The infliction of Corporal punishment a second time under one and the same sentence is illegal. The cuplrit is therefore, to be considered as having expiated his offence when he shall have undergone, *at one time*, as much of the corporal punishment to which he has been sentenced, as, in the opinion of the Medical Officer in attendance, he has been able to bear.'[39]

Although flogging was still considered necessary to maintain discipline, the number of lashes awarded was much reduced, and from 1837 onwards 200 was the maximum. Moreover a general feeling was growing condemning such brutal methods, and medical officers condemned it more than most. Robert Jackson was one who wrote—'There is not an instance in a thousand that the cat o' nine tails has made a soldier what he ought to be,—there are thousands where it has rendered those who were forgetful or careless rather than vicious, insensible to honour and abandoned to crime.'[40]

But there was one form of punishment which created anger and dismay amongst medical officers. This was the instruction that they must personally carry out the branding of deserters. This barbarous practice consisted of driving into the skin of the left side of the chest two inches below the armpit small metal spikes in the form of the letter D and then colouring the marks.[41] It had been found that these marks were being obliterated by artificial and other means by the men who had been branded, and a more permanent marking was necessary. The order raised such a storm of protest that it had to be cancelled. Medical officers pointed out that they were looked up to by the men for their sympathy and understanding, they were regarded as relievers of pain and not as tormentors. But they were not altogether absolved from responsibility as the following extract from Regulations shows:—'The punishment of marking a deserter with the letter D (in terms of the 11th clause of the Military Act) is to be inflicted on the parade in the presence of the men, and under the personal superintendence of a medical officer. The operation is to be performed with an instrument recommended for the purpose, a pattern of which is lodged in the office of Military Boards, and the punishment is to be inflicted in the Cavalry by the Trumpet-Major, and in the Infantry by the Drum-Major or Bugle-Major, who are to be instructed by the Regimental Medical Officers how to apply the instrument properly but effectually, as well as the substance, whether ink or gunpowder, with which the mark is to be coloured.'[42]

Military prisons were being built around 1848 and to each was attached a medical officer taken from the half pay list. Their exertions in the advancement of prison hygiene had a marked influence in the more humane treatment of military offenders.

Surgeon Van Millingen in his *Army Medical Officers Manual* published in 1819 suggested a more efficient method of dealing with the evacuation of casualties during battle. Although in many regiments there was an indeterminate arrangement by which wounded men would be carried out of the firing line by the regimental drummers and other details not engaged in actual combat, there was no regulated plan, and this often led to a haphazard arrangement by which the wounded men's comrades removed them to the regimental aid post, thus creating a loss of fighting strength and an excuse for the faint hearted to leave the combat area.

Millingen suggested the formation of a Hospital Corps of Ambulance. It is true that in the West Indies in 1795 a Royal Hospital Corps had been formed for duty in general hospitals in peace but this had become extinct within six months. The personnel now suggested was an ambulance field company on the scale of 20 for every 1,000 men in the field or 60 for an infantry brigade. Each man carried one half of a stretcher which could be fitted together by a wooden traverse carried above the knapsack. There were two types of ambulance transport. A 'Long Car' constructed on the lines of an Irish jaunting car with twenty-four lightly wounded sitting sideways and provided on the scale of one per regiment; while for the lying cases there were spring ambulances. The wounded were carried from the front line by the drummers and pioneers of the regiment to a regimental aid post where they were taken over by a Hospital Ambulance Corps with one of the regimental assistant surgeons in charge, and removed by hand carriage to the brigade hospital which was located out of musket fire range. Here the regimental surgeons of the brigade and two regimental assistant surgeons were concentrated leaving the second regimental assistant surgeon of each unit to go into action with the regiment. Wounds were dressed and hæmorrhage controlled before evacuation by the ambulance waggons and long cars to the divisional hospital situated out of hostile artillery range where the brigade staff surgeon and his two assistant surgeons performed any essential operations. The scheme is made plain by the plan below.

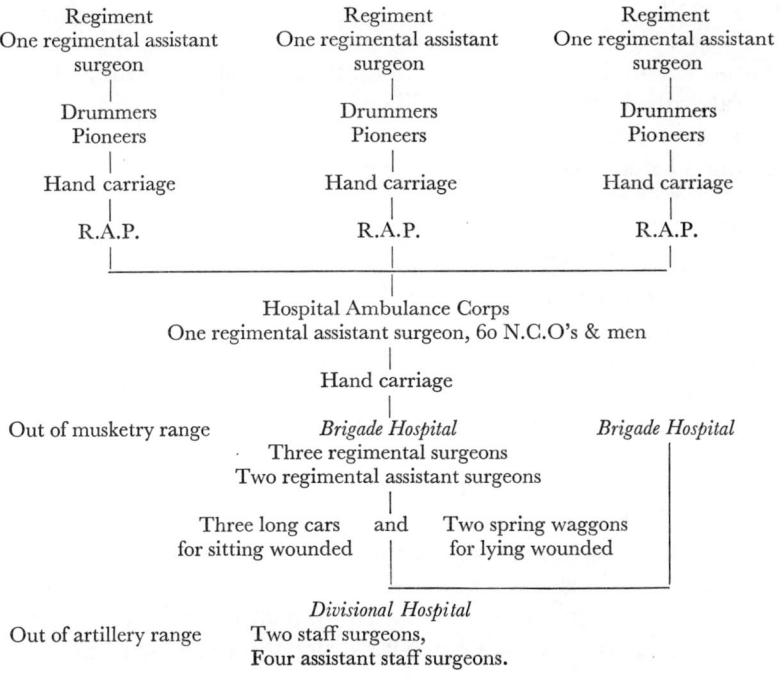

447

It was a workable plan, but the weak point of Millingen's scheme arose from the fact that the Ambulance Corps personnel who were employed in the battle zone were withdrawn in inactive periods to act as trained orderlies in the general hospitals. This meant that when moved to the fighting area their place in the general hospitals had to be taken by untrained men from regiments, and this at a time when the hospitals would be most heavily engaged in treating battle casualties. Moreover the post-Waterloo period when the scheme was put forward coincided with reductions in man power and financial restraint. Any innovations was doomed to failure, and Millingen's followed the general pattern.

On other administrative matters this officer had views to express. He deprecated the appointment of military commandants in general hospitals who are, he said, 'unacquainted with the nature of their administration and of the purveying department'.[43] He agreed with the regulation that a military officer should pay a daily hospital visit to check abuses and listen to complaints, for medical officers should never be employed on duties which included the punishment of patients or orderlies. Although he says it was their duty to maintain discipline, 'a medical officer who aims at the character of martinet, loses the confidence and affection of the men, and becomes an object of ridicule to the officers'.[44]

Millingen was a reformer who was not afraid to put his views in print, but it was nearly half a century before an ambulance corps came to be officially adopted.

McGrigor issued in 1827 an operational memorandum entitled 'General instructions for the guidance of medical officers, heads of staffs and others in charge of departments.' It was in fact the first Standing Orders ever issued for active service conditions and was based naturally on the field medical organisation of the Peninsular War. But the orders for the medical staff officers taking part in an assault landing are so precise and so relevant to all similar operations that we venture to give them in detail. They read thus: 'The staff surgeon attached to the brigade which first lands together with any hospital attendants allocated to him will be stationed centrally, and will notify his position at once to the commanding officers of regiments, to the deputy inspector of the division, and to the staff surgeons of adjacent brigades. Casualties after treatment will be removed by waggons provided on application to the brigade commander and evacuated to a pre-arranged location made by the deputy inspector.' The divisional deputy inspector who was responsbile for supervising the regimental and brigade hospitals was instructed to liaise with the brigade surgeons to ensure that the supply of medical equipment from stores or hospital ships was adequate. The waggons for evacuation of casualties were to be strictly used for that purpose only and staff surgeons were to see that they were not utilised for private baggage. This misappropriation of waggons appears to have been a constant temptation and the senior medical officer was specifically ordered never to fail when passing any waggons earmarked for casualties to examine them closely to ensure no unathorised baggage was carried.

After further orders on the inspection of hospital ships and transports, and the apothecaries' medical stores, the purveyor's duties are more clearly defined than those we are so far familiar with. The purveyor, said the memorandum, was responsible for the hospital equipment carried in each transport and for the cleanliness, ventilation and equipping of hospital ships. Once ashore, his duty was to see that medical comforts, food supplies, and cooking utensils were carried on the waggons, and that stretcher bearers were available to remove the wounded to the hospital. Both medicines and surgical materials for the Ordnance Medical Department and the Royal Navy were supplied on occasion by the Department, while sick and wounded sailors were to be admitted to military hospitals and given the same rations plus any extras which they usually received.

In a previous chapter the reader may remember that the question of excessive profits made by Mr. Garnier and the Apothecary General was under examination by the Committee of Inquiry which was set up in 1809 to investigate the state of the Medical Department. It will be convenient here to remind the reader that up to 1783 the surgeons of regiments received medicine money by deductions from the soldiers' pay and after that date a medicine allowance from Government was fixed at an annual rate. In 1796 this practice was stopped and medicines were provided in kind from public funds, a policy which at once led to so great an increase in the quantities consumed that in a period of twelve years up to 1809 over £700,000 had been expended and that consequently Garnier on the basis of 10 per cent had amassed a very considerable fortune. The Treasury became worried to the extent that an attempt was made to try and persuade him to sell the patent which he held by granting an annuity of £2,500 to his wife. To this Garnier agreed, but for some reason it was never implemented, and when he died in 1819 he was still in full possession of his patent. After his death, his deputy Calvert Clarke was told to continue for a year while an attempt was made to find an acceptable solution, and in due course several alternative suggestions were put forward for medicines to be provided by the Society of Apothecaries, or by contract, or by a private druggist. The other Service departments all had their supplies from one or other of these sources; the Navy by contract, the Army in Ireland and the H.E.I.C. from the Society of Apothecaries, and the

Ordnance Medical Department whose budget only amounted to £1,500 a year, from a private druggist.

Under the existing system the Department possessed its own Elaboratory and a Medical Depot in London, institutions which McGrigor wished to abolish, both on expense grounds (the London Depot alone cost £588 a year), and because medical officers were not qualified to assess the quality of drugs with any degree of efficiency. Of the various alternatives suggested Treasury preferred the Apothecary Society's offer of providing medicines at a profit of 15 per cent because they could be relied upon to supply drugs of a high standard as well as providing large quantities at short notice; furthermore they had their own Elaboratory. Be this as it may a decision to change the system was continually put off year after year until Clarke died in 1842. He had held his temporary appointment for twenty-three years! The new method of supply involved the usual Government compromise; the Society of Apothecaries was to supply half the medicines and two different drug firms the other half. It was doubtless intended in this way to play off one supplier against the other.

To McGrigor's energy and forethought we owe the formation of the Friendly Society, and the Army Medical Officers' Benevolent Society. The Friendly Society was originally named 'The Society for the benefit of the Widows of the Officers of the Hospital and Regimental Staff of His Majesty's Army' and was instituted on 1st January 1816. Originally the intention was to provide for members' orphans as well as their widows, but on actuarial advice this additional idea was dropped, and in consequence of this exclusion of orphans the Army Medical Officers Benevolent Society was formed.

When appealing for funds for the Friendly Society either by donations or annual subscriptions from officers, the committee 'hoped that the opulent in the Department will remember this Fund in their testamentary dispositions'.[45] But the Secretary of State for War subsequently forbade such pressure.

In the first year when over £1,000 was raised, amongst notable benefactors were the Worshipful Society of Apothecaries, Sir James Fellows a retired regimental surgeon, and Sir Lucas Pepys the former Physician General. The first annuitant was the widow of a hospital assistant who received an annual payment of £20 in 1821. By 1840 the Society's capital was over £17,000 and the yearly income nearly £2,000.

The Officers Benevolent Society was instituted at a meeting held at Medical Department Headquarters at 5 Berkeley Street on the 8th June 1820 with McGrigor in the chair. The first allocation of grants commenced in 1826 when £100 was distributed among nine children of regimental and assistant surgeons. By this time there were nearly 450 subscribers, and as the funds gradually accumulated the amount dispensed increased until in 1843 it had reached the sum of £415 annually. These encouraging results were amply confirmed in the years to come, and at the time of writing dependents receive grants amounting in all to some £1,500 yearly. McGrigor's initiative must receive every credit for launching a project which has so materially alleviated distress and provided educational aid for the families of officers who would otherwise have suffered hardship and deprivation.

It was on the 6th February 1851 at the advanced age of eighty-one and after fifty-seven years of active employment that Sir James McGrigor retired, full of years and of honours. His desire to be made a baronet which he had expressed so freely to the Duke of Wellington in 1815 was fulfilled in 1831, and he was made K.C.B. in 1850. His military honours included the medal of the Imperial Ottoman Order of the Crescent conferred by the Sultan of Turkey after his services in Egypt in 1801, the Portuguese Order of the Ancient and Most Noble Order of the Tower and Sword 'for his great merit and his services in the field during the recent campaign in the Peninsula' and Knight of Guelph a Hanoverian Order conferred on him after Waterloo. His academic distinctions were numerous. Fellow of the Royal Society in March 1816, and Fellow of the Royal Society of Edinburgh; L.L.D., Edinburgh; F.R.C.P., London and Edinburgh. Both Edinburgh and Aberdeen conferred on him the Freedom of their Cities and his Alma Mater thrice elected him as Rector of the University. He was Honorary Physician to George IV, William IV and Queen Victoria, and was one of the founders of the Aberdeen Medico-Chirurgical Society.

It is said that when seventy-five years of age he asked leave to retire but the Duke of Wellington replied 'No, no, Mac, there is plenty of work in you yet.' But now in his eighty-second year he felt it was high time to make way for a younger man. The event was a memorable one. In the presence of a gathering of friends a deputation of medical officers led by Inspector General Skey presented him with a farewell address signed by more than 500 of his brother officers which recounted many of the improvements in the service which were the outcome of his forethought and proficiency.

As befitted his long and distinguished career his retirement did not pass unnoticed by the Government, and in the Army Estimates for 1851 it was stated, 'In the Army Medical Department the Service has lost by the retirement, not, I am happy to say, by the death of Sir James McGrigor, an officer to whom the public is much indebted,' and the Lords of the Treasury in fixing his pension expressed their high approbation of his 'long, able and most meritorious services'.

He made London his home after his retirement and we are told that 'the urbanity of his manners, the benevolence of his disposition, and the simplicity of his heart drew around him for the remaining years of his eventful life a large circle of friends'. He died on the 2nd April 1858 in his eighty-eighth year, and was buried in Kensal Green Cemetery.

There are several permanent memorials in his honour. In 1865 a statue was erected in the grounds of the Royal Hospital at Chelsea which now stands in the forecourt of the Royal Army Medical College at Millbank in London. The subscribers to this included the Duke of Cambridge who was then Commander-in-Chief, fourteen generals, and many other combatant officers. In his native Aberdeen a stone obelisk in the Duthie Park also commemorates his outstanding services. When Wellington College was founded McGrigor was assigned one of the niches reserved for the reception of statues or busts of the principal officers, the contemporary statesmen, and the personal friends of the Duke. In the R.A.M.C. Headquarter Officers Mess hangs his portrait by Sir David Wilkie and his name is also perpetuated by the McGrigor Barracks at Aldershot and by the Anatomical and Pathological Museum and Library at the Royal Army Medical College the basis of which was his own personal gift of 1,500 volumes. Of outstanding importance for the benefit of medical officers' widows is the Army Medical Friendly Society and the Army Medical Benevolent Society for their dependants which after nearly 150 years still continue to distribute charitable sums to the necessitous. But one of the highest tributes in which McGrigor would have rejoiced was the statement that 'He rendered the most effective service to his country by appointing to the Army gentlemen of high professional attainments.'

REFERENCES

[1] P.R.O., W.O. 26/41, p.199.
[2] Wellington MSS Torrens to Wellington. 17th Feb. 1813.
[3] P.R.O., W.O. 7/109.
[4] There were articles in this indent of May 1811 which shows us something of the appliances, the dressings, and the medicines which had to be supplied. Some 10,000 bandages, 100 sets of splints, 400 lbs. of tow, 200 sheets which were used for fractures, 200—18 tailed bandages, 50 trusses, 100 stump pillows, 4 strait waistcoats, 48 urethra syringes, long and short bearers (stretchers) in bundles, as well as hospital utensils, dressing trays, and fumigating lamps. Amongst drugs cinchona bark was demanded in quantity, and there were four kinds of this drug in use, namely cinchona lanc.cort.contret; cinchona lanc.crass. pulv; cinchona flav.pulv; cinchona flav.crass.pulv. The active principle quinine was isolated from cinchona bark in 1820 by two Frenchmen, Pelletier and Caventou.
[5] Gibney. *Eighty Years Ago*, p. 96. Bellair's London (1896).
[6] Gibney. *Eighty Years Ago*, p. 96. Bellair's London (1896).
[7] Gibney. *Eighty Years Ago*, p. 95. Bellair's London (1896).
[8] Fortescue, vol. XI, book XVI, chapter 1, p. 10. MacMillan, London (1910).
[9] Six wives to every hundred men.
[10] Fortescue says the men at the Tower drank the filthy water from the shore below the fortress. vol. XI, book XVI, chapter 1, p. 12. MacMillan, London (1910).
[11] It is interesting to note that tinned meat was first supplied in this year.
[12] Lord Howick quoted the following statistics in 1837 (*Hansard* XXXVII 7th April 1837) Troops in West Africa—571, deaths 441.

[13] The reader is referred to the Introduction to Johnstone's Roll of Commissioned Officers in the Medical Services of the British Army R.A.M. College.

[14] P.R.O., W.O. 7/108.

[15] *Fifth Report Military Inquiry* 1808.

[16] *Johnstone's Roll*. Introduction p. xxxv.

[17] *Fifth Report Military Inquiry*, p. 158.

[18] *Johnstone's Roll*, Introduction, p. xliii. Aberdeen University Press (1917).

[19] McGrigor. *Autobiography*, p. 94. Longman, Green, Longman & Roberts, London (1861).

[20] Gore. *Our Services under the Crown*, p. 163. Balliere, Tindall & Cox, 1879.

[21] Gore. *Our Services under the Crown*, pp. 163-164. Balliere, Tindall & Cox, 1879.

[22] Lloyd and Coulter. *Medicine and the Navy*, vol. IV, p. 15. Livingstone, London (1961).

[23] McGrigor. *Autobiography*, p. 197. Longman, Green, Longman & Roberts, London (1861).

[24] McGrigor. *Autobiography*, p. 197. Longman, Green, Longman & Roberts, London (1861).

[25] This does not include medical officers serving in India or those of the Ordnance Medical Department.

[26] United Kingdom 25, Ireland 9, Canada 7, Nova Scotia 6, Windward and Leeward Islands 25, Jamaica 13, Gibraltar 6, Malta 4, Ionian Islands 8, West Africa 1, Cape of Good Hope 8, Mauritius 5, Ceylon 14.

[27] Kempthorne. 'The Army Medical Service 1816-1825', Journal *R.A.M.C.*, vol. LX, p. 301.

[28] *Lancet* 22nd September 1849, pp. 321-326.

[29] *Lancet*, 24 August 1850, p. 240.

[30] *Lancet* (1828) 684. Lloyd G. Stevenson (1953). *Military Service and Licensing in British Surgery*. Bull. Hist. Med. 426; *Medicine and the Navy*. vol. IV, p. 22.

[31] Quot. Stevenson. op. cit.

[32] P.R.O., W.O. 43/57.

[33] Longmore Pamphlets, vol. IX, Muniment Room, R.A.M. College.

[34] See Chapter XV.

[35] Kempthorne. 'The Army Medical Service 1816-1825', Journal *R.A.M.C.*, vol. LX, p. 300.

[36] Marshall and Tulloch. *Statistical Report on the sickness, mortality and invaliding in the West Indies*, p. 44. (1836).

[37] The exact figures are as follows:

Cost of general and regimental hospitals	£52,478	
Cost of medicines and instruments	£16,165	15s.
Total cost	£68,643	15s.

Hospital stoppages: £61,676. Cost to Government: £6,967 15s.

[38] On full diet the scale in 1838 was meat 12oz., bread 16oz., potatoes 8oz., oatmeal 3oz. or rice 2oz., barley ¾oz., sugar 1oz., salt ¼oz., table beer 1 quart. Barley was used for making meat broth.

[39] *Queen's Regulations*. 1st July 1844, para. 30 and 31.

[40] Jackson 1824. *A view of the Formation, Disipline and Economy of Armies*, p. 145. Stockton, Morrison, London (1824).

[41] This instrument can be seen at the R.A.M.C. Historical Museum.

[42] *Queen's Regulations*, 1st July 1844, para. 32.

[43] Van Millingen. *Army Medical Officers Manual*, p. 59. Burgess & Hill, London (1819).

[44] Van Millingen. *Army Medical Officers Manual*, p. 182. Burgess & Hill, London (1819).

[45] Minute Book of The Officers' Benevolent Society, Muniment Room, R.A.M. College.

Chapter 15

ASIA AND AFRICA (1824–1853)

In this chapter we recount the Campaigns which were fought in the second quarter of the 19th century. These events will take us as far afield as Burma, West Africa and South Africa, Afghanistan, China, and India.

First Burma War 1824

We come now to the first campaign undertaken in Burma which in the year 1824 was under the harsh and tyrannical rule of the King of Ava. In his arrogance the King had violated the Indian frontier in the neighbourhood of Chittagong in south eastern Bengal, followed by further incursions into Assam. This led to a declaration of war by India on the 24th February 1824. Little or nothing was known of the country except reports from merchants who had penetrated up the Irrawaddy river, and from two or three British officers who had gone on missions to the court of Ava. It was thought the Burmese army was some 30,000 to 40,000 strong, armed with firearms, spears and swords, with artillery comprising a vast number of guns of varying calibres. Their chief method of warfare was based on the building of strongly constructed teak stockades. The principal means of communication was by water, the Irrawaddy being the great river on which the towns of Rangoon, Prome, and Amarapura were sited. Roads were mere tracks through swamp and jungle and impassable in the rains.

The force gathered for the invasion of Burma comprised some 11,000 men under the command of Major General Sir Archibald Campbell. This included three British infantry regiments, the 1st Madras Europeans, native infantry from Madras, and artillery. As it was decided that operations would be mainly dependent on penetration of the main rivers the expedition was timed to arrive at the beginning of the rainy season when it was thought that the flotilla of ships,[1] sloops, cruisers, and forty smaller craft which accompanied the force could navigate the 400 to 500 miles from Rangoon to Ava in some six weeks.

The medical preparations were confined to the employment of the regimental hospitals each with their surgeons and assistant surgeons in the case of British units and the medical officers of the Honourable

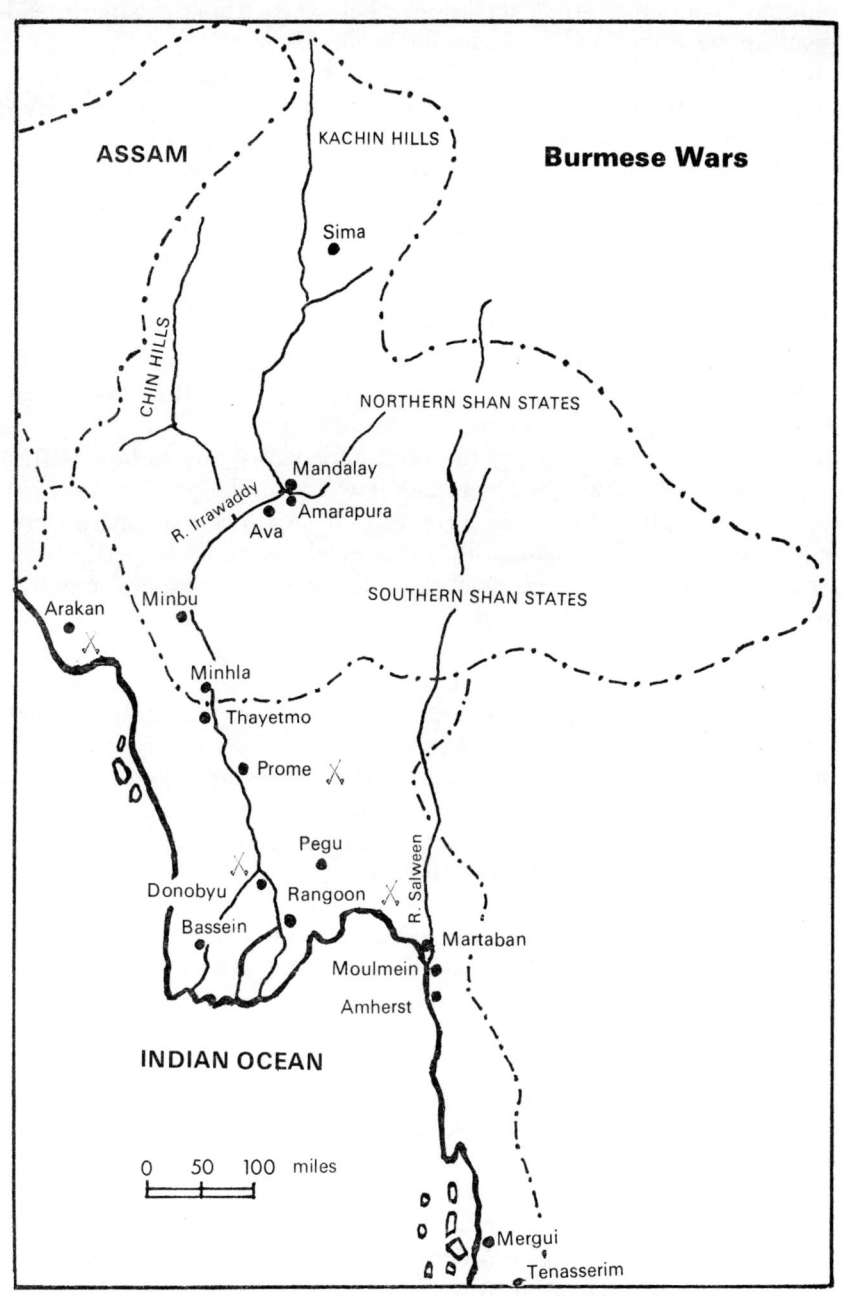

ASSAM

KACHIN HILLS

Burmese Wars

Sima

CHIN HILLS

NORTHERN SHAN STATES

Mandalay

R. Irrawaddy

Amarapura

Ava

Arakan

Minbu

SOUTHERN SHAN STATES

Minhla

Thayetmo

Prome

Pegu

R. Salween

Donobyu

Rangoon

Bassein

Martaban

Moulmein

Amherst

INDIAN OCEAN

0   50   100   miles

Mergui

Tenasserim

East India Company's service for Indian troops. There were also naval surgeons with the flotilla, and in all between thirty and forty medical officers accompanied the expedition. There was at first no superintending surgeon appointed as senior medical officer of the force but Dr. Howard H.E.I.C. arrived later to take up this appointment.

On the 11th May 1824 the naval flotilla and the transports arrived off Rangoon and effected a landing. As the local natives had fled, no supplies of fresh meat and vegetables were procurable, and the troops had to rely on meat salted rapidly before leaving India, hard biscuit, and a ration of spirits. The next few weeks were occupied in attacking and driving out the Burmese from the stockades they had erected in the vicinity of the city. This included a heavily fortified post on the river at Kemmendyne after an initial repulse had caused some 120 casualties. The monsoon had already begun and it was not long before the men began to fall sick with dysentery and malaria. Mosquito breeding was soon at its height. The salt meat became half putrid in the heat; the biscuit became mouldy from the rain, and scurvy due to lack of fresh vegetables was added to fever and bowel complaints. Scurvy made wounds difficult to heal, and leech bites from which the native troops especially suffered developed into fearful ulcers and frequently led to amputation. Clad in their scarlet tunics, with their stocks and their tight cross belts, the men were quickly bathed in sweat and exhausted after any exertion. Within a few months of landing sickness had played such havoc that each of the European regiments had two to three hundred men under treatment in the regimental hospitals and men were dying at the rate of four to six daily. In the space of two months there were 103 inches of rain, and under these depressing conditions it was only Campbell's insistence on keeping the troops occupied by constant attacks on the enemy round Rangoon which kept their morale from deteriorating into despair. Invariably in these engagements they stormed the stockades and drove out the Burmese with heavy casualties and little loss to themselves. By August the main Burmese army had learnt a lesson from their constant defeats and had retired to Donobyu on the river 50 miles north of Rangoon. After reinforcements in the shape of three native battalions from Madras had helped to make good his losses from sickness, Campbell was able to act further afield, and at Hlegu after a preliminary reverse when panic seized the sepoys and several British officers were killed and wounded, a succession of stockades were successfully stormed and the Burmese fled incontinently, thoroughly disheartened at their lack of success.

Sickness continued to decimate the force and by October only 1,300 Europeans were fit for duty. The regimental hospitals were so poorly accommodated and overcrowded that some transports lying in the river were converted into hospital ships. However the end of the monsoon in November brought better weather and better health. A greater variety of food was provided by the arrival of traders from India, and instead of the constant salt meat and rice such articles as butter and meat could be purchased although the former was 8s. and mutton or goat 24s. a pound.

With the end of the monsoon the Burmese under a new general made a vigorous attempt to recapture Rangoon but failed, and Campbell then took the offensive. On the 9th December the stockades were stormed and 200 guns captured at the cost of only 250 casualties including 230 wounded; this was followed by further successes on the 15th December when the enemy was driven out of their last stronghold with heavy loss. The whole character of the war now changed. The local inhabitants swarmed back into Rangoon; fresh meat and vegetables quickly made their appearance; buffaloes and carts were produced and transport could be organized. After further reinforcements including three British and eight native battalions had arrived from India more extensive operations were now possible.

In the meantime on the eastern frontiers of India a force from Calcutta had driven the enemy from the hills of Assam and the swamps of the Arakan, not without difficulty and casualties, and with heavy losses from sickness. Between May and September 1824 the European units buried 259 men out of a strength of 1,500, and at the end of September there were 400 redcoats and 3,600 sepoys in hospital. When eight months of active operations had ended the British had lost 600 dead from dysentery and malaria out of an average strength of 1,000, and not half the survivors were alive after a further four months. Fortescue says these losses were not in fact much worse than those sustained by the troops in the West Indies where a British battalion had to be renewed every two years and where this was looked upon as inevitable. But this kind of warfare was new to the Government of India, which so far had only been used to fighting in the plains.

Campbell now divided his force into a river and a land column and in February 1825 commenced his advance through dense teak forests and jungle. Doolie bearers were employed to carry along the sick and wounded, and the regimental hospitals accompanied the land column, their equipment loaded on whatever animals and transport the local facilities could provide. On two occasions the wounded were lost owing to a panic amongst the bearers. After severe fighting at Donobyu, Prome was entered on the 24th April 1825 and envoys were received from the King of Ava, but there was no hope of reaching Ava itself before the rains came, so Campbell decided to remain in cantonments at Prome. The troops here were well housed, well supplied, and on friendly terms with the natives, but even so the Europeans lost one seventh of their number sick between June and October. The situation however was very different from the deplorable conditions which had prevailed in Rangoon the previous year, and in that city itself the sick rate was not now excessive, while a convalescent depot which had been established at Mergui in the better climate of the Tenasserim coast had brought great benefit to the invalids. Nevertheless within the first eleven months after landing at Rangoon nearly one half of the Europeans died, a large number from amœbic dysentery and its complications of hepatitis and liver abscess. Many dysentery cases relapsed, and this can be readily understood when treatment by calomel was the usual remedy, for without ipecacuanha the sufferers could have experienced little relief.

After a so-called armistice had come to nothing, a large Burmese host attacked Prome in November 1825 and was repulsed and subsequently completely overthrown. This was achieved with a total casualty list of only 150 killed and wounded, a remarkable achievement of courage and endurance carried out under tropical conditions. Drenched with sweat, parched with thirst, and riddled with malaria, the men unhesitatingly carried all before them.

The war however was not yet over and cholera which broke out both in the land column and the flotilla added to their troubles. On arrival at Minhla a treaty was signed but as this was again unfulfilled, Campbell denounced it. In these negotiations the part that one of the regimental surgeons was constrained to play is worth recording. Dr. Sandford was surgeon to the Royals, and while travelling by boat from Prome to Rangoon with a brother officer both were captured while having a siesta on the bank. Taken to the prison at Amarapura they were threatened with death by disembowelling, but Sandford by successfully treating the King for an illness was dealt with less harshly, and eventually was used as an envoy to carry messages to General Campbell; much to the astonishment of the Burmese he returned to his captors with the reply.

Campbell now attacked and routed the enemy in Minhla, but not until February 1826 was the final battle of the Burma War fought, and the King of Ava compelled to accept defeat. It had taken nearly two years fighting against a skilful enemy, and Campbell deserves great credit for his strong will, his high moral courage, his persistence and his leadership.

At Rangoon in May 1826 the expedition re-embarked for India; the remnants of both the British and the native battalions riddled with disease, 'many of them literally skin and bone and living skeletons'.[2] If it was dysentery and malaria which struck down the troops during the rains it was cholera which attacked them in the dry season, and in the country at large this disease in six months killed more than all the casualties received in action. 'We had no parades or any duty but the digging of graves, until the best part of the regiment was under the sod.'[3] As the sick were embarked they underwent almost unbelievable want of care and attention. 'There was no carriage or transport for the invalids; some were carried down to the wharf by the Burmese, two in a basket, others crawled down on hands and knees. I saw one poor sinner going along at a snail's pace on his back, feet foremost, kicking his bundle before him, so anxious to get away.'[4]

Wilson[5] accounted for the heavy mortality in Burma as due to the exposure and hardship endured under severe conditions of heat and tropical rains—bivouacking unsheltered in mud and water, marching through inundated fields, fed on unwholesome and insufficient food. In the view of Major Tulloch the statistician of the Army Medical Department the future lessons to be learnt to diminish disease were to commence operations in the dry season when the conditions were best for taking the field, and to advance rapidly through the unhealthy area of the Irrawaddy delta near Rangoon to the upper reaches of the river where operations could be carried out with less damage to health. With tactics such as these and with independent food supplies Tulloch's opinion is that a moderate force should be able to accomplish what on this occasion both in Burma and in the Arakan took the combined efforts of 20,000 men.

In the state of medical knowledge at the time nothing could be done to prevent the onset of malaria and dysentery. But the hard drinking which went on, although the sole consolation which the soldiers enjoyed to make them forget their hardships and suffering, undoubtedly helped to ruin their resistance and encouraged the liver complications which amœbic dysentery brought in its train. Some statistics we quote will show the extent of the losses from disease. The admissions to hospital each year amounted to 3,540 per 1,000 of strength, which means that on the average every man of the force was admitted to hospital three and a half times. The annual mortality was 483 per 1,000 of strength, and of these 446 died from disease. Of the 89 cases of cholera 48 died, a 54 per cent mortality. Amongst the original British regiments, there were 1,311 deaths in a strength of 2,716 and of these 1,215 were killed by disease, 60 were killed in action and 36 died of wounds.

There were two deaths of A.M.D. surgeons, Cowen and Leich, while four H.E.I.C. surgeons lost their lives. The services rendered by the medical officers under these trying conditions were not forgotten by the Governor General of India and we are told that Superintending Surgeon Howard and the officers of the Medical Department were suitably recognized by His Lordship in Council.

First Ashanti War 1824-26

Our last reference to the West Coast of Africa was at the termination of the Seven Years War in 1763 when the effect of the climate was so deadly that hardly anyone survived. The years which followed showed no abatement in this tragic loss of lives and it truly lived up to its reputation of being the white man's grave.

Gore[6] gives an account of the conditions in the disease ridden climates of Sierra Leone, the Gold Coast and Gambia. Freetown the capital of Sierra Leone was named from the negro slaves who settled there after their discharge following the American War of Independence. His review covers a period of fifty years from 1816 to 1865. Previous to 1816 there are no reliable data, although the explorer Mungo Park was in Gambia in April 1805 with forty-four Europeans of whom all but four had died by October.

The Corps of Foot which constituted the garrison in the early years of the 19th century had a strength of 540 British troops. They lived in the most squalid conditions in dilapidated and unhealthy huts and dwellings and consumed rations of salt beef and pork. Malaria, dysentery, cholera, guinea worm, yellow fever, and scurvy decimated the ranks. In 1816, 6 officers and 115 men died and 32 were invalided; in 1817, out of a strength of 242, 3 officers and 62 men died and 23 were invalided; in 1818, 2 officers and 33 men died out of 102 and 10 were invalided, and in 1819, 18 died out of 54. Those still alive returned to the United Kingdom as it was considered impossible to retain white troops under such deadly conditions. As a replacement, the West India Regiment some 500 strong with some British officers arrived from Jamaica and served in the Colony until 1825. In 1822 the first definite outbreak of yellow fever occurred, the origin of which was put down to 'sui generis'; but yellow fever had prevailed in the south of Spain from 1819 to 1821 and an American vessel arrived from the West Indies with several cases of undiagnosed fever on board. But these coloured troops stationed in Sierra Leone, the Gold Coast, and Gambia, were much less prone to disease with a death rate of only 6·9 per cent compared to the white troops 23·4 per cent.

Between 1822 and 1825 the Royal African Corps was formed in England and 20 officers and 511 men arrived as a first instalment to replace the West India Regiment. It was composed of men who were jailbirds and whose punishment was commuted. They were dispatched to almost certain death. One report refers to them as the 'very dregs of the army', with 'riot and debauchery marking their footsteps'. Deputy Inspector Nichols the P.M.O. at the time described them as reckless, dissipated, and intemperate, with much excessive drinking. To show the extent of depravity and crime no less than one hundred punishments by lashes were awarded within one period of twelve months. Those who survived for two years gave every appearance of being completely prostrated by debauchery and disease, with enlarged spleen and liver. A detachment at anchor for three months off the Gambian coast en route to Sierra Leone lost 73 men out of 91.

In the year of their arrival out of a strength of 44 officers in all West African stations 28 died and 9 were invalided; 17 women out of 54 died. Within a short period two P.M.O's lost their lives and between 1824 and 1834 there were nine Governors.

In 1828 new barracks were built and fresh provisions took the place of the salt beef and pork. Living conditions were considerably improved but this seemed to have little effect upon the sick wastage. Quinine was freely used for treatment of fever, and preparations of mercury were popular.

In 1824 the first Ashanti War broke out, for the rise of the Ashanti nation as warriors was a menace to the trading ports on the Gold Coast of which Cape Coast Castle was the most important. When hostilities broke out the Royal African Corps assisted by local native levies were committed to the fighting. In the bush warfare which continued for some two years, fortune favoured first one side and then the other, but apart from the fighting it was fever and dysentery which decimated the troops while smallpox carried off the natives.

In this type of bush warfare front line medical aid depended entirely on equipment transported by native porters. From the forward area sick and wounded were borne in litters along the forest tracks to the hospital which must have existed at Cape Coast Castle. This was certainly at full stretch, for in 1824 on the Gold Coast there were 844

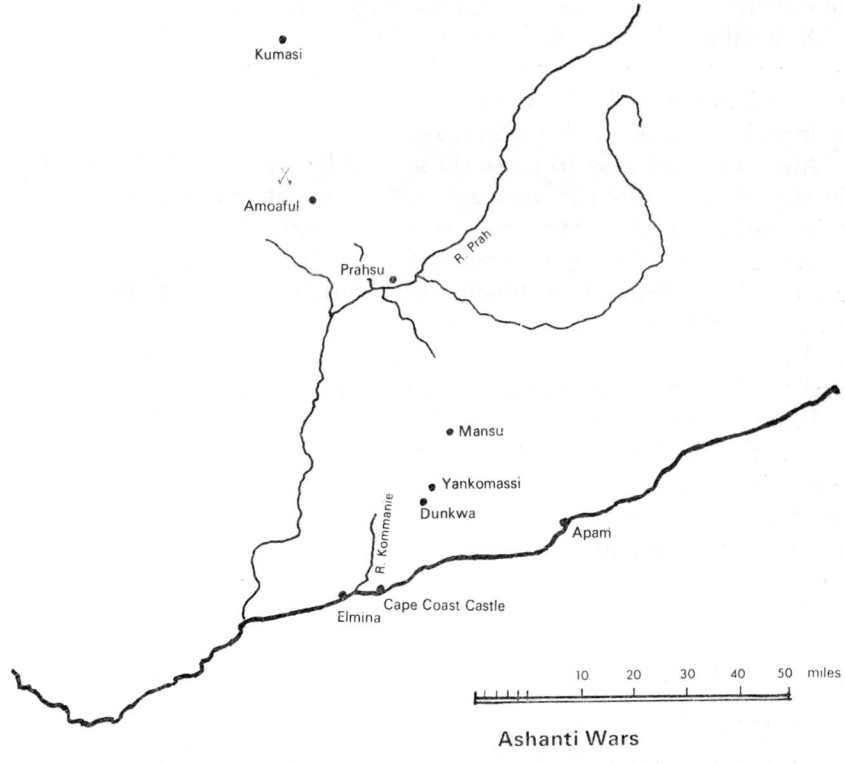

Ashanti Wars

461

admissions and 221 deaths, and in the following year 603 admissions and 136 deaths, a mortality rate of 26·2 and 22·5 per cent respectively. Although there were relatively few battle casualties one of the victims of the fighting was Assistant Surgeon Tedlie, A.M.D. At the battle of Dodowah fought in August 1826 the Ashantis were finally decisively beaten and peace resulted which lasted for fifty years.

In the Sierra Leone area in the year 1825 there were 247 deaths in 1,008 hospital admissions (24·5 per cent), and in Gambia 160 deaths in 317 admissions (50 per cent). An experiment was then tried of sending out young recruits from Chatham who would at least be free from the drunken excesses of the old soldiers. They were separately stationed on the Isles of Los, a location which had a 'salubrious aspect' and was away from the 'miasmal exhalations' which were considered the cause of sickness on the mainland. Here it was confidently expected that they would be safe from fever, but this expectation was doomed to disappointment; the death dealing but unsuspected mosquito was just as prevalent here as in Sierra Leone. To the dismay of the authorities, within a period of eighteen months (June 1825 to December 1826), out of a strength of 108 healthy young soldiers, 48 were dead, 21 invalided, 29 unfit from fever, and only 10 fit for duty. The experiment was not repeated.

A naval squadron which lay off Sierra Leone suffered fewer losses as the seamen to some extent avoided the mosquitoes, while they are reported to have benefitted enormously from the use of prophylactic quinine in doses of 3 to 6 grains daily.

After the years 1827 to 1829 still showed heavy losses the War Office in 1830 shrank from the uneviable task of sending men to almost certain death, and European troops were withdrawn. Thereafter the West India Regiment alone garrisoned the West Coast. Before we weary the reader with statistics let us finally mention that out of 1,658 Europeans sent out to the Royal African Corps between 1822-1830, 1,298 perished, and of the 360 who were invalided, 123 died on the passage to England, and 57 of the remainder were discharged unfit for service.

From the time of the arrival of the West India Regiment the picture again altered for the better as they were more immune to these endemic diseases and in the ten years 1839 to 1849 the ratio of deaths per 1,000 varied between 34 in the best years to 127 in the worst yellow fever years. Mortality appeared to be in inverse ratio to the rainfall. By 1860 the annual admission ratio per 1,000 had fallen to 615. In this period of 50 years there were eight yellow fever epidemics in each of which three of the medical officers died each year, and in no other country did medical officers endure such risks to life and health.

South Africa

We have previously mentioned the capture of the Cape of Good Hope from the Dutch in 1806 and we must now refer to the activities of the Medical Department in Cape Colony during the period after its capture. As was often the case when new territories were added to the Empire the military medical authorities played a conspicuous part in the creation and the administration of the medical institutions which were either newly formulated or taken over from their former enemies. In Cape Town Deputy Inspector John Arthur M.D., Physician to the Forces was Principal Medical Officer with a number of junior medical staff officers who in addition to their duties in the military hospital in Cape Town looked after the Somerset Hospital for natives, the jail and the leper asylum. Arthur himself became President of the Supreme Medical Council, a Government body which administered medical affairs, and which in due course became the Colonial Medical Committee, a body also largely controlled by officers of the Department.

To the Colony came two officers of whom we must take note. In 1816 Hospital Assistant James Barry arrived, a remarkable character about whom we shall have more to say subsequently, while five years later came Andrew Smith a Hospital Assistant who was destined to reach the highest rank in the Department. During the sixteen years which Smith was to spend in the Colony he built up a reputation as a naturalist of great prominence, as an explorer, and more remarkable still as a semi official Government political officer. This hard headed Scot came to acquire such an outstanding knowledge of natives and their affairs that he was strongly pressed to accept the appointment of Lieutenant Governor of Natal. In a man so sincere and conscientious Smith's military duties were always carefully attended to, but he was passionately devoted to his role as a naturalist, and his journeys in South Africa were of historical interest, not only because he explored new territory, but because his expeditions had a strong political motif in discussions with native chiefs near and far. As Smith's peace time military duties were not exacting Deputy Inspector Arthur seems to have readily agreed to him carrying out a role so unusual for a mere hospital assistant.

Smith made three journeys into the interior of Cape Colony much of it in unexplored territory. The first in 1828 took him to Namaqualand some 400 miles north of Cape Town, the second was in 1832 to the Zulus in Natal, and the third in 1834 when he set out on a journey to the Transvaal and the Matabele tribes which lasted for two years. These journeys were often hazardous because of native hostility especially from the Zulus, while unlike some of the previous missions in the Transvaal which had never returned he came through them unscathed.

Apart from their diplomatic success, (one report was described as 'An able, comprehensive and statesmanlike document'[7]) these expeditions gave Smith an unrivalled opportunity of following his bent as a naturalist, and in his last journey he collected upwards of 5,000 specimens of newly discovered or rare quadrupeds, birds, and other animals, together with some 500 drawings of native tribes, and their life customs. He also found time to inaugurate a South African Museum in Cape Town and became its Superintendent; edited a Quarterly Journal of Science, and wrote accounts on the origins and history of the Bushmen, and a description of the birds inhabiting the 'South of Africa'. All these activities resulted in his being elected a member of the Zoological and the Horticultural Societies of London. Between the intervals of exploration Smith carried out his military duties as regimental medical officer or as civil surgeon at Grahamstown and Cape Town.

After sixteen years in South Africa he was recalled for duty at home and sailed for England in January 1837. He had acquired distinction as naturalist, anthropologist, and explorer, altogether an unique experience for a young army doctor.

Kaffir Wars 1834 and 1846

Ever since Britain's capture of Cape Colony the Dutch and British settlers had been gradually extending their territory towards the east with the inevitable result that there were continual clashes with the Kaffir tribes, and in 1834 and again in 1846 this led to open war. In 1834 some 15,000 Kaffirs invaded Colony territory, cutting off and murdering many settlers in their farms before they were able to make good their escape. There were less than 800 British troops on the spot mostly of the 75th Foot, but luckily there was an able commander in the shape of Colonel Harry Smith.[8] After raising a force of 850 more burghers to reinforce his regular force, Smith straightaway took the offensive and by his energetic and active intervention succeeded within a month in driving back the hostile tribes. General D'Urban the Governor decided that signal punishment must be inflicted, and Smith invaded Kaffraria with 3,000 men which now included the 72nd Foot and some 2,000 burghers. Dividing his men into columns, the territories of the various chiefs were overrun and with the rounding up of their cattle the rebellion collapsed. By September 1835 a treaty was concluded which annexed to Cape Colony all the lands between the Great Fish and Kei rivers.

In this type of bush warfare the necessary medical care for the columns was provided by the regimental establishments; medical and surgical panniers and tentage were carried on horseback or in waggons, while the returning commissariat ox-waggons evacuated the sick and wounded to the field hospital opened at Grahamstown. Casualties were few and the health excellent; between April and June 1835 only seventeen wounded had to be treated, and Deputy Inspector Murray the P.M.O. reported that during the short campaign not a single officer or soldier had to leave the field on account of sickness.

The Kaffir war of 1846 was a much more serious and prolonged affair

464

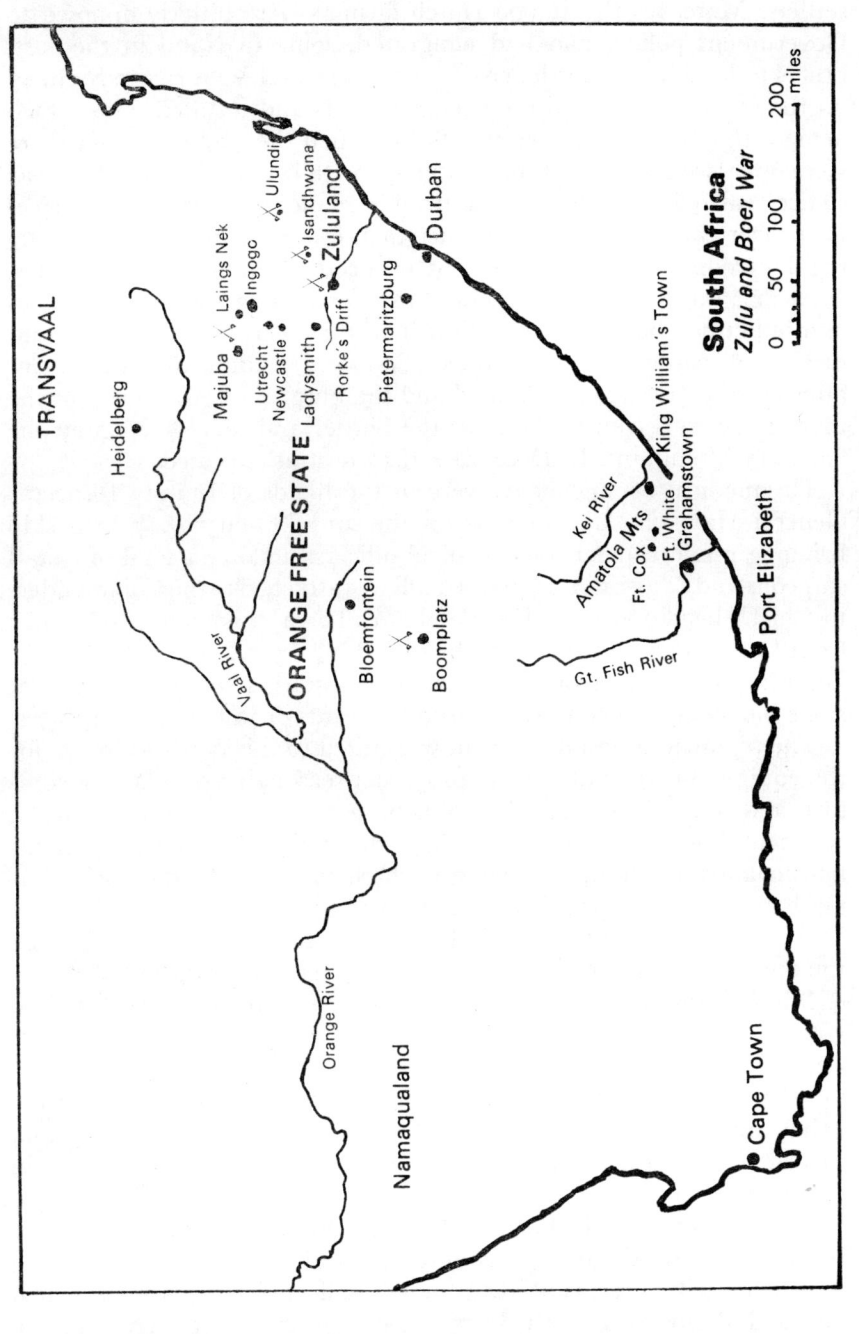

TRANSVAAL

Heidelberg

ORANGE FREE STATE

Vaal River

Orange River

Bloemfontein

Boomplatz

Namaqualand

Cape Town

Port Elizabeth

Gt. Fish River

Grahamstown

Ft. White

Ft. Cox

Amatola Mts

Kei River

King William's Town

Durban

Pietermaritzburg

Zululand

Isandhwana

Ulundi

Ingogo

Laings Nek

Majuba

Utrecht

Newcastle

Ladysmith

Rorke's Drift

South Africa
Zulu and Boer War

0   50   100   200   miles

for it dragged on until 1852. Over the years there had been periods of unrest when raiding tribes continued to steal cattle and to murder the settlers. Moreover the 10,000 Dutch farmers were bitterly opposed to Government policy, and had emigrated, some to Natal in the east, others to land in the north across the Orange and Vaal rivers. Security on the frontier depended on a series of forts and fortified posts which acted as bases for offensive operations. When the war broke out there were only two regular battalions to cope with it but as soon as the War Office realized the extent of the trouble reinforcements arrived piece-meal over the years until at its height there were in all some 10,000 regular troops engaged[9] supplemented by settlers and loyal native levies.

At first the Kaffirs had successes in overrunning the waggon trains and inflicting about 100 casualties; soon they were burning farms and driving off cattle with the settlers valiantly defending themselves, but after martial law was proclaimed and the burghers were called out the invaders were driven back across the border and sought refuge in the Amatola Mountains. In December 1847 hostilities ceased.

The medical arrangements were in the hands of Deputy Inspector General Hall who had arrived on the 2nd January 1847 in a ship bringing reinforcements of 9 medical officers, making a total of 6 staff surgeons and 12 assistant surgeons. Hall was attached to the Commander-in-Chief's headquarters at King William's Town; this involved a journey from Cape Town during which he was shipwrecked. With the G.O.C. he visited all the forts and regimental hospitals, some of the latter in stone barracks, others in wattle and daub huts or in tents or marquees.

The regimental hospital system was suited to this type of warfare for the equipment was sufficient to provide a reasonable standard of comfort, and the numbers of sick and wounded were never more than the regimental officers could cope with, so that only the long term patients and invalids had to be evacuated to the field hospital again located at Grahamstown. The medical arrangements imposed no strain on the Department as casualties were light and the health good, but Hall called the operations 'tiresome, unprofitable and inglorious warfare'.[10]

Midway through the campaign Lieut General Smith returned to command operations and the Boers hailed his advent with joy as they remembered the energy and determination he had displayed in suppressing the Kaffir War of 1834. Smith released on terms of good behaviour those Kaffir chiefs who had been imprisoned and created British Kaffraria as a Kaffir reserve with a strong force of troops in occupation.

Then in July 1848 the Boers beyond the Orange river revolted as they refused to accept the British claim to the Orange Free State and Smith took Hall with him as P.M.O. of a small column of troops which defeated Pretorius and his Boers at Boomplatz. There were some 50 casualties including 46 wounded, and Hall reports 'We are able to dress them all on the field, and this house, which is about three quarters of a mile from where the action commenced I took possession of and got all the men under cover before sunset.'[11] At the termination of hostilities a General Order issued from Bloemfontein on the 15th September 1848 included the words 'This record of meritorious service attaches to Dr. Hall D.I.G.H. and to the medical officers generally, whose care of the wounded could not be exceeded.'[12]

After two years of peace the Kaffirs in 1850 broke out afresh. Smith took the field in March 1851 and throughout the year mobile columns attacked the enemy on all sides. But there were setbacks and losses in various petty engagements. Assistant Surgeon Stewart was killed and Assistant Surgeon Catty wounded. Fort White and Fort Cox were attacked and some 40 casualties sustained. Sixteen men of the 45th Foot were surprised and murdered. These reverses encouraged not only the enemy but also the Hottentots in the Colony itself who rose in revolt and went on a campaign of murder and pillage. With these troubles on all sides Smith was faced with a baffling problem but with a force now numbering some 9,000 men in all he intensified his offensive with the fixed intention of harassing the enemy without respite until they could bear no more. Under his forceful leadership the chiefs' mountain fast-nesses were penetrated one by one after incredible exertions and the Kaffirs broken up by fire and sword. By January 1852 many had been slain and 30,000 cattle captured. As the Boers still refused to give any assistance, all the work fell on the regular troops, and in these operations in mountainous country the hardship and fatigue was severe. The rain which sometimes turned to sleet and a bitter wind which blew from the snow capped mountains chilled the men to the bone when they had but one blanket to cover themselves with in their small bivouac tents. A further year's harassing operations was necessary before in December 1852 the war came to an end.

On the medical side little of importance occurred as the wounded were few in number and the troops were healthy. What sick there were suffered chiefly from fever and bowel diseases, some of it due to enteric (typhoid) fever, and rheumatism in the winter months from exposure. In the treatment of the wounded the introduction of anaesthetics was a milestone and Surgeon Irwin of the 27th Foot was present at the first amputation performed by Dr. Atherstone the civil surgeon at Grahams-town, the first it was said outside Europe and America. In the field a regimental mule carried a pair of field panniers while the heavier equipment was brought forward in a special ox-waggon set aside for medical use. Stretcher bearers there were none, and men were carried out of action by their comrades. Evacuation behind the regimental hospitals was performed by commissariat waggons to the field hospitals.

Before the end of the campaign Hall had left the Colony on his transfer to India and had been replaced by Deputy Inspector General

Melvin. That he had performed his task with ability and success is shown by the glowing tribute paid to him by Sir Harry Smith who had now been made Governor of the Colony. 'The C.-in-C. cannot permit Dr. Hall to leave the Army under his command or relinquish the important office he has filled with such advantage to the service and credit to himself without a strong and deep felt expression of his regret at parting with so valuable and talented an officer—a feeling in which the whole Army participates; nor can His Excellency convey to Dr. Hall this public testimony of his work without adding his personal feelings of regret and tendering to him his grateful acknowledgments for that unceasing attention to which he is so much indebted to him personally. Exclusive of this officer's great professional ability he is one of the most able officers of his Department in the field His Excellency has ever associated with.'[13]

Although as already stated there was no great strain on the Medical Department either from casualties or from sickness, the medical officers' duty was not only severe but hazardous. They were continually on the move with the columns or visiting the different forts and outposts. Four were killed, Loch of the 7th Dragoon Guards, Howell of the 9th Foot, Campbell of the 73rd and Stuart of the Cape Mounted Rifles, while Catty of the 6th Foot was wounded. Campbell and four other officers of the regiment were cut off, killed, and mutilated by Kaffirs in operations near the river Kei.

For their attention to the wounded three medical officers were mentioned in despatches: Assistant Surgeon George of the 12th Lancers, Surgeon Booth of the 73rd, and Staff Assistant Surgeon Campbell.

First Afghan War 1838-42

It is not within the scope of this history to recount the political implications which influenced Lord Auckland, the Governor General of India, to decide on the invasion of Afghanistan in 1838. Suffice it to say that Dost Mohammed the ruler of that country at Kabul had usurped the throne from the rightful holder Shah Sujah who was living under British protection in India. Dost Mohammed was a strong and forceful ruler while Shah Sujah his rival was weak and irresolute and had but little following. He was however supported by Ranjit Singh the ruler of the Sikh kingdom in the Punjab, and Auckland who although diligent and conscientious lacked the power of decision, allowed himself to be influenced by General Fane the Commander-in-Chief in India.

The force to invade Afghanistan and place Shah Sujah on the throne comprised a Bengal and a Bombay Division. The Bengal Division under Major General Cotton had set out from Ferozepore with an enormous host of followers. The Commissariat arrangements were unable to produce all the thousands of camels required to transport the huge quantities of personal baggage and camp furniture which characterized Indian warfare. For his personal baggage the superintending surgeon had eight camels, one of the brigadiers had sixty! Even slipper baths were not excluded from their belongings. Vast numbers of camels died from lack of forage and the desertion of the camel drivers.

The Bombay Division with a fighting strength of 5,000, and also swollen by thousands of followers disembarked at Karachi and marched north by way of the river Indus. Both Divisions were united at Sukkur on the Indus in January 1839, the combined strength amounting to 15,000 fighting troops, including two cavalry and four British infantry regiments, 6,000 Indian auxiliaries under Shah Sujah, and some 80,000 followers.

The medical arrangements were controlled in each Division by a Superintending Surgeon who was supported by a field surgeon and a medical storekeeper, all H.E.I.C. service. Each regimental hospital was equipped on the liberal scale customary in Indian warfare with three medical officers in British and two medical officers including one H.E.I.C. medical officer in Indian units. Sixty beds were provided in each, a 12 per cent bed cover, and transport required sixty camels. No field hospital as such appears to have been mobilised but the field surgeon was detailed for duty with a regimental hospital selected to act as a field hospital. Thirty-five years before in the Mahratta War Wellesley had insisted that a reserve of junior officers should be formed to staff any field hospital it might be necessary to open, but this lesson appears to have been forgotten. Doolies for the carriage of the sick and wounded were supplied by the Commissariat Department on a scale of 10 per cent, and their allotment in the field was controlled by the Superintending Surgeon who kept a proportion under his own control.

Dr. Kennedy H.E.I.C. who was the Superintending Surgeon of the Bombay Division later wrote an account of the campaign,[14] and he tells us that for the march up the Indus the sick were carried in four flat bottomed boats each holding 40 patients, with the field surgeon and two assistant surgeons in charge—a floating hospital as he described it. For the Bengal Division, the Superintending Surgeon was Dr. Atkinson H.E.I.C., and after the divisions had joined forces at Sukkur on the Indus a depot hospital was established here under Dr. Don the medical storekeeper of the Bombay Division. This remained open throughout the campaign.

The next stage was the march of the 1st (Bengal) Division under General Cotton to the Bolan Pass some 170 miles on the road to Quetta. The route was constantly threatened by marauding tribesmen, and was short of water; the transport arrangements were hopelessly deficient but no thought was given to reduce the number of followers or the baggage, and with the death of thousands of camels carrying supplies, the troops were soon reduced to half rations. The temperature in the

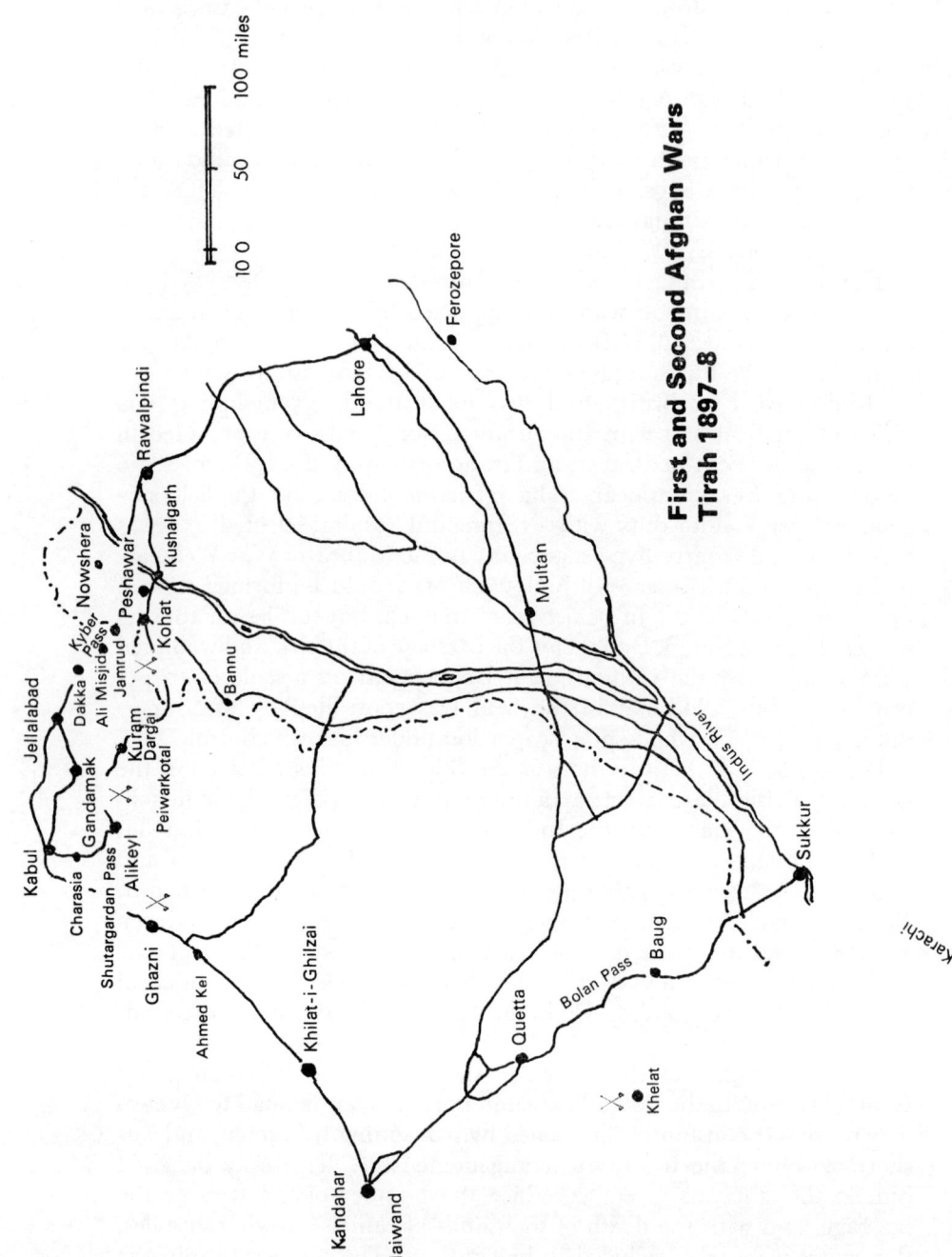

First and Second Afghan Wars
Tirah 1897–8

10 0   50   100 miles

Ferozepore

Lahore

Multan

Rawalpindi

Kushalgarh

Indus River

Peshawar

Nowshera

Khyber Pass

Dakka

Ali Misjid

Jamrud

Kohat

Bannu

Dargai

Kurram

Jellalabad

Charasia

Gandamak

Kabul

Shutargardan Pass

Alikeyl

Peiwarkotal

Ghazni

Ahmed Kel

Khilat-i-Ghilzai

Kandahar

Maiwand

Baug

Bolan Pass

Quetta

Khelat

Sukkur

Karachi

Bolan Pass was anything over 100°F in March and heatstroke amongst European officers and men occurred at every stage. Although these pressing difficulties slowed down the advance, Quetta, which then boasted only a mud village, was reached on the 26th March. Here twenty days' supplies had confidently been expected, but practically none were forthcoming, and Cotton found it impossible to move further. So the force sat immobile awaiting starvation until on the 20th April General Keane with the 2nd (Bombay) Division and Shah Sujah's auxiliaries arrived together with a supply train. In spite of the exposure to heat and the hardships of the journey the health had not suffered unduly and Kennedy reports that in his Division he had only 77 sick Europeans and 42 natives on his hands, which was just over 4 per cent for the former, and just over 2 per cent for the latter. There were a few wounded from the skirmishes with the Baluchi tribesmen and there were constant losses of camels. Quetta itself was cool and pleasant with many fruit orchards, and Kennedy remarks, 'To one who like myself had not seen European trees and fruit for nearly twenty-nine years the sight was refreshing and exhilarating in the extreme.'[15]

The Divisions now took the road to Kandahar after 130 sick had been left in Quetta in the care of a section of the field hospital. The march proved difficult with the precipitous Kojak Pass to negotiate, a scarcity of water and shortage of food; all this in a temperature of 100° F; on one day 90 men went to hospital and 50 horses died; dead camels lay in heaps. On the advice of Dr. Atkinson camel kajawahs were used in place of the doolies, and proved much more effective. This was a wooden frame $4\frac{1}{2}$ feet long and $3\frac{1}{2}$ feet broad with room for two patients; one was slung on each side, so each camel carried four patients. Ten pairs were authorized for British, and five for Indian regiments.

Kandahar was reached on the 25th April after some 40 casualties had been incurred, many camp followers had been murdered, the cavalry had lost one fifth of its horses, and 20,000 camels had died since leaving Sukkur. The expedition had taken over three months to cover some 350 miles and there now followed a halt of two months for the replenishment of supplies.

Although the health of the army in the uplands of Afghanistan gave no cause for anxiety it was on the lines of communication that the convoys and their escorts suffered. Apart from the perils of the road, the stifling heat and the lack of sanitation at the staging posts caused a great deal of sickness. In the month of May the temperature rose to 120°F. in the tents, and 6 out of 14 European officers died as well as hundreds of soldiers and camp followers. At Shirkapur near Sukkur two officers were found dead in their beds 'their bodies turning as black as charcoal'. An Indian battalion escorting a convoy lost 6 officers, 100 sepoys, and 300 followers, and the single fly tents in which they lived did little to lessen the burning rays of the sun. Apart from heatstroke and exhaustion, dysentery and some outbreaks of cholera laid them low.

But in spite of these hazards thousands of camels carrying grain supplies managed to get through, and on the 27th June, Keane marched out from Kandahar on the road to Kabul, leaving behind a section of the field hospital to care for the sick unable to march. The troops were still on half rations and equally serious from the British soldiers' point of view was the failure of the spirit ration[16] although many officers considered it to be a blessing in disguise for its deprivation led in their opinion to increased bodily power and resistance to disease as well as improved discipline. Dr. Atkinson attributed to its absence the quicker healing of wounds.

When Ghazni was reached there were only three days' rations left and unless the army was to perish the town must be taken at once. It was a formidable fortress, but Afghanistan is the land of treachery and by its help Keane's task was made easier. A nephew of Dost Moham-med who had disaffected gave away the information that the Kabul gate was unguarded, and on the 23rd July the gate was blown in and the town stormed and captured at the cost of 17 killed and 165 wounded. The assault was undertaken by the British infantry alone, and nothing could have excelled the spirit displayed by the troops. On visiting the regimental hospitals of the 2nd (Queens) and the 17th Foot, Dr. Kennedy tells us, 'I was surprised to find them cleared of sick. The gallant fellows had all but risen in mutiny on their surgeons, and insisted on joining their comrades; none remained in hospital but the hopelessly bedridden who literally could not crawl; and even of these a portion, who could just stand and walk, were dressed, and made to look like soldiers, to take the hospital guard; no effective man could be kept away.'[17]

For the assault the General Order states: 'The Superintending Surgeon will arrange for having a portion of the field hospital established in the vicinity of the batteries; but in a hollow of the mountain and out of range of fire.' The site was a tented one a mile south-east of the town and Staff Surgeon Pinhey the Field Surgeon was assisted in his operations by the regimental surgeons of the 2nd and 17th Foot and the assistant surgeon of the Poona Horse. The others went in with the assault, and the medical officers of the artillery and engineers formed an aid post near the guns. That the R.M.O's were well up to the front line is vouched for by Havelock's account of the attack, for he found the stout hearted doolie bearers so far forward that they were obstructing the advance of the support party and enduring 'the fire of screened and hidden marksmen in the ramparts'. Some wounded who had been collected near the citadel after the town had been taken were unexpectedly attacked by Afghans and many were butchered before they were driven off. With the fall of the city, Kennedy exultantly reckons that there was £25,000 in prize money to be distributed. A proposal that all the sick and wounded should remain behind was vetoed by the Superintending Surgeons who considered it dangerous to split up the field hospital further, and it was then decided to leave only the worst cases with three assistant surgeons to look after them and carry along the remainder, some 250 in number, with the column.

With the capture of Ghazni food supplies were assured and the march at once resumed. On the 7th August Kabul was entered only to find that Dost Mohammed had fled, and Shah Sujah made his formal entry. The troops of the Bengal Division from Forezepore had marched 1,500 miles. Little opposition had been encountered, and since entering Afghanistan the health had greatly improved for the heat at this height was not oppressive, and food was good and plentiful.

The main objective having been attained the field hospital was broken up and the Bombay Division now only some 1,500 strong left Kabul, and during its return march to India a small force which included the 2nd (Queen's) and the 17th Foot were diverted to the capture of Khelat which was stormed on the 13th November 1839 at a cost of 31 killed and 107 wounded. When the Division arrived at Quetta there were only 7 per cent of Europeans and 6 per cent of sepoys in hospital, but it was a different story when they came to Baug on the lines of communication. 'There was little of the elation of men returning from a successful campaign. Death in fact was busy in their ranks. That dreadful scourge the cholera had made its appearance. Dr. Forbes . . . was the first victim, . . . the malady then spread with frightful rapidity,' and later, 'It was no longer possible to bring in those who died. The jungle and the road were strewn with corpses. I rode a little way into the town and about the camp. Many Europeans were lying on the ground intoxicated. In front of the agency they were digging a large pit, another outside the wall. They had thrown thirteen of the dragoons into one and at least as many of the artillery into the other. At least a hundred died that night.'[18] Kennedy who returned with the division describes it as the most distressing and untoward event of the whole campaign.[19] He was convinced the disease was contagious.

During his year at Sukkur Dr. Don had to treat many cases of sickness in the mud hospital which he had constructed. After the rains nine tenths of the garrison had gone down with malaria and at one staging post on the lines of communication an Indian battalion had 1,526 admissions and 90 deaths within six months; this site had been selected in spite of Kennedy's protests and he complains bitterly of the way medical proposals went unheeded. At the same time he was a genial and popular officer, and after his return he received an appreciative reference in orders and wrote a departmental order congratulating his officers on having won the approbation of higher authority on the way their duties had been performed. A discovery which pleased him was finding the root of the orchis plant, salep or salop, which when boiled down formed a finer jelly than arrowroot and has already been noticed as a popular light diet for invalids.

In Kabul, where the occupation, although an uneasy one continued for two and a half years, it was considered peaceful enough to allow wives and families to join their husbands. As time went on disaffection amongst the tribes gradually increased with Dost Mohammed still a powerful enemy hovering in the background. Sir John Macnaghton who acted as political adviser to Shah Sujah was entirely ignorant of any military principles and dispersed the troops in isolated forts where if danger occurred they would be overwhelmed piecemeal. Kabul was dominated by the fort of Bala Hissar but through Shah Sujah's wishes it was never occupied, and because of this serious omission the troops were housed in hutted cantonments in defiance of the military commander's advice. Keane was now replaced by Lieutenant General Elphinstone, a Peninsular veteran 75 years of age who was in poor health and disliked for his strict disciplinary measures which emphasised his morose nature. To keep the tribes quiet Macnaghton adopted the fatal policy of bribing them to silence, with the result that they soon realised that the more rebellious they became the more blackmail money they could extort.

During the summer of 1841 a new brigade including the 44th (Essex) Regiment had arrived and Sale's brigade which was relieved had attempted to return to India by the northern route through Peshawar. Because of opposition it had been unable to get further than Gandamak, and attempts to recall it met with no success. By November 1841 matters in Kabul had become critical; the Afghans were everywhere in open hostility, the outlying garrisons were cut off and destroyed, and both Macnaghton and Sir Alexander Burnes the agent were shortly afterwards treacherously murdered. The troops were besieged in their cantonments in Kabul, the tragic result of not occupying the Bala Hissar, and by a succession of blunders the food supplies and all the medical stores were lost to the Afghans, so that the plight of the sick in the regimental hospitals became pitiful.

Elphinstone was now faced with the difficult choice of fighting his way out of Kabul by immediately taking the road to Jalalabad and Peshawar, or of capitulating to the Afghans. Many officers would have preferred the former, but worn out by anxiety and ill health and hindered by the presence of the wives and families the General chose to agree to the specious promises of the Afghans to grant them safe conduct back to India. But by continually inventing excuses the wily Afghans delayed Elphinstone's departure until January 1842 when snow lay on the ground and it was bitterly cold. On the 6th of that month 4,500 fighting men, some women and children and 1,500 followers left the capital for the journey of 100 miles to Jalalabad through wild mountain roads and passes. The only British element was the 44th Foot and one troop of Horse Artillery, the remainder being native infantry, while there was a convoy of 600 to 700 sick of all units to encumber the slow moving column. Confusion and delays existed from the start and in two days only 10 miles were covered. In the narrow defiles through which the long column threaded its way attacks by tribesmen commenced and there were daily scenes of massacre. Defending themselves gallantly day after day until their ammunition ran out, food supplies failed, and exhaustion overtook them, officers and men sold their lives dearly. The regimental surgeons[20] brought their sick and wounded along as best they could amidst the confusion, and did what little was possible for them without medicines or dressings. But on the 10th January near Tezin four of them[21] lost their lives in the slaughter of that day when the last of the sepoys perished and the sick and wounded inevitably shared the same fate. Dr. Duff, the Superintending Surgeon who had relieved Atkinson was severely wounded in the hand, and endured an amputation at the wrist with a penknife, the only instrument available; weakened by his wound he fell behind and was cut down. Cardew was mortally wounded and laid on the last gun carriage to die. When they entered the Jagdalak Pass there remained only some 350 men mostly of the 44th Foot, and of this number only 20 officers and 45 rank and file survived when they emerged. Here Surgeon Harcourt of the 44th was killed. The last remnants made a final stand at Gandamak where Assistant Surgeon Primrose of the same regiment met his end. The few who survived including Dr. Harper all perished at Fatiabad, all that is except Dr. Brydon who alone and desperately wounded rode into Jalalabad. 'On 13th January the garrison . . . saw from its walls a solitary white faced horseman struggling on towards the fort. Slowly and painfully as though horse and man were in an extremity of mortal weakness the solitary mounted man came reeling tottering on.' Truly Brydon was described as 'the remnant of an army'.[22]

Brigadier General Sale's brigade had succeeded in reaching Jalalabad in November 1841 and since then had been under siege. In spite of many difficulties in procuring enough food and forage to survive the constant Afghan attacks these were always successfully repulsed, and relief arrived in April 1842 when a force under General Pollock pushed through by the way of the Khyber Pass. Assistant Surgeons Robertson and Barnes of the 13th Foot were deservedly mentioned for their meritorious services during the siege.

After delay due to transport difficulties and the presence of much dysentery amongst his troops, General Pollock in September forced his way through to Kabul, and released some eighty officers and others who had been kept as hostages. Elphinstone himself had succumbed from dysentery but the sick left behind in the city under the charge of the medical officers had suffered no harm. The Afghans had retaken Ghazni and slaughtered the garrison there, but General Nott with the 40th and 41st Foot stood firm at Kandahar and fought their way through enemy territory to Kabul where the two forces were finally united. The time had now come to shake the dust of the Afghan capital off their feet, and on the 11th October 1842 the army took the road to India via the Khyber Pass and the First Afghan War came to an end.

The statistics available cover only the early part of the campaign. Those for the Bombay Division alone are given in Kennedy's final report which covers the period of fourteen months from the 1st November 1838 to the 31st December 1839. Admissions to British hospitals numbered 4,648 and deaths 273, and to Indian hospitals 7,041, and deaths 135. Amongst the deaths were four medical officers. The strength of the Division after leaving Sukkur is given as 1,850 British and 1,820 Indian troops and if these figures are taken, the average rate per 1,000 for admissions for the period covered is 2,512 for British and 3,868 for Indian troops, and deaths for British are 147·5 and for Indian 74 per 1,000.

Another set of statistics commencing in January 1839 and ending on the arrival in Kabul in August 1839 covers the whole force. In British units there were 5,336 admissions in a strength of 2,684, which gives a rate of 1,990 per 1,000, and there was a death rate of nearly 100 per 1000. Surprisingly, the admissions for Indian troops who rarely suffered from bowel diseases or malaria to the same extent was almost equal at 1,680 per 1,000, but the death rate at 35 per 1000 was almost two thirds less. In the highlands the health was reasonably good in spite of the hardships of the march, and undoubtedly the heaviest incidence of disease occurred along the lines of communication where the sanitary conditions at the fouled ground of the staging posts was abysmally low. Here dead camels cumbered the ground, flies swarmed, and much dysentery occurred, with outbreaks of cholera from time to time as well as heatstroke, malaria and jaundice. As to the drinking habits of the British soldiers it is perhaps not surprising that too much rum and arrack was consumed and drunkenness however deplorable became a solace for the hardships they were called upon to endure. Borne down by the unchanging monotony of marching day after day and week after week to cover the 1,500 miles which some units travelled; contending with the heat, the dust, and the sand; loaded with 60 pounds of kit, living on insufficient food, and at times tortured by thirst, can it be wondered at that they eagerly turned to the consolation which alcohol afforded to wipe out their physical and mental weariness. Let it be remembered too that enlistment was for life and that there was no escape from this environment. No wonder the soldier rejoiced in the excitement which action brought and even the sick made light of their disabilities to join in the fray.

The officers of the Army Medical Department who took part in this campaign were twenty-seven in number. All were regimental medical officers but Assistant Surgeon Ross was also medical storekeeper of the Bengal Division. The three medical officers of the 44th (Essex Regiment), Surgeon Harcourt, and Assistant Surgeons Balfour and Primrose all perished in the march from Kabul, and two others died of disease. The H.E.I.C. suffered much more heavily and at least 13 medical officers lost their lives, 8 in action and 5 from disease.

China War 1839-1842

Our history now takes us to the China War of 1839, otherwise known as the Opium War. In the year 1833 the East India Company's monopoly of trade with China was broken and business with Canton thrown open to all merchants. The sale of opium to China brought India enormous profits, but the Chinese authorities wished to exclude the drug owing to its deleterious effects on the nation's health. This however did not stop the parties interested trading in the commodity, and as Fortescue puts it, 'The Chinese at large yearned for it, the British merchants were very eager to sell it, and the minor Chinese officials were very ready to admit it upon receiving a share of the gain.'[23]

The dispute was prolonged for some years and culminated in the expulsion of British merchants from Canton and the attack by a Chinese flotilla on two British frigates in the Canton river; vast quantities of opium were seized and the factories blockaded. Lord Auckland the Governor General of India was ordered by the British Government in 1840 to prepare an expedition to uphold the right after two centuries for British merchants to continue to trade with China, for their exclusion was an insult which could not be endured; the so-called Opium War was thus only one factor in a larger issue.

Initially a force including three British regiments[24] sailed from India with an escort of men of war and arrived off Macao on the 31st June 1840 where the British community expelled from Canton had taken refuge. A blockade of the Canton river was begun, but the troops themselves were landed at Ting-hai on the island of Chusan which was some 1,000 miles further up the coast off the mouth of the Yangtse-Kiang river. After this initial move months of inactivity followed which was marked by severe outbreaks of disease. For political reasons the buildings in the town were not used and the men were housed in tents pitched on low paddy fields surrounded by stagnant water which was putrid and stinking from quantities of dead animal and vegetable matter. The sole supply of drinking water was drawn from the irrigation channels. 'Under a sun hotter than ever experienced in India, the men on duty were buckled up to the neck in full dress coatees. Bad provisions, low spirits and despondency drove them to drink, and, in consequence of there being no camp followers, fatigue parties of Europeans were daily detailed to carry provisions and stores from the ships to the tents and to perform all menial employments.'[25] Fever and bowel infections swept through the ranks, and within six months the force of 2,500 men had had 3,239 admissions to hospital and 445 deaths. Malaria was the cause of 2,654 admissions and 91 deaths; diarrhoea 829 admissions and 70 deaths; and dysentery 759 admissions and 218 deaths; there were also 255 cases of continuous fever most of which were doubtless due to typhoid infections. To try and improve matters the 26th Foot (Cameronians) moved into the town in September, when their 400 sick were 'stretched pale and emaciated' on the floor of a large ill adapted building in Ting-hai. But it is doubtful whether the town with its narrow squalid streets and stagnant canals was much preferable to the paddy fields. Anyhow the plague was not stayed. 'On many a morning three to seven victims were carried out to be buried.'[26] This magnificent battalion originally 900 strong could at length only muster 110 weakened soldiers fit for duty. The 18th (Royal Irish) who occupied a joss house on high ground suffered less and had a death roll of 52, compared with 268 in the 26th, and 142 in the 49th.

Camping amidst this squalor and filth was not solely to blame for the illhealth, for the food was appalling. The meat, hurriedly salted in India, soon became semi putrid in the heat, and Surgeon Maclean[27] of the 18th tells us that the colonel of the regiment was such a hard man and indifferent to his men's health that he insisted that none of this semi putrid meat was to be wasted but consumed to the last cask, although all this time the seamen of the Royal Navy were eating fresh beef two or three times a week. By these harsh methods, says Maclean, he condemned his men to scorbutic dysentery, which, added to malaria and typhoid fever, destroyed the health of the regiment in a few weeks.

Dr. King of the Bengal Army who was Superintending Surgeon made strong representations on this appalling loss of life, a loss which he considered was largely due to the ignorance and obstinacy displayed by those commanding officers who refused to listen to the introduction of sanitary measures of any kind. King's advice was consistently ignored.

The blockade of Canton utterly failed to have any effect upon the Chinese Government and it was obvious further steps had to be taken. Accordingly every fit man to bear arms was summoned from Chusan, and with the arrival of a sepoy battalion from India and with the help of marines from the fleet the Canton river was entered and several forts on its banks captured. Although this forced the Chinese authorities to open talks, they proved entirely evasive; and the only concrete gain and one which was to have future important consequences was the occupation of the island of Hong Kong.

In March 1841 General Gough arrived from India to take command bringing with him Dr. French as Superintending Surgeon in place of Dr. King who, disgusted with the lack of co-operation displayed by the

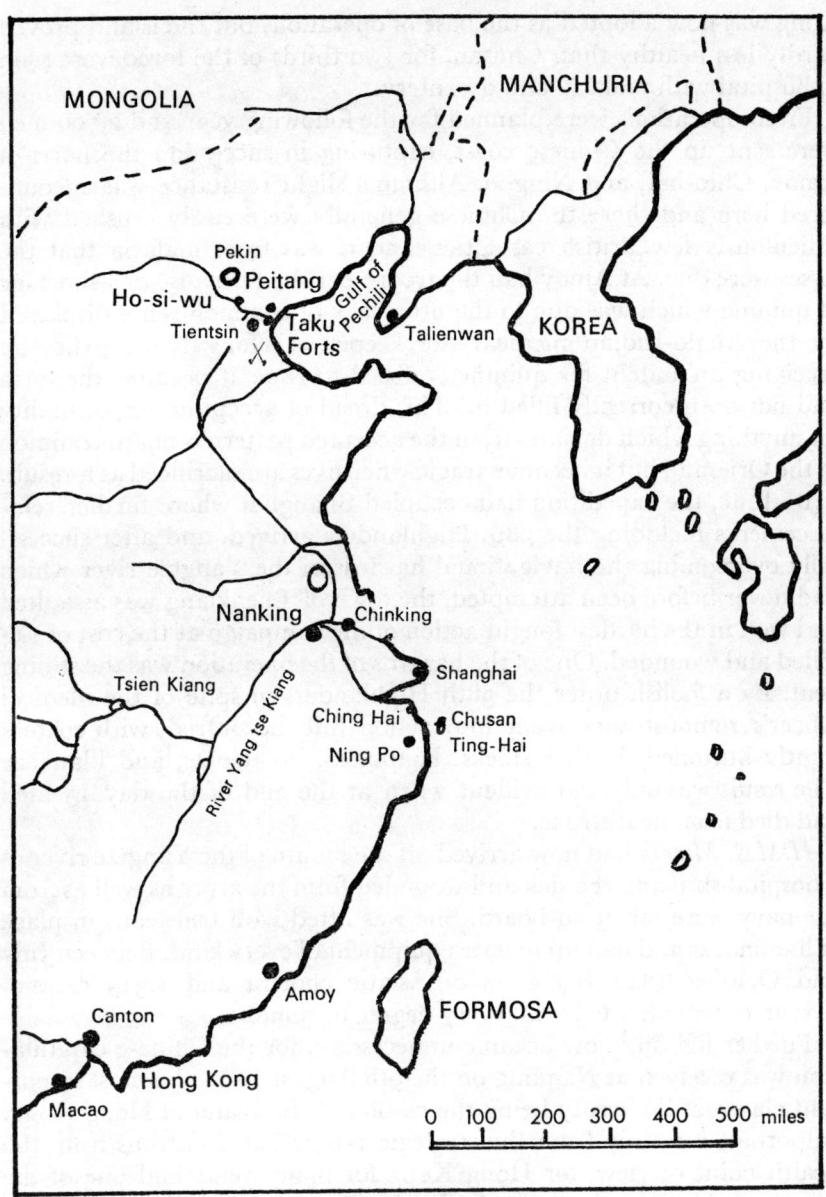

MONGOLIA

MANCHURIA

Pekin
Peitang
Ho-si-wu
Tientsin
Taku
Forts
Gulf of Pechili
Talienwan

KOREA

Nanking
Chinking
Tsien Kiang
River Yang tse Kiang
Shanghai
Ching Hai
Ning Po
Chusan
Ting-Hai

Amoy

FORMOSA

Canton
Hong Kong
Macao

0 100 200 300 400 500 miles

The China Wars 1839–42 1857–60

senior commanders, was, no doubt not unhappily, evacuated sick to India. Gough's attitude to health problems proved to be quite different, and French's advice was welcomed and carefully listened to.

Canton itself was now successfully stormed in May 1841 by a force of 3,500 men at the small cost of 14 killed and 91 wounded, and its fall resulted in an indemnity being paid by the government of China. Hong

Kong was now adopted as the base of operations but the island proved hardly less healthy than Chusan, for two thirds of the force were soon in hospital with malaria and dysentery.

Fresh operations were planned for the following year and 2,700 men were sent up the Chinese coast, capturing in succession the ports of Amoy, Chin-hai, and Ningpo. Although slight resistance was encountered here and there the Chinese generally were easily crushed with ridiculously few British casualties, and it was from malaria that the losses were due. At Amoy half the troops perished because of a shortage of quinine which was due to the utter lack of common sense displayed by the Anglo-Indian medical storekeeper at Hong Kong, who, on receiving an indent for quinine, refused to issue it because the form had not been correctly filled in! This dread of accepting responsibility for anything which deviates from the accepted pattern is not uncommon in the Oriental, but it becomes tragic when lives are sacrificed as a result.

By June, the expedition had occupied Shanghai where further reinforcements including the 98th Highlanders arrived, and after successfully overcoming the navigational hazards of the Yangtze river which had never before been attempted, the town of Tsienkiang was assaulted and won in the hardest fought action of the campaign at the cost of 144 killed and wounded. One of the hazards of the operation was the stifling heat. By a foolish order the 98th Highlanders in spite of the medical officer's remonstrance went into action fully accoutred, with coatees tightly buttoned, leather stocks, knapsacks, greatcoats, and blankets. The result was only too evident when at the end of the day 15 men had died from heat stroke.

H.M.S. Minden had now arrived off the mouth of the Yangtze river as a hospital ship and the sick and wounded from the army as well as from the navy were taken on board. She was fitted with bedsteads in place of hammocks and had up to date equipment of every kind. Between July and October 1842 107 cases of Asiatic cholera and 1,313 cases of dysentery were treated with every degree of comfort.

Further fighting now became unnecessary, for the Chinese capitulation was received at Nanking on the 9th August 1842, the most important clause of the treaty being the cession of the island of Hong Kong. Important certainly from the strategic aspect but disastrous from the health point of view, for Hong Kong for many years had one of the worst records for sickness in the British Empire. Sirr called it 'an unhealthy, pestilential, unprofitable and barren rock.'[28]

From the sanitary point of view Maclean considered the campaign as one of the most disgraceful in our military history and half the force lost their lives due to the utter disregard of the simplest precautions. He said that in his opinion if newspaper correspondents had been permitted to accompany the expedition, the scandal aroused would have led to reforms which would have obviated some of the breakdowns which later occurred in the Crimean War. Three medical officers were amongst those who lost their lives.

Hong Kong proved a costly acquisition as in spite of good barracks and hospitals the men continued to sicken and die. In July 1847 the 95th Foot buried 47 men and had 299 sick out of 450; in August a further 47 died, and to prevent further deterioration in health the whole unit was moved into vessels anchored in the harbour. Even this failed to stem the plague. In the following year the same luckless regiment between 1st June and 30th September buried a further 88 soldiers while 173 more were sick. The anopheles mosquito bred freely in the flooded hill terraces where rice was grown but this cause was still unknown, and one popular theory was that the disease was caused by 'disintegrated granite'.

First Sikh War 1845-1846

Since the death of Ranjit Singh in 1839 there had been anarchy and chaos in the Punjab amongst the various factions of the Sikh nation. Then the murder of Shere Sing the reputed son of Ranjit Singh resulted in the rise to power of a faction which was hostile to the Indian Government. General Sir Hugh Gough the Commander-in-Chief sensing the danger to some of the Sikh states which were under British protection took the precaution of reinforcing the frontier garrisons of Ferozepore, Ludhiana, and Ambala. On the 11th December 1845 the Sikhs crossed the Sutlej with hostile intent and Gough advanced from Ambala to meet them with a force of between 11,000 and 12,000 men.

The battles of the First Sikh War were fought against a brave and resolute enemy and it was chiefly the fire power of the regular forces backed up by the indomitable fighting spirit of the British soldier which brought victory. The battles of Mudki, Ferozeshah, Aliwal, and Sobraon were all fought within a period of three months between December 1845 and February 1846, and in the campaign three British cavalry regiments and ten British infantry regiments were engaged apart from Indian units.

In the initial stages the field medical organization in the hands of the Honourable East India Company was woefully deficient. There was a superintending surgeon in administrative control, a field surgeon, and a medical storekeeper,[29] but no field hospital was provided, and the regimental hospitals had to bear the whole brunt of treating the casualties. Evacuation in the field was carried out entirely by doolies and 75 were apportioned to each British regiment.

At the battle of Mudki, where there were 812 casualties, a shortage of doolies due to many having been left behind in the rapidity of the approach march added to delays in bringing in the wounded. Both the superintending surgeon and the field surgeon lent a hand in the regimental hospitals, and when the force followed up the enemy defeat

First and Second Sikh Wars (1845–6) (1848–9)

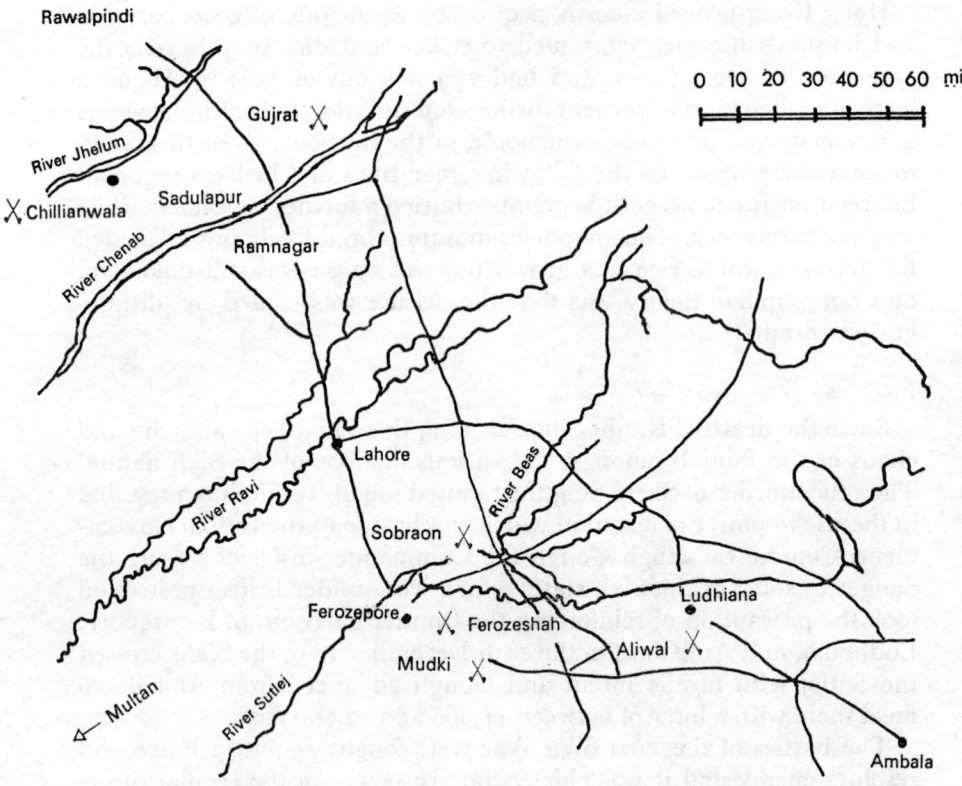

and took with them the regimental hospitals, they remained behind at Mudki to continue their work in a temporary hospital hastily formed with improvised equipment. In spite of the lack of proper facilities, Lieutenant Edwards, one of the patients, testified to the comfort and cleanliness and the attention he received from both surgeons and subordinates. In this fiercely fought battle Sir Robert Sale the Q.M.G. was mortally wounded, one of the divisional commanders was killed, and two brigadiers wounded. Assistant Surgeon Graydon of the 50th Foot was struck down while dressing the wounds of a gunner under fire and died later.

With an army now 18,000 strong Gough attacked the Sikh position at Ferozeshah on the 21st December and defeated the enemy after a desperate conflict which lasted for two days. Our losses were 700 killed and 1,720 wounded,—the 62nd Foot being heavily engaged lost half their strength. Again there was no field hospital to help the overwhelmed regimental surgeons, and with both the superintending and the field surgeons still engaged in treating the casualties left at Mudki there was no-one to direct operations. Nearly all the doolie bearers bolted from panic; the severely wounded lay uncollected on the battle-field all night; while the walking wounded straggled back to Ferozepore some 15 miles distant. By commendable exertions the Commissariat Department collected fresh bearers, elephants, and bullock carts, by whose help the wounded were eventually brought in, although Surgeon Taylor of the 29th Foot says that some lay on the field for three days as all the baggage and tents had been left at Mudki.

To illustrate the chaos which resulted from the lack of any medical direction we quote from a private letter written by a regimental surgeon and sent to the *Lancet* by George Guthrie of Peninsular fame. 'I have just brought in the wounded of our regiment to this station (Ferozepore) where there is a commissariat and some accommodation. They are 175 in number. I am here single handed . . . the labour I have undergone is excessive . . . I am one of four (officers) three of whom are absent . . . How can I be expected to practice scientific surgery surrounded by 175 wounded men all clamouring and beseeching for assistance? I have no time to do anything satisfactorily. I have however managed to do four amputations today, and dressed the greater number of serious cases, including two amputations I brought off the field, and am weary of the bloody work. We had in the field with us a quantity of water, some brandy, wax candles and a fair proportion of medical and surgical stores, and followed close in rear of the regiment, till the men began to drop around us chiefly with wounds from cannon shot . . . We halted under a tree . . . and the hospital soon became a dreadful scene of mangled bodies. The men of the band brought in the wounded and we were getting on well when a great misfortune befell us.' The writer then describes how they were inundated by wounded from every unit; many of his doolie bearers were stolen by the cavalry; all their water was soon consumed. When it grew dark they were ordered to rejoin the regiment but they lost their way and blundered into fire from the Sikh lines. The few doolie bearers left threw down the hospital stores and bolted; the wounded lying on the field had to be abandoned, and were afterwards massacred in cold blood.

The absence of a field hospital was more acutely felt than at Mudki for the losses were three times as heavy. Eventually the Governor General himself took a hand and arranged for the wounded to be moved into the barracks of the 23rd Foot at Ferozepore where a commissary was appointed to attend to the feeding. Overcrowding was inevitable and hospital gangrene was soon rife. The only A.M.D. casualty was Assistant Surgeon Gahan of the 31st Foot who died from secondary hæmorrhage after amputation of the thigh.

On the 29th January followed another victory at Aliwal where a force of 12,000 horse and foot was commanded by Sir Harry Smith. This was a fine achievement at a cost of only 589 casualties and had an encouraging effect upon the morale of the sepoy battalions. A minor engagement before the battle had resulted in the baggage train and wounded being cut off by the Sikhs with the loss of all the wounded. Here Assistant Surgeon Banon of the 62nd Foot who was in charge fell into enemy hands and was kept in irons for twelve days; after great suffering and constant peril he was finally released on the advance to Lahore.

Learning from previous mistakes there was now a most welcome improvement in the field medical arrangements; the staff and equipment of a field hospital had been brought up and this was opened at Ludhiana under the field surgeon's direction. The official despatch says: 'Owing to the judicious arrangements of Dr. Murray the Field Surgeon, every wounded officer and soldier was placed under cover and provided for soon after dark; and to the zeal displayed by this able and persevering medical officer and to the several regimental surgeons are the wounded and our country deeply indebted.'[30]

Sobraon which took place on the 9th February 1846 was the decisive battle of the war and a complete British victory. Our casualties were heavy, amounting in all to 2,283 including nearly 2,000 wounded, and the losses fell more equally on British and Indian units alike; the sepoys fought well and the Gurkhas especially distinguished themselves.

The effective medical arrangements were repeated here with Dr. Macleod new H.E.I.C. Superintending Surgeon. A tented field hospital was established behind the front and the wounded treated by a team of surgeons before they were removed to the main hospital centre which had grown up at Ferozepore. General Gough in his despatch said: 'Superintending Surgeon B. Macleod, M.D, has been indefatigable in the fulfilment of every requirement of his important and responsible situation. I am entirely satisfied with his exertions and their results.'[31]

In discussing the surgery of this campaign Surgeon McGrigor emphasised the desirability of performing primary amputation which could however only be effected when there was ample surgical potential. 'The necessity,' he says, 'for promptitude was well exemplified by what occurred in some regiments where hardly an amputation succeeded when performed at a late period. In all engagements, in India at least, the sooner a limb is lost after it has been wounded the greater will be the chance of success. Hence the necessity for a field hospital is an important point which will not, it is hoped, be overlooked in future wars.'[32] A similar point was made by Mr. Guthrie who wrote an outspoken commentary on the great loss of life which must have resulted from the absence of any field hospital with its operating staff. Whether this was due to lack of planning by higher authority or by financial stringency in the matter of hospital equipment or medical stores, or the feeling that the regimental hospitals with their generous standard of equipment would be able to cope it is impossible to say. It was not until the disaster at Ferozeshah brought the matter officially to light under the eyes of the Governor General himself that the neglect was rectified. As we have seen, the policy of denuding the regimental establishment of officers to staff the temporary field hospitals broke down, and the field surgeon whose responsibility it was to perform the major operations was unable to cope singlehanded and had to be assisted by the superintending surgeon. Both moreover were immobilised at Mudki. This *ad hoc* arrangement could not compete with the two major engagements fought within three days of each other in different localities, and many of the wounded consequently lost the benefit of early amputation. In the hurly burly of action it was always difficult and often impossible for the regimental officers to perform capital operations, and only a team of surgeons working in a field hospital could devote the requisite attention to surgery. Moreover the regimental surgeon was always torn between remaining with his regimental headquarters during the fight or remaining behind and treating the wounded in the regimental hospital. McGrigor had no doubts on the subject. 'The duty' he says, 'of the regimental surgeon is to be with the wounded, no matter whether they be in the field or at a depot near at hand, until all capital operations are performed.'[33] But not all commanding officers agreed with this and many preferred to retain the surgeon at regimental headquarters and leave operations to less skilled assistant surgeons.

The failure of the Company's medical organization to provide efficient treatment for British casualties had a disturbing effect on the British Government and the Director General decided that a senior A.M.D. officer must be present in future to safeguard their interests. Deputy Inspector Franklin was consequently appointed to supervise the arrangements for any future operations which included British units.

In the First Sikh War twenty-nine officers of A.M.D. took part in the campaign as regimental medical officers and of these, two lost their lives.

Second Sikh War 1848-1849

In 1848 the Sikhs broke out again in open rebellion after the murder of two political officers at Multan. The town was stormed by Government troops and occupied in January 1849 at the cost of over 1,000 casualties. That the medical preparations won approval is recorded in General Whish's despatch which reads 'Superintending Surgeon Dempster had uniformly and successfully applied his talents and assiduity to the promotion of the health and comfort of the sick and wounded, and been ably supported by the medical officers of every corps and department'. Hostilities then broke out in the northern Punjab and to deal with this threat General Gough concentrated at Lahore an army of some 20,000 men.

As a result of the lessons of the First Sikh War the field medical organisation was now on an ample scale, and associated with Dr. Renny of H.E.I.C. the Superintending Surgeon, Deputy Inspector Franklin of A.M.D. was present throughout. Field hospital beds were provided on a scale of 3 per cent for 6,400 British troops, (200 beds) and 1·4 per cent for 13,600 Indian troops, (200 beds), this bed cover being in addition to each regimental establishment of 60 beds, (6 per cent), making a total of 9 per cent for British and 7·4 per cent for Indian troops.

At Ferozepore a main hospital base was established with reserves of medical officers and subordinate staff, and a medical supply depot containing six months supply of medical comforts and wine for 5,000 British troops. For the carriage of sick and wounded there were 383 doolies with over 2,500 bearers, together with country carts and charpoys (native beds) for use either for carriage in the field or as hospital beds. Hospital tentage was conveyed on elephants.

After minor actions at Ramnagar and Sadulapur Gough attacked an army of 30,000 Sikhs at Chillianwala and had to fight the most stubborn battle of the war, the result of which was indecisive. The casualties amounted to 2,300 including 1,641 wounded, the greater proportion falling on the Queen's regiments. The 24th Foot lost 518 of all ranks.

For this operation the field hospital was moved up to Ramnagar, and for the battle itself a section of twenty-five beds was at first pushed across the river Chenab at Sadulapur, and subsequently opened up in the battle zone. The fighting was so intense that the doolie bearers who generally showed a great deal of courage refused to collect the lying cases and they had to be left on the field until nightfall, while the field hospital section was temporarily thrown out of action by the rout of a cavalry brigade. For the surgeons the night was one of incessant labour while the rain descended in torrents, but the resources at Ramnagar were ample[34] and 504 surgical cases were dealt with, 284 of whom were Europeans.

Gough was now reinforced, and with an army 24,000 strong was ready to strike a decisive blow. Thus at the battle of Gujrat on the 21st February 1849, a Sikh army of 60,000 men suffered a disastrous defeat. The tactics employed differed from previous battles. The heavy guns on this occasion battered the Sikh position for two and a half hours until the enemy guns were mastered. Then the infantry, still covered by our artillery, attacked and swept all before them. The cavalry were then let loose and pursued the enemy for miles. All the wounded were treated in the field hospital pitched in tents behind the artillery park.

The enemy were followed up as far as Rawalpindi, and to this flying column was attached a field hospital with equipment for 300 to 400 beds, a field surgeon, and 11 assistant surgeons, with 91 doolies under 2 medical officers for the carriage of cases. It had in fact only sick to deal with as the Sikhs had had enough and the final surrender took place on the 14th March 1849.

In the northern Indian climate which is dry and cold in the winter the health was good. Between the 1st November and the 31st March only 7 per cent of British and 4 per cent of Indian troops were evacuated to the base hospital at Ferozepore.

With Inspector Franklin there were twenty-eight regimental officers of the Army Medical Department employed in this campaign, and Renny, Franklin, and Macrae the Field Surgeon, were mentioned personally in despatches by General Gough, who added, 'the medical officers of the army generally have been most unwearied and praiseworthy'.

Clearly the lessons of the First Sikh War had been taken to heart; the medical services were well directed and the field organisation all that could be desired.

Scinde 1842-43

We pass now to the conquest of Scinde by Sir Charles Napier in 1842. The country was in the hands of a despotic body of Baluchi nobles, or Amirs, who had consented very unwillingly to a treaty permitting the passage of troops through their country on the occasion of the First Afghan War and subsequently to the occupation of Karachi and free navigation on the Indus. The hostile designs of the Amirs led to war and the force which Napier led against them amounted in all to some 3,500 men including one British unit, the 22nd (Cheshire) Regiment. The area was largely desert and the first operations involved a four days march through an ocean of loose sand where the guns had to be dragged by fatigue parties of infantry in addition to teams of twenty-five camels which were yoked to each. All transport was by camel, and the sick, luckily few in the fine winter climate, were carried on kajawahs.

Two battles were fought at Miani and at Hyderabad at a cost in all of over 500 casualties including some 400 wounded who were dealt with entirely on a regimental basis. Superintending Surgeon Dalrymple of H.E.I.C. was the senior medical officer at Miani to whose 'activity and zeal' Napier referred in his despatch. At the successful battle of Hyderabad which followed 'the exertions of the officers of the medical service under Inspecting Surgeon Bell' were described as 'very laudable'.[35] The next three months were spent in hunting down the enemy in the desert in the terrific heat of summer. Marching was only done at night, the men remaining in their tents during the day with wet towels round their heads; even so there were many casualties from the sun and on one day alone thirty-three British soldiers died. But in the end Napier's success in conquering Scinde with such a tiny force under conditions of appalling hardship did much to restore the prestige of the army after the disasters of the First Afghan War.

Leadership in the field was matched by Napier's success as an administrator during the next four years as Governor of the province, and he was worshipped by his men for the interest he took in their health and their living conditions. Owing to the prevalence of malaria and cholera the country proved a veritable death trap to Europeans and sepoys alike. Malaria was impossible to prevent while the all prevailing anopheles mosquito lurked unsuspected as the cause, and Napier points this out in a letter to the Commander-in-Chief in 1843. 'I can tell you as much about sickness as the doctors. Malaria has long been watched by me in various countries . . . the cause is known to be decayed vegetable matter. Nothing in the power of Government can prevent it; while the Indus overflows its banks and rain falls, malaria will be present in Scinde.'[36] There were numerous instances to prove his words. In August 1844 the 78th (Seaforth Highlanders) arrived at Sukkur on the Indus and in seven months the regiment lost from malaria 3 officers, 532 other ranks, 68 women and 134 children. 'Some lingered for weeks, some for days. It was not infrequent to hear of the death of a man to whom one had spoken but half an hour previously. The hospital was filled with upwards of 800 men under treatment. Quinine alone appeared to give them any relief, and their eagerness for it was pitiable to behold.'[37] This was malignant malaria in its severest form and after the damage was done and it was too late Sukkur was abandoned as a station. The lessons of the First Afghan War when so many died at this very station might have been taken to heart before condemning British troops to a similar fate. But such is ever the way.

From malaria we turn to cholera which in 1846 broke out in Karachi. In the course of a week the 86th Regiment (2nd Royal Ulster Rifles) lost 208 men (apart from women and children), and in the course of seven months there were 1,838 admissions and 918 deaths in a community numbering 8,566. Surgeon Alexander Thom described the scene in his hospital on the 16th June. 'As the night closed in a scene presented itself such as few minds can conceive or pens depict. The floors were literally strewed with the livid bodies of men labouring under the pangs of premature dissolution, surrounded by crowds of attendants trying to alleviate their hopeless sufferings. Many were brought in with the cold and clammy damp of death, as if sudden obstruction of every vital function had taken place, and the fountain of life had been arrested by an invisible but instantaneous shock. For these all human aid was in vain. Others were struggling with all the violence of strong men against the agony produced by the spasmodic action of the muscles of the body, and their yells and cries, commingling in fearful discordance with the subdued groans and gaspings of those nearer the closing scene, were truly heart rending . . . the places of those who continued to fall victims to the disease were too often occupied by men who had lately been their attendants. Indeed, it not infrequently happened that the soldier's attendant was found lying in the agonies of the disease beside the pallet of his dying charge.'[38] In this devastating epidemic which attacked 410 persons the death rate rose to over 50 per cent. The little that could be done to alleviate the symptoms of such a disease as Asiatic cholera is given in Surgeon Thom's report. Bleeding of course was a 'sine qua non' but was carried out only in the early and never in the later stages, while internally, a variety of drugs were tried, mostly with little effect. Calomel 10 to 20 grs. was given with 1 to 2 grs. of opium; or two drops of croton oil to rouse biliary function; or again diacetate of lead $\frac{1}{8}$ to 1 gr. in severe cases, with $\frac{1}{2}$ or $\frac{1}{4}$ gr. acetate of morphia every one or two hours; or hydrocyanic acid 1 drop hourly. As stimulants, brandy, wine, beer, ammonia, ether, and camphor were administered. Locally, patients were treated by friction, heat, vesication by scalding water, turpentine, and mustard. To supplement the overwhelmed hospital staff Napier had given orders that 3 officers, 9 sergeants, and 100 men were to be camped near each regimental hospital and divided into three reliefs, each on duty for six hours at a time.

Asiatic cholera has sent many thousands of British troops and their families to their death throughout the length and breadth of India, and it is right that our readers should realize the scenes however horrifying which accompanied such outbreaks. Not until the cause of cholera had been discovered over forty years later could any effective preventive measures be undertaken to lessen this deadly scourge.[39]

In his efforts to improve living conditions Napier swept away the low mud huts, dark, windowless, and unventilated, which for too long had housed the British soldier. The stench of these in the morning he says is horrible. At Hyderabad and Karachi new barracks were built 30 feet high with thick walls and windows for ventilation. These 'are expensive no doubt; so are sick soldiers; so are dead soldiers.'[40] When five years later he became Commander-in-Chief in India he laid down the standard allotment of 1,000 cubic feet of space to every person in barracks. Of the injurious effects of drink he held the strongest views. The soldier's daily ration of two 'drams' of rum was equal he says to on third of a quart bottle, and he was in the habit of drinking one glass before and one after breakfast as a pick me up before the day's work. Dr. Robertson of the 13th Foot said that whenever it was impossible to get spirits the hospitals were empty, and quoted the case of the siege of Jalalabad where there was not a sick man until they were relieved and the spirits arrived. There is too the evidence of the First Afghan War when after the rum ration failed medical opinion was convinced that the general health and the discipline vastly improved. A surgeon in the American War put it in another way. 'When a soldier is poor in money he abounds in health.'[41]

It may be easy enough in the light of modern knowledge to criticise many of Napier's sanitary orders in detail especially in the handling of a cholera epidemic, but his persistent and successful exertions for the welfare of the army deserve that his name be held in perpetual memory.

The Gwalior War of 1843 must be dismissed in a few words. This Mahratta state situated in Central India was the victim of a dispute about the succession, and six British regiments were here involved. There were two battles fought simultaneously at Maharajpore and Panniar on the 29th December by Sir Hugh Gough the Commander-in-Chief in Bengal and Sir John Grey respectively. At Maharajpore the Mahrattas put up a stiff fight and casualties amounted to 797 of whom 648 were wounded, half of them borne by the 39th and 40th Foot. In the absence of any planned field hospital an extemporised one was set up on the scene of action, and three of the regimental surgeons assisted each other in dealing with the wounded. When the army moved away these were left under guard until after Gwalior fell, when they were dispatched to Allahabad by doolies and native carts and thence by steamer to Calcutta.

Superintending Surgeon Andrew Wood and Field Surgeon Alexander Chalmers both of the Company's service were mentioned in despatches and also one A.M.D. officer, Assistant Surgeon Stephens of the 63rd serving on the C.-in-C's staff.

Second Burma War 1852

After a lapse of nearly thirty years, trouble arose in Burma when the British residents at Ava were treated with indignity and British traders in Rangoon were subjected to interference and oppression. The Commodore of the British squadron ordered all British residents on board his flagship and blockaded the mouth of the Irrawaddy river. After some minor naval actions it was decided to send two infantry brigades from India under Major General Godwin, and escorted by a naval flotilla the force arrived in April 1852, six weeks before the breaking of the rains. Dr. Montgomerie. H.E.I.C., was the Superintending Surgeon and brought with him a fully equipped field hospital and a staff of 5 assistant surgeons, all conveyed in the hospital ship *Tubal Cane*.

The campaign of 1852 was fought under similar conditions to that of 1824 in swamp and jungle and in stifling heat. Inevitably there were many victims of disease, but the lessons of thirty years before had not been thrown away and there was an increasing appreciation of sanitary problems and some genuine and well directed effort toward their solution. For housing purposes sectional wooden huts were sent from Moulmein, and in striking contrast to 1824 when the ration was semi putrid salt meat, the troops were now well fed; salt meat had been abandoned in the tropics since 1838 and fresh beef on the hoof was now supplied with fish, poultry, fruit and vegetables freely available from the bazaars. The problem of clothing had however never been fully tackled and the unsuitable tight coatee and the leather stock which had

proved such an encumbrance in China ten years before were still retained; but trousers were of drill, dyed blue, and some head protection
achieved by winding pugri cloth around the headdress.

Active operations commenced by the bombardment of Rangoon and
the destruction of the stockade, and in the landing that followed there
were 17 killed and 132 wounded. But April was the hottest month of the
year and the heat caused many casualties. Two officers died soon after
landing, while 'here and there others were to be seen on the ground
. . . the medical officers and their subordinates administering
relief by pouring water over the patients'.[42] Cholera too had already
made its appearance at Martaban on the coast and now struck with
deadly effect. At night the 51st (K.O.Y.L.I.) bivouacked amidst the
burning ruins of the town surrounded by heaps of dead bodies giving
out an intolerable stench; upwards of 50 men were seized with
cholera and 42 were dead by morning. After the hospital ship
had been towed up the river to Rangoon, the field hospital was disembarked and set up in a temple. Here Assistant Surgeon Joseph
Fayrer, H.E.I.C.[43] was in charge, and when the G.O.C. arrived complaining that he had not been met by a commissioned officer and mur-
mured something about neglect of duty, Fayrer was equal to the
occasion and indignantly denied that there had 'been any neglect and
that all officers and men had worked very hard,' a fact which the
General had to admit when he went round the hospital. On leaving he
embraced Fayrer and confessed he was 'much obliged for his kindness
to my sick and wounded . . .'[44]

Bassein and Pegu were next captured and there followed a period of
inaction when dysentery, malaria and cholera decimated the units;
one sepoy battalion had 300 men on the sick list, and at Martaban out
of 2,000 men, 1,200 were in hospital. To relieve this overcrowding a
convalescent depot was established at Amherst a more healthy site south
of Moulmein. An expedition now steamed up the Irrawaddy river and
temporarily occupied Prome, but Godwin had not sufficient troops for
permanent occupation owing to the heavy sick wastage, and operations
had therefore to be held up pending the arrival of reinforcements in
September which brought the total strength to some 20,000 men.
Prome was again occupied, but all attempts to bring the enemy to
battle in the open were in vain. Eventually a column of some 1,250
men was organized to attack Donobyu, and advanced through thick
jungle in steaming heat with cholera depleting the ranks. After enduring these hardships for twenty-four days the enemy stockade was
stormed and captured at the cost of 120 killed and wounded, and 100
victims from cholera. All were evacuated along jungle paths by doolies
until river transport on the Irrawaddy took them to Rangoon. Meanwhile a local revolution had broken out in the Burmese capital of Ava
and fighting ceased in the spring of 1853 after the war had lasted just

a year. Peace was proclaimed on the 30th June and the whole of southern Burma passed into our hands.

The First Burma War with its phenomenal death roll was one of the most costly in lives and one of the worst found expeditions ever fought by the Indian Government. On this occasion conditions were greatly improved. The troops in Rangoon were hutted, the food was good, the hospitals well equipped, and the men according to the standards of the time well cared for. But contemporary medical knowledge could do little to overcome the wastage caused by fever, dysentery, and cholera.

The table below gives the rates of sickness and the mortality for the two years 1852 and 1853.

Year	Regiments	Mean strength during the year	Mean number constantly sick in hospital	Admissions into hospital during the year	Deaths
1852	18th 51st 80th	1635	169·25	4,328	376
1853	18th 51st 80th	1703	220·25	4,687	436

These figures show that on average every soldier was admitted to hospital between two and a half and three times each year. The mortality was extremely heavy being 236 per 1,000 in 1852, and 256 per 1,000 in 1853. Amongst individual units the 18th Foot had 16 other ranks killed and lost 302 from disease; the 51st, 289 from disease, and the 80th, 221.

In referring to the prevailing diseases, the figures are based on the five year period 1852 to 1856. This shows that dysentery and diarrhœa were the cause of the largest number of hospital admissions amounting to 4,945 cases and 481 deaths, of which number dysentery accounted for 3,255 cases and 441 deaths, a mortality rate of 13·5 per cent. There were 4,362 admissions for fever and this includes intermittent fever or malaria (1,696), common continued fever (1,387), and remittent fever (1,299). Evidently the malaria cases were well controlled for only twelve deaths occurred. Cholera was of course the most deadly of all infections and of the 785 cases, 235 perished or 29·9 per cent.

Amongst the ten regimental medical officers of A.M.D. who served in this campaign one was wounded, and another present was Assistant Surgeon Thomas Crawford who afterwards became Director General. Assistant Surgeon Joseph Fayrer of the H.E.I.C. was destined to be one of the most famous of the many outstanding doctors of the Indian Medical Service, and began his army career in the British Ordnance Medical Department.

REFERENCES

[1] Included as a novelty was a small steam vessel, the first ever used in British warfare.

[2] Bell. *Rough Notes of an Old Soldier*, p. 247. Day & Son, London 1867.

[3] Bell. *Rough Notes of an Old Soldier*, p. 232. Day & Son, London 1867.

[4] Bell. *Rough Notes of an Old Soldier*, p. 248. Day & Son, London 1867.

[5] Wilson. *Narrative of the Burmese War*.

[6] Gore, A. A. West Africa. *Annual Report of the Health of the Army for 1867*, p. 404.

[7] Michie (1877). *Memoir of Sir Andrew Smith*, p. 7. Alnwich Blair, London (1877).

[8] Later Sir Harry Smith

[9] Two cavalry regiments and eleven infantry battalions.

[10] Mitra. *Life of Sir John Hall*, p. 161. Longmore, Green, London (1811).

[11] Mitra. *Life of Sir John Hall*, p. 233. Longmore, Green, London (1811).

[12] Mitra. *Life of Sir John Hall*, p. 238. Longmore, Green, London (1811).

[13] Mitra. *Life of Sir John Hall*, p. 278. Longmore, Green, London (1811).

[14] Kennedy (1840). *Narrative of the Campaign of the Army of the Indus 1838-9*.

[15] Kennedy (1840). *Narrative of the Campaign of the Army of the Indus 1838-9*, vol. I, p. 227.

[16] The rum ration was 2 'drams' a day apparently 8 ounces, and normally an unlimited amount of arrack could be bought in the regimental bazaar.

[17] Kennedy (1840). *Narrative of the Campaign of the Army of the Indus 1838-9*, vol. III, pp. 46-7.

[18] *Dry leaves from young Egypt*—quoted by Kempthorne. Journal *R.A.M.C.*, vol. LVI, p. 61. The deaths were in fact 2 officers and 56 other ranks out of a strength of 700.

[19] Kennedy (1840). *Narrative of the Campaing of the Army of the Indus 1838-9*, vol. II, p. 158.

[20] The surgeons had drawn lots as to who should be left behind. Assistant Surgeon Primrose of the 44th was one of these but unfortunately for himself exchanged with the Embassy surgeon.

[21] Duff, Bryce, Cardew and Metcalfe, all of H.E.I.C.

[22] Dr. Willaim Brydon served with distinction in the Indian mutiny during the siege of Lucknow and received the C.B.

[23] Fortescue. Vol. XII, chapter XXXV, pp. 302-3. MacMillan, London (1910).

[24] 18th, 29th, 49th Foot.

[25] Dr. Macpherson. *Two years in China*.

[26] Morrison. Journal *R.A.M.C.*, vol. LIV, pp. 398-393.

[27] Maclean. *Memories of a Long Life*. Constable, Edinburgh (1895).

[28] Sirr. *China and the Chinese*, p. 389.

[29] The medical storekeeper in Indian formations was a Commissioned British medical officer.

[30] Sir Harry Smith. Despatches, 30th January 1846.

[31] Gough's Despatches.

[32] W. L. McGrigor. *History of the Sikhs*.

[33] W. L. McGrigor. *History of the Sikhs*.

[34] A field surgeon, 13 assistant surgeons, a medical storekeeper, 2 uncovenanted physicians, a sub-assistant surgeon, 2 apothecaries, 3 stewards, 10 hospital apprentices, 6 native doctors.

[35] Kempthorne. 'The Army Medical Services in India 1840-53', Journal *R.A.M.C.*, vol. LVI, p. 225.

[36] Napier. *Life of Sir Charles Napier*.

[37] Napier. *Life of Sir Charles Napier*.

[38] Kempthorne. 'The Army Medical Services in India 1840-53', Journal *R.A.M.C.*, vol. LVI, p. 228.

[39] The cholera bacillus was identified by Koch in 1884.

[40] Napier. *Life of Sir James Napier*.

[41] Parkes. Pamphlet No. 11, Muniment Room, R.A.M.C. College.

[42] Laurie. *Our Burmese Wars*.

[43] Later Sir Joseph Fayrer.

[44] Kempthorne. 'The Army Medical Service in India 1840-53', Journal *R.A.M.C.*, vol. LVI, p. 309.

APPENDICES

Appendix to Chapter 2

A

'Charles R.

'Whereas, for the preventing of the great and uncertain charge of the Apothecaries' bills of physic and internal medicines for sick soldiers, we have thought fit to allow forty shillings a year to Richard Whittle for providing of physic and internal medicines besides the forty shillings for each company allowed to the Surgeon of the Regiment of Our Foot Guards for external medicines yearly, which said allowance of forty shillings yearly for physic or internal medicines is to commence from the twentieth of September last. Our Will and Pleasure, therefore, is that you take notice thereof, and give it in orders, that when the non-commissioned officers and private soldiers respectively shall be sick, the said Richard Whittle may be applied to for internal medicines, as well as hurt men are to apply to the Surgeon of the Regiment for external medicines, when they need the same.'

'Given at Our Court at Whitehall, the
24th day of January, 1673.

'By His Majesty's Command
'Arlington.'

'To our Trusty and Well-beloved
Colonel John Russell, or other the
Officer in Chief commanding Our
Regiment of Foot Guards under his command.'

B

'Charles R.

'Whereas, for preventing of the great and uncertain charge of Apothecaries' bills of physic and internal medicines for sick soldiers. We have thought fit to allow twenty shillings a year for each Regimental Company of three score soldiers besides officers, to the respective Surgeons of Regiments, from the twentieth of September last, for providing and furnishing of physic, and internal medicines, as well as there has been and is forty shillings yearly, for each such company allowed to the said Surgeons for external medicines for the respective requirements in which they serve. Our Will and Pleasure therefore is, that you take notice thereof, and that you give it in orders, that when the non-commissioned officers or private soldiers of your Regiment

497

shall be sick or wounded, the Surgeon of your Regiment do provide physic or internal medicines, as well as external medicines for them.'

'Given at Our Court at Whitehall,
the 24th day of January, 1673.

'By His Majesty's Command,
'Arlington.

'To our Trusted and Well-beloved
Colonel Sir Charles Littleton,
or the Officer in Chief commanding
Our Most Dear Brother James,
Duke of York's Regiment.'

C

'William Rex
'Our will and pleasure is that the Establishment for the Marching Hospital to attend our Army in Ireland to commence from 1st March 1689/90. In the second year of our Reign, from which time the former Establishment for the Hospital in that Kingdom is to cease and determine.

	At per diem each
A Governor or Director	10. 11½
Two Physicians whereof one to be Physician General to the Army	£1 0. 0.
The Chirurgeon General to all the Army	£1 0. 0.
Another Master Chirurgeon	10. 0.
Eight Chirurgeon's Mates	3. 0.
Two Chaplains whereof one to be Chaplain to the General	6. 8.
To the Apothecary General to the Army	10. 0.
Another Master Apothecary	8. 0.
Three Apothecaries' Mates	3. 0.
Three Purveyors	6. 0.
Two clerks to keep the accounts of the Hospital	5. 0.
Clerk for the beds and furniture	4. 0.
Conductor for the Waggons	5. 0.
Three cooks	3. 0.
Two persons to look after the bread and beer	3. 0.
Twenty nurses as Tenders to look after the sick persons	2. 6.

Total cost £12 7s. 8½d. a day or £4,518 1s. 8d. a year.

'A third Royal Warrant was signed at Whitehall on 14th March 1690 which added "from the 1st day of April next" one chaplain to the hospitals in Ireland and established "twelve waggons with four horses to attend our Marching Hospital, twelve waggoners at one shilling and sixpence, twelve boys at eightpence, and one smith at two shillings and sixpence per diem".

The daily allowance per horse for maintenance was one shilling and three-pence.

'This added £4 15s. 2d. a day or £734 15s. 1od. a year, and the grand total was £5,247 17s. 6d.'

D

'The Fixed Hospital which was later to become the General Hospital had the following staff:

	At per diem each
A Governor or Director	10 11½
Two Physicians	£1 o. o.
Two Master Chirurgeons	10. o.
Ten Chirurgeons' Mates	3. o.
One Master Apothecary	8. o.
Three Apothecaries' Mates	3. o.
Three Purveyors	6. o.
Two clerks to keep the accounts of the hospital	5. o.
Clerk for beds and furniture	4. o.
Three cooks	3. o.
Two persons to look after the bread and beer	3. o.
Thirty nurses	2. 6.

The total daily pay of the staff came to £12 6s. 7½d. a day or £4,500 18s. 4d. a year.'

Appendix to Chapter 5

A

REGULATIONS AND ORDERS FOR A REGIMENTAL INFIRMARY

Every soldier, when taken sick, must be sent to the infirmary, a portable chair should always be in readiness at the main-guard, to carry such as are ill; but, if not so, a corporal and 2 men should assist him.

The orderly corporal of the company must bring the pay with the sick men; and take care that the patient has a cap and shirt, and search him, that he may not carry into the infirmary money, cards, dice, spirits or tobacco; nor is any clean linen to be brought, or foul fetched away, except by a sergeant or corporal. If the sick man's mess is put in, his mess-mates must allow him his proportion in money for the remainder of the week; and what is deficient must be advanced to make good his pay to the pay-day following, –s. –d. per week is to be the infirmary allowance till further orders. Sergeants, corporals, drummers, musicians to pay the same. A sergeant or corporal of the companies who have any man in the regimental infirmary are ordered to carry their linen every   and   ; on which last day they must also carry their subsistence and pay it to the sergeant attending the infirmary. If any soldier, while a patient in the infirmary, does not quietly submit to the rules of the house, and directions of the doctor, he is to be confined in the black-hole, as soon as cured, for 24 hours; if notoriously refractory he should be tried by a regimental court martial. If a patient in the infirmary should break out from there, he shall, when recovered, be sent to the black-hole for 10 days.

A sergeant or corporal of a company must visit the sick in the infirmary twice every week, to know what linen they want; and he must bring nothing to any patient but wearing apparel, without the surgeon's or his mate's permission. If any soldier should be detected in carrying spirituous liquors to the sick in the infirmary, or is aiding or assisting thereto, he shall be punished by the sentence of a court martial. If any sergeant or corporal is a patient in the infirmary he must be aiding or assisting to the doctor, in keeping order and decency among the patients, and in detecting any mean practices committed in the infirmary, for if either sergeant or corporal connives at any thing improper to be brought in or does not discover it to the surgeon, he shall be reduced to the pay and duty of a private soldier.

The sergeant attending the infirmary must keep an exact account of the pay of each ward; see it properly expended by the nurse, according to the doctor's directions, give receipts for coals, candles, and sheeting, and close the account every half week; that any man who is to be discharged on . . . may have his overplus divided when he is dismissed.

A corporal of a company must attend every   and   afternoon to receive the recovered men; and every man discharged the infirmary must be duty free for 3 days, or more, at the discretion of the surgeon.

The account of money disbursed, and the dividend for each man must be given every   morning to the surgery that the commanding officer may inspect it when he pleases, and the sergeant must give a distinct copy of that account to the sergeant or corporal who relieves him: which relief must be weekly.

No sick soldier can have his wife employed as one of the nurses, and if any of the nurses' husbands are taken ill, such nurse must be dismissed, or her pay discontinued till the recovery of her husband; but married men of good character who live near the infirmary and have careful wives, if they are taken ill, may be allowed to remain in their lodgings at the discretion of the surgeon.

When any man is taken ill with small pox, or any other pestilential disorder, he should immediately, upon the discovery of the disease, be sent to as private and remote lodgings as can be had, and all soldiers prevented from visiting him, lest the visitors catch such distempers, and communicate the infection. The sentry posted at an infirmary must suffer no one to enter, unless accompanied by a corporal or the people attending it; he is also to prevent the sick from coming out, or leaving their ward to trouble the kitchens. The sentry may be taken off at 10 (except anything extraordinary requires his being continued,) and planted again at daybreak. Any of the men who have slight complaints may attend the surgeon at a place appointed, in the morning, when corporals are to give in their report of the sick. The surgeon must make a report to the commanding officer whenever any of these orders are not complied with, that the offender may be punished for neglect.

B

Characters	Name	From 1762	To 1763	
I. Director at £1 5s. od.	William Young	Feb. 10th	May 14th	
Physicians £1 0s. od.	W. Cadogan	Feb. 10th	May 14th	
	M. Morris	Feb. 10th	May 14th	
	R. Huck	Nov. 7th	May 14th	vice Cadogan sick.
Surgeons 10s. od.	J. Hunter	Feb. 10th	May 14th	
	F. Tomkins	Feb. 10th	May 14th	
	W. Maddox	Feb. 10th	May 14th	
	W. Young	Sep. 6th	May 14th	
Apothecaries 10s. od.	H. Smith	Feb. 10th	May 14th	
	M. Obryan	Feb. 10th	May 14th	
	W. Hamilton	Feb. 10th	May 14th	
	A. Robinson	Feb. 10th	May 14th	
	E. Taylor	Feb. 10th	May 14th	
	A. McDonald	Feb. 10th	May 14th	
	W. Rogerson	Feb. 10th	May 14th	
	M. Croker	Feb. 10th	May 14th	
	J. Digby	Dec. 4th	. . . .	died that day
	N. Jenty	Apr. 13th		Remains in Portugal on his own affairs.
Surgeons Mates 5s. od.	T. Armstrong	Feb. 12th		died that day
	T. Deveil	Sep. 26th		died that day
	R. Scott	Feb. 10th	May 14th	
	D. Griffith	Feb. 10th	May 14th	
	S. Hayes	Apr. 13th		left on duty in Portugal
	B. Cluck	Feb. 10th	May 14th	
	E. Golding	Feb. 10th	May 14th	
	M. Clarck	Feb. 10th	May 14th	
	J. Kingston	Feb. 10th	May 14th	Remains in Portugal on his own affairs.

II. List of Servants belonging to the Hospital:

Matron	Mrs. Sullivan		2s. 6d.
Quartermaster	D. O'Neil		2s. 6d.
Assistant Storekeeper	H. Andrews		1s. od.
Head Nurses	Mary Fenton		1s. od.
	Ann Milross		1s. od.
Cooks (3)		each	1s. od.
Washerwomen (4)		each	1s. od.
Nurses (18)		each	6d.

Appendix to Chapter 7
A

Medical Works recommended for the Regimental Medical Officer

Cullen's *Outline of Disease*.
Lind on *Scurvy*.
Pringle and Monro on *Soldiers' Diseases*.
Zimmerman on *Dysentery*.
Cullen's *Nosology*.
Le Roy on *Prognostics*.
Simmons and Hunter, and other authors on *Venereal Disease*, which 'is so
      universal in the army'.
Bell on *Ulcers of the Legs*.
Mudge on *Catarrhal Affections*.
Reid on *Phthisis*.
Treatises on *Small pox and Measles*.
Cheselden on *Anatomy*.
Cullen on *Materia Medica*.
The London Dispensary.
Haller's *Physiology*.
Clarke's *Treatise on Fevers*.
Warner on *Eye Diseases*.
Heister and Bell, Wiseman and Pott on *Operative Surgery*.
Bell and Pott on *Rupture*
Ranby on *Gun Shot Wounds*
Smilies on *Midwifery*.
Leak on *Puerperal Fever*.
Cavallo on *Medical Electricity*.
The London Medical Journal.

B

Weekly account of expenditure of the Regimental Hospital   31st Regiment

Days		No. of patients	Rate of diet High Low		Meat lbs. ozs.		Bread lbs. ozs.		Tea pints	No. of men on stoppage	£ s. d.
Sunday	15	18	14	4	7	0	15	0	22	18	13s. 6d.
Monday	16	18	17	1	8	8	17	4	19	18	13s. 6d.
Tuesday	17	18	16	2	8	0	16	8	20	18	13s. 6d.
Wednesday	18	18	14	4	7	0	15	0	22	18	13s. 6d.
Thursday	19	19	13	6	6	8	14	8	25	19	14s. 3d.
Friday	20	19	14	5	7	0	15	4	24	19	14s. 3d.
Saturday	21	20	17	3	8	8	17	12	23	20	15s. 0d.
Seven Days		130	105	25	52	8	111	4	155	130	£4 17s. 6d.

Expenditure

			£ s. d.
Meat	52 lbs 8 ozs.	@ 3¼d.	14s. 2½d.
Bread	111 lbs 4 ozs.	@ 1½d.	13s. 10¾d.
Tea	155 pints	@ 1½d.	19s. 4½d.
Extra Milk	2 quarts	@ 3½d.	7d.
26 Eggs		@ 2d.	4s. 4d.
Hog's Lard	1 lb	@ 1/3d.	1s. 3d.
Soap			1s. 6d.
Vegetables, salt and pepper, for 130 patients @ ½d.			5s. 5d.
Extra Bread	6 lbs	@ 1½d.	9d.
Vinegar and stationery			3s. 0d.
Washing			7s. 0d.
Hospital sergeant and 2 orderlies wages			9s. 11d.

	£4 1s. 2¾d.
Stoppages at 9d. per head daily	£4 17s. 6 d.
Surplus	16s. 3¼d.

C

Scale of diet of a General Hospital

	Full	*Half*	*Low*	*Milk*	*Remarks*
Breakfast	1pt oatmeal or rice gruel	do.	do. with wine or sugar at discretion of surgeon	1pt milk	Mutton, fish, chicken broth, wine, porter, cyder, brandy, tea, potatoes or vegetables
Dinner	1lb bread 1lb meat 1 quart small beer	1lb bread ½lb meat 1 quart small beer	1pt broth ½lb bread barley or rice water	1pt broth 1lb bread	to be allowed to such part-icular patients whose cases the attending
Supper	1pt broth	1pt broth	1pt oatmeal or rice gruel	1pt milk	surgeon may think will require such indulgences.

Appendix to Chapter 10

A

Sick returns for 1810

Date	Strength	Sick present in regimental hospitals	Sick absent in general hospitals	Total	Percentages
9th January	30,220	927	7,826	8,753	28·9
15th January	29,920	1,046	7,441	8,487	28·3
1st February	29,576	1,184	6,687	7,871	26·6
1st March	28,546	605	5,365	5,970	20·9
1st April	31,548	909	4,971	5,880	18·6
8th May	31,720	993	4,388	5,381	16·9
1st June	31,573	1,180	3,871	5,051	15·9
1st July	31,851	777	3,090	3,867	12·1
8th July	31,753	797	2,978	3,775	11·9
1st August	32,571	472	3,681	4,153	12 7
1st September	34,816	579	4,746	5,325	15·3
1st October	37,930	259	6,966	7,225	19·0
15th November	41,855	1,018	6,298	7,316	17·4
8th December	41,562	919	6,959	7,878	18·9

B

Sick returns for 1811

Date	Strength	Sick present in regimental hospitals	Sick absent in general hospitals	Total	Percentage
8th January	41,120	1,031	6,218	7,249	17·6
1st February	42,768	901	5,250	6,151	14·4
1st March	42,822	882	4,767	5,649	13·2
1st April	45,481	184	5,976	6,160	13·5
1st May	47,542	731	8,814	9,545	20·0
1st June	46,345	662	11,730	12,392	26·7
1st July	48,733	394	11,744	12,138	24·9
5th August*	77,297	1,478	17,486	18,964	24·5
1st September	54,009	1,488	12,280	13,768	25·5
1st October	53,797	1,720	12,517	14,237	26·4
8th October	55,706	942	16,131	17,073	30·6
15th October	55,310	1,645	16,139	17,784	32·1
10th November*	80,738	2,967	18,422	21,389	26·5
7th December*	80,360	2,291	17,490	19,781	24·6

* Includes Portuguese

Appendix to Chapter 11

A

Sick returns for 1812

Date	Strength	Sick present in regimental hospitals	Sick absent in general hospitals	Total	Percentage
1st January	49,699	1,410	10,345	11,755	23·6
1st February	50,217	999	11,758	12,757	25·4
1st March	49,693	813	10,361	11,174	22·5
1st April	49,173	519	12,026	12,545	25·5
1st May	50,712	788	14,379	15,167	29·9
1st June	51,283	1,068	11,788	12,856	25·0
1st July	53,276	605	12,697	13,302	24·9
1st August	53,035	1,163	17,283	18,446	34·7
1st September	51,294	1,454	16,575	18,029	35·0
2nd October	50,512	1,902	16,803	18,705	37·0
29th November	53,648	1,946	17,594	19,540	36·4
15th December	57,952	1,946	17,317	19,263	33·2

B

Sick returns for 1813

Date	Strength	Sick present in regimental hospitals	Sick absent in general hospitals	Total	Percentage
1st January	58,748	2,802	14,896	17,698	30·1
7th February	55,112	4,907	11,219	16,126	29·3
7th March	55,176	4,310	9,906	14,216	25·6
11th April	52,870	3,393	7,535	10,928	20·7
9th May	55,519	1,962	7,123	9,085	16·4
11th June	54,835	995	7,892	8,887	16·2
16th July	53,490	1,217	11,288	12,505	23·6
15th August	52,029	1,133	13,033	14,166	27·2
8th September	55,161	2,228	11,852	14,080	25·5
15th October	55,938	1,701	11,611	13,312	23·8
11th November	57,399	2,060	11,388	13,448	23·4
23rd December	57,472	2,158	12,623	14,781	25·7

C

An order published in 1813 lays down the regulations for military hospitals.

(1) *General Hospitals*
- (a) Separate wards of buildings laid down for
    - (i) Continued fever
    - (ii) Dysentery
    - (iii) Surgical cases, including cases of chronic ulcers and inter-mittent fever (presumably malarial and not considered contagious)
    - (iv) Convalescents.
- (b) Diets
    - (i) Full diet, with 1lb. of meat and 1lb. bread, 5oz. rice, sugar, salt, vegetables and $\frac{1}{2}$ pint wine.
    - (ii) Half diet, as above except $\frac{1}{2}$lb. meat, and no wine.
    - (iii) Low. $\frac{1}{4}$lb. meat, $\frac{1}{2}$lb. bread, 1 oz. rice, tea, sugar, salt, $\frac{1}{2}$ pint milk.
- (c) Returns
    - (i) A return of principal diseases.
    - (ii) A meteorological statement from P.M.O.'s, including state of civilian health.
    - (iii) Monthly board on purveyors and apothecary accounts.
- (d) Examination of hospital mates for Commissions. They were enlisted with only twelve months attendance at a public hospital and lectures on professional subjects. Orderlies and messengers were recruited from civilian Spanish and Portuguese and for sick officers civilian female nurses were used.

(2) P.M.O.'s of stations had to report on medical topography and civilian health with steps for its improvement. They were responsible for clinical records and prescription books.

(3) Purveyors were responsible for cleanlinness of hospital except for sick wards which were responsibility of the M.O.'s. They dealt with equipment, supplies, diets and pay. They could only receive orders from the P.M.O. and not from M.O.'s in charge of wards, and were also responsible to the Purveyor-in-Chief for accounts.

(4) Apothecaries and dispensers were under the P.M.O. and physicians and surgeons were ordered occasionally to taste the prescriptions made up. Quarterly returns were made to the Apothecary-in-Chief.

D

Table 1

Admissions, Discharges and Deaths in the General and Regimental Hospitals in the Peninsula between 21st December 1811 and the 20th June 1814

	1 Remained	2 Admitted	3 Total treated	4 Discharged	5 Of which were transferred	6 Died	7 Remaining
Remained in general hospitals 20th December 1811	4,260						
Admitted between 21st December 1811 and 20th December 1812		95,075		85,003	23,652	6,931	
Admitted between 21st December 1812 and 20th December 1813		46,715		43,189	13,964	5,267	
Admitted between 21st December 1813 and 20th June 1814		22,013		22,936	4,855	2,474	
Remaining in general hospitals							2,263
General hospital total	4,260	163,803	168,063	151,128	42,471	14,672	2,263
Regimental hospitals	1,978	176,067	178,045	173,544	52,571	3,841	660
Total:	6,238	339,870	346,108	324,672	95,042	18,513	2,923

Table 2

General Abstract of Admissions, Discharges and Deaths in the Regimental Hospitals in the Peninsula between 21st December 1811 and the 20th June 1814

Diseases	Admitted Totals	Discharged
Continued fever	40,244	38,817
Intermittent	22,914	22,680
Remittent	3,961	3,905
Typhus	1,795	1,346
Pneumonia	4,027	3,909
Hepatitis	290	270
Rheumatism	4,933	4,868
Ophthalmia	1,875	1,878
Catarrh	1,552	1,614
Dysenteria	7,526	7,085
Diarrhoea	15,677	15,649
Phthisis pulmonalis	271	240
Syphilis	4,912	4,830
Vulnus (wounds)	20,886	19,931
Ulcers	12,167	11,901
Chronic disease	542	548
Various	30,445	31,973
Punishment	2,070	2,100
Total admitted	176,067	173,544*
Remained on 20th December 1811	1,978	
Remaining 20th June 1814		660
		174,204
Died		3,841
	178,045	178,045

*Of this number 52,571 were transferred to general hospitals.

Table 3

Causes of Death in Regimental Hospitals

Continued fever	1,504
Typhus	551
Remittent	66
Intermittent	59
Pneumonia	137
Dysenteria	431
Diarrhoea	86
Phthisis	90
Wounds	505
Various	104
Hepatitis	23
Enteritis	29

Table 4

The total number of cases treated in all regimental and general hospitals in 1812, 1813 and 1814 and the principal causes of deaths.

	1812	*1813*	*1814*	*Total*
Number treated	176,180	123,019	53,073	352,272
Discharged cured	119,798	79,010	34,591	233,399
Transferred	39,757	29,090	12,825	81,672
Died	7,193	6,866	2,909	16,968
Chief causes of death				
Dysentery	2,340	1,629	748	4,717
Continued fever	2,020	1,598	387	4,005
Typhus	999	971	307	2,277
Wounds	905	1,095	699	2,699
Intermittent fever (malaria)	148	139	4	291
Chronic disease	102	58	15	175
Various	97	71	35	203
Diarrhoea	79	106	34	219
Remittent fever	67	65	18	150
Pneumonia	58	133	96	287
Phthisis	49	158	72	279
Hospital gangrene	35	446	122	603
Tetanus	4	23	24	51

Table 5

Principal admissions to Regimental Hospitals

---

(1) Continued fever

1812	16,923	
1813	18,294	40,224
1814 June	5,007	

(2) Typhus fever

1812	331	
1813	1,309	1,795
1814 June	155	

(3) Remittent fever

1812	1,826	
1813	1,699	3,961
1814 June	436	

(4) Intermittent fever

1812	13,759	
1813	8,203	22,914
1814 June	952	

(5) Dysentery

1812	3,241	
1813	3,420	7,526
1814 June	865	

(6) Pneumonia

1812		
1813		4,027
1814		

(7) Rheumatism

1812		
1813		4,933
1814		

Table 6

Return of capital (major) operations performed in the general hospitals at Toulouse from 10th April to 28th June 1814.

Wounds	Number	Died	Discharged to duty	Transferred to Bordeaux
Head	95	17	25	53
Thorax	96	35	14	47
Abdomen	104	24	21	59
Upper extremity	304	3	96	205
Lower extremity	498	21	150	327
Compound fractures	78	29	—	49
Wounds of spine	3	3	—	—
Wounds of joints	16	4	—	12
Amputations:				
arm 7 ⎫ 48	48	10	—	38
thigh and leg 41 ⎭				
Total	1,242	146	306	790

Secondary Operations

	Number	Died	Transferred to Bordeaux
Amputation of upper extremity	15	3	12
Amputation of lower extremity	37	18	19
Operation of taking up the femoral artery	1	1	—
Trephine	4	3	1
Shoulder joint	1	1	—
Total	58	26	32

Index

INDEX

513

INDEX

515

INDEX

Printed by Willmer Brothers Limited, Birkenhead